Essentials of Oral and Maxillofacial Surgery

Essentials of Oral and Maxillofacial Surgery

Edited by

M. Anthony (Tony) Pogrel
DDS, MD, FRCS, FACS
Professor and Chair
Associate Dean for Hospital Affairs
Department of Oral and Maxillofacial Surgery
University of California, San Francisco
USA

Karl-Erik Kahnberg
DDS, PhD, DrOdont
Professor Emeritus, Oral and Maxillofacial Surgery
Institute of Odontology
The Sahlgrenska Academy
University of Gothenburg
Sweden

Lars Andersson
DDS, PhD, DrOdont
Professor, Oral and Maxillofacial Surgery
Chairman, Department of Surgical Sciences
Faculty of Dentistry
Health Sciences Center
Kuwait University
Kuwait

WILEY Blackwell

Library of Congress Cataloging-in-Publication Data
Essentials of oral and maxillofacial surgery / edited by M. Anthony (Tony) Pogrel, Karl-Erik Kahnberg, Lars Andersson.
        p. ; cm.
    Includes bibliographical references and index.
    ISBN 978-1-4051-7623-1 (pbk.)
    I. Pogrel, M. Anthony, editor of compilation.   II. Kahnberg, Karl-Erik, editor of compilation.   III. Andersson, L. (Lars), 1950- editor of compilation.
    [DNLM: 1. Oral Surgical Procedures–methods.   2. Stomatognathic System–surgery. WU 600]
    RK501
    617.6'05–dc23

                     2014001169

A catalogue record for this book is available from the British Library.

Wiley also publishes its books in a variety of electronic formats. Some content that appears in print may not be available in electronic books.

Cover image: © Yegor Tsyba/iStockphoto
Cover design by Garth Stewart

Set in 9.5/12 pt Palatino LT Std by Toppan Best-set Premedia Limited, Hong Kong

1   2014

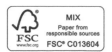

Contents

Part 1 Basic Principles   1

Section Editor: Tony Pogrel

Part 2 Dentoalveolar Surgery   61

Section Editor: Lars Andersson

Part 3 Implant Surgery   125

Section Editor: Karl-Erik Kahnberg

List of Contributors

Adel Al-Asfour BDS, BA (Chapter 8)
Associate Professor
Department of Surgical Sciences
Faculty of Dentistry, Health Sciences Center
Kuwait University
Kuwait

Ala Al-Musawi DDS, BA (Chapter 5)
Assistant Professor
Department of Surgical Sciences
Faculty of Dentistry, Health Sciences Center
Kuwait University
Kuwait

Jens O. Andreasen DDS, Odont. Dr.h.c. (Chapters 11 and 28)
Consultant
Department of Oral and Maxillofacial Surgery
Section for Rare Oral Diseases
Rigshospitalet
Copenhagen, Denmark

Ashraf Ayoub PhD, FDS RCS, FDS RCPS, BDS, MDS (Chapter 4)
Professor of Oral & Maxillofacial Surgery
Glasgow University Dental Hospital & School
Glasgow, UK

Selçuk Basa DDS, PhD (Chapter 13)
Department of Oral and Maxillofacial Surgery
Marmara University
Istanbul, Turkey

Brian Bast DMD, MD (Chapter 27)
Associate Clinical Professor
Residency Program Director
Department of Oral and Maxillofacial Surgery
University of California, San Francisco
San Francisco, California, USA

R. Bryan Bell DDS, MD, FACS (Chapter 21)
Attending Surgeon and Director of Resident
Education,
OMFS Service
ACS Cancer Liaison Physician
Legacy Emanuel Hospital and Health Center
Clinical Associate Professor of Oral and Maxillofacial
Surgery
Oregon Health and Science University
Head and Neck Surgical Associates
Portland, Oregon, USA

John Beumer III DDS, MS
Professor and Chair
Division of Advanced Prosthodontics, Biomaterials,
and Hospital Dentistry
University of California, Los Angeles – School of
Dentistry
Los Angeles, California, USA

Krishnamurthy Bonanthaya MBBS, MDS, FDSRCS, FFDRCS
(Chapter 29)
Professor, Oral and Maxillofacial Surgery
Bangalore Institute of Dental Sciences
and
Consultant Surgeon
Bhagwan Mahavir Jain Hospital
Bangalore, India

Peter Carrotte BDS, MDS, LDS.RCS(Eng), MEd, MHEA
(Chapter 12)
Senior Clinical Teacher and Honorary Associate
Specialist
Department of Restorative Dentistry
University of Glasgow
Glasgow, UK

Allen Cheng DDS, MD (Chapter 19)
Department of Oral and Maxillofacial Surgery
University of California, San Francisco
San Francisco, California, USA

Lim K. Cheung BDS, PhD, FFDRCS, FDSRCPS, FRACDS, FDSRCS
(Edin), FRACDS(OMS), FHKAM(DS), FCDSHK(OMS), FFGDP(UK)
(Chapter 30)
Chair Professor
Discipline of Oral and Maxillofacial Surgery
Faculty of Dentistry
University of Hong Kong
Hong Kong, SAR, China

Radhika Chigurupati DMD, MS (Chapter 29)
Associate Clinical Professor of Oral and Maxillofacial
Surgery
Department of Oral and Maxillofacial Surgery
Boston University
Boston, Massachusetts, USA

Hannah Daile P. Chua DMD, MA, MDS (OMS), MOSRCS, PhD
Assistant Professor
Discipline of Oral and Maxillofacial Surgery
Faculty of Dentistry
University of Hong Kong
Hong Kong, SAR, China

William Chung DDS, MD (Chapter 27)
University of Pittsburgh Medical Center
Pittsburgh, Pennsylvania, USA

Cameron M.L. Clokie DDS, PhD, FRCDC
Professor and Director of Graduate Program in Oral
and Maxillofacial Surgery and Anaesthesia
University of Toronto
Toronto, Ontario, Canada

Bernard J. Costello DMD, MD, FACS (Chapter 27)
Chief, Division of Craniofacial and Cleft Surgery
Associate Professor and Program Director
Department of Oral and Maxillofacial Surgery
University of Pittsburgh School of Dental Medicine
Pittsburgh, Pennsylvania, USA

Christer Dahlin DDS, PhD, Dr Odont (Chapter 15)
Associate Professor
Department of Biomaterials
Institute for Clinical Sciences
Sahlgrenska Academy, University of Gothenburg
Gothenburg, Sweden
and
Department of Oral and Maxillofacial Surgery
NÄL Medical Centre Hospital
Trollhättan, Sweden

Nagi Demian DDS, MD
Assistant Professor
Department of Oral and Maxillofacial Surgery
University of Texas Health Science Center – Houston
Houston, Texas, USA

Thomas B. Dodson DMD, MPH (Chapter 7)
Professor and Chair
Department of Oral and Maxillofacial Surgery
University of Washington
Seattle, Washington, USA

Carlo Ferretti BDS, MDent (MFOS), FCD (SA), MFOS
(Chapter 30)
Senior Specialist
Department of Maxillofacial and Oral Surgery
and
Chris Hani Baragwanath Hospital
Faculty of Health Sciences,
University of the Witwatersrand
Johannesburg, South Africa

Earl G. Freymiller DMD, MD
Clinical Professor
Section of Oral and Maxillofacial Surgery
UCLA School of Dentistry
Los Angeles, California, USA

Takashi Fujibayashi DDS, PhD (Chapter 22)
Visiting Professor
Department of Oral and Maxillofacial Surgery
Kanagawa Dental College
Yokosuka, Japan

Nicholas M. Goodger BSc, BDS, MBBS, PhD, FDSRCS(Eng),
FFDRCSI, FRCSEd, DLORCS(Eng) (Chapter 20)
Consultant Oral and Maxillofacial Surgeon
East Kent Hospitals University NHS Foundation Trust
Kent and Canterbury Hospital
Canterbury, UK

Gosta Granstrom MD, DDS, PhD
Professor of Otolaryngology, Head and Neck Surgery
Department of Otolaryngology, Head and Neck
Surgery
Sahlgrenska Academy, University of Gothenburg
Gothenburg, Sweden

Firdaus Hariri BDS, MDS (OMS)
Consultant and Lecturer
Department of Oral and Maxillofacial Surgery
Faculty of Dentistry
University of Malaya
Kuala Lumpur, Malaysia

Richard H. Haug DDS (Chapter 28)
Carolinas Center for Oral Health
Charlotte, North Carolina, USA

Andrew Heggie MBBS, MDSc, BDSc, FRACDS(OMS)
(Chapter 29)
Associate Professor, Oral and Maxillofacial Surgery
Department of Plastic and Maxillofacial Surgery
Royal Children's Hospital of Melbourne
Parkville, Australia

Christopher W. Hendy BDS, FDSRCS(Eng), LRCP, MRCS,
FRCSEd (Chapter 20)
East Kent Hospitals University NHS Foundation Trust
Kent and Canterbury Hospital
Canterbury, UK

Alan S. Herford DDS, MD (Chapter 1)
Chairman
Department of Oral and Maxillofacial Surgery
Loma Linda University
Loma Linda, California, USA

C. Michael Hill MDSc, FDSRCS, MSc, BDS
Consultant and Honorary Senior Lecturer in Oral and
Maxillofacial Surgery
Cardiff Dental Hospital
Cardiff, UK

Anders Holmlund DDS, PhD Professor (Chapter 33)
Department of Oral and Maxillofacial Surgery
Institution of Odontology
Karolinska Institutet/Karolinska University Hospital
Huddinge, Sweden

Mehran Hossaini DMD (Chapter 9)
Health Sciences Associate Clinical Professor
Department of Oral and Maxillofacial Surgery
University of California, San Francisco
San Francisco, California, USA

Vesa T. Kainulainen DDS, PhD
Assistant Professor
Institute of Dentistry
University of Oulu
Oulu, Finland

Sanjiv Kanagaraja DDS, PhD (Chapter 8)
Consultant/Assistant Professor
Department of Oral and Maxillofacial Surgery
University of Göteborg
Göteborg, Sweden

Reha Kışnışçı DDS, PhD (Chapter 13)
Department of Oral and Maxillofacial Surgery
Ankara University
Ankara, Turkey

Goran Kjeller PhD (Chapter 24)
Associate Professor
Department Oral and Maxillofacial Surgery
Institute of Odontology
Sahlgren's Academy
Gothenburg University
Göteborg, Sweden

Paul Koshgerian DMD (Chapter 28)
University of Louisville School of Dentistry
Department of Surgical and Hospital Dentistry
Louisville, Kentucky, USA

Fabio Kricheldorf DDS, MSc (Chapter 6)
Professor of Oral and Maxillofacial Surgery
and Chairman
Department of Surgical Sciences, Faculty of Dentistry
University of Joinville
Joinville, Santa Catarina, Brazil

Tomoari Kuriyama DDS, PhD (Chapter 4)
Honorary Clinical Instructor and Research Fellow
Department of Oral and Maxillofacial Surgery
Graduate School of Medical Science
Kanazawa University
Kanazawa, Japan
and
Private practice
Toyama, Japan

David K. Lam DDS, MD, PhD, FRCDC
Assistant Professor
Department of Oral and Maxillofacial Surgery
University of Toronto
Toronto, Ontario, Canada

Anh Le DDS, PhD
Professor and Chair
Department of Oral and Maxillofacial Surgery
University of Pennsylvania
Philadelphia, Pennsylvania, USA

Michael A.O. Lewis PhD, BDS, FDSRCPSG, FRCPath,
FDSRCS(Eng), FDSRCS(Ed), FFGDP(UK) (Chapter 4)
Professor of Oral Medicine
Cardiff University
Cardiff, UK

John Lo BDS, MDS (OMS), MOSRCS, FHKAM (DS), FCDSHK
(OMS)
Assistant Professor
Discipline of Oral and Maxillofacial Surgery
Faculty of Dentistry
University of Hong Kong
Hong Kong, SAR, China

Leif Lysell DDS, Odont Dr (Chapter 9)
Associate Professor
Faculty of Odontology
Malmö University
Malmö, Sweden
and
Private practice
Kristianstad, Sweden

Carlo Maiorana MD, DDS (Chapter 18)
Professor and Chairman
Oral Surgery and Implantology
Dental Clinic Fondazione Cà Granda
University of Milan
Milan, Italy

Chantal Malevez MD, DDS
Specialist in Oral and Maxillofacial Surgery
Professor Emeritus
Free University of Brussels (ULB)
and
Consultant Department of Maxillofacial Surgery
Children's Hospital
Brussels, Belgium
and
Consultant at the EOIC
Brussels, Belgium

Joann Marruffo DDS, MS
Maxillofacial Prosthodontist
Private practice
Houston, Texas, USA

James McCaul PhD, FRCS(OMFS), FRCS(Glasg), FDSRCPS
Consultant Oral and Maxillofacial/Head and Neck
Surgeon
Bradford Teaching Hospitals NHS Foundation Trust
Bradford, UK

Mark McGurk BDS, MD, FDS RCSEng, FRCS Ed, DLO RCS
(Chapter 25)
Professor
Department of Oral and Maxillofacial Surgery
King's College
London, UK

Charles McNeill DDS (Chapter 32)
Professor Emeritus and Director
UCSF Center for Orofacial Pain
Department of Oral and Maxillofacial Surgery
University of California, San Francisco
San Francisco, California, USA

John Gerard Meechan BSc, BDS, PhD, FDSRCS, FDSRCPS
(Chapter 3)
Senior Lecturer in Oral Surgery
School of Dental Sciences
Newcastle University
Newcastle upon Tyne, UK

Marc Christian Metzger MD, DMD, PhD (Chapter 27)
Department of Craniomaxillofacial Surgery
University Hospital Freiburg
Freiburg, Germany

Colin Murray PhD, FDS RCS(Edin), BDS, FDS(Rest Dent)
RCS(Edin), FDS RCPS(Glas) (Chapter 12)
Professor in Restorative Dentistry/Honorary
Consultant
Head of Clinical Dentistry Section and Head of
Restorative Group University of Glasgow
Glasgow, UK

Joe Niamtu
Private practice
Cosmetic Facial Surgery
Richmond, Virginia, USA

Kyösti S. Oikarinen DDS, PhD
Professor and Head of Oral and Maxillofacial Surgery
Institute of Dentistry
University of Oulu
Oulu, Finland

Andrew Ow BDS, MDS(OMS), FRACDS, MOSRCS, AdvDip(OMS)
Assistant Professor
Department of Oral and Maxillofacial Surgery
National University of Singapore
Singapore

Zachary S. Peacock DMD, MD
Assistant Professor
Department of Oral and Maxillofacial Surgery
Massachusetts General Hospital and Harvard School
of Dental Medicine
Boston, Massachusetts, USA

Arne Petersson DDS, Odont Dr (Chapter 2)
Department of Oral and Maxillofacial Radiology
Faculty of Odontology
Malmö University
Malmö, Sweden

Lars Rasmusson DDS, PhD (Chapter 14)
Professor of Maxillofacial Surgery
Head of Department of Oral and Maxillofacial Surgery
The Sahlgrenska Academy
University of Gothenburg
Gothenburg, Sweden

Tara Renton BDS, MDSc, PhD, FDS, RCS, FRACDS (OMS), ILTM
(Chapter 9)
Professor in Oral Surgery
King's College London Dental Institute
London, UK

Johan P. Reyneke B Ch D, M Ch D, FCMFOS (SA), PhD
(Chapter 30)
Honorary Professor
Department of Maxillofacial and Oral Surgery
Faculty of Health Sciences
University of the Witwatersrand
Johannesburg
South Africa
and
Clinical Professor
Department of Oral and Maxillofacial Surgery
University of Oklahoma
Oklahoma City, Oklahoma, USA
and
Clinical Professor
Department of Oral and Maxillofacial Surgery
University of Florida
Gainesville, Florida, USA
and
Private practice, Sunninghill Hospital
Sunninghill, Johannesburg, South Africa

Richard C. Robert DDS, MS
Clinical Professor
Oral and Maxillofacial Surgery
University of California Medical Center
San Francisco, California, USA
and
Private practice, Oral and Maxillofacial Surgery
South San Francisco, California, USA

Simon N. Rogers BDS, MBChB, FDSRCS, FRCS
Professor, Regional Maxillofacial Unit
University Hospital Aintree
Liverpool, UK
and
Evidence-based Practice Research Centre (EPRC)
Faculty of Health
Edge Hill University
Ormskirk, UK

†Bo Rosenquist BSc, DDS, PhD (Chapter 16)
Associate Professor of Oral and Maxillofacial
Surgery
Head of the Head and Neck Division
Department of Oral and Maxillofacial Surgery
University Hospital of Lund
Lund, Sweden

Patricia A. Rudd PT, DPT, CCTT (Chapter 32)
Assistant Clinical Professor
UCSF Center for Orofacial Pain
Department of Oral and Maxillofacial Surgery
University of California, San Francisco
San Francisco, California, USA

George K.B. Sándor MD, DDS, PhD, Dr. Habil, FRCDC,
FRCSC, FACS
Professor of Tissue Engineering
Regea Institute for Regenerative Medicine
University of Tampere
Tampere, Finland
and
Dosent in Oral and Maxillofacial Surgery
University of Oulu
Oulu, Finland

Henning Schliephake MD, DDS, PhD
Professor and Chair
Department of Oral Maxillofacial Surgery
George Augusta University
Göttingen, Germany

Rainer Schmelzeisen MD, DMD (Chapter 27)
Professor and Chairman
Department of Craniomaxillofacial Surgery
University Hospital Freiburg
Freiburg, Germany

Brian L. Schmidt DDS, MD, PhD, FACS (Chapters 19, 23
and 31)
Professor
Department of Oral and Maxillofacial Surgery and
Director of the Bluestone Center for Clinical Research
New York University School of Dentistry
New York, NY, USA

Ralf Schon MD, DMD (Chapter 27)
Associate Professor
Department of Craniomaxillofacial Surgery
University Hospital Freiburg
Freiburg, Germany

Petr Schutz MD (Chapter 27)
Consultant
Head of Oral and Maxillofacial Surgery Unit
Dental Center, Farwaniya Hospital
Ministry of Health
Kuwait

Lars Sennerby DDS, PhD (Chapter 14)
Professor of Clinical and Experimental Oral
Implantology
Department of Biomaterials
Institute for Clinical Sciences
Sahlgrenska Academy
University of Gothenburg
Gothenburg, Sweden
and
Clinica Feltre
Feltre, Italy

Bethany Serafin DMD (Chapter 28)
Valley Village Oral Surgery Associates
Baltimore, Maryland, USA

Arun B. Sharma BDS, MSc
Health Sciences Clinical Professor
Division of Prosthodontics
University of California, San Francisco – School of
Dentistry
San Francisco, California, USA

Jeremy Sherman BDS, MBChB, FRCS, FDRCS, FRCS Ed
(Chapter 25)
Consultant Maxillofacial Surgeon
Department of Oral and Maxillofacial Surgery
Queen Elizabeth II Hospital
Welwyn Garden City, UK

Vivek Shetty DDS, Dr Med Dent
Professor
Section of Oral and Maxillofacial Surgery
University of California, Los Angeles
Los Angeles, California, USA

Ryan J. Smart DMD, MD (Chapter 7)
Resident
Department of Oral and Maxillofacial Surgery
Massachusetts General Hospital
Boston, Massachusetts, USA

Srinivas M. Susarla DMD, MD, MPH (Chapter 7)
Resident
Department of Oral and Maxillofacial Surgery
Massachusetts General Hospital
Boston, Massachusetts, USA

Wayne K. Tanaka DDS, FACD, FICD (Chapter 1)
Associate Professor, Predoctoral Program Director
Department of Oral and Maxillofacial Surgery
Loma Linda University
Loma Linda, California, USA

Peter Tarnow MD, PhD
Chairman, The Craniofacial Unit
Department of Plastic Surgery
Sahlgrenska University Hospital
Gothenburg, Sweden

Mitsuhiro Tsukiboshi DDS, PhD (Chapter 11)
Private practice, general dentistry
Aichi, Japan

Sina Uçkan DDS, PhD (Chapter 13)
Department of Oral and Maxillofacial Surgery
Başkent University
Ankara, Turkey

Kalyan Voruganti BDS
Senior House Offi cer
Regional Maxillofacial Unit
University Hospital Aintree
Liverpool, UK

Anders Westermark DDS PhD (Chapter 33)
Associate Professor
Department of Maxillofacial Surgery
Karolinska University Hospital
Stockholm, Sweden

Nils Weyer MD, DMD (Chapter 27)
Department of Craniomaxillofacial Surgery
University Hospital Freiburg
Freiburg, Germany

David W. Williams BSc(Hons), PhD (Chapter 4)
Reader in Oral Microbiology
School of Dentistry
Cardiff University
Cardiff, UK

Mark Eu-Kien Wong DDS
Chairman and Program Director
Department of Oral and Maxillofacial Surgery
University of Texas Health Science Center – Houston
Houston, Texas, USA

Leena P. Ylikontiola DDS, MD, PhD
Assistant Professor
Institute of Dentistry
University of Oulu
and
Co-ordinator of Cleft Lip and Palate Program
Oulu University Hospital
Oulu, Finland

Li-wu Zheng DDS, MD, PhD
Assistant Professor
Discipline of Oral and Maxillofacial Surgery
Faculty of Dentistry
University of Hong Kong
Hong Kong, SAR, China

Preface

Shortly after the successful launch of our international reference textbook *Oral and Maxillofacial Surgery* in 2010, we had the idea of abstracting and distilling the essential elements of the textbook and adding new sections to produce a textbook suitable for dental students and trainees worldwide. This textbook is the result of those efforts. It is designed to fulfill the curricular needs in oral and maxillofacial surgery for all dental students and it will also fulfill most of the needs of trainees in oral and maxillofacial surgery and allied disciplines. We have maintained the same team of international authors as in the larger textbook. We hope this textbook portrays the excitement we feel in the development of our specialty over the past 20 years and gives a flavor of some of the anticipated achievements of the next few years.

This book is dedicated to our teachers and mentors (we stand on the shoulders of giants) as well as the dedication and sacrifices of our wives Ann, Ingrid, and Karin.

M. Anthony (Tony) Pogrel   Karl-Erik Kahnberg   Lars Andersson

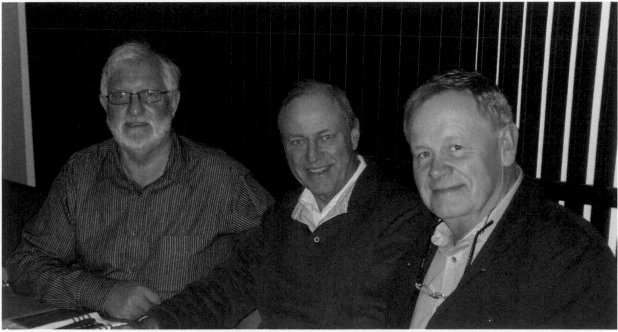

Editors at editorial board meeting, Gothenburg, Sweden, March 2013

About the companion website

This book is accompanied by a companion website:

www.wiley.com/go/pogrel/oms

The website includes:

- 89 interactive multiple-choice questions
- Powerpoints of all figures from the book for downloading

Part 1: Basic Principles

(Section Editor: Tony Pogrel)

Chapter 1

Patient Evaluation

The goal of preoperative evaluation is to reduce patient risk and the morbidity of surgery, and is based on the premise that it will modify patient care and improve outcome.

The Joint Commission for the Accreditation of Healthcare Organizations (JCAHO) requires that all patients receive a preoperative anesthetic evaluation and the American Society of Anesthesiologists (ASA) has approved Basic Standards for Preoperative Care which outline the minimum requirements for a preoperative evaluation. Preoperative patient assessment is important in order to develop a safe and appropriate surgical and anesthetic plan.

Obtaining a patient history

The importance of an accurate, detailed history cannot be overemphasized because it provides the framework on which the clinician builds an accurate diagnosis and treatment plan. An inaccurate or incomplete evaluation may lead to a delay in treatment, unnecessary testing, or misdiagnosis.

It is often helpful to review previous medical records. This can provide important information and save time during the interview process. The patient should be asked to describe the history of the present illness (HPI). Information should be gathered regarding onset, intensity, quality, location, duration, radiation, and any exacerbating or relieving factors. Constitutional symptoms that relate to the present illness should also be noted. Examples of pertinent positives and negatives with regard to the chief complaint may include fever, chills, loss of weight, weakness, etc.

The past medical history (PMH) alerts the clinician to any coexisting illnesses that may have an impact on any planned surgeries. A family history (FH) may reveal risk factors for patients as well as the possibility of inherited illnesses such as hemophilia or malignant hyperthermia.

The social history (SH) of a patient should include information regarding their social support system and also any habits such as tobacco, alcohol, or illicit drug use. These habits may adversely affect healing and also increase a patient's risk for undergoing a planned surgical procedure.

A review of systems (ROS) is a comprehensive method of inquiring about a patient's symptoms on an organ system basis. The review of systems may reveal undiagnosed medical conditions unknown to the patient.

Physical examination

During the physical exam the clinician further reinforces or disproves impressions gained during the history-taking portion. Vital signs are recorded at the beginning of the physical exam. These include blood pressure, pulse rate, respiratory rate, and temperature. The patient's general appearance should be noted.

For a complete description of examination techniques the reader is advised to consult textbooks on physical diagnosis.

Comorbidities/systemic diseases

The clinician needs to assess potential risk factors and understand their effect on treatment. Changes in heart rate, rhythm, blood pressure, preload, afterload, and inotropy may occur during surgery and these can have deleterious effects, especially in patients with comorbidities. The risks for complications are greatest when caring for patients who are

Essentials of Oral and Maxillofacial Surgery, First Edition. Edited by M. Anthony Pogrel, Karl-Erik Kahnberg and Lars Andersson.
© 2014 John Wiley & Sons, Ltd. Published 2014 by John Wiley & Sons, Ltd.
Companion website: www.wiley.com/go/pogrel/oms

already medically compromised. Many significant untoward events can be prevented by careful preoperative assessment along with attentive intraoperative monitoring and support.

Cardiovascular system

Cardiac disease

Cardiac complications following non-cardiac surgery constitute an enormous burden of perioperative morbidity and mortality. More than one million operations annually are complicated by adverse cardiovascular events, such as perioperative myocardial infarction or death from cardiac causes. Common cardiac risk factors include diabetes, hypertension, family history of heart disease, hypercholesterolemia, and obesity. Certain populations of patients, such as the elderly, diabetics, or women, may present with more atypical features.

Methods for evaluating a patient's cardiac risk preoperatively include a careful history, including exercise tolerance, physical examination, and electrocardiogram (EKG). Based on this information, various risk indices, guidelines, and algorithms can assist the clinician in deciding which patients can undergo surgery without further testing and which patients may benefit from further cardiac evaluation or medical therapy prior to surgery. Risk assessment involves evaluating patients' comorbidities and exercise tolerance, as well as the type of procedure to be performed to determine the overall risk of perioperative cardiac complications. Exercise tolerance is a major determinant of cardiac risk and need for further testing. Beta blockade has shown clear benefits in risk reduction whereas revascularization procedures, such as coronary artery bypass grafting, have not been shown to be useful in reducing non-cardiac surgical risk.

Hypertension

Hypertension is a common disease which can increase perioperative cardiac risk. Hypertension has been associated with an increase in the incidence of silent myocardial ischemia and infarction. The Joint National Committee on Prevention, Detection, Evaluation and Treatment of High Blood Pressure recently revised their definition. Hypertensive patients with left ventricular hypertrophy are at a higher perioperative cardiac risk than non-hypertensive patients.

Controversy exists regarding whether to delay a surgical procedure in a patient with untreated or poorly controlled hypertension. Aggressive treatment of high blood pressure does diminish long-term risk. A study often quoted as the basis for delaying surgery for patients with a diastolic blood pressure greater than 110 mmHg actually demonstrated no major morbidity in that group of patients. Other authors have found little association between blood pressures less than 180 mmHg systolic or 110 mmHg diastolic and postoperative outcomes. Patients with severe hypertension are more prone to perioperative myocardial ischemia, ventricular dysrhythmias, and lability in blood pressure. For patients with blood pressures greater than 180/110 mmHg there is no absolute evidence that postponing surgery will decrease the cardiac risk. For patients without end-organ changes, such as renal insufficiency or left ventricular hypertrophy, it may be appropriate to proceed with surgery. However, patients with a markedly elevated blood pressure and new onset of a headache should have surgery delayed for further medical treatment. Patients with hypertension may have a contracted intravascular volume and therefore have an increased susceptibility to vasodilator effects of commonly used sedative and anesthetic agents. For elective surgery it is best to have the patient's blood pressure optimized prior to surgery.

Risk factors for hypertension include smoking, hypercholesterolemia, increasing age, family history of cardiovascular disease, and diabetes. Untreated hypertension commonly causes coronary heart disease, cardiomegaly, congestive heart failure, and end-organ damage. When evaluating a patient with hypertension, it is important to determine the presence of end-organ damage (heart, lung, and cerebrovascular systems). An elevated systolic blood pressure may be a better predictor of postoperative myocardial ischemia than elevated diastolic blood pressure.

Pulmonary system

Pulmonary complications are a major cause of morbidity for patients undergoing a surgical procedure. They occur more frequently than cardiac complications with an incidence of 5–10% in those having major non-cardiac surgeries. Perioperative pulmonary complications include atelectasis, pneumonia, bronchitis, bronchospasm, hypoxemia, and respiratory complications. For patients with an upper respiratory illness, surgery should be delayed if possible for at least 2 weeks after resolution of the illness. Studies have indicated a 10% incidence of severe complications, respiratory as well as cardiac arrest, pneumonia, and prolonged intubation due to increased sputum, when surgery is performed on patients with an active upper respiratory tract infection.

During the presurgical evaluation, the clinician should obtain information about exercise tolerance, chronic cough, or unexplained dyspnea. On physical exam, findings of rhonchi, wheezing, decreased breath sounds, dullness to percussion, and a prolonged expiratory phase are important. Preoperative pulmonary function tests are usually reserved for patients undergoing lung resection or those undergoing major surgery who have unexplained pulmonary signs and symptoms after a history and physical examination.

Obesity

A patient is considered obese when their body weight is 20% or more above ideal weight. Obesity can be measured by the body mass index (BMI) which is derived by dividing the weight in kilograms by the height in meters squared (BMI = Wt/ht^2).

A BMI greater than 30 suggests increased morbidity due to stroke, heart disease and diabetes. At a minimum, these conditions indicate the need for close evaluation of the patient's airway and cardiac and pulmonary status. Even with an adequate airway, ventilation may be difficult because of the patient's size and a tendency toward hypoxemia. There may also be significant cardiovascular changes.

On the other hand, the clinician should not dismiss a low BMI, especially with evidence suggesting an eating disorder. Nutritional deficiency may be present along with significant cardiac changes, fluid and electrolyte imbalances, delayed gastric emptying, and severe endocrine abnormalities.

Imaging

A patient's presentation will dictate which films are required. Radiographs such as plain films, cone beam or fan beam computed tomography (CT), nuclear scans, and arteriography are helpful in various circumstances. The risks associated with these studies should be weighed against the added benefit from them.

Laboratory studies

Some institutions have preadmission screening test algorithms based on factors such as age of the patient (Table 1.1). Preoperative laboratory tests should be ordered based on defined indications such as positive findings on a history and physical exam. A thorough history and physical examination can be used to identify those medical conditions that might affect perioperative management and direct further laboratory testing. A study by Golub *et al.* reviewed the records of 325 patients who had undergone preadmission testing prior to surgery. Of these 272 (84%) had at least one abnormal screening test, while only 28 surgeries were canceled or delayed. Only three patients potentially benefited from preadmission testing, including a new diagnosis of diabetes in one and non-specific EKG changes in two. Another study

Table 1.1 Sample preadmission screening test algorithm. (EBL, estimated blood loss; HTN, hypertension; IVDA, intravenous drug abuse; LMP, last menstrual period; ABG, arterial blood gases; CBC, complete blood count; PT, prothrombin time; PTT, partial thromboplastin time; LFTs, liver function tests; CXR, chest X-ray; EKG, electrocardiogram; HCG, human chorionic gonadotropin; UA, urinalysis; PFTs, pulmonary function tests; T/S, type and screen.)

CIRCLE APPROPRIATE LABS TO ORDER												
Preoperative condition	ABGs	CBC	PT/PTT	Lytes	BUN/Creat	Blood/Glucose or Accucheck	LFT	CXR	EKG	Hcg preg/UA	PFTs	T/S
Possible EBL >500 ml		X										X
Neonates		X										
Age: >40 yr									X			
Age: >75 yr		X			X				X			
Cardiovascular disease/chronic HTN		X			X			X	X			
Use of diuretics, digoxin				X*	X				X			
Severe pulmonary disease/prethoracotomy	X	X						X	X		X	
Malignancy/radiation/chemotherapy		X, plt	X	X								
Hepatic disease		X, plt					X					
Chronic alcoholism		X, plt	X	X	X		X		X			
Renal disease (dialysis)		X	X*	X*				–/+	–/+			
Bleeding disorder/anticoagulant therapy		X,plt*	X*									
Diabetes				–/+	X	X*			>30 yr			
Possible pregnancy/gyn surgery										X*		

Note: Not all diseases are included. Therefore, the physician should use own judgment regarding patients having diseases that are not listed.

In patients with stable medical conditions, labs and EKGs within the last 3 months, and CXR within the last year, will be acceptable. X Items should be done within 72 hours of surgery.

*Urine pregnancy test if LMP >21 days with possibility of pregnancy or menstruating females <18 years of age, all women undergoing tubal ligation and all women having a hysterectomy who are in their reproductive years or who are experiencing the first year of menopause.

Table 1.2 American Society of Anesthesiologists physical status classification.

Status	Disease state
ASA class 1	No organic, physiologic, biochemical, or psychiatric disturbance
ASA class 2	Mild to moderate systemic disturbance that may not be related to the reason for surgery
ASA class 3	Severe systemic disturbance that may or may not be related to the reason for surgery
ASA class 4	Severe systemic disturbance that is life threatening with or without surgery
ASA class 5	Moribund patient who has little chance of survival but is submitted to surgery as a last resort (resuscitative effort)
Emergency operation (E)	Any patient in whom an emergency operation is required

by Narr *et al.* demonstrated minimal benefits from routine testing and proposed that routine laboratory screening tests were not required in healthy patients.

Assessing anesthetic/surgical risk

Once the clinician has gathered information by interviewing and examining the patient, they can classify them according to the American Society of Anesthesiologists (ASA) Classification of Physical Status (Table 1.2). Patients with a lower ASA classification represent a lower surgical risk than do patients with severe systemic disease. This system is commonly used and is helpful in identifying risk factors so that modifications in the treatment plan can be undertaken. The surgical procedure influences the scope of preoperative evaluation required by determining the potential range of physiologic flux during the perioperative period.

Office vs inpatient

Once the clinician has gathered pertinent information during the preoperative work-up, they must decide where best to perform the surgical procedure.

Safety continues to be the guiding factor in deciding where various types of procedures should be performed. Options available include office surgery, ambulatory surgery centers, and traditional hospital-

based locations. Many variables are considered when deciding on whether to perform a surgery in the office or perform the surgery elsewhere, including the size and severity of the surgery.

Patient factors should also be an important part of the decision on where to perform the procedure. Patients with poorly controlled medical conditions such as morbid obesity or poorly controlled hypertension should be carefully evaluated, and appropriate preoperative testing should be performed to determine their surgical risk. Patient factors such as increased age, an operating time longer than 120 minutes, cardiac diagnoses, peripheral vascular disease, cerebrovascular disease, malignancy, and immunodeficiency can place patients at higher risk for immediate hospital admission.

Advantages of performing surgery in a hospital setting include the addition of another health care provider to administer anesthetic during the surgical procedure. Imaging techniques such as ultrasonography, CT, and chest radiographs are readily available, as are blood chemistries to rapidly diagnose and treat complications. Also, procedures such as interventional radiology, for such things as embolization, are available. Ultimately the decision on where to perform a surgery depends on both the surgeon and informed patient considering the type and length of the procedure, patient health factors, and safety.

Summary

The process of preoperative evaluation is essential in assessing the medical condition of patients, evaluating their overall health status, determining risk factors, and educating them. The goal of preoperative evaluation is to reduce patient risk and the morbidity of surgery.

Recommended reading

Golub R, Cantu R, Sorrento JJ, *et al.* (1992). Efficacy of preadmission testing in ambulatory surgical patients. *The American Journal of Surgery*, **163**, 565.

Herford AS, Tanaka WK. (2010) Patient evaluation. In: *Oral and Maxillofacial Surgery* (eds, Andersson L, Kahnberg K-E, Pogrel MA). Oxford, Wiley-Blackwell.

Narr BJ, Hansen TR, Warner MA. (1991) Preoperative laboratory screening in healthy Mayo patients: cost-effective elimination of tests and unchanged outcomes. *Mayo Clinic Proceedings*, **66**, 155.

Chapter 2

Radiographic Imaging in Oral and Maxillofacial Surgery

Introduction

The most common radiographic examinations of oral and maxillofacial surgery patients are intraoral and panoramic radiographs. However, today computed tomography (CT) and magnetic resonance imaging (MRI) are common examinations in imaging of many different conditions. A useful investigation is one in which the result – positive or negative – will alter management or add confidence to the clinician's diagnosis. It is important to try to minimize the radiation dose to the patient (particularly children). CT can potentially give significant absorbed doses to the patient. The trend today is to use a low-dose technique for CT, but this can be at the expense of the image quality and its use depends on the clinical problem.

Computed tomography (CT)

CT is a digital technique providing images of thin slices of the patient with a variable thickness. The slice thickness can be less than 1 mm by use of very small X-ray detectors and a fan-shaped X-ray beam transmitted through the patient. By simultaneously scanning several slices of the body (multislice CT), the scan time can be reduced significantly and the smallest details can be imaged within short scan times. Multislice CT enables a wide range of clinical applications and, through the use of computer software, three-dimensional (3D) images can be produced. Images can be viewed in the axial, coronal, or sagittal planes depending on the diagnostic task. This is referred to as multiplanar reformatted (MPR) imaging. Images can also be viewed in any other plane decided by the operator. CT has the advantage over other radiographic techniques that it eliminates superimposition of images of structures outside the area of interest. It has an inherent high-contrast resolution and differences between tissues that differ in physical density by less than 1% can be distinguished. For image display, each pixel is assigned a CT number (Hounsfield units – HU) representing density. The density of air is defined as $-1000\,HU$, water as $0\,HU$ and bone tissue has more than $+400\,HU$. To allow the observer to interpret the image, only a limited number of HU are displayed. A clinically useful gray scale is achieved by setting the window level and window width on the computer console to a suitable range of HU, depending on the tissue being studied. The term "window level" represents the central HU of all the numbers within the window width. The window width covers the HU of all the tissues of interest and these are displayed as various shades of gray.

Cone-beam computed tomography (cone-beam CT)

This technique has been commercially available since the early years of the present century. Cone-beam CT is based on volumetric tomography, in contrast to conventional fan-beam CT where slices are scanned. From this, volume slices can be reconstructed in various planes. One advantage with cone-beam CT compared to conventional CT is the lower radiation dose. The radiation dose is reduced by up to 98% compared with conventional CT and is comparable to 2–28 average panoramic radiographs. The dose varies substantially, however, depending on the device, imaging field and selected technique factors. The scan time is relatively short (around 10 s) and the resolution is high (i.e. around 0.125 mm) and approaches that of fan-beam CT. The software is usually adapted to maxillofacial imaging and is real-time interactive, for example for implant planning.

Essentials of Oral and Maxillofacial Surgery, First Edition. Edited by M. Anthony Pogrel, Karl-Erik Kahnberg and Lars Andersson.
© 2014 John Wiley & Sons, Ltd. Published 2014 by John Wiley & Sons, Ltd.
Companion website: www.wiley.com/go/pogrel/oms

In both cone-beam CT and conventional CT, artifacts are produced by metal objects and it is important to try to avoid exposing metal fillings and crowns.

Magnetic resonance imaging (MRI)

MRI does not use ionizing radiation, but rather uses magnetic fields to align protons in the body, which can then be recorded electronically as they revert to their baseline orientation, and reformatted to build up an image. There are, however, some contraindications since the presence of ferromagnetic metals is a potential hazard. Patients with magnetic or paramagnetic metallic foreign objects, pacemakers, and metal clips must not be examined. Pregnancy is a relative contraindication.

The advantage of MRI is that it offers the best resolution of tissues of low inherent contrast and it has an excellent soft tissue contrast resolution. Disadvantages are relatively long imaging times and patients who suffer from claustrophobia cannot be examined. Open MRI scanners are sometimes used for claustrophobic patients but the images are of low resolution and are usually unsuitable for head and neck imaging.

MRI physics is complex and an understanding of the basic concepts is important in order to manipulate the scan parameters to improve the quality of the images.

Impacted teeth

A preoperative examination of an impacted tooth usually consists of two intraoral radiographs exposed at different angles (Fig. 2.1 a and b) or a panoramic radiograph. Using intraoral films in three different projections gives an insight into the true anatomy of third molars when the radiographic appearance was compared to the clinical observation. Intraoral and panoramic radiographs are usually sufficient to show

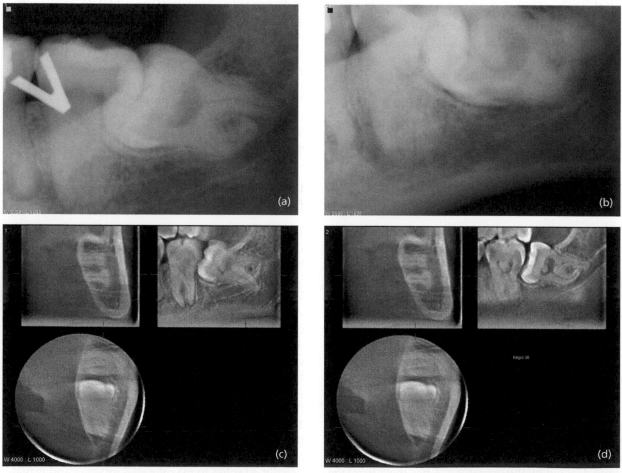

Fig. 2.1 Impacted lower third molar in a mesioangular position. (a) Periapical radiograph taken with +10° vertical angulation of the X-ray tube. Two mesial roots (one straight and one curved) and one distal root are seen. (b) Periapical radiograph taken with −10° vertical angulation of the X-ray tube. The mandibular canal seems to be buccal to the curved root. (c) Cone-beam CT with 1 mm thick sections. Upper left image is a cross-section of the mandible through the roots. The mandibular canal is seen below the mesial roots, lingual to the buccal root and buccal to the lingual root. Upper right image is a sagittal view of the buccal part of the tooth and the straight mesio-buccal root is shown. Lower section shows an axial view of the tooth, which is situated close to the lingual compact bone. (d) Same as (c), but the section is lingually placed. The curved mesio-lingual root is shown in the sagittal view.

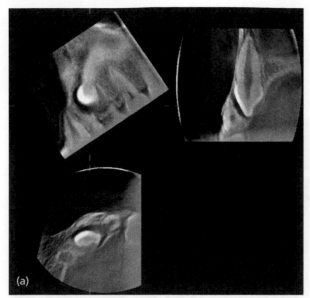
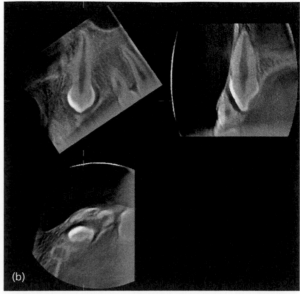

Fig. 2.2 Cone-beam CT examination of a non-erupted maxillary canine causing resorption of the root of the lateral incisor. The crown of the canine is situated palatal to the root of the incisor. (a) Upper left, sagittal view. Upper right, cross-section of the jaw. Lower, axial view. (b) Same as (a), but the 1 mm thick section is placed more palatal in the sagittal section. The root tip of the canine is curved mesially.

the relationship between the roots of the third molar and the mandibular canal. However, narrowing of the canal, increased radiolucency ("dark band") and interruption of the radiopaque border of the mandibular canal can justify a CT examination. Cone-beam CT has been shown to have a high diagnostic accuracy in predicting neurovascular bundle exposure during extraction of impacted mandibular third molars. Figure 2.1 c and d show an example of an impacted mandibular third molar with a complicated root anatomy examined with cone-beam CT.

CT is also valuable when examining impacted teeth in other regions. Cone-beam CT has been shown to be indicated for localization of impacted maxillary canines and has demonstrated root resorption better on the adjacent incisors compared to conventional radiography. Figure 2.2 shows a cone-beam CT examination of a non-erupted maxillary canine causing resorption of the root of the lateral incisor.

Pathological conditions – inflammatory lesions, cysts, benign and malignant tumors

The aims of the radiographic examination are to give information that leads to the most probable diagnosis and to the optimal treatment. The examination must cover the whole pathological area in at least two dimensions. A combination of different radiographic techniques can lead to a more certain diagnosis, but it should always be kept in mind that the treatment also must be affected positively by the extended examinations in order to be justified. There are some

radiological signs that always must be looked for when interpreting radiographs of pathological conditions, such as:

- location and size;
- periphery and shape;
- internal structures;
- effects on surrounding structures.

Inflammatory lesions

There are several lesions that present as a radiolucent area in the jaws. Inflammatory lesions located in the periapical area are by far the most common changes. It is not possible to differentiate radiologically between a radicular cyst and apical periodontitis. Radicular cysts tend to be larger than periapical granulomas, but a large variation in size has been shown for both types of lesions. This is not a diagnostic problem for small periapical radiolucencies as endodontic treatment has a high success rate and the prevalence of true cystic lesions is low. At follow-up after endodontic treatment and periapical surgery it is important to standardize the radiographic examination regarding projection and density/contrast of the image to be able to compare different examinations. An example is given in Figure 2.3 where the projection was changed between the two radiographs taken on the same occasion and it appears that the size of the periapical bone destruction has changed.

Cone-beam CT should be considered when no detectable pathology is found in periapical radiographs and clinical tests indicate pathology, as more periapical lesions are found with cone-beam CT. This is especially important in patients with chronic

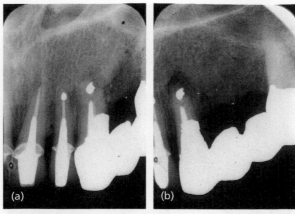

Fig. 2.3 Evaluation of healing after apical surgery of the upper left canine. Radiographs in (a) and (b) are taken at the same occasion, but with different projections. The apical bone destruction has a different appearance depending on the change of projection.

maxillary sinusitis, as a dental cause may be found in up to 40% of patients with chronic maxillary sinusitis.

Radiographs of the paranasal sinuses are not indicated routinely when sinusitis is suspected. Panoramic radiography should not be used for the detection of small osteolytic lesions in the maxillary sinus and soft tissue changes can be difficult to detect in panoramic radiographs depending on whether the surrounding structures are projected into the maxillary sinuses. CT is more rewarding than conventional radiography in the examination of the paranasal sinuses. Low-dose, high-resolution CT is recommended when medical treatment has failed, when complications arise, or if malignancy is suspected. Figure 2.4 shows a case of chronic maxillary sinusitis examined with panoramic radiography and low-dose CT.

Cysts and benign tumors

Radicular cysts are the most common cysts found in the jaws, followed by dentigerous cysts and keratocystic odontogenic tumors (KCOT). Large cysts in the region of the maxillary sinus may be difficult to image with conventional radiographs and CT is usually indicated to see the extension of the cyst (Fig. 2.5). Dentigerous cysts and KCOTs are usually incidental findings in panoramic radiographs, with KCOT predominantly found in the mandible (Fig. 2.6).

Malignant tumors

Primary malignant bone tumors are uncommon in the jaws. Squamous cell carcinoma is the most common head and neck cancer and it may invade the underlying bone. The typical appearance on a panoramic radiograph of a malignant lesion involving the jaw bone is bone destruction with a border that is ill defined. Figure 2.7 shows an example of a carcinoma

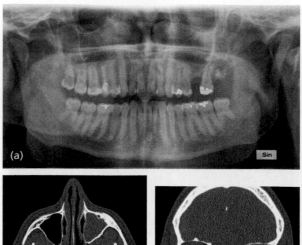
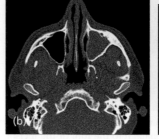
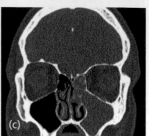

Fig. 2.4 A patient with chronic maxillary sinusitis. Panoramic radiography (a) and low-dose CT (b, c) were performed. (a) Panoramic radiograph showing root fragments of the upper left third molar with periapical bone destruction. The maxillary sinuses are difficult to evaluate. (b) Axial CT showing complete radiopacification of the left maxillary sinus. The bony walls are slightly sclerotic. (c) Coronal reconstruction showing the same picture as (b).

of the maxillary sinus involving the upper jaw detected on a panoramic radiograph. Rapidly growing malignant lesions destroy the alveolar bone but usually no root resorption is present. A typical sign is that the teeth may appear to be floating in space: "floating teeth".

The radiographic examination of malignant tumors often comprises CT and MRI to determine the extent of the tumor and to evaluate cervical lymphadenopathy. Post-treatment examinations are usually performed to evaluate the effect of treatment. A combination of CT and positron emission tomography (PET) has been introduced and PET/CT is now widely used as an advanced clinical tool for the diagnosis, staging, and restaging of cancer, and for the assessment of tumor therapy. A combination of MRI and PET is also becoming available. PET is a functional study where a radiolabelled isotope of glucose is given intravenously and areas of high metabolic activity can be recorded. The uptake is recorded by a nuclear imaging system and is normally merged with CT or MRI imaging for improved localization.

Temporomandibular joint (TMJ)

Imaging of TMD patients plays a minor role in the management of these patients as it has been shown that the treatment outcome is not affected by the radiological findings. Despite the success of conservative care, however, some patients do not improve and TMJ surgery may be indicated. In these cases

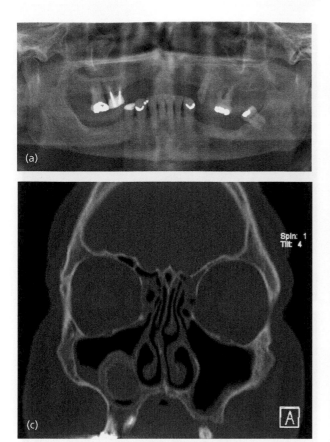

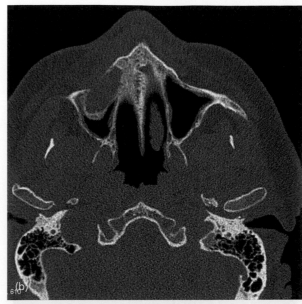

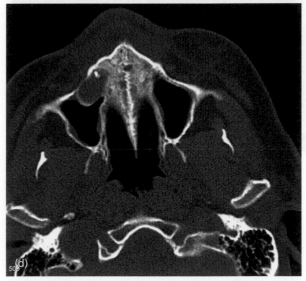

Fig. 2.5 Patient with a fistula in the maxillary right canine region. Buccal swelling and symptoms of sinusitis. He mentions that a tooth was extracted in the region about 10 years ago when he had similar symptoms. The final diagnosis was proved to be residual cyst. (a) Panoramic radiograph which is difficult to interpret. (b) CT with an axial section showing well-defined bone destruction in the right maxillary canine region. (c) Coronal section showing the cystic lesion with thickened bone around the cyst. Soft tissue swellings are seen in the maxillary sinus. (d) Axial CT taken 10 years earlier, when the patient had symptoms of sinusitis. A cystic lesion is seen around the root tip of the right maxillary canine. The tooth was later extracted.

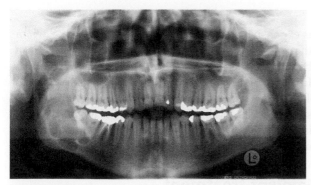

Fig. 2.6 Panoramic radiograph showing a multilocular bone destruction in the right mandibular ramus area. The patient had no symptoms and the cyst was detected in bitewing radiographs taken by his dentist. The tentative radiological diagnoses were ameloblastoma or keratocystic odontogenic tumor (KCOT). The diagnosis from the pathologist's report was KCOT.

radiography is indicated, as well as in patients with trauma, tumors, ankylosis and developmental anomalies. Further, radiographic examination of patients with polyarthritic conditions, such as rheumatoid arthritis, can be recommended to evaluate the degree of joint destruction. Bone scanning with [99m]technetium phosphate isotopes might be indicated to determine the level of growth activity in condylar hyperplasia.

There are different techniques for imaging the TMJ: panoramic radiography, plain radiography, conventional and computed tomography, arthrography, and MRI. Panoramic radiography is not a reliable method for accurately showing the shape of the mandibular condyle and the temporal component is poorly visualized. Plain radiography of the TMJ

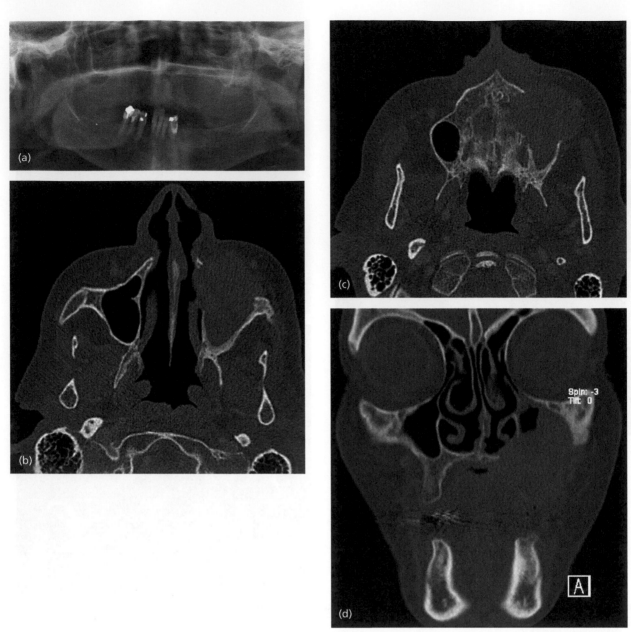

Fig. 2.7 The patient complains of pain in the upper left jaw. A swelling of the left cheek is noticed. (a) Panoramic radiography shows an ill defined bone destruction in the area of the left maxillary sinus and the edentulous jaw seems to be involved in the bone destruction. (b, c) Contrast-enhanced axial CT sections showing bone destruction of the anterior and medial walls of the maxillary sinus and of the alveolar bone. The tumor is expanding buccally into the cheek. (d) Coronal section showing complete destruction of the jaw. The superior bony wall to the orbit seems intact.

depicts the mineralized part of the joint, but superimposition of adjacent anatomic structures can make interpretation difficult. Conventional tomography improves the depiction of the bone structures. However, minor bony changes will not be shown in conventional tomography. CT imaging provides exquisite detail for bony abnormalities, such as ankylosis, fractures (Fig. 2.8), osseous tumors and arthrosis and 3D images can be produced; 3D reconstructions of a patient with condylar aplasia are shown in Figure 2.9.

MRI has replaced arthrography and can provide information about disk position, joint fluid, bone marrow changes, and bone structure at multiple levels of the joint. MRI is the prime diagnostic imaging technique in TMD patients. The technique, however,

is expensive and there are no studies showing when the results of the MRI examination will result in a better treatment outcome for the typical TMD patient. Imaging of the TMJ is definitely indicated prior to TMJ surgery and the preferred method is MRI if the soft tissue should be shown and CT if the hard tissue is of prime interest. In cases of tumors the methods often are combined.

Implant treatment

Panoramic radiography is the first choice for the radiological appraisal before implant treatment. The technique is, however, dependent on proper positioning of the patient during exposure and objects located outside the center of the sharply depicted plane are reproduced with distortions. Reliable measurements have been found for digital panoramic radiography, but both over and underestimation of vertical linear measurements have been found in other studies of panoramic radiography. The inherent errors in panoramic radiography should always be kept in mind whenever an exact assessment of a distance is required. Panoramic radiography is inferior to CT in visualization of the mandibular canal and in measurements related to the mandibular canal. Today, CT has almost totally replaced conventional tomography. There is equal accuracy so cone-beam CT should be preferred as this technique gives lower radiation dose compared to multislice CT and has a superior array of software for dental implant and related planning procedures. However, when a completely edentulous patient is examined several exposures with cone-beam CT with a narrow field size are necessary (Fig. 2.10). CT is indicated whenever the bone volume

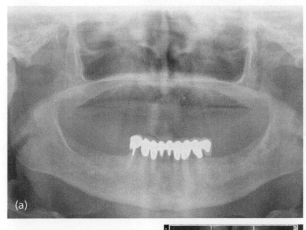

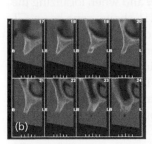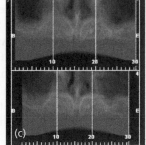

Fig. 2.10 Multislice CT examination for planning of implant treatment of an edentulous maxilla. (a) Panoramic radiograph. The bucco-palatal bone width of the maxilla was judged to be questionable. (b) 3 mm thick paraxial reconstructions made perpendicular to the alveolar bone (cross-sections) of the left side from the incisor to the premolar region. The images are produced in scale 1:1. B = buccal, L = lingual. (c) 3 mm thick panoramic reconstructions. The number of the vertical lines can be identified in the paraxial sections in order to locate the section.

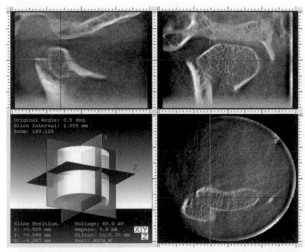

Fig. 2.8 Cone-beam CT of a fracture of the condylar neck after a bicycle accident. Upper left, sagittal view; upper right, coronal view; lower right, axial view. The condylar fragment has been dislocated medially and inferiorly. The images are taken with 3D Accuitomo (Morita Corp.)

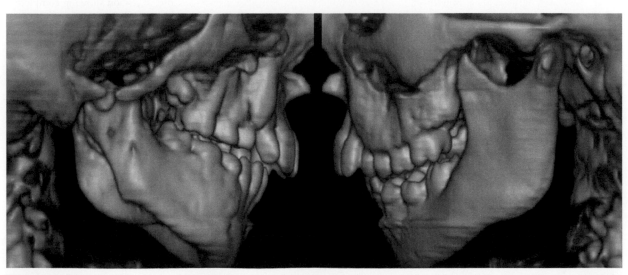

Fig. 2.9 CT 3D reconstructions of a patient with hemifacial microsomia and aplasia of the right condyle. The patient is missing the ear and a defective zygomatic arch is seen on the right side. The left side has developed normally.

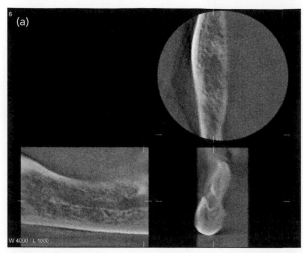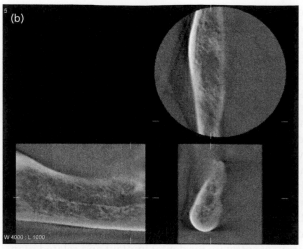

Fig. 2.11 Cone-beam CT of the mandible to visualize the mandibular canal. Images are produced in scale 1:1. (a) Anterior section showing the mental foramen (coronal section, lower right). (b) Posterior section in the molar region showing the mandibular canal (coronal section, lower right).

must be evaluated accurately and when localizing the mandibular canal. Figure 2.11 shows cone-beam CT of the mandibular canal. Another indication for CT is when evaluating bone grafting procedures in relation to implants, as two-dimensional radiographs underestimate bone resorption. Postoperative follow-up examinations after implant treatment are usually performed with intraoral radiographs taken in a standardized way.

Recommended reading

Endo K, Oriuchi N, Higuchi T, *et al.* (2006) PET an PET/CT using ^{18}F-FDG in the diagnosis and management of cancer patients. *The International Journal of Clinical Oncology*, **11**, 286–96.

Limchaichana N, Petersson A, Rohlin M. (2006) The efficacy of magnetic resonance imaging in the diagnosis of degenerative and inflammatory temporomandibular joint disorders: a systematic literature review. *OralSurgery, Oral Medicine, Oral Pathology, Oral Radiology and Endodontology*, **102**, 521–36.

Petersson A. (2010) Radiographic imaging in oral and maxillofacial surgery. In: *Oral and Maxillofacial Surgery* (eds, Andersson L, Kahnberg K-E, Pogrel MA). Oxford, Wiley-Blackwell.

Reddy MS, Mayfield-Donahoo T, Vanderven FJ, Jeffcoat MK. (1994) A comparison of the diagnostic advantages of panoramic radiography and computed tomography scanning for placement of root form dental implants. *Clinical Oral Implants Research*, **5**, 229–38.

Scarfe WC, Farman AG, Sukovic P. (2006) Clinical applications of cone-beam computed tomography in dental practice. *Journal of the Canadian Dental Association*, **72**, 75–80.

Tantanapornkul W, Okouchi K, Fujiwara Y, *et al.* (2007) A comparative study of cone-beam computed tomography and conventional panoramic radiography in assessing the topographic relationship between the mandibular canal and impacted third molars. *Oral Surgery, Oral Medicine, Oral Pathology, Oral Radiology and Endodontology*, **103**, 253–9.

Chapter 3

Local Anesthesia

Mode of action of local anesthetics

Local anesthetic drugs achieve their action at the voltage-gated sodium channel. In simple terms they inhibit sodium entry into nerve cells. As the entry of sodium into the nerve cell during the firing cycle is the chief driver producing depolarization, blockade of sodium transfer causes inhibition of neural activity.

It should be pointed out that the sodium channel is not a singular structure and that at least nine different variations have been identified. In theory this means that very selective local anesthetics could be developed. At present the local anesthetics used clinically are not specific for peripheral sensory nerves and can affect transmission in any excitable tissue such as motor nerves, central nervous system, and cardiovascular tissue.

Techniques of local anesthesia for oral and maxillofacial surgery

There are a number of different techniques that can provide local anesthesia in and around the mouth and jaws. These include methods that are used elsewhere in the body such as topical anesthesia, infiltration, and regional block techniques; however, there are methods that are unique to the mouth and jaws, such as intraosseous, intraligamentary, and intrapulpal injections.

Topical anesthesia

Topical anesthesia can be useful when applied to the oral mucosa. It may be employed prior to local anesthetic injections in the mouth to lessen the discomfort of needle penetration.

Topical anesthetics for intraoral use are available in a number of formulations including creams, ointments and sprays. The local anesthetic agents most commonly used as topical anesthetics in the mouth are lidocaine and benzocaine. Oraqix® is a combination of lidocaine and prilocaine specifically designed for intraoral topical anesthesia.

Advances in topical anesthesia (for example the development of Oraqix® and incorporation of drugs into liposomes) have meant that some intraoral soft tissue procedures can be performed using topical anesthesia as the sole agent; however, anesthesia of the teeth and jaws is not at present possible by this method.

Infiltration anesthesia

Infiltration anesthesia is useful in providing localized skin and mucosal anesthesia and can also be used to provide anesthesia for some teeth and part of the jaws. It is the technique of choice in the maxilla for dental pulpal anesthesia and can also be used for this purpose in the mandible of children for anesthesia of the deciduous dentition. It can be successful in the incisor teeth in the adult mandible and there is increasing evidence that some formulations (as described in the following paragraphcan be effective when infiltrated in the molar region of the mandible.

When used intraorally, access to the point of needle penetration is easiest when the patient has the mouth only partly open. The technique is performed by inserting the needle through reflected mucosa at the depth of the buccal sulcus; if bone is contacted the needle should be withdrawn slightly so that it is supraperiosteal. A supraperiosteal location is recommended as injection below the periosteum is painful at the time of injection and may cause postinjection discomfort. Following aspiration 1.0–2.0 mL of

Essentials of Oral and Maxillofacial Surgery, First Edition. Edited by M. Anthony Pogrel, Karl-Erik Kahnberg and Lars Andersson.
© 2014 John Wiley & Sons, Ltd. Published 2014 by John Wiley & Sons, Ltd.
Companion website: www.wiley.com/go/pogrel/oms

solution is deposited at a rate of 30 s/mL. This rate is slower than many practitioners use. Slow injection has a number of advantages. It reduces discomfort and increases success. In addition, a slow rate of injection may lessen the effects of systemic problems.

This method allows about 45 minutes of anesthesia of the dental pulps when a solution containing a vasoconstrictor (such as lidocaine with epinephrine) is used; soft tissue anesthesia is longer and the patient may have subjective anesthesia of the soft tissues for 1.5–2 hours.

Regional block anesthesia

Several regional block techniques are described to anesthetize structures in the jaws.

Mandibular anesthesia

There are a number of methods used to anesthetize the lower jaw, teeth and associated structures (for example, articaine 4% with 1 in 100 000 adrenaline). It should be remembered that midline structures (such as lower central incisor teeth) often receive bilateral supply; therefore, these may not be satisfactorily anesthetized by a single regional nerve block.

Inferior alveolar nerve block (Halstead technique)

This method anesthetizes the teeth and bone on one side of the mandible along with the soft tissues on the buccal aspect anterior to the mental foramen. The Halstead method achieves its effect by deposition of the solution in the pterygotemporal space on the medial aspect of the mandibular ramus, specifically in the region of the mandibular foramen. When successful this technique anesthetizes the inferior alveolar nerve, which supplies the teeth on the same side of the mandible, the bone of the mandible to the midline and the soft tissues of the lower lip to the midline as well as the reflected and attached gingivae from the premolar teeth to the midline. In addition, this injection usually anesthetizes the lingual nerve that supplies the anterior two-thirds of the tongue on one side.

The technique is illustrated in Figure 3.1. The patient has the mouth open wide and the operator places the thumb of the non-syringe hand in the mouth on the coronoid notch of the mandible; the index finger is extraoral at the same height on the posterior border of the ramus. The syringe is advanced to the point of needle penetration across the lower premolar teeth of the opposite side. The point of penetration of the needle is between the internal oblique ridge of the mandible (which was palpated by the operator's thumb before resting on the coronoid notch) and the pterygomandibular raphe (which is visible). The height of needle penetration is halfway up the operator's thumb nail. A long 35 mm needle no narrower

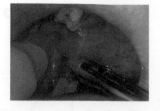
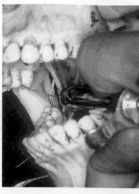

Fig. 3.1 The position of the needle during the Halstead approach to the inferior alveolar nerve. Source: Meechan, 2002. Reproduced with permission of Quintessence Publishing Co Ltd.

than 27 gauge is used and advanced until bone is contacted; this is usually around 25 mm of needle insertion. After contacting bone the needle is withdrawn slightly, aspiration performed and 1.5–2.0 mL of solution deposited slowly.

Two common problems with this method are either contacting bone too soon (after 5–10 mm of insertion) or failure to touch bone. The former (actually due to striking the internal oblique ridge of the mandible) is corrected by withdrawing the needle away from the bone, but not completely out of mucosa, and swinging the barrel of the syringe over the mandibular teeth of the side being anesthetized. The needle is then advanced about 25 mm and swung back again over the opposite premolar teeth; the rest of the injection is completed as described in the preceding paragraph. This is a modification of the indirect method of performing an inferior alveolar nerve block. If bone is not contacted after about 30 mm of insertion, the needle should be withdrawn until approximately 15 mm is still in tissue and the syringe swung over the molar teeth of the side not being injected, and then advanced until bone is contacted. Failure to contact bone may lead to injection into the parotid gland, affecting the intraparotid portion of the facial nerve, leading to hemifacial paresis.

When a vasoconstrictor solution, such as lidocaine with epinephrine, is used this technique will anesthetize the hard tissues including the teeth for around 45 minutes; however, subjective soft tissue numbness may be apparent for up to 3 hours. When the so-called long-acting solutions are employed anesthesia of the teeth can last for 6–8 hours.

Gow-Gates technique

In addition to the anesthesia of the inferior alveolar nerve this method may anesthetize the lingual, long buccal, mylohyoid and auriculotemporal nerves. This may be of value in countering accessory nerve supply to the teeth and jaw. This approach deposits solution more superiorly than the Halstead technique and that is the reason why more branches of the mandibular

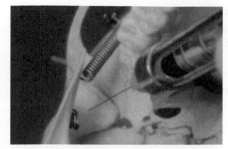

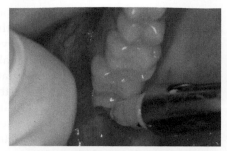

Fig. 3.2 Syringe position for the Gow-Gates mandibular block. Source: Meechan *et al.* 1998. Reproduced with permission of Oxford University Press.

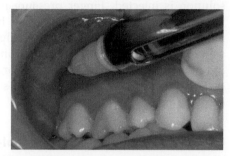

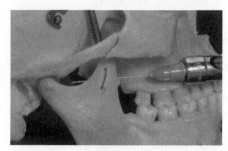

Fig. 3.3 The position of the syringe for the Akinosi–Vazirani mandibular block. Source: Meechan *et al.* 1998. Reproduced with permission of Oxford University Press.

nerve are affected by this injection. The target is the mandibular condyle (Fig. 3.2). As with the Halstead approach the patient has the mouth open wide. The syringe is advanced in a plane parallel to a line visualized between the corner of the mouth and the inter-tragal notch. The syringe, fitted with a long needle, is introduced into the mouth across the maxillary canine tooth of the opposite side to that being injected and advanced across the palatal cusps of the maxillary second molar on the side to be injected. This technique is often more successful in anesthetizing teeth than the Halstead approach. This may be the result of affecting nerves other than the inferior alveolar nerve that might supply the teeth.

Akinosi–Vazirani technique

This technique (Fig. 3.3) differs from the methods described earlier in two respects. Firstly, it is administered with the patient's mouth closed and so is useful in individuals who cannot fully open their mouth and is helpful in individuals with large or uncontrollable tongues when it is difficult to get access to the insertion point of a Halstead block. Secondly, there is no bony end-point for needle insertion. As is normal for all of the methods used to anesthetize the mandibular nerve, a long needle no narrower than 27 gauge is required. The syringe is introduced intraorally in the buccal sulcus along a plane level with the mucogingival junction of the maxillary mucosa. It is advanced at this level towards the posterior aspect of the maxilla until the hub of the needle is adjacent to the distal surface of the maxillary second molar. At this point the needle will have entered the mucosa and reached the correct depth of

insertion. Aspiration is performed and 2.0 mL of solution injected slowly. If the anterior aspect of the mandibular ramus is contacted the barrel of the syringe can be swung more laterally or the patient instructed to move their lower jaw over to the side being injected. This method anesthetizes the inferior alveolar nerve, lingual nerve, nerve to mylohyoid, and occasionally the long buccal nerve.

Mental and incisive nerve block

This injection anesthetizes the teeth and jaw from the premolars anteriorly as well as the soft tissues of the lower lip and chin to the midline on one side. Anesthesia of the first molar tooth is achieved in some cases. It relies on the deposition of solution around the mental nerve as it exits the mental foramen and the entry of solution into the foramen to block the incisive branch that supplies the lower anterior teeth on the same side. The usual method is intraoral although an extraoral approach may also be used. The needle is inserted at the depth of the buccal sulcus between the premolar teeth and advanced to a zone below the premolar apices. Around 1.5 mL of solution should be deposited and after injection the tissues should be massaged to encourage entry of solution into the mental foramen.

Long buccal nerve block

If the long buccal nerve has not been anesthetized by the methods which are described under the heading Regional block anesthesia (for example, if the Halstead technique was used) then this nerve must be anesthetized separately if required. The area supplied is the buccal gingivae and mucosa and part of the cheek in the mandibular molar region. The nerve can be anesthetized by either buccal infiltration in the zone of interest or by a regional block. The regional block is achieved by depositing 0.5 mL of solution in the region of the coronoid notch of the mandible (the point at which the thumb rests during the Halstead technique).

Maxillary anesthesia

Several regional block techniques are used in the maxilla. These are described as follows.

Maxillary nerve block

There are intraoral and extraoral approaches to the maxillary nerve block. The intraoral methods are the tuberosity approach and the greater palatine foramen approach. The maxillary nerve block anesthetizes the teeth and bone of the maxilla on one side together with the buccal and palatal mucosa, the skin and mucosa of the upper lip, the lower eyelid, and the lateral aspect of the nose.

Tuberosity approach
This is administered by depositing solution high in the buccal sulcus in the plane of the distal surface of the maxillary second molar tooth. The needle is advanced at an angle of 45° superiorly, posteriorly and medially to a depth of 30 mm, at which point 2.0 mL of solution is deposited following aspiration.

Greater palatine foramen approach
This technique involves inserting a needle into the pterygopalatine fossa via the greater palatine foramen. The patient has the mouth open wide and the greater palatine foramen is identified as a depression medial to the distal surface of the second maxillary molar tooth. The needle is inserted into the greater palatine foramen and advanced at an angle of 45° superiorly and posteriorly to a depth of 30 mm. At this point 2.0 mL of solution is deposited.

Posterior superior alveolar nerve block

This injection anesthetizes the maxillary molar teeth, associated bone and buccal gingivae. In those individuals with a middle superior alveolar nerve the first molar will not be satisfactorily anesthetized with this method as the mesio-buccal root of this tooth is supplied by that nerve (see Maxillary molar nerve block). The technique is identical to that described for the tuberosity approach to the maxillary nerve except that needle penetration is only 20 mm.

Maxillary molar nerve block

This is an adaptation of the posterior superior alveolar nerve block. It is designed to anesthetize the maxillary molar teeth by countering any accessory supply to the mesio-buccal pulp of the first molar from the middle superior alveolar nerve. During the injection the patient has the mouth half closed. The operator's finger palpates the zygomatic process of the maxilla intraorally and advances the finger posteriorly towards the maxillary tuberosity. The needle penetrates mucosa high in the buccal sulcus between the finger and the distal surface of the zygomatic process and advanced about 10 mm into the space above the buccinator attachment. At this point aspiration is performed and 2.0 mL of local anesthetic solution is injected. Finger pressure is maintained throughout the injection. Following injection, the patient is asked to close the mouth slightly and the solution, which has created a swelling above the buccinator, is massaged in a superior, medial and distal direction towards the posterior superior alveolar foramen.

Middle superior alveolar nerve block

This injection anesthetizes the premolar pulps as well as the mesio-buccal pulp of the maxillary first permanent molar tooth. The technique is performed by delivering a buccal infiltration at the apex of the second premolar tooth.

Anterior superior alveolar nerve block

The anterior superior alveolar nerve supplies the maxillary incisor and canine teeth on one side of the jaw. It can be anesthetized either by an infraorbital nerve block (described under Infraorbital nerve block) or by a buccal infiltration in the region of the apex of the canine.

Infraorbital nerve block

The infraorbital nerve can be approached either from the intraoral or the extraoral sides. The intraoral approach (Fig. 3.4) involves inserting a long needle high into the buccal sulcus between the premolar teeth and advancing towards the infraorbital foramen, which is being palpated extraorally by the operator's non-syringe hand. At this point 1–1.5 mL of solution is deposited following aspiration.

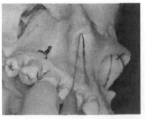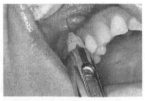

Fig. 3.4 The intraoral approach to the infraorbital nerve block. Source: Meechan, 2002. Reproduced with permission of Quintessence Publishing Co Ltd.

This injection anesthetizes the teeth and associated bone from the second premolar to the central incisor (although the latter may obtain some collateral supply from the opposite side). In addition the gingivae adjacent to these teeth and the mucosal and skin surfaces of one half of the upper lip and part of the skin on the lateral aspect of the nose are affected.

Greater palatine nerve block

This method anesthetizes the soft tissues of the palate from the foramen anteriorly to the canine region. The nerve can be anesthetized at any point by a palatal infiltration; however, the true block involves injection of 0.5 mL of solution in the region of the greater palatine foramen. The soft tissues of the hard palate up to the canine region on one side will be anesthetized. In addition this technique can be effective in countering any palatal supply to the maxillary teeth. Duration of anesthesia is not as long as with mandibular blocks. Indeed both palatal infiltration and blocks provide a similar duration of around 45 minutes of soft tissue anesthesia.

Nasopalatine nerve block

This method anesthetizes the tissues of the hard palate adjacent to the incisor teeth bilaterally. It is performed by injecting 0.2–0.5 mL of solution adjacent to the incisive papilla.

Anterior middle superior alveolar nerve block

This technique relies on the slow delivery of solution and is best achieved using a computer-controlled local anesthetic delivery device. The method works by entry of local anesthetic solution into the cancellous bone of the maxilla via multiple foramina in the hard palate. It anesthetizes the soft tissues of the palate and the teeth from the premolars anteriorly on one side. The needle is inserted halfway between the palatal midline and the premolar palatal gingival margin and 1.0 mL of solution is injected very slowly.

Palatal anterior superior alveolar nerve block

This technique achieves anesthesia of the teeth and anterior hard palate mucosa by the deposition of around 1.0 mL of local anesthetic solution into the nasopalatine foramen and thence into the cancellous bone of the anterior maxilla. As was the case with the anterior middle superior alveolar nerve block injection, the technique is most readily achieved using a computerized local anesthetic delivery device as a slow rate of delivery is required for patient tolerance. This technique can achieve pulpal anesthesia of the canine and incisor teeth bilaterally and on occasion may also anesthetize the premolar teeth.

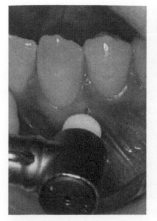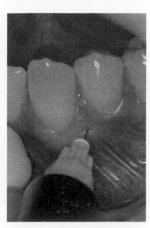

Fig. 3.5 The intraosseous injection showing preparation of the needle site with a perforator and then needle insertion. Source: Meechan, 2002. Reproduced with permission of Quintessence Publishing Co Ltd.

Supplementary intraoral techniques of local anesthesia

Intraosseous anesthesia

This method (Fig. 3.5) can be used in either jaw and, although it can be employed as a primary technique, it is normally reserved as a supplementary injection when conventional measures fail to produce adequate anesthesia of the pulps of teeth. The method is as follows. Firstly the buccal gingiva around the tooth of interest is anesthetized by a small-dose (0.2–0.5 mL) buccal infiltration. A perforation through soft tissue and cortical bone is made using a perforator matched to the needle (these are provided in customized systems) or with a small round dental bur. The point of penetration is 2 mm below the intersection of two imaginary lines. These are: a line joining the lowest part of the buccal gingival margin of the tooth of interest and its posterior neighbor; and a line at 90° to the former line that bisects the interdental papilla. If the point 2 mm below the intersection of these two lines is in reflected mucosa a point more coronal in attached gingiva is chosen. Once the perforation has reached cancellous bone the perforator or bur is replaced with a needle and 1.0 mL of solution injected slowly intraosseously. As intraosseous deposition of solution is equivalent to intravenous entry, slow deposition and dose limitation are important with this technique.

Intraligamentary (periodontal ligament) anesthesia

This is regarded as a specific version of an intraosseous technique (Fig. 3.6). Like the method described within Intraosseous anesthesia it can be used as a primary method of anesthesia but it is considered a supplementary method when tooth pulpal anesthesia is problematic. There are specialized syringes designed specifically for this method; however it is equally effective with conventional delivery systems.

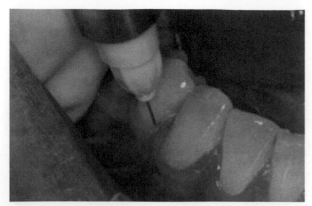

Fig. 3.6 The intraligamentary injection. Source: Meechan, 2002. Reproduced with permission of Quintessence Publishing Co Ltd.

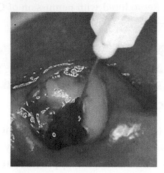

Fig. 3.7 An intrapulpal injection in a molar tooth. Source: Meechan *et al.* 1998. Reproduced with permission of Oxford University Press.

Normally a 30 gauge needle is used. It is inserted to the point of maximum penetration at the mesio-buccal aspect of the root of the tooth (each root for a multirooted tooth). The needle becomes wedged at the crest of the interdental bone and will not traverse far into the periodontal space. Delivery of solution (0.2 mL per root) is performed slowly with controlled pressure. The method obtains anesthesia by entry of the local anesthetic solution into the cancellous space of the bone via the perforations in the cribrifom plate of the socket. As the number of these perforations is low in anterior mandibular sockets the technique is not very successful in lower incisor teeth.

Intrapulpal anesthesia

This method (Fig. 3.7) has limited indications, as exposure of the tooth pulp is essential. It is unique among the techniques described here as the presence of a local anesthetic solution is not essential for success: saline has been shown to be as effective. The key to success is delivery of solution under pressure. This can be achieved with a needle that fits tightly into the pulpal exposure, by advancement of the needle into the pulp canal until it is wedged or by placing an obturator such as a cotton wool bud around the needle during injection. This is the most localized form of anesthesia described here and in theory could be used to anesthetize one pulp canal of a multirooted tooth.

Various drugs are available for local anesthesia in and around the jaws. These can be classified in a number of ways. The main categorization is by chemical structure. Local anesthetics are divided into two groups by their composition. These are the esters and the amides. The local anesthetics in current use as injectable agents are amides. The ester procaine is only used in those patients who are proven to be allergic to amides and such cases are very rare. Topical anesthetics such as benzocaine and tetracaine (amethocaine) are esters. There are two major differences between esters and amides; these relate to metabolism and the production of allergy. Esters are metabolized in plasma. Most amides primarily undergo hepatic metabolism, although prilocaine also undergoes some breakdown in the lungs. Articaine is an exception: although it is an amide, its primary metabolism occurs in the plasma.

In addition to categorizing local anesthetics by their chemical structure they can also be classified with respect to their duration of action into conventional and long-acting agents. Conventional agents may provide better operative anesthesia; however, long-acting agents may be preferred for postoperative pain control, especially in combination with general anesthesia. In order to achieve their long-acting effect such agents must be employed as regional blocks.

Lidocaine

Lidocaine is the gold standard drug to which all others are compared. When used as a plain solution in concentrations up to 2% it provides short-lasting soft tissue anesthesia. Such a formulation does not provide acceptable anesthesia of the dental pulps. When a vasoconstrictor is added to 2% lidocaine then satisfactory anesthesia is provided for the teeth. The vasoconstrictor most commonly employed is epinephrine (adrenaline) usually in the concentration range of $1:200\,000$ ($5\,\mu g/mL$) to $1:80\,000$ ($12.5\,\mu g/mL$).

Mepivacaine

Mepivacaine, when injected at a concentration of 2% in combination with $1:100\,000$ epinephrine, provides similar anesthesia to 2% lidocaine with epinephrine. It is also provided as a plain 3% solution and this provides better anesthesia than 2% lidocaine when a vasoconstrictor-free solution is required.

Prilocaine

Prilocaine is used as a plain 4% solution or as a 3% formulation in combination with the vasoconstrictor felypressin (a synthetic analog of vasopressin). The 3% formulation is a useful alternative to 2% lidocaine with epinephrine if an epinephrine-free solution is indicated.

Articaine

As mentioned earlier, articaine is unique among the amides in that initial metabolism occurs in plasma and thus, having a shorter plasma half-life, it is safer systemically than the other amides. This means that it can be used in higher concentration and so most articaine formulations are 4% with epinephrine in either 1:100000 or 1:200000 concentrations. There are some concerns, however, that local anesthetic drugs used in high concentration may increase the chances of localized toxicity leading to long-lasting anesthesia, paraesthesia or dysesthesia when used for regional blocks (see later). An advantage of the 4% articaine solution is that it is superior to 2% lidocaine solutions in providing anesthesia of the mandibular teeth following infiltration in the adult mandible. There is some evidence that buccal infiltration with 4% articaine is as effective as inferior alveolar nerve blockade with 2% lidocaine in providing anesthesia of the adult mandibular teeth.

Etidocaine

Etidocaine in a concentration of 1.5% with 1:200000 epinephrine has been used in oral surgery. It has a longer duration of action than 2% lidocaine with epinephrine 1:100000 when used as a regional block but is not as effective as lidocaine with epinephrine when used for infiltration anesthesia.

Bupivacaine

Bupivacaine is a long-lasting local anesthetic. When used as a supplementary intraoral injection during general anesthesia, this drug has been shown to reduce the number of analgesics required for postoperative pain control following oral surgery. It is presented in a number of formulations ranging from 0.25–0.75% with and without epinephrine (usually 1:200000).

Levobupivacaine

This is a single isomer of bupivacaine and has the advantage of being less cardiotoxic. It has been shown to be as effective a local anesthetic as bupivacaine and, like the latter drug, its use as an intraoral injection during general anesthesia can reduce postoperative analgesic requirements following oral surgery. It is available in concentrations ranging from 0.25–0.75%.

Ropivacaine

Like levobupivacaine this is a single isomer with reduced cardiotoxicity compared to bupivacaine.

There is a suggestion that it may be as effective with and without a vasoconstrictor; when used intraorally, however, the presence of epinephrine increases efficacy. It is available in concentrations ranging from 0.2–1.0%.

Complications of local anesthesia in the orofacial region

In addition to failure of local anesthesia there are a number of complications that can occur following the use of local anesthetics in the orofacial region. These can be separated into localized and systemic complications.

Localized complications

Localized complications can arise either as a result of physical damage from the needle or chemically as a result of the local anesthetic.

Nerve damage

Nerve damage can occur following regional block techniques. The nerve that is most commonly affected is the lingual nerve. The mechanism is unknown but there is an assumption that this can be due to physical trauma from the needle, which can result in altered sensation lasting for a few weeks. Normal sensation should recover in most cases following such trauma. The deposition of local anesthetic into the nerve bundle should be avoided as this can cause damage, both as a result of the physical disruption and chemically.

As mentioned earlier, the concentration of the local anesthetic has been implicated in the production of long-lasting paresthesias. Certainly *in vitro* the survival of nerve cells decreases as the local anesthetic concentration rises. There is some circumstantial evidence from both North America and Europe that local anesthetics in the concentration of 4% are associated with more paresthesias (particularly of the lingual nerve) than 2% and 3% solutions, although other investigations have failed to confirm this.

If nerve function does not return to normal within a few weeks the prognosis is poor. Surgical exploration does not generally reveal any obvious defect and nerve repair is not possible, in contrast to the treatment of surgically damaged nerves.

Motor nerve paralysis

Local anesthetics are not specific for peripheral sensory nerves and motor function can be affected. Facial nerve function may be affected if solution is injected into the substance of the parotid gland. Fortunately any paralysis produced is temporary. This may occur during the delivery of mandibular block techniques but can be avoided when using the Halstead method if bone is palpated before solution is delivered. This should ensure that the needle is not advanced beyond the posterior border of the mandibular ramus. The most serious consequence is loss of the blink reflex and thus the patient must have some form of eye protection until the effect wears off.

Trismus

Mandibular block techniques involve deep penetration of the needle and this may cause minor bleeding. If this occurs in the medial pterygoid muscle it can lead to muscle spasm and the inability to fully open the mouth. Although this problem does resolve it may take a few weeks to do so.

Intravascular injection

Intravascular injection can cause both localized and systemic complications. The use of an aspirating technique should reduce the chances of intravascular injection. Localized problems may result from intra-arterial injection. It is more difficult to penetrate an artery compared to a vein; however, it is not impossible and a variety of adverse effects may ensue. Entry or contact of an artery is painful and arteriospasm may produce localized vascular shutdown, which appears as blanching. Injecting local anesthetic into an artery that has an intracranial course can result in a number of spectacular sequelae. Vision may be affected. Both diplopia and loss of vision have been recorded following intraoral injections. Hearing loss has also been noted. The most dramatic effect reported is hemiparesis. This could result from the phenomenon known as reverse carotid flow. This occurs when local anesthetic is injected into a branch of the external carotid artery under pressure. This can send some of the agent to the carotid bifurcation resulting in transport of some anesthetic intracranially via the internal carotid. Such an effect has been demonstrated in animals following injection into the facial artery. This rare complication can be reduced by aspirating and injecting slowly.

Systemic complications

The following systemic complications caused by the injected agent can occur after the injection of local anesthetics: allergy, infection, toxicity, and drug interactions. These are discussed under their respective headings. Other systemic complications such as syncope are unrelated to the injected solution.

Allergy

Allergic reaction to the amide group of local anesthetics is extremely rare. Many individuals who claim to be allergic are found not to be so after formal testing. Nevertheless any individual complaining of non-localized swelling, rash, or breathing difficulty following injection should be tested, as the full range of allergic reactions, including anaphylaxis, has been reported after intraoral injections. Ester allergy is more common. Some local anesthetic cartridges (carpules) contain latex in their plungers or diaphragms and these should be avoided in patients with severe latex allergy. Older local anesthetic formulations contained preservatives related to paraben and this could cause allergic reactions in susceptible patients; however, most modern formulations are preservative-free.

Infection

Sensible precautions are essential during the administration of local anesthesia to prevent contaminating the patient and to avoid transfer of infection between operator and patient. The use of safety-type syringes, which eliminate resheathing of used needles, has been shown to reduce the chances of needle-stick injury. The use of such equipment is recommended.

Toxicity

As many local anesthetics contain an anesthetic and a vasoconstrictor it is, in theory, possible to have a toxic reaction to either component; however, as a result of their relative concentrations, a patient is more likely to suffer a toxic reaction to the anesthetic. The systems most susceptible to toxicity are the central nervous and cardiovascular systems. Most serious cases of overdose are the result of central nervous system effects. A toxic reaction to the anesthetic initially manifests as overexcitation, such as excessive talking and tremors. The later stages are signs of central nervous system depression ultimately leading to unconsciousness, and fatality can result from respiratory depression. The management is to stop the injection, monitor vital signs, and provide basic life support.

Overdose of epinephrine presents as anxiety, headache, and palpitations. If this occurs the patient should be sat upright and administered oxygen.

Systemic toxicity from local anesthetics can be the result of intravascular injection, use of excessive doses, or inability of the patient to metabolize the drug. Intravascular injection should be avoided by use of an aspirating technique. This is essential. Some workers report positive aspirates in over 20% of mandibular block injections.

Overdose of local anesthesia can occur, particularly in children. The maximum dose is related to the patient's weight. This means that overdose and an ensuing toxic reaction is more likely to occur in children.

Hepatic disease will reduce the metabolism of local anesthetics and this must be considered when deciding maximum doses for patients with such conditions.

Drug interactions

Interactions may occur between concurrent medication and local anesthetics or vasoconstrictors. There is no concurrent medication that absolutely contraindicates the use of local anesthetics or vasoconstrictors; however, there are times when a dose reduction is required. The main group of drugs that necessitate dose reduction are the cardiovascular drugs. In theory all antihypertensive medications can interact with epinephrine, for example beta-adrenergic blocking drugs can result in unopposed rises in systolic blood pressure, and calcium channel blockers and diuretics may increase epinephrine-induced hypokalaemia. Similarly beta-adrenergic blocking drugs can increase the toxicity of local anesthetics by reducing hepatic blood flow, which inhibits metabolism.

As well as prescribed medication, drugs of abuse such as cocaine and methamphetamine, can interact with epinephrine and avoidance or dose reduction of epinephrine-containing anesthetics is wise for patients who have recently used this drug (usually within the preceding 48 hours).

Although there are no absolute contraindications to the use of particular local anesthetics resulting from drug interactions there are some medical conditions where the use of an epinephrine-containing solution should be avoided. These include unstable angina, severe cardiac dysrhythmias, untreated pheochromocytoma and untreated hyperthyroidism.

Local anesthesia during pregnancy

The use of local anesthesia is not contraindicated in the pregnant patient. Nevertheless, it should be noted that all local anesthetics will cross the placenta. This is not problematic for most agents at the doses used in routine dentistry but warrants caution when higher amounts are considered. The local anesthetic drugs vary in the degree in which they diffuse across the placenta. Prilocaine diffuses the most. The drug that produces least concentration in the fetus is bupivacaine; however, it has been demonstrated in animal models that this agent produces cardiovascular collapse at lower plasma concentrations in the pregnant animal compared to non-pregnant controls. Theoretically, prilocaine can cause methemoglobinemia, particularly in the fetus, but this has not been reported clinically at the doses used for dentistry. The vasoconstrictor felypressin has some oxytocic activity; however, the dose that would induce labor equates to about 100 carpules of a dental local anesthetic.

Recommended reading

Gow-Gates GAE. (1973) Mandibular conduction anaesthesia: a new technique using extraoral landmarks. *Oral Surgery, Oral Medicine, Oral Pathology and Oral Radiology*, **36**, 321–8.

Jung IY, Kim JH, Kim ES, Lee CY, Lee SJ. (2008) An evaluation of buccal infiltrations and inferior alveolar nerve blocks in pulpal anesthesia for mandibular first molars. *Journal of Endodontics*, **34**, 11–13.

Kanaa MD, Whitworth JM, Corbett IP, Meechan JG. (2006) Articaine and lidocaine mandibular buccal infiltration anesthesia: a prospective randomised double-blind crossover study. *Journal of Endodontics*, **32**, 296–8.

Meechan JG. (2010) *Practical Local Dental Anaesthesia*, 2nd edn. New Malden, UK, Quintessence Publishing Co Ltd.

Meechan JG. (2010) Local anesthesia. In: *Oral and Maxillofacial Surgery* (eds, Andersson L, Kahnberg K-E, Pogrel MA). Oxford, Wiley-Blackwell.

Meechan JG, Robb ND, Seymour RA. (1998) *Pain and Anxiety Control for the Conscious Dental Patient*. Oxford, Oxford University Press.

Chapter 4

Dentofacial Infection

Introduction

Inflammation, infection, and pus formation were first described in Egyptian papyri. Inflammation is a reaction of the tissues to irritation as in an invasion by pathogenic microorganisms. These reactions tend to destroy and limit the spread of infectious agents and repair the damaged tissues. The inflammatory process involves fluid and cellular exudates in an attempt to destroy and engulf the invading microorganism.

Dentoalveolar abscess

The acute dentoalveolar abscess is a localized suppurative inflammation which involves the teeth and the supporting periodontal structures (Fig. 4.1). The pathogenic microorganisms, which are predominantly anaerobes, normally gain entry to the periapical tissue through the necrotic pulp of carious teeth or via the gingival crevice of the periodontal ligament. The most typical clinical features are severe pain and exquisite tenderness on percussion or touching the tooth during mastication. The pain is due to the local release of inflammatory mediators such as kinins and histamines, and fluid exudates causing increased pressure in the confines of the underlying alveolar bone. Pyrexia and lymphadenopathy can be common symptoms associated with this infection. Prompt evacuation of pus by either extracting the tooth or removing the infective pulp reduces the internal pressure and the patient's pain.

The fate of the acute dentoalveolar abscess depends on the number and the virulence of the invading microorganisms, as well as the resistance of the patient. The spread of the infection will be governed by the position of the tooth in the alveolus and relationship of the apices of the infected teeth to muscle attachments and their relative proximity to the lingual and buccal surfaces of the jaw bones.

Infection originating from a dental abscess may spread to involve the deeper tissues of the head and neck region, once the abscess has broken through the surface (usually buccally) of the alveolar bone. On the other hand, the invading microorganisms may be destroyed by the natural local resistance of the body, prescription of antibiotics, and removal of the source of infection by extraction or endodontic means. The lesion would then resolve. However, in some instances, lack of appropriate treatment may lead to the development of a chronic dentoalveolar abscess where the lesion never heals by itself but persists as a lesion of low-grade virulence, characteristic of the typical granuloma. Chronic dentoalveolar abscesses and periapical granulomas are generally asymptomatic unless, or until, reignited in an acute phase. Only the development of an acute exacerbation would lead to the cardinal signs of inflammation such as tenderness, pain, redness, and swelling. Sinus formation, either intraorally or extraorally, is not an infrequent feature of this chronic infection. The chronic lesion has the potential to stimulate epithelial cells and initiate the development of a dental cyst.

Radiographic appearance

In the acute phase, the earliest changes are thinning of the periodontal space followed by loss of apical lamina dura, then radiolucency with ill-defined margins. Chronic abscesses or apical granuloma are usually associated with a well-circumscribed radiolucency.

Site and spread of infection

Bone, muscle, aponeurosis or fascia, neurovascular bundles, and skin, can act as barriers against spread

Essentials of Oral and Maxillofacial Surgery, First Edition. Edited by M. Anthony Pogrel, Karl-Erik Kahnberg and Lars Andersson.
© 2014 John Wiley & Sons, Ltd. Published 2014 by John Wiley & Sons, Ltd.
Companion website: www.wiley.com/go/pogrel/oms

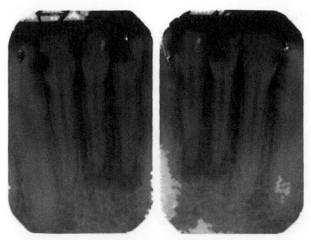

Fig. 4.1 Radiograph of dental abscess. Courtesy of Glasgow Dental Hospital and School.

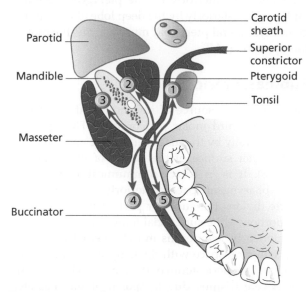

Fig. 4.2 Direction of spread of infection, and the fascial spaces involved, from the lower third molar site.

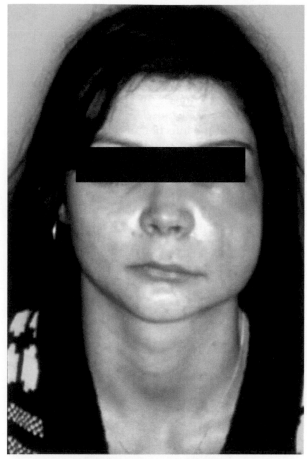

Fig. 4.3 Clinical infection of the upper teeth spreading to the canine fossa. Courtesy of Glasgow Dental Hospital and School.

of infection. However, none of these tissue barriers or boundaries is so restrictive or containing that they necessarily prevent the spread of infection into contiguous anatomic spaces (Fig. 4.2). The following are the most common routes for the spread of infection from dentoalveolar infections:

* upper lip;
* canine fossa;
* infraorbital region;
* buccal space (5 in Fig. 4.2);
* palate;
* submasseteric (3 in Fig. 4.2);
* retropharyngeal;
* lateral pharyngeal (1 in Fig. 4.2);
* pterygomandibular space (2 in Fig. 4.2);
* infratemporal fossa;
* parotid space;

* buccinator space (4 in Fig. 4.2);
* suprahyoid region:
  - submandibular space;
  - submental space;
  - sublingual space.

Upper lip

Infection at the base of the upper lip originates from the upper anterior teeth. It spreads on to the orbicularis muscle from the labial sulcus between the levator labii superioris muscle and the levator angularis oris muscle.

Canine fossa

Spread of infection to the canine fossa usually originates from maxillary canine or upper premolar teeth, often presenting above the buccinator muscle attachment. These swellings obliterate the nasolabial fold (Fig. 4.3).

This space is in close proximity to the lower eyelids, and therefore early management is mandatory to avoid circumorbital infection. There is a risk of spread cranially via the external angular vein which may become thrombosed.

Buccal space

The attachment of the buccinator muscle to the base of the alveolar process can control the spread of infection in the region of the mandibular and maxillary molars. The infection spreads intraorally superficial to the buccinator muscle in front of the anterior border of the masseter muscle. Therefore the clinical manifestation of the infection of this space is characterized by swelling confined to the cheek (Fig. 4.4). However, infection may spread superiorly towards the temporal space, inferiorly to the submandibular space or posteriorly into the masseteric space. In some cases infection may spread to the surface of the skin, leading to fistula formation (Fig. 4.5).

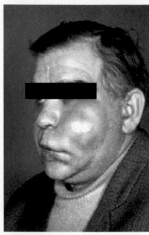

Fig. 4.4 Clinical infection of the buccal space. Courtesy of Glasgow Dental Hospital and School.

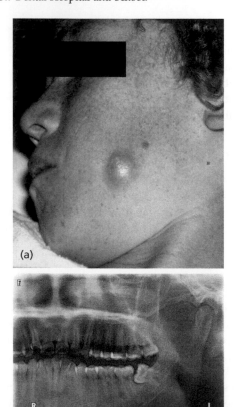

Fig. 4.5 Cheek infection secondary to spread of infection from an upper molar. Courtesy of Glasgow Dental Hospital and School.

Palate

The palate is usually involved by infection originating from the maxillary lateral incisor or the palatal roots of the posterior teeth. The infection spreads from the apices of these teeth, perforating the palatal alveolar bone, and pus accumulates below the palatal mucoperiosteum (Fig. 4.6). Since the tissue is tightly bound down in this area, infection at this site is often very painful. It is important to be aware that, although the lateral incisor is the commonest source of palatal abscess, most lateral incisor abscesses present labially.

Pterygomandibular space

Infection in this space is manifested by trismus due to the involvement of the pterygoid muscles. This space is bounded medially by the medial pterygoid muscle and laterally by the medial surface of the mandible, anteriorly by the pterygomandibular raphe, and posteriorly by the deep lobe of the parotid gland. The lateral pterygoid muscle forms the roof of this space (Fig. 4.7).

Submasseteric space

The commonest source of infection in this space is from lower third molar pericoronitis. This space is bound laterally by the masseter muscle and medially by the outer surface of the ramus of the mandible (Fig. 4.8). It is in direct communication with the lateral pharyngeal space posteriorly. The temporalis muscle divides the superior part of this space into two portions – the superficial temporal space, which is bounded by temporalis muscle medially, and the deep temporal space with the temporalis muscle laterally and the periosteum of the temporal bone medially. Severe trismus due to spasm of the masseter muscle is a characteristic feature of involvement of this fascial space.

Infratemporal space

Extension of infection from maxillary molars can pass into this space. Infection may also spread from the

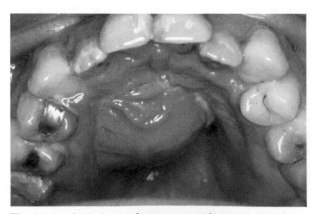

Fig. 4.6 A palatal abscess from an upper lateral incisor. Courtesy of Glasgow Dental Hospital and School.

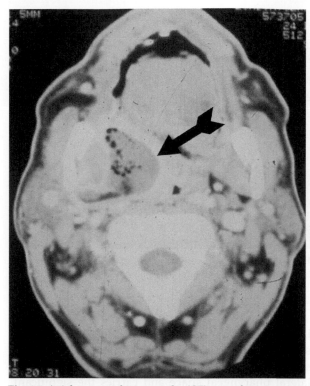

Fig. 4.7 Axial computed tomography (CT) scan of pterygomandibular space infection. Courtesy of Glasgow Dental Hospital and School.

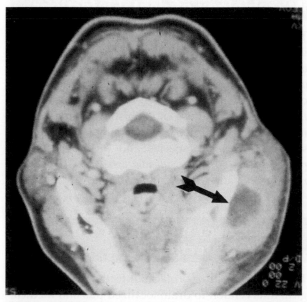

Fig. 4.8 Axial CT scan of a submasseteric abscess. Courtesy of Glasgow Dental Hospital and School.

pterygomandibular, parotid or lateral pharyngeal region to the infratemporal space. The patient then complains of pain, particularly with mouth opening, some dysphagia, and difficulty with lateral mandibular movements. This space is located behind the zygomatic bone posterior to the maxilla and medial to the insertion of the medial pterygoid muscle. The infratemporal space is bounded superiorly by the greater wing of the sphenoid and is in close proximity to the inferior orbital fissure with a possible risk of spread of infection to the orbit.

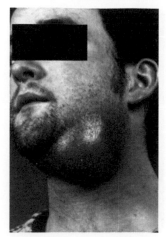

Fig. 4.9 Clinical picture of submandibular space infection. Courtesy of Glasgow Dental Hospital and School.

Parotid space

Involvement of this space may be an extension of infection from the middle ear or the mastoid region. Infection from the masseteric or the lateral pharyngeal space may also spread to the parotid region. Therefore, the most characteristic feature of involvement of this space is swelling of the parotid gland region below the ear lobe. This space contains several important structures which may be affected by infections. These include the 7th cranial nerve, auriculotemporal nerve, facial vein, the parotid lymph node, and, more deeply, the external carotid with its branches.

Submandibular space

This space is located below the mylohyoid muscle, medial to the ramus and body of the mandible. It is bounded anteriorly by the attachments of the anterior belly of the digastric muscle and posteriorly by the posterior belly of digastric muscle and stylomandibular ligament. Infection from the posterior mandibular teeth may pass lingually below the attachment of the mylohyoid muscle into this space. Clinically, swelling of the submandibular regions tends to obliterate the angle of the mandible, causing pain and redness of the skin overlying this region. Dysphagia is usually a marked symptom (Fig. 4.9).

Submental space

This space lies between the two anterior bellies of the digastric muscle. Anteriorly and laterally this space is bounded by the body of the mandible (Fig. 4.10). It is contained superficially by the platysma muscle and deeply and superiorly by the mylohyoid muscle. The infection of this space usually arises from mandibular anterior teeth where the infection perforates the lingual cortex; swelling of the submental region is a characteristic clinical feature. The skin over the swelling is stretched and hardened, and the patient experiences considerable pain and difficulty with

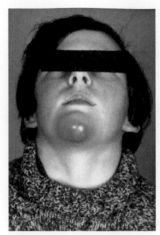

Fig. 4.10 Clinical picture of submental abscess. Courtesy of Glasgow Dental Hospital and School.

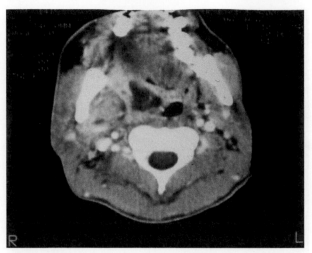

Fig. 4.11 Axial CT scan of pharyngeal space infection. Courtesy of Glasgow Dental Hospital and School.

swallowing. The infection may progress buccally causing swelling in the labial sulcus and over the chin.

Sublingual space

Infection spreads into this space as the result of perforation of the lingual cortex above the attachment of the mylohyoid muscle. This space is bounded superiorly by mucous membrane and inferiorly by the mylohyoid muscle. The genioglossus and geniohyoid muscles form the medial boundary. Laterally, this space is bounded by the lingual surface of the mandible. Infection in this space will raise the floor of the mouth and displace the tongue medially and posteriorly. The tongue displacement may compromise the airway and immediate intervention may be required. Dysphagia and difficulty in speech are also common.

Pharyngeal space

This space is located on the lateral side of the neck, bounded medially by the superior constrictor muscle of the pharynx and posterolaterally by the parotid space. Infection in this space may originate from mandibular molars or third molar pericoronal suppuration. This could also be a site of spread of infection from the parotid space or fascial space around the body of the mandible. The lateral pharyngeal space contains the carotid sheath, glossopharyngeal nerve, accessory nerve, and the hypoglossal nerve, as well as the sympathetic trunk. Therefore, spread of infection into this space carries the significant danger of spread into a descending neck infection and involvement of the mediastinum. Clinically, stiffness of the neck, swelling of the lateral wall of the pharynx, medial displacement of the tonsils, dysphagia, and trismus are among the characteristic clinical features of involvement of this space (Fig. 4.11).

Retropharyngeal space

This space is located between the posterior wall of the pharynx and the prevertebral fascia. This space is in direct communication with the base of the skull superiorly and the mediastinum inferiorly. It has the same characteristic clinical features as infection of the lateral pharyngeal space and carries the significant complication of a descending neck infection.

Microbiology of dental infections

There is usually a polymicrobial cause for oral/dental infection comprising facultative anaerobes, such as viridans group streptococci and the *Streptococcus anginosus* group, with predominantly strict anaerobes, such as anaerobic cocci, *Prevotella* and *Fusobacterium* species. The use of sophisticated non-culture methods has identified a wider range of organisms such as *Treponema* species and anaerobic Gram-positive rods such as *Bulleidia extructa*, *Cryptobacterium curtum*, and *Mogibacterium timidum*.

Management of patients with orofacial infection

The management of orofacial infection involves surgical intervention to drain localized pus and medical support for the patient.

1. *Incision and drainage.* This could be carried out either intraorally or extraorally depending on the location of the infection (Fig. 4.12). Aspiration of pus prior to incision allows a more accurate sampling method as it reduces contamination and helps preserve anaerobic bacteria. Fluctuation of the swelling indicates the presence of pus and is defined as fluid transmission using bi-digital palpation.
2. *Antibiotics.* Antibiotics can be provided empirically or a specific antibiotic given based on culture and sensitivity tests. Penicillin has the potential to be the first-line agent in the treatment of odontogenic

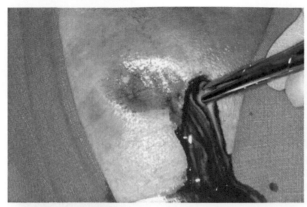

Fig. 4.12 Clinical picture of extraoral incision and drainage of a submandibular abscess. Courtesy of Glasgow Dental Hospital and School.

infections. Most other beta-lactam antibiotics, including fourth-generation cephalosporins, are not found to have greater effectiveness than penicillin. Amoxicillin is a useful broad-spectrum drug in this context although many clinicians prefer the specific anti-anaerobic effect of metronidazole.

3. *Analgesics.* Analgesics provide temporary relief of pain until the causative factors of infection have been brought under control. The choice of analgesic should be based on the patient's suitability. Non-steroidal anti-inflammatory drugs are used in mild to moderate pain. Opioid analgesics, such as dihydrocodeine and pethidine (meperidine or Demerol), are used for severe pain. Paracetamol (acetaminophen), ibuprofen and aspirin are adequate for most mild pain secondary to dental infection. Analgesics need to be given with care, especially when narcotics are used, as they carry the risk of depression of respiration.
4. Identification and elimination of the source of infection. Identification is achieved by both clinical and radiographic assessment. Elimination of the source is by root canal therapy, extraction or periradicular surgery.

Ludwig's angina

Bilateral involvement of the submandibular, submental, and sublingual spaces with a suppurating infection may lead to diffuse cellulitis, classically called Ludwig's angina. This is demonstrated by induration of the swollen skin of the neck, tenderness, elevation of the floor of the mouth, trismus, and dysphagia. The tongue usually shows a varying degree of edema.

The infection of Ludwig's angina may be secondary to the spread of infection from mandibular teeth or penetrating injury to the floor of the mouth. Ludwig's angina is a life-threatening condition which demands emergency treatment. The treatment procedure consists of:

1. Protection of the airway.
2. Hospitalization and administration of intravenous antibiotics and fluids.

3. Incision and drainage extraorally of the submandibular and submental space with through-and-through drainage when necessary.
4. Relief of pain. This is achieved by incision and drainage in addition to the administration of analgesics.

Identification and treatment of the causative factor, often extraction of an infected lower tooth, is necessary after dealing with the acute condition. Emergency cricothyroidotomy or tracheostomy may be necessary to deal with respiratory obstruction. A tracheostomy may have to be made low down to avoid the infected area and may have to be carried out while the patient is awake due to a tendency to lose the airway in the supine position.

Osteomyelitis

Osteomyelitis means the spread of infection through the soft tissue component or marrow of the bone which may include periosteum, neurovascular bundles, narrow spaces of the spongy bone, and the Haversian systems of the cortical bone. It is more common in the mandible than in the maxilla due to the less profuse nature of the blood supply and the density of the cortical plates of the mandible. The most common cause of suppurative osteomyelitis is an odontogenic infection.

The patient complains of a deep-seated pain and swelling due to the ongoing inflammatory edema and spread of infection in the bone. The associated teeth are tender to percussion and may be loose. There may be regional lymphadenitis and alteration of sensation of the lower lip due to the involvement of the inferior alveolar nerve and pressure from the inflammatory process. The acute inflammatory reaction involving fluid exudate into the medulla of the mandible causes this pressure effect on the nerve and may also cause thrombosis of vessels leading to necrosis and sequestrum (dead bone) formation.

Depending on the signs and symptoms, osteomyelitis can be classified into acute, subacute, and chronic forms. Radiographic changes do not appear immediately in the acute suppurative form of osteomyelitis as it may take about 2 weeks for the trabecular pattern of bone to change and areas of radiolucency to start to appear, usually accompanied by a periostitis. If the acute osteomyelitis is not treated effectively this will lead to chronic suppurative osteomyelitis. The infection may be a manifestation of lowered patient resistance; this sometimes occurs in immunosuppressed patients on medication or those suffering from an impaired immune defense, as in acute leukemia, human immunodeficiency virus (HIV) infection, poorly controlled diabetes mellitus or malnutrition.

Damage to the jawbones secondary to radiation, osteosclerosis or trauma may be a predisposing cause of chronic osteomyelitis. Clinically, the disease is dominated by pain and the development of intraoral

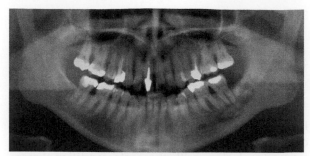

Fig. 4.13 Radiograph of osteomyelitis. Courtesy of Glasgow Dental Hospital and School.

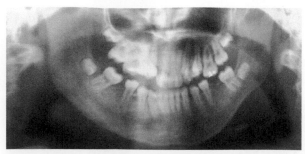

Fig. 4.14 Panoramic radiograph showing subperiosteal bone formation in Garré's osteomyelitis of the right mandible. Courtesy of Glasgow Dental Hospital and School.

and/or extraoral sinuses. Induration of soft tissues overlying the infected segments of the jawbones is marked and the distension of the periosteum with pus or inflammatory exudate which may cause trismus and difficulty swallowing. Regional lymph nodes are usually tender and enlarged. Pathological fracture may develop if the inferior border of the mandible is damaged by the infection process. The radiographic picture of chronic osteomyelitis is loss of detail of the trabecular pattern of the osseous architecture giving the bone a mottled or moth-eaten appearance (Fig. 4.13). The ischemic or necrotic islands of bone tend to sequestrate, appearing more radiopaque than the surrounding bone and these form a sequestrum of necrotic bone. In younger persons subperiosteal new bone formation appears adjacent to the diseased area. This new bone, known as involucrum, tends to be structureless or granular in appearance radiographically and may surround the necrotic sequestrum and pus lying within the bone.

Management of osteomyelitis involves:

1. Culture and sensitivity testing to provide specific antibiotic therapy which generally tends to be given intravenously and for a prolonged period (several weeks);
2. Drainage and debridement, including sequestrectomy;
3. Removal of source of infection and, if necessary, decortication of the mandible;
4. Possible resection and reconstruction of the affected bone after infection is controlled.

Chronic sclerosing non-suppurative osteomyelitis (Garré's osteomyelitis)

This is a chronic form of osteomyelitis with characteristic deposition of bone, subperiosteally and endoperiosteally, in response to an inflammatory process often initiated by a dental infection of low virulence. It affects the mandible in young individuals. Clinically, the condition has the appearance of a nodular, firm swelling related to the inferior border of the mandible. The florid proliferative periostitis is characteristic of this condition in addition to the multilayers of bone formation giving the "onion skin"-like appearance radiographically (Fig. 4.14).

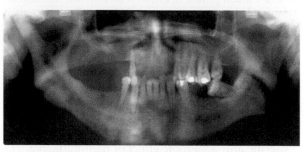

Fig. 4.15 Panorex radiograph of diffuse sclerosing osteomyelitis of the right mandible. Courtesy of Glasgow Dental Hospital and School.

Computed tomography (CT) scanning may help to identify the cause of infection but normally there is no sequestration of the expanded bone.

This condition may persist over a long period of time. A corticotomy and exploration of the damaged bone may be helpful. Appropriate antimicrobial therapy is required to deal with the infection. However, relapse is common. The bone gradually remodels over 6–12 months. A focus of infection is rarely identified. The condition tends to slowly resolve as patients reach adulthood but may require lengthy steroid therapy which downregulates the inflammatory process.

Diffuse sclerosing osteomyelitis of the mandible

This is an inflammatory disease of the mandible whose cause and pathogenesis is still largely unknown. The disease can occur at any age but rarely in young children and often lasts for years with recurrent pain and swelling. The radiographic appearance is variable with areas of diffuse rarefaction and some sclerosis (Fig. 4.15). Organisms cannot usually be cultured from the lesion, although it has been claimed that with meticulous culturing techniques, organisms, including *Actinomyces* species and *Eikenella corrodens*, can be recovered. However, many believe that the disease may be due to an autoimmune process. Various therapies have been suggested including antibiotics, anti-inflammatories, corticosteroids, hyperbaric oxygen, and intravenous bisphosphonate therapy. Only partial success has been claimed, and surgical treatment may be necessary, consisting of either debridement of the lesion or decortication, or even resection of the mandible. Recurrence often occurs, though ultimately the condition often burns itself out leaving a dense sclerotic mandible.

Osteoradionecrosis

This is a type of bone necrosis which occurs following radiotherapy to the jaw region and often becomes secondarily infected. Radiotherapy induces endarteritis obliterans, which reduces vascularity and renders the bone vulnerable to infection. Once secondary infection develops it spreads through the bone but sequestration is delayed in these cases. Patients who have had radiotherapy are potentially at risk of developing this type of osteomyelitis and the mandible is particularly at risk if it has received more than 55 Gy of radiation. Extraction and other surgical procedures should be carried out as atraumatically as possible. Primary closure of the socket and pre- and postoperative antibiotic treatment, antiseptic mouthwash and good oral hygiene are essential. The use of hyperbaric oxygen to increase the blood supply of the affected bone has proven successful in the management of these cases as have other new and experimental treatments. Better collimation of the beam of radiation and protection of tissues adjacent to tumors have reduced, although not eliminated, this unpleasant sequela.

Osteonecrosis secondary to bisphosphonate therapy

Bisphosphonates reduce pain and bone destruction due to metastatic disease, particularly in patients with multiple myeloma, breast and prostate carcinoma. The medication inhibits bone resorption by reducing osteoclastic activity. Long-term administration of high-dose intravenous bisphosphonates may lead to osteonecrosis of the jawbones. This is mainly due to a reduction of the vascularity, which together with inhibition of osteoclastic activity, reduces bone turnover. Both are required to protect the bone from the risk of necrosis and superadded infection. There is a lesser risk of this condition occurring in patients taking oral bisphosphonates to prevent osteoporosis.

The mandible is most often affected and the disease usually arises after dental treatment (Fig. 4.16). The patient may present with either a non-healing extraction socket or exposed bone which does not respond to conservative management and antibiotic therapy. Extraction of infected or periodontally involved teeth should be carried out before the administration of bisphosphonates, if at all possible. Surgery should be avoided whenever possible. It has been suggested that the assessment of the bone's reparative ability can be assessed by measuring the terminal polypeptide chain (CTX). Perioperative and postoperative antibiotics are essential for extractions.

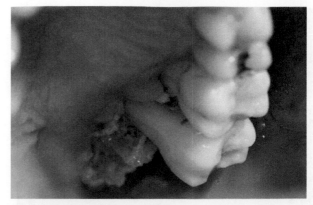

Fig. 4.16 Bisphosphonate-related osteonecrosis of the jaws (BRONJ), maxillary tuberosity region. Courtesy of Glasgow Dental Hospital and School.

Chlorhexidine mouthrinse pre- and postextraction are also considered valuable. In non-urgent cases the risk may be reduced if the bisphosphonate is withheld for 3 months prior to surgery. This must, however, be done only in consultation with the physician prescribing the drug. Other inhibitors of bone turnover, such as denosumab, may well have similar affects in the relationship to osteonecrosis, and concomitant steroid therapy may increase the risk as with bisphosphonates.

Cavernous sinus thrombosis

Thrombosis of the cavernous sinus is an extremely serious condition which may occur secondary to an acute infectious process of the dental, nasal, and orbital regions. The cavernous sinus is a fold between the inner and the outer layer of dura matter. It is lined by endothelial cells and drains venous blood from the brain. Each sinus extends from the superior orbital fissure anteriorly, through the apex of the petrous part of the temporal bone posteriorly. There are two general mechanisms by which infection may reach the cavernous sinus through the venous network of the dentofacial region. The first is the facial, or afferent system, which comprises the facial vein which communicates with the superior ophthalmic veins, since these veins are in direct communication with the cavernous sinus through the superior orbital fissure. The second mechanism is the pterygoid venous plexus, or the efferent system. Infection may reach the pterygoid venous plexus in a retrograde fashion through the posterior facial vein or the internal maxillary vein. Infection from the pterygoid venous plexus would reach the cavernous sinus via the inferior ophthalmic vein or the veins of the foramen ovale and lacerum (Fig. 4.17).

The signs and symptoms of cavernous sinus thrombosis are those related to venous obstruction, and involvement of the nerves within the vicinity of the cavernous sinus (the occulomotor nerve, trochlear nerve, and the ophthalmic and maxillary divisions of the trigeminal nerve). Edema of the retina,

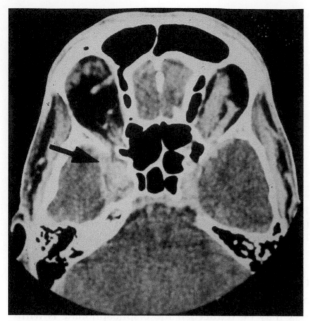

Fig. 4.17 Axial CT scan showing cavernous sinus thrombosis (arrowed). Courtesy of Glasgow Dental Hospital and School.

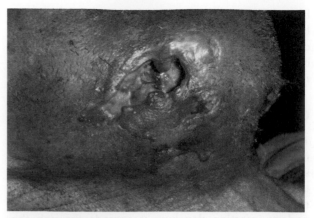

Fig. 4.18 Necrotizing fasciitis of the submandibular region. Courtesy of Glasgow Dental Hospital and School.

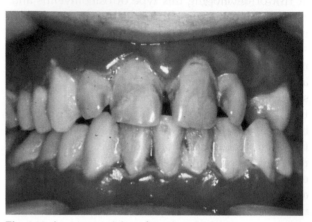

Fig. 4.19 Acute necrotizing ulcerative gingivitis.

eyelids and bridge of the nose, as well as ocular swelling are the main characteristics of cavernous sinus thrombosis. This is due to distension of the tissues behind the eyeball. Involvement of the cranial nerves in the septic condition causes ptosis of the upper eyelid, dilatation of the pupil of the eye, and restriction of eye movement. In addition, the patient may show symptoms of septic shock which includes pyrexia, profuse sweating, vomiting, and coma. Treatment of this condition should be prompt. The patient should be admitted to hospital, the airway should be maintained, and fluids should be administered. Antibiotics should be administered immediately and adequately. Anticoagulant therapies are used to prevent extension of the thrombus and interference with the venous drainage of the brain. Drainage of pus should be carried out as soon as possible. Permanent cranial nerve damage, brain damage, and death have been reported following a septic cavernous sinus thrombosis of dental origin.

Necrotizing fasciitis

This is a rapid spreading infection of the skin causing necrosis of the subcutaneous tissue. A combination of aerobic and anaerobic microorganisms is responsible for this condition which occurs most often in diabetic or otherwise immunocompromised patients. A dental source of infection is rare but possible (Fig. 4.18).

Clinically, there is loss of skin due to the necrosis of the underlying subcutaneous tissue. Other areas of the skin may appear erythematous, edematous, rapidly changing to purplish and black in color. The patient requires aggressive and immediate surgical intervention. The necrotic tissue requires wide excision to healthy margins. Intravenous fluid support is

given together with a combination of clindamycin, penicillin, and metronidazole until alternative therapy is chosen following culture and sensitivity. Death has occurred from this condition.

Acute necrotizing ulcerative gingivitis

Acute necrotizing ulcerative gingivitis (ANUG) is unique in clinical presentation and course. Its clinical presentation is distinctive from all other periodontal diseases. ANUG is characterized by a rapidly progressive ulceration typically starting at the tips of the interdental papilla, spreading along the gingival margins, and going on to acute destruction of the periodontal tissue with severe pain, interdental necrosis, and bleeding (Fig. 4.19).

The etiology of ANUG is not fully understood. However, spirochetes and *Fusobacterium* species are thought to be associated with the etiology. Other oral strict anaerobes, including *Prevotella* species, may also be involved in the disease. Pre-existing gingivitis, nutritional deficiency, tobacco smoking, psychological stress, and immunosuppression have been implicated as predisposing factors.

The clinical presentation of ANUG comprises a punched out ulcer, which is involved primarily with the tips of interdental papillae and the labial or lingual margin, or both. Involvement may be a single tooth, a group of teeth or throughout the mouth, but the condition is rare in edentulous patients. The mandibular anterior region is most frequently affected.

The edge of the ulcer is usually defined by erythema and edema and often the lesion itself is covered by a grey pseudomembranous slough. The affected area often becomes highly sensitive to touch, and produces a constant radiating, gnawing pain, which is intensified by hot food or mastication. Spontaneous gingival bleeding upon exposure to the slightest stimuli can occur. In addition ANUG is often accompanied by a distinct halitosis and foul taste.

Mild to moderate cases may manifest as local lymphadenopathy with a slight elevation in body temperature. However, in its most severe form, high fever, increased pulse rate, leukocytosis, headache, loss of appetite, lassitude, and insomnia can all result.

ANUG may subside spontaneously, although the disease has the potential to cause progressive destruction of periodontium and denudation of dental root with systemic complications.

The patient's clinical history and symptoms are often sufficient information to permit diagnosis. If there is uncertainty, ANUG can be confirmed rapidly by microscopic examination of a Gram-stained smear taken from an area of ulceration and should reveal numerous fusobacteria, medium-sized spirochetes and acute inflammatory cells.

Initial management should involve a thorough mechanical cleaning and debridement of the teeth in the affected area. The use of hydrogen peroxide mouthwashes, both to provide mechanical cleaning and also to serve as an oxidizing agent, has been recommended, although the benefit of such treatment is not universally accepted. The importance of local measures cannot be overemphasized, but symp-toms will improve more rapidly if the patient is also given a systemic antimicrobial agent. Metronidazole (200 mg 8-hourly or after meals), or penicillin, prescribed for 3 days will usually produce a dramatic improvement within 48 hours. In the long term, good oral hygiene therapy prevents further gingival damage.

Actinomycosis

This is a chronic suppurative granulomatous infective process which is characterized by the development of swelling in the region of the face and neck. It is normally a soft tissue infection but can occasionally involve bone. The causative microorganism is *Actinomyces israelii* which is present in the normal oral flora in the spore form.

Damage to the tissue, resulting from either lower tooth extractions or jaw fractures, creates a condition of low oxygen tension in which the organism becomes invasive. The condition starts as a swelling, which may occur up to several weeks after the trauma, usually within the submandibular region. The swelling appears first as a firm and indurated lesion and the overlying skin is usually inflamed, firm, but may have a bluish color. Within the swelling multiple abscesses may form with sinuses draining fluid containing yellow granules (sulfur granules) which appear microscopically as a mass of Gram-positive mycelia and polymorphs (Fig. 4.20). Radiographic examination may reveal little destruction of affected bone as the infection is essentially one of the soft tissue. Penicillin is the drug of choice in addition to adequate incision and drainage. The organism is penicillin-sensitive but it takes time for the antibiotic to penetrate the granulomatous reaction of the body. Antibiotic treatment must be continued for at least 6 weeks. Surgical removal of any infection will facilitate the recovery.

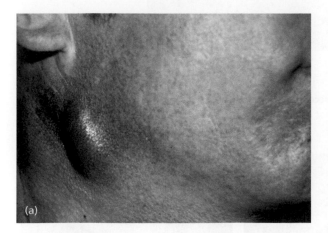
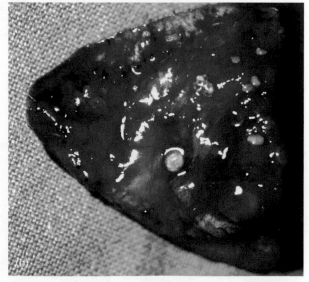

Fig. 4.20 Mandibular actinomycosis showing (a) a raised firm and inflamed swelling and (b) sulfur granules in the resected specimen. Courtesy of Glasgow Dental Hospital and School.

Mycobacterium infection of the oral mucosa and jawbones

This is a specific granulomatous condition which is caused by *Mycobacterium tuberculosis*. This condition is rare but tends to be more common in developing countries. The tongue is the organ most commonly affected by this condition (Fig. 4.21). The lesion may be primary (often from infected milk), usually presenting as enlarged nodes in the neck, or can be secondary to pulmonary tuberculosis (when the causative organism is coughed up in infected sputum). *Mycobacterium tuberculosis* is present in the sputum and gains access to the deeper parts of the oral mucosa as the result of minor trauma following dental extractions or due to abrasion of the mucous membrane. The invading microorganism may also gain access to the jawbones and cause a tuberculosis osteomyelitis. Clinically, the affected lesion will be a swelling with multiple draining sinuses. Looseness of the teeth and sequestration of the affected bone may be clinically apparent. With new subperiosteal bone formation, an involucrum is rarely observed. Enlargement of the submandibular and cervical lymph nodes (a condition known as scrofula), which are rubbery in consistency, with erythematous overlying skin, is a characteristic of infection with *Mycobacterium bovis*; in time an extraoral sinus develops.

Histological examination shows caseation (a "cheesy" form of necrosis) in the center of the granu-loma. The presence of tuberculous bacilli in the specimen, appearance of the primary focus in the chest radiograph, and a biopsy of the lesion will confirm the diagnosis. Management of this case will include medical treatment and surgical intervention. Isonicotinic acid hydrazide (INH), para-aminosalicylic acid (PAS), and rifampicin are still the drugs of choice. Incision and drainage of the localized abscess and sequestrectomy of dead bone are indicated. In addition, extraction of the affected teeth and the surgical excision of the involved cervical lymph nodes may be recommended.

Syphilis

This is a chronic infectious disease which is caused by the spirochete *Treponema pallidum*. Though now rare, primary (the chancre), secondary (skin rashes, lymphadenopathy, mucous patches, and snail track ulcers), and tertiary (gumma or syphilitic leukoplakia) may be found in the oral cavity (Fig. 4.22). The first and second stages are highly infectious. Bony changes may occur in the tertiary stage of syphilis. The periosteum is a common site for the development of gumma, with the midline of the palate being classically involved, leading in time to oronasal fistula. This appears radiographically as peeling of the periosteum away from the underlying bone and the formation of sclerotic bony margins at the periphery. Gumma may extend to the underlying bone and

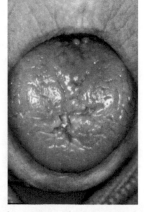
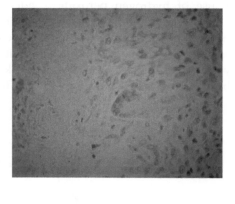

Fig. 4.21 Tuberculosis of the tongue. The lesion in this case is secondary to pulmonary TB and coughing up infected sputum. Courtesy of Glasgow Dental Hospital and School.

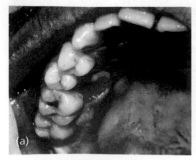
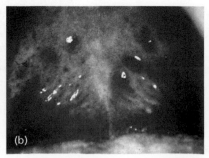
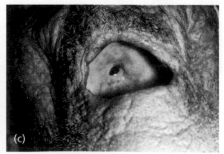

Fig. 4.22 Photos of (a) primary chancre, (b) secondary snail track ulcers of the soft palate, and (c) tertiary gumma of the palate. The chancre and snail track ulcers are highly infectious. Courtesy of Glasgow Dental Hospital and School.

cause syphilitic osteomyelitis. The condition is diagnosed by the identification of the *Treponema pallidum* using dark field microscopy, serological tests, and biopsy of the granulomatous tissue. Long-term penicillin is the drug of choice in addition to local measures to deal with damaged soft tissue, sequestrated bone, and involved teeth. The fourth stage of syphilis is rare; it affects the cardiovascular system causing aortic aneurysms or aortic valve incompetence. The central nervous system may be involved which may lead to dementia or spinal cord disease.

Congenital syphilis is rare because treatment during pregnancy eradicates the infection. The characteristic features of an infected baby include saddle-nose deformity, tapering widely separated incisors (Hutchinson's teeth), domed-shaped molars (Moon's or mulberry molars), and papules at the angle of the mouth, which heal forming radiating scars (rhagades).

Antibiotic prophylaxis

Antibiotic prophylaxis has had a positive impact on the incidence of infection after certain types of surgery. However, the clinician should not overestimate the effects of antibiotic prophylaxis and must recognize its limitations. Systemic prophylactic antibiotic should not be used routinely and should be tailored to the individual patient.

Benefit and risk of antibiotic prophylaxis

Antibiotic prophylaxis is highly effective in reducing the likelihood of infection. However, it has the potential risk of toxic and allergic reactions, drug interactions, alteration in the composition of normal host flora, and may promote an emergence of resistant bacteria. The cost of the antibiotic is also a matter that needs to be considered. In cases where the risk of infection is extremely low, an antibiotic provides little additional reduction in the incidence of infection. Such cases, therefore, do not need prophylactic antibiotic treatment.

Principles of antibiotic prophylaxis

The benefits versus the risk and the effectiveness versus cost should be considered for antibiotic prophylaxis. The most important factor to consider is the patient's host defense activity. In cases where the host immunity is significantly compromised or the surgical site may have reduced resistance to infection (e.g. a history of radiation therapy or poor blood supply), then antibiotic prophylaxis may be indicated.

Choice of antibiotic

The effectiveness of a prophylactic antibiotic is reliant on its efficacy against the predicted bacterial microorganisms most likely to cause infection, the extent of its tissue penetration, a lack of host toxicity, and its ability to cause a minimal disturbance to the intrinsic body microflora. An antibiotic with a narrow spectrum of activity should be chosen. Cost effectiveness should also be taken into consideration. In the case of oral wound, it is the penicillin class of antibiotic that fulfills these requirements. First-generation cephalosporin antibiotics may be adequate for cutaneous or antral contamination.

Dose of antibiotic and duration of administration

The dosage of the prophylactic antibiotic should be the same or greater than that for therapeutic use. It should be remembered that the dose of the antibiotic is primarily determined by the serum level of the drug and the minimum inhibitory concentration (MIC) for the pathogen involved. If the surgical wound has a poor blood supply or the host defense mechanism is compromised, then a high dose of the antibiotic should be administered.

The timing of administration is critically important because the concentration of the antibiotic should be at its therapeutic level at the time of incision, during the surgical procedure, and, ideally, for a few hours postoperatively. An antibiotic administered preoperatively does exhibit a greater prophylactic effect than one administrated postoperatively. Although many practitioners prescribe antibiotic postoperatively, it does not accomplish the true purpose of prophylactic antibiotic treatment. Oral antibiotics should be administrated 30 minutes to 1 hour prior to the start of the operation. Intravenous or intramuscular antibiotics should be administrated within 30 minutes of the incision time. Antibiotics should not be administered more than 2 hours prior to surgery. An additional dose of an intraoperative antibiotic should be administrated to maintain an adequate serum concentration of the antibiotic during surgery if the operation is prolonged.

In the case of immunocompetent patients, if the surgery involves bacterial contamination that may occur only during the operation, antibiotic coverage during the operation may be sufficient and additional postoperative antibiotic may be unnecessary. In contrast, in circumstances where recontamination is suspected, use of an antibiotic postoperatively is recommended. Patients who have any factor that depresses the host defense mechanism or impedes wound healing have a great risk of recontamination during the healing period. In these cases, use of an antibiotic until evidence of biological wound sealing appears, is advocated.

Prophylaxis for wound infection on specific surgical procedure

There is some disagreement over the effectiveness of prophylactic antibiotic use for different surgical procedure. Although this section presents the guidelines for indication of antibiotic prophylaxis, actual use and regimen must be tailored to individual cases.

- *Endodontic procedures.* In pulpectomy, use of antibiotic prophylaxis is generally unnecessary regardless of the host's immunity level. However, antibiotic prophylaxis is advocated in cases of removal of infected necrotic material from the root canal of immunocompromised patients (e.g. treatment of asymptomatic (chronic) periapical lesions). In these situations the endodontic procedure itself can act as a trigger for acute infection.
- *Tooth extraction and other dentoalveolar surgery.* Most routine surgical procedures performed by dentists in healthy patients, such as tooth extraction, apicectomy, periodontal surgery, endodontic surgery, biopsy, do not require prophylactic antibiotics. Also, despite being a subject of controversy, third molar surgery (removal of impacted third molar in the mandible) does not require antibiotic prophylaxis. However, in cases of an immunocompromised host, prophylactic antibiotic treatment is recommended. The use of systemic antibiotics is also recommended where oroantral communication occurs. Use of antibiotics should be considered in cases of dental implant treatment. In situations where the maxillary sinus or the nasal cavity is exposed, prophylactic antibiotics should be used.
- *Removal of oral benign tumors and cysts in the jaw.* Indication of antibiotic prophylaxis follows the same principles as those of common dentoalveolar surgery. An extensive operation may require the use of prophylactic antibiotic.
- *Management of soft tissue trauma.* In cases of fresh wounds caused by simple traumatic injury within the mouth, antibiotic prophylaxis is unnecessary. Antibiotic prophylaxis is also unnecessary in simple and fresh extraoral lacerations made with relatively clean objects. However, in cases of blunt traumatic wounds, gunshot wounds, bite wounds caused by human or animal, lacerations from dirty objects, traumatic injuries with delayed treatment, or contact with the saliva or any oral contaminants, use of antibiotic prophylaxis is recommended.
- *Management of fracture.* Fresh simple fractures of the condyle, ramus, and body of the mandible, with no saliva contamination, can be treated without antibiotic prophylaxis if treated through an extraoral approach. However, if treatment is performed through an intraoral incision, if treatment is delayed or if there is a pathologic fracture, the use of antibiotic prophylaxis is recommended. Antibiotic prophylaxis is also advocated in cases of compound fracture of the mandible, maxillary fractures involving the nasal cavity or paranasal sinuses.
- *Orthognathic surgery.* Orthognathic surgery performed via an extraoral approach is considered a clean procedure and antibiotic prophylaxis is unnecessary. However, if the surgery is undertaken transorally or if salivary or antral communication is anticipated, use of prophylactic antibiotics may be advocated.

Recommended reading

Ayoub A. (2010) Dentofacial infection. In: *Oral and Maxillofacial Surgery* (eds, Andersson L, Kahnberg K-E, Pogrel MA). Oxford, Wiley-Blackwell.

Flynn T. (2000) Surgical management of oral infections. *Atlas of Oral and Maxillofacial Surgery Clinics of North America*, **8**, 77–100.

Kuriyama T, Lewis AOM, Williams DW. (2010) Infections of the oral and maxillofacial region. In: *Oral and Maxillofacial Surgery* (eds, Andersson L, Kahnberg K-E, Pogrel MA). Oxford, Wiley-Blackwell.

Lyons A, Ghazali N. (2008) Oral bisphosphonate induced osteonecrosis, risk factors, prediction of risk using CTX testing, prevention, and treatment. *British Journal of Oral and Maxillofacial Surgery*, **46**, 653–61.

Marx RE, Johnson RP, Kline SN. (1985) Prevention of osteoradionecrosis: a randomized prospective clinical trial of hyperbaric oxygen versus penicillin. *The Journal of the American Dental Association*, **111**, 49–54.

Rega AJ, Aziz SR, Ziccardi VB. (2006) Microbiology and antibiotic sensitivities of head and neck space infections of odontogenic origin. *Journal of Oral and Maxillofacial Surgery*, **64**, 1377–80.

Chapter 5

Armamentarium for Basic Procedures

Basic instrumentation for soft tissue procedures

Basic soft tissue instrumentation consists of a scalpel for making incisions (Fig. 5.1), toothed and non-toothed forceps (Figs 5.2, 5.3, 5.4) for grasping tissues and arresting bleeding vessels, Allis-type clamps (Fig. 5.5) for appropriately holding biopsy specimens and tissue margins, retractors (Figs 5.6, 5.7) as well as a range of forceps ranging from smaller mosquito-type forceps to larger Kelly and Schnidt-type forceps (Fig. 5.8), needle-holding forceps (Fig. 5.9), and appropriate scissors (Figs 5.10, 5.11, 5.12). All of these instruments can be combined to make an appropriate soft tissue instrument tray.

Basic hard tissue instrumentation

For surgery involving the mandible or maxilla, the basic soft tissue instrumentation is required, and additionally, one requires periosteal elevators (Figs 5.13, 5.14) to raise periosteum from bone, periosteal retractors (Figs 5.6, 5.15), curettes (Fig. 5.16) and rongeurs (Fig. 5.17) for removing and scraping bone, and bone files (Fig. 5.18) for smoothing the bone.

Drills

An appropriate drill for removing bone (Fig. 5.19) will be either gas-powered or electric-powered and will not exhaust gas or air through the tip of the handpiece, since this gas can force debris and bacteria into the bone and can even cause an air embolus. Any gas used to power the drill should exhaust back along the tubing into the operatory or into a scavenging device. For preference, drills should have an automatic irrigation system built into them which is linked to the drill control and can be used in conjunction with a sterile irrigant solution. Burs should be appropriate bone-cutting burs rather than burs intended to cut enamel and dentin.

Dental elevators

Elevators are often used in conjunction with dental forceps to remove teeth and roots. The general principle in the use of the elevators is that the surrounding alveolar bone is used as a fulcrum for the action of the elevator rather than the adjacent tooth, unless it is intended to also remove the adjacent tooth. If the alveolar bone is used as a fulcrum and it is crushed by the elevator, this bone should be removed with a curette or bone file. Elevators that have a right-angle point of elevation can exert significantly higher forces on the mandible than those with an in-line direction of elevation. Care should be taken with such instruments (e.g. Cryer's elevators) since fracture of the mandible is possible if these instruments are used inappropriately. Similarly, instruments with a so-called T-bar handle can exert even more force on the mandible, and particular care should be used with these instruments (e.g. Winter's elevators). Examples of dental elevators are illustrated in Figures 5.20, 5.21, 5.22, 5.23, 5.24, 5.25, 5.26 and 5.27.

Dental forceps

Dental forceps essentially come in two types. The first is the in-line forceps where the handle of the forceps is in line with the dental arch. To a certain extent, these forceps are safer but rely on the inherent

Essentials of Oral and Maxillofacial Surgery, First Edition. Edited by M. Anthony Pogrel, Karl-Erik Kahnberg and Lars Andersson.
© 2014 John Wiley & Sons, Ltd. Published 2014 by John Wiley & Sons, Ltd.
Companion website: www.wiley.com/go/pogrel/oms

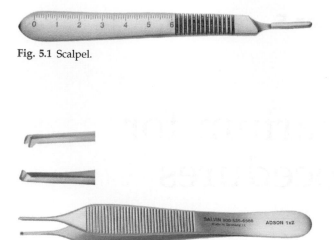

Fig. 5.1 Scalpel.

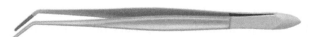

Fig. 5.2 Toothed forceps.

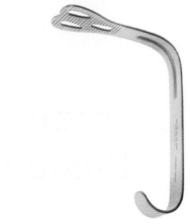

Fig. 5.7 Weider retractor.

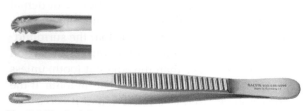

Fig. 5.3 Non-toothed forceps.

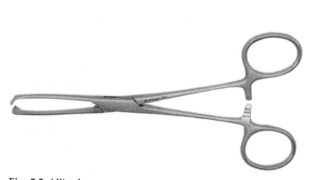

Fig. 5.4 Toothed forceps.

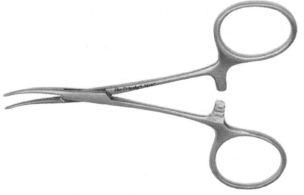

Fig. 5.8 Mosquito and Kelly-type forceps.

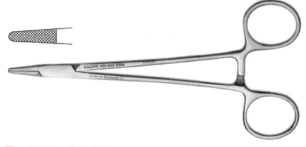

Fig. 5.9 Needle holders.

Fig. 5.5 Allis clamp.

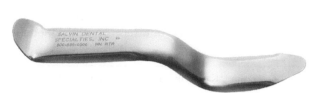

Fig. 5.6 Minnesota retractor.

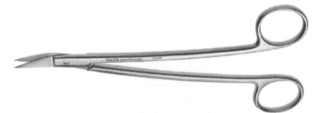

Fig. 5.10 Dean scissors.

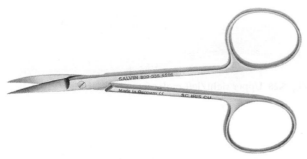

Fig. 5.11 Iris scissors.

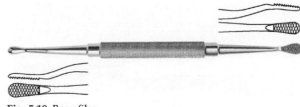

Fig. 5.18 Bone files.

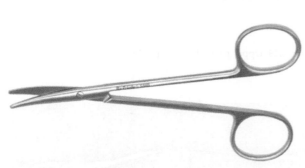

Fig. 5.12 Metzenbaum scissors.

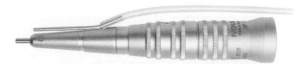

Fig. 5.19 Surgical drill.

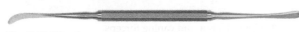

Fig. 5.13 Woodson periosteal elevator.

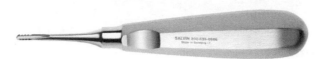

Fig. 5.20 Straight elevator.

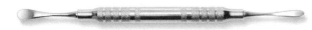

Fig. 5.14 Molt #9 periosteal elevator.

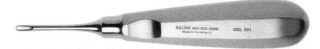

Fig. 5.21 Straight elevator.

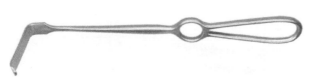

Fig. 5.15 Langenbeck retractor.

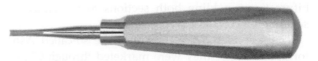

Fig. 5.22 Coupland's chisel.

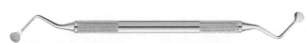

Fig. 5.16 Curettes.

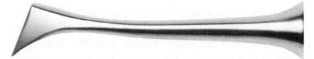

Fig. 5.23 Cryer's elevators.

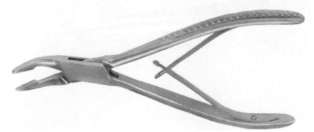

Fig. 5.17 Rongeurs.

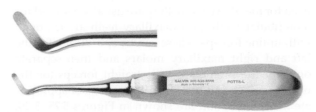

Fig. 5.24 Potts elevators.

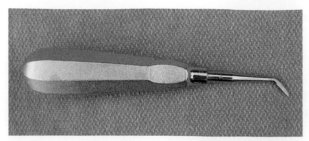

Fig. 5.25 Crane's elevators.

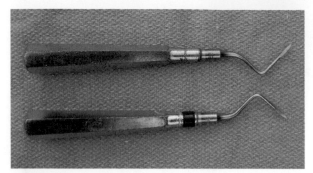

Fig. 5.26 Root pick elevators.

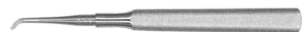

Fig. 5.27 Warwick-James elevator.

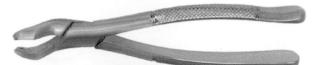

Fig. 5.28 Upper right/left molar forceps: 53 R/L.

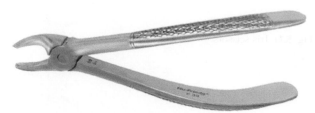

Fig. 5.29 Upper premolar forceps: 150.

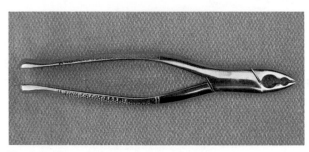

Fig. 5.30 Upper incisor and canine forceps.

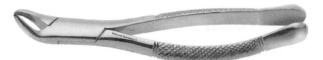

Fig. 5.31 Lower premolar in-line forceps: 151.

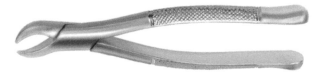

Fig. 5.32 Cowhorn forceps.

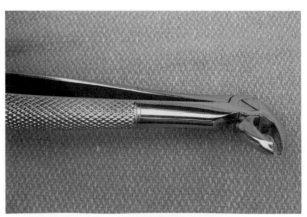

Fig. 5.33 Ash pattern lower molar forceps.

strength in the surgeon's wrist. A particular example of an in-line forceps is the cowhorn forceps, which is meant to be placed between the bifurcation of the roots of a lower molar and will either remove the molar intact or will split the molar through the bifurcation, enabling both sections to be removed separately.

The second type of forceps is the so-called Ash forceps (because they were marketed through Claudius Ash and Sons, dental supply house), and these are forceps that have a handle that comes out at a right angle to the arch. Potentially, these forceps can create much greater force on the tooth, through the principle of levers. It is possible to fracture the mandible with these instruments, so care must be taken. There are different Ash forceps for lower molars, premolars, and incisors. Many dentists, however, prefer to use premolar forceps for the molars, grasping the mesial root only so that either the whole tooth will be removed, or if it splits, the mesial root will be removed making the distal root easier to remove on its own. Although Ash-type forceps are sometimes used for maxillary teeth, they are usually reserved for mandibular teeth, and maxillary teeth are removed with in-line forceps. These can be specifically for the left and right maxillary molars and then separate ones for the premolars and straight forceps for the upper canines and incisors. Illustrations of appropriate instrumentation are shown in Figures 5.28, 5.29, 5.30, 5.31, 5.32, 5.33 and 5.34.

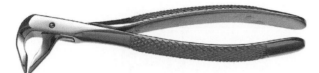

Fig. 5.34 Ash pattern lower premolar incisor and canine forceps.

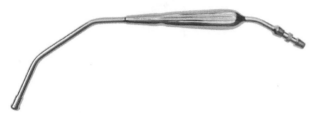

Fig. 5.35 Yankauer suction tip.

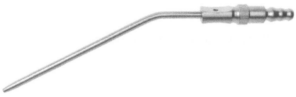

Fig. 5.36 Surgical suction tip.

Ancillary instrumentation

In addition to the instrumentation already shown, additional instrumentation required for most surgical procedures includes:

1. Suction, which is normally electric or vacuum driven, and suitable suction tips that work well intraorally are illustrated in Figures 5.35 and 5.36.
2. Cautery, diathermy, or electrosurgical instrumentation is often required for surgical procedures for both cutting and coagulation. There are technical differences between these systems. In a monopolar diathermy system (Fig. 5.37) there is a small active electrode and a large indifferent electrode, which takes the form of plate in contact with the body. The small active electrode is the diathermy tip but its effect is not localized as it spreads towards the indifferent electrode. By altering the waveform the tip can predominately cut or coagulate. In a bipolar system (Fig. 5.38) both tips of a pair of forceps are insulated from each other and form the two electrodes. The current and tissue damage is localized to the tissue between the forceps tips and does not spread and there is no large indifferent electrode in another part of the body. Because of this there is no current passing through the rest of the body so it is safe for patients with pacemakers etc. Desiccation is a cauterizing process whereby a single

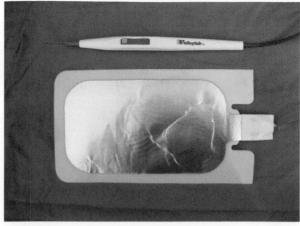

Fig. 5.37 The active electrode (tip) and indifferent electrode (plate) in a monopolar diathermy system.

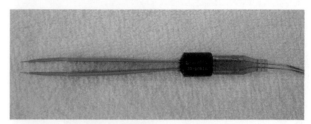

Fig. 5.38 The insulated tips of a bipolar diathermy system. Each tip is a separate electrode.

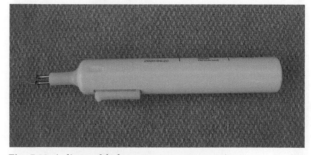

Fig. 5.39 A disposable low-power cautery unit.

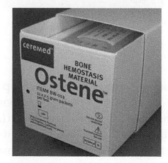

Fig. 5.40 Bone wax.

wire has an area of high resistance so it can become hot at that point and cauterize. Desiccation instruments tend to be of lower power and energy levels and are often disposable (Fig. 5.39).
3. Bone wax (Fig. 5.40) is also often used when bleeding is encountered during intraosseous surgery. It

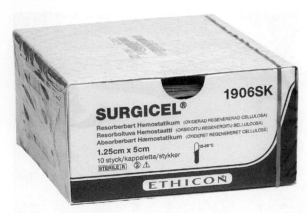

Fig. 5.41 Surgicel®.

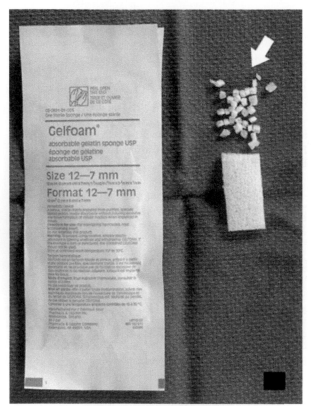

Fig. 5.42 Gelfoam®.

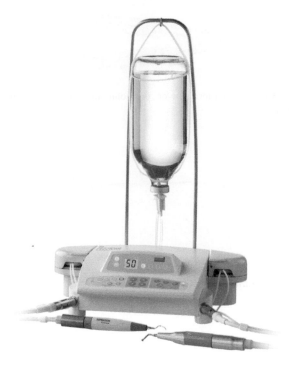

Fig. 5.43 Piezoelectric bone-removal system.

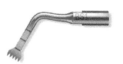

Fig. 5.44 Piezoelectric bone-removal system.

can be squeezed into the cancellous spaces of the bone and will cause hemostasis. Bone wax is non-resorbable, whilst fibrillar collagen (Avitene™) used for the same purpose, is resorbable. In a dental socket where bleeding is a problem, one normally uses a material such as Surgicel® (Fig. 5.41) or Gelfoam® (Fig. 5.42).

New innovations in surgical instrumentation

Although over the years many different systems have been suggested for removing bone, none has super-

seded the dental drill. More recently, a piezo instrument using high-frequency vibration to remove bone has been advocated (Figs 5.43, 5.44). Initially, these instruments lacked power and could only remove small areas of relatively thin bone. However, new generations of these instruments are expected to have greater power and more flexibility to change the frequency and wavelength of the vibrations to achieve a more efficient cutting action. It is claimed that the heat generated and peripheral damage produced are much less than with a dental drill, and, therefore, with further improvements, they may have a place in bone removal in oral and maxillofacial surgery.

Sterilization of instruments

Many instruments used today are disposable single-use instruments, and no attempt should ever be made to reuse these instruments. In theory, the more single-use instruments are used, the better the chain of sterility.

For instruments that are not single use and must be reused, they must be sterilized between surgical procedures. This involves removal of all organic and inorganic debris from the instrument, and this can be

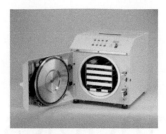

Fig. 5.45 Steam autoclave.

done manually but is better performed by ultrasonic cleaning. Following ultrasonic cleaning, the instruments should be packaged in appropriate bags and sterilized. For most instruments, autoclaving to a temperature of 134°C for 3 minutes, or 121°C for 15 minutes will sterilize instruments of all known bacteria and viruses (Fig. 5.45). To be effective, however, the steam must penetrate through to the instruments, and the package must not be blocked by other packages that prevent the full effects of the steam to be effective.

For more delicate instruments, ethylene oxide can be used for sterilization, but this is not universally available and usually takes up to 24 hours for instruments to be available following ethylene oxide sterilization, since time must be allowed for the ethylene oxide to disperse following appropriate sterilization.

Radiation is used to sterilize some instruments, but more often, it is used to sterilize alloplastic grafts including bone grafts. Bone grafts sterilized by radiation may maintain more activity than those sterilized by ethylene oxide.

Lower-temperature autoclaves that are combined with formaldehyde are available and do ensure sterilization at a lower temperature for some instruments.

There is no known reliable method of removing or sterilizing prions from surgical instruments, and in the present state of knowledge, if one is operating on a patient with known or suspected prion disease, all instruments must be appropriately disposed of following the procedure, and no effort must be made to reuse the instruments. Most authorities have regulations in place for how and where to perform surgery in a patient with suspected prion disease.

Recommended reading

Al-Musawi A. (2010) Armamentarium for basic procedures. In: *Oral and Maxillofacial Surgery* (eds, Andersson L, Kahnberg K-E, Pogrel MA). Oxford, Wiley-Blackwell.

Vercellotti T, De Paoli S, Nevins M. (2001) The piezoelectric bony window osteotomy and sinus membrane elevation: introduction of a new technique for simplification of the sinus. *International Journal of Periodontics and Restorative Dentistry*, **21**, 561–7.

Chapter 6

Basic Surgical Principles

Aseptic technique

Since the late 1800s, when bacteria were first recognized, the concept in surgery has turned from accepting pathogenic agents, and hoping that the body can overcome them, to attempting to eliminate them from the surgical field. In hospitals, most operations are carried out using a truly aseptic technique. All instruments are sterile, having been autoclaved, or all organisms eliminated by some other physiochemical means. In addition, the operating room itself is surgically clean, and all trays, etc., on which instruments rest are sterile. The surgeon wears sterile gloves and a sterile gown, and a mask, head covering, and shoe covers or separate footwear that is only worn in the operating room. An aseptic technique is employed whereby sterile and non-sterile objects do not contact each other so that there is a continuous chain of sterility; the only organisms that come in contact with the patient are their own endogenous organisms. In this way, infections should not occur, and, in theory at least, antibiotics and other chemotherapeutic agents should be unnecessary if no exogenous infecting agents are introduced. In practice this type of sterility, although ideal, is imperfect. Infections do still occur in the operating room for a variety of reasons and antibiotics do still need to be employed in many cases.

The rules for carrying out invasive surgery in the operating room environment of a hospital are fairly standard and clear cut. The rationale in a dentist's, or oral surgeon's office, is, however, less clear cut. For many years, dentistry and relatively minor oral surgical procedures were carried out in an outpatient office without the use of gloves, cap, or mask and with only a clean gown or coat. This changed in the 1980s when new generations of pathogenic organisms were identified including hepatitis B and hepa-

titis C viruses, and human immunodeficiency virus (HIV). Following this, to protect both the dentist and the patient, dentists started to wear gloves, caps, and masks.

At the present time, there is no standard for the level of asepsis to be practiced in a dental office or for oral surgery performed in an outpatient setting. In all cases, dentists will now wear caps, masks, and gloves, but in most cases they will continue to wear their outside shoes. Gowns are often worn but are often not sterile but rather cleaned and laundered and changed between patients. Gloves are normally sterile for invasive procedures but are generally non-sterile for non-invasive procedures. Aseptic technique is not strictly followed in most cases, and, although all instruments are sterile and are normally placed on a sterile surface, they may on occasion come in contact with non-sterile instruments and techniques. For this reason, the chain of sterility is less secure in an office environment, and thus antibiotics tend to be used more frequently, and often prophylactically.

Principles of surgical incisions

Incisions are most often made with a surgical scalpel, and for oral and maxillofacial surgery, the #15 blade with its rounded tip is the most popular, although the #11 blade with its pointed tip and the #12C blade with its smaller rounded tip are popular for some procedures with some surgeons. Incisions should be made with one single firm movement using the palm of the hand as a support for the scalpel handle to avoid undesirable instability.

Incisions can also be made with electrosurgery or a laser, or even combined instruments such as a scalpel blade with electrosurgery capacity built into

Essentials of Oral and Maxillofacial Surgery, First Edition. Edited by M. Anthony Pogrel, Karl-Erik Kahnberg and Lars Andersson.
© 2014 John Wiley & Sons, Ltd. Published 2014 by John Wiley & Sons, Ltd.
Companion website: www.wiley.com/go/pogrel/oms

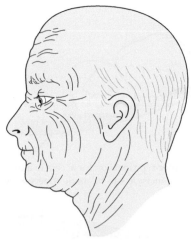

Fig. 6.1 The relaxed skin tension lines of the face which are the sites of choice for surgical incisions. In general, they run at right angles to the underlying muscles.

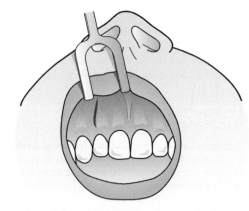

Fig. 6.2 A straight vertical incision intraorally for access to a variety of soft tissue and bone lesions.

it, although these latter instruments are often expensive, somewhat unreliable, and not widely used. Electrosurgical cutting, although it produces a relatively bloodless field, does so at the expense of surface cauterization and does produce more wound breakdown, scarring and wound contracture, and so is generally not employed in esthetic areas.

Skin incisions around the face are best sited either in established skin creases, the site of future skin creases (in young patients), or in the relaxed skin tension lines (RSTL) (Fig. 6.1). These lines generally run at right angles to the direction of the underlying musculature and are roughly equivalent to the original lines described by Langer in 1861, which he produced by puncturing the skin of fresh cadavers with a dagger. He then observed how much the incision gaped compared with the direction of the wound. Although there are differences between these and the relaxed skin tension lines, or even the so-called lines of minimal tension of Converse, they all follow the same general principles. If incisions are placed in this way, they will produce minimal scarring and the best esthetic results. One also needs to be cognizant of any underlying nerves, particularly the branches of the facial nerve. Incisions made on the oral mucosa are generally full thickness over the mandible and maxilla and go down to bone.

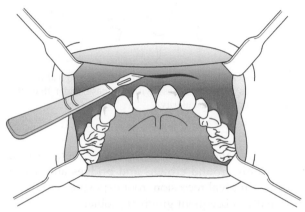

Fig. 6.3 A horizontal sulcular incision suitable for access to periapical pathology and sinus procedures.

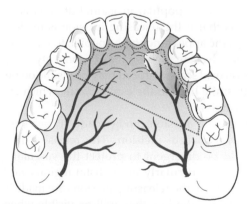

Fig. 6.4 An intrapapillary or sulcular incision used to give access to the palatal surface of the alveolus.

Types of intraoral incisions

1. The straight vertical incision is shown in Figure 6.2, and produces the most esthetic result with minimal scarring. It is indicated for obtaining access to deeper lesions, for tunneling procedures, and for many minimally invasive intraoral procedures. Access, however, is limited.
2. The straight horizontal incision in the buccal sulcus, as shown in Figure 6.3, is often indicated for management of periapical pathology, impacted teeth,

tumors, and sinus procedures. It does, however, tend to produce more scarring than a vertical incision.
3. The intrapapillary incision, sulcular incision, or gingival margin incision is carried out using a scalpel at a reverse bevel and sectioning the interdental papillae and some of the supracrestal and transeptal fibers of the periodontal ligament. It is shown in Figure 6.4 and gives excellent access with minimal scarring and can be used buccally,

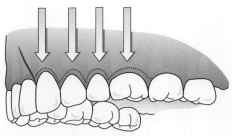

Fig. 6.5 A gingival margin incision incorporating a releasing incision which is wider at its base than its apex to protect the vascularity of the flap (arrows). If the releasing incision is in the esthetic zone of the mouth, the esthetics may be compromised.

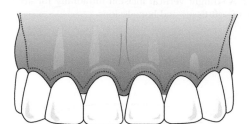

Fig. 6.6 A releasing incision at each end of a gingival margin incision gives excellent access with the base wider than the apex to protect the vascularity.

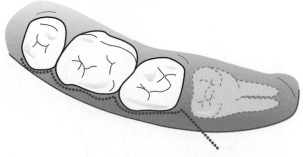

Fig. 6.7 The Winter-type incision for access to a third molar. An anterior releasing incision can be made if necessary.

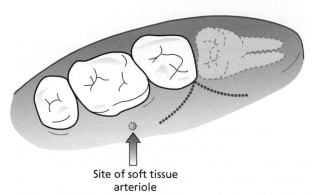

Site of soft tissue
arteriole

Fig. 6.8 An alternative third molar incision down the external oblique ridge of the mandible, down to the disto-buccal line angle of the second molar and then down into the vestibule. This does not involve access to the gingival sulcus of adjacent teeth.

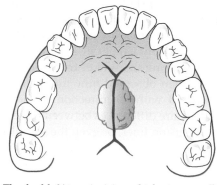

Fig. 6.9 The double Y-type incision which gives excellent access for a palatal torus or similar lesion.

palatally, and lingually. However, there can be problems around crowns and bridges and it can cause gingival recession, root exposure, and occasionally subsequent gingival problems.

4. The gingival margin incision can be combined with a releasing incision at an angle of about 70° to allow improved access to a bony lesion but maintain adequate vascularization of the flap (Fig. 6.5). This is a popular incision, but one disadvantage is that if the releasing incision is made anteriorly, the appearance of the papilla that is included in the releasing incision may become atypical, and the vertical scar produced may be visible on people with smile lines in the esthetic zone which expose the gingiva.

5. A releasing incision can be made at each end of a gingival margin incision. The releasing incision should be divergent to protect the vascularity of the flap, particularly in its distal regions, and the further back the releasing incisions are made in the oral cavity, the less they will be visible when the patient smiles (Fig. 6.6). It is a general rule of all soft tissue flaps that the base should be wider than the apex to protect the vascularity.

6. Incisions for third molars are generally a Winter type incision, which comes down the external oblique ridge to the disto-buccal line angle of the second molar and then continues around the gingival margin of the first and second molar, occasionally with a releasing incision anteriorly if necessary (Fig. 6.7). This gives good access but it can be difficult to suture the papillae and can cause gingival recession on occasions. An alternative incision for third molars runs down the external

oblique ridge to the disto-buccal line angle of the second molar and then proceeds as a releasing incision down into the sulcus terminating around the posterior edge of the first molar so as not to encounter a small arteriole which is often present opposite the first molar (Fig. 6.8).

7. For lesions such as a palatal torus, a double Y-type incision down to bone is often indicated. This incision leaves a good blood supply for the palatal mucosa and allows excellent access to the torus which can then be removed with a combination of drills and chisels (Fig. 6.9).

Following the initial incision, if the deeper soft tissues are to be incised, this can be done with either a sharp or a blunt technique. A sharp technique will employ a scalpel or dissecting scissors and involves a thorough knowledge of the anatomy of the area to avoid damaging important structures. In some cases, a #15 scalpel blade laid on its side and used in a scraping motion can be a compromise method of quickly going through tissue layers but leaving adequate opportunity to visualize important structures. With a blunt technique, a pair of mosquito, or similar, forceps is placed in the tissue layer closed, is then opened, and then withdrawn and closed outside the body. In this way, an incision is gradually widened (with sharp dissection or excision of structures where necessary) without damaging or crushing structures. The mosquito forceps should not be closed within a cavity since important structures may be trapped between the blades.

When access is being gained to the bone of the mandible or maxilla, periosteal elevators will need to be employed to gain access to the bone itself. Periosteum should be retracted with care with a periosteal elevator, bearing in mind that as the subject ages a greater proportion of the blood supply to the bone comes from the periosteum, particularly in the mandible, and, therefore, it should be preserved wherever possible.

Principles of soft tissue biopsy

A biopsy entails obtaining material suitable for establishing a tissue diagnosis. In principle, a biopsy can be either incisional, where a representative portion of a lesion is removed for examination, or it can be excisional, where the whole lesion is removed.

Biopsy can be performed with a scalpel, electrosurgery, laser (Fig. 6.10), tissue punch (Fig. 6.11), or a combination. A scalpel is most frequently employed, and once a portion of the lesion has been excised, care must be taken when handling the tissue so as not to crush or distort the tissue. This means that forceps must be used judiciously in securing the specimen. The use of a scalpel, however, does enable the soft tissue to be sutured back with minimal distortion. If a tissue punch is used, there is usually less distortion of the specimen, but since the punch is circular, a round defect is produced which is more difficult to close and often has to be left open to granulate. Nevertheless, a tissue punch, either 3 mm or 5 mm in diameter, is an excellent way to obtain a palatal biopsy since the punch can be taken down to palatal bone with ease to obtain a full-thickness specimen. In most cases, the punch is used to sever the lesion laterally from the surrounding tissue and a pair of forceps is then used to retract on the specimen which can be dissected from the underlying bed with scissors or periosteal elevator as appropriate. Although electrosurgery or laser can be used to obtain a biopsy specimen for pathological examination, this is generally not preferred since the electrosurgery or laser will both cause coagulation or vaporization damage to the

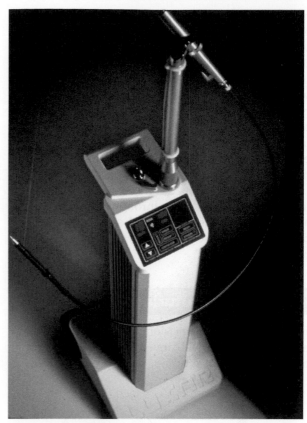

Fig. 6.10 A surgical carbon dioxide laser which can be used for soft tissue surgery, but in practice has limited use and has not replaced the surgical scalpel. Courtesy of Luxar.

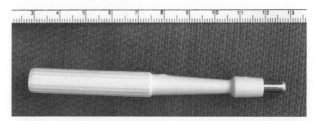

Fig. 6.11 A dermatological tissue punch which can be very useful for obtaining deep biopsy specimens, particularly from the palate where the punch can be inserted down to palatal bone.

bed of the tissue which makes examination of the margins more difficult and problematic.

Biopsy of the mucosal surface of the lip

Excisional biopsy of lesions such as irritation fibromas, mucus retention cysts, and other minor pathology of the lips, is common. Although these are often viewed as very straightforward lesions to remove, there is morbidity associated with them since the lips are such sensitive and minutely controlled organs. Most of the lesions occur on the lower lip since it is much more often traumatized than the upper lip. If the lesion is removed via a longitudinal incision, this produces the least scarring but can interfere with the small branches of either the facial nerve or the mental nerve in the lips. It is sometimes surprising how often excision of a small mucocele can leave the patient with either a slight weakness of part of that area of the lower lip or a small area of paresthesia due to interference with minor nerve branches. Interference with the 7th nerve is usually not a problem in normal movements but only becomes apparent when a tighter lip seal is required such as blowing a musical instrument or blowing against closed lips when some escape of air will be noted. These problems become more frequent the closer one is to the commissure.

In order to minimize the risk of this occurring, incisions should be made through the mucosa only and any further tissue removal should be by blunt dissection to cause minimal trauma to any nerve branches (Fig. 6.12).

Principles of suturing

Following surgical incision, a wound classically needs to be closed. The conventional way to carry this out is by means of suturing, although other systems, such as stapling or the use of tissue adhesives, are available. Suturing with a needle and thread tends to get the best apposition of the tissues and leave the most acceptable scarring. Instruments used for this purpose are needle holders, tissue forceps, and scissors. There are many types of suture material and needles available. Today most sutures are already swaged to the needle so threading a needle is no longer required except in exceptional circumstances.

Types of sutures

There are many different types of suture material available for different uses. Differences between sutures include:

1. Sutures are either resorbable or non-resorbable. If they do resorb, they take differing lengths of time to do so.
2. Sutures are either monofilament or multifilament (also referred to as braided sutures).

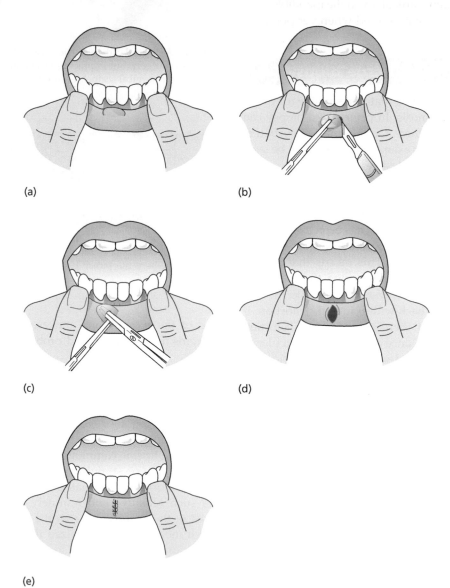

(a)

(b)

(c)

(d)

(e)

Fig. 6.12 The vertical incision for removal of a lip lesion.

Monofilament sutures tend to stay cleaner and leave less suture marks on the tissues but are harder to knot, more likely to become unknotted, and more likely to irritate the tongue and cheeks. Conversely, braided sutures are easy to knot, tend to lie flat so are non-irritant but are harder to keep clean and have a tendency to "wick", meaning they attract moisture and, therefore, bacteria, etc. A combination of the two would be preferable, and some synthetic sutures are available as a braided suture, which is then coated with a liquid layer of the suture material to provide an impervious outer sheath over a braided suture, which can provide the optimal suture material.

Individual types of sutures include:

- Catgut. This is a biological product generally made from sheep intestine, which is a proteinaceous product. Plain catgut sutures are monofilament and resorb in 5–7 days. Resorption takes place because of enzymatic action and so they often do invoke an inflammatory response. By treating the catgut with chromic acid (chromic catgut), the handling properties are improved, the inflammatory response is less, and the suture takes about 2 weeks to resorb. Chromic catgut is often felt to be an ideal material for many types of intraoral suturing. The possibility of transmission of prion disease by catgut sutures taken from sheep has not been totally eliminated.
- Polyglycolic acid and polyglactin sutures are very similar and are a totally synthetic product which resorbs in about 6 weeks, mainly by hydrolysis, and is available as multifilament, monofilament, coated multifilament, and also in a variety of colors.
- Polydioxanone (PDS) and polyglyconate are again synthetic sutures which resorb in around 120 days and, therefore, have little place in oral and maxillofacial surgery except in the few instances where long-term resorption is an asset. This may be in areas such as the alar cinch suture used in LeFort orthognathic surgery. Since they are synthetic, they can again be made either monofilament, multifilament, coated multifilament, and also in a variety of colors.
- Silk is a natural product from the silkworm used as a non-resorbable suture material and is always braided. It is very easy to knot and lies flat easily but does have to be removed – food does tend to stick to it, and if not kept clean, it will cause wicking and possible infection. On the skin, it will leave suture marks if not removed after a few days.
- Cotton is a natural material which is non-resorbable and multifilament and is occasionally used on the mucosa. It knots easily but does tend to wick.
- Nylon and polypropylene are synthetic monofilament suture materials which are non-resorbable. They can be made extremely fine and are very non-irritant, so are often used for microsurgery and skin suturing. Polypropylene, in particular, may be the most benign suture to use on the skin, leaving the least suture marks behind.

Examples of the above sutures are shown in Figure 6.13.

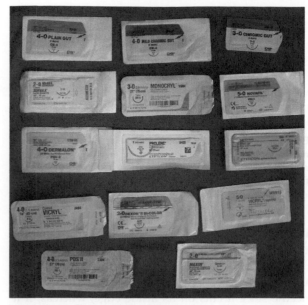

Fig. 6.13 A selection of the different types of suture that are available today for intraoral use.

Uses for the various suture materials

A resorbable material is generally used in the oral cavity so that sutures do not need to be removed. Since only single-layer suturing is normally appropriate intraorally, this is normally with a 3-0 or 4-0 thickness material, and plain catgut, chromic catgut, polyglycolic acid or polyglycolide–lactide are normally appropriate. Extraorally, tissues are often closed in layers, and as such, the appropriate material determines the layer. Fascia can normally be repaired with an intermediate resorption time material such as polyglycolic acid or polyglycolide–lactide, but chromic catgut may also be appropriate. Muscle layers requires a material that will retain its strength for 2–3 weeks, and again polyglycolic acid or polyglycolide–lactide are appropriate. For the subcutaneous tissues, a suture is required which will maintain its strength for around 14 days, and again chromic catgut, polyglycolic acid or polyglycolide–lactide are appropriate. For the skin, a 5-0 or 6-0 nylon is appropriate, or a running subcuticular suture, which is normally carried out with a longer-term resorbable solid suture, is appropriate. Monocryl, polydioxanone, or polyglyconate would be appropriate for this purpose.

Types of needles

Needles normally come ready-swaged to the suture and vary in their length, diameter of a circle (most of them are some proportion of the circumference of the circle), but some come in other shapes such as a J shape. A round-bodied needle is non-cutting and is generally used on friable internal organs. A cutting needle is triangular in cross-section with one edge sharpened to cut through the tissues. A cutting needle

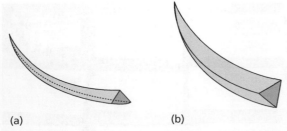

(a)   (b)

Fig. 6.14 The contours of (a) a forward-cutting and (b) a reverse-cutting needle. The reverse-cutting needle is usually more applicable in the oral cavity since it will not cut through the tissues.

is necessary for mucosa and skin and also some of the fascial layers of the head and neck.

If the needle is bent so that the cutting edge is on the inside of the circle, it is called a forward-cutting needle since it cuts on its inside edge; whereas, if it is bent so that the cutting edge is on the outside of the circle, it is called a reverse-cutting needle since it cuts away from the direction the needle is passed. In most oral surgical procedures, the reverse-cutting needle is preferred, since a forward cutting needle will cut through the tissues too often (Fig. 6.14).

Today, many needles combine the best of all properties with a reverse-cutting tip and then a round bodied needle so that the reverse-cutting portion makes the initial incision into the tissues, and then the round-bodied portion of the needle passes through the tissues without causing any further damage. These combined needles go by a number of different names such as taper cut.

Suturing techniques

Once the suture has been passed through the tissues, it must be tied in a knot. Knots can be tied with an instrument or with the hands, but in each case, the principle is the same. In general, a monofilament suture will require more knots than a braided suture since it is more likely to become untied. In most cases, the knot needs to start with a double overhand or double thumb knot, which is essentially a simple thumb knot with an extra twist on it, so that it is less likely to "give" or "slip" (Fig. 6.15). One more thumb knot is then thrown, and if this is in the same direction as the first knot, it will form a surgeon's knot which will not "give", but if it is thrown in the opposite direction, it will form a granny knot which can loosen or be tightened (Fig. 6.16). This can be an advantage on occasions when one wishes to adjust a knot to exactly the right position and tension. However, the final knot that is thrown must convert the previous knot to a reef or square knot so that when it is tightened the knot will not loosen. Thus, there are variations in the technique, but in all cases, the first knot thrown must be able to hold the tissues in position whilst the second knot may be a square knot if

Fig. 6.15 A single overhand, or single thumb knot.

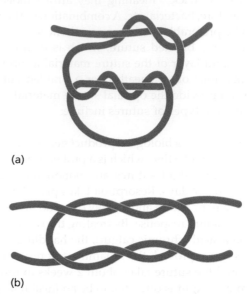

(a)

(b)

Fig. 6.16 (a) Conversion of a double thumb knot to a square or reef knot which will not slip. (b) Conversion of a single thumb knot to a granny knot which can be adjusted. When it has been adjusted to the correct position it will require a third thumb knot to convert the last two into a reef or square knot.

the position of the first knot is ideal or can be a granny knot if further tension is required, but the final knot must convert the next-to-final knot to a reef or square knot.

As far as suturing techniques are concerned, the most frequent sutures used are simple interrupted sutures, and although there are no absolute rules, placing around three sutures per centimetre of length is a good compromise between having too many sutures and, therefore, too many stitch marks and too many possibilities of infection, versus not having enough sutures and having a widened scar. By making the base of the suture wider than the skin or mucosal puncture marks, a slightly everted wound edge is produced, which will flatten as it matures to blend with the adjacent skin or mucosa (Fig. 6.17).

Variations include both the horizontal and vertical mattress sutures which are generally employed intraorally to obtain a watertight closure (Fig. 6.18). The vertical mattress suture, in particular, not only obtains a watertight closure but produces an everted suture line with a lot of tissue in contact to have the maximal chance of healing well. In particular, vertical mattress sutures can be used when suturing over a dead space such as a cyst cavity or an oroantral fistula. A horizontal mattress suture produces a watertight suture line.

Continuous sutures can be either locking or non-locking (Fig. 6.19). They are generally non-locking on

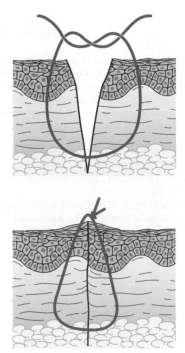

Fig. 6.17 Interrupted sutures placed six to the inch, or three to the centimeter. Note the deep pass of the needle is wider than superficially to cause eversion of the wound edges.

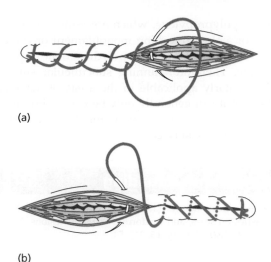

(a)

(b)

Fig. 6.19 (a) A locking (suitable for intraoral use) and (b) a non-locking (suitable for cutaneous use) continuous suture.

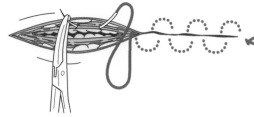

Fig. 6.20 The concept of a running subcuticular suture which is inserted in the white line of the dermis and advances by 3 mm with each pass of the needle but starts 1 mm behind the last pass needle on the opposite side of the wound. Various systems are available for starting and completing a running subcuticular suture, but, in general, the knot is tied on the skin. Ideally, these sutures are left in place for at least 3 weeks to ensure the thinnest scar.

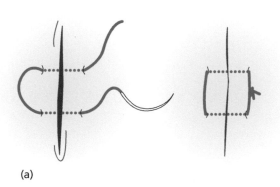

(a)

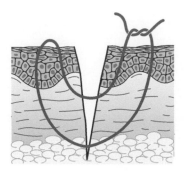

(b)

Fig. 6.18 (a) Horizontal mattress suture. (b) Vertical mattress suture. The horizontal mattress suture will provide a watertight seal, while the vertical mattress suture will provide excellent wound apposition with the best possibility of healing, particularly in a site where healing may be compromised, e.g. over a dead space.

the skin for added cosmesis, but in the oral cavity they can be locked for better closure and better water-proofing of the suture line. The risk with a continuous suture is that if it does break, the whole suture is rendered worthless; whereas, with separate inter-rupted sutures, the loss of one suture may not com-promise the whole suture line.

A running subcuticular suture (Fig. 6.20) is an excellent skin closure technique providing the correct principles are adhered to. The running subcuticular suture needs to be inserted at the white line of the epidermal-dermal junction, and each needle pass needs to be 2–3 mm but backing up 1 mm on the previous needle pass on the opposite side of the wound. If a non-resorbable material such as nylon is used, the suture needs to come to the surface every 2 cm to facilitate removal, but if a resorbable suture has been employed, this is not necessary. Running subcu-ticular sutures have the advantage that they can be left in for the optimal time for collagen strength across the suture line, which is about 3 weeks, without causing unacceptable stitch marks or infection which would occur if any type of suture was left in the skin for 3 weeks. Running subcuticular sutures can be in nylon or polypropylene, which are removed after 3 weeks, or a slow resorbing monofilament or coated multifilament suture, such as polydioxanone or polygluconate. Therefore, running subcuticular sutures are particularly applicable in the areas of maximal cosmesis but can generally only be used with linear incisions. They are normally augmented with adhesive strips on the surface.

Recommended reading

Borges AF, Alexander JE. (1962) Relaxed skin tension lines, Z-plasties on scars, and fusiform excision of lesions. *British Journal of Plastic Surgery*, **15**, 242–54.

Converse JM. (1964) Introduction to plastic surgery. In: *Reconstructive Plastic Surgery* (ed., Converse JM,). Philadelphia, PA: WB Saunders, 42–3.

Langer K. (1978) On the anatomy and physiology of the skin. I. The cleavability of the cutis. (Translated from Zur Anatomie und Physiologie der Haut. I. Uber die Spaltbarkeit der Cutis. (1861) Sitzungsbericht der Mathematisch-naturwissenschaftlichen Classe der Kaiserlichen Academie der Wissenschaften, 44, 19). *British Journal of Plastic Surgery*, **31**, 3–8.

Langer K. (1978) On the anatomy and physiology of the skin. II. Skin tension by Professor K. Langer, presented at the meeting of 27 November 1861. *British Journal of Plastic Surgery*, **31**, 93–106.

Pogrel MA, Kricheldorg F. (2010) Basic surgical principles. In: *Oral and Maxillofacial Surgery* (eds, Andersson L, Kahnberg K-E, Pogrel MA). Oxford, Wiley-Blackwell.

Chapter 7

Complications Associated with Dentoalveolar Surgery

Bleeding

Etiology and prevalence

Postoperative bleeding is a side-effect of dentoalveolar procedures. In healthy patients, postoperative bleeding is typically minimal and self-limited by the clotting processes. It is important to distinguish active bleeding from surgical site oozing. Patients will often complain of excessive bleeding because they have noticed blood in their saliva. Oozing should resolve within 36–72 hours postoperatively, should respond to pressure, and is generally a nuisance for the patient. In contrast, patients with an active bleed will often complain of their mouth filling with blood immediately after removing a gauze dressing or other local pressure measure.

Risk factors and prevention

Among the most important steps in the management of excessive postoperative bleeding is recognition of the at-risk patient. During the preoperative assessment, a detailed history should be obtained, including a history of disorders associated with coagulation, e.g. hemophilia, von Willebrand disease, use of medications such as antiplatelet agents like aspirin and clopidogrel (Plavix), vitamin K antagonists like warfarin (Coumadin), or heparin or its derivatives, e.g. enoxaparin (Lovenox) or fondaparinux (Arixtra), an individual or family history of bleeding with surgical procedures, excessive bleeding upon loss of deciduous teeth, and, in females, a history of menorrhagia.

As the average age of oral surgical patients increases due to prolonged life, practitioners will encounter a greater number of anticoagulated patients. Appropriate adjuvant therapy, such as discontinuation of anticoagulant medications, factor infusions, or use of clot-stabilizing medications, should be considered in patients with risk factors for bleeding or known bleeding diatheses. Of note, patients taking clopidogrel, aspirin and other non-steroidal anti-inflammatory medication do not need to stop their medications prior to routine dentoalveolar procedures.

Patients on warfarin pose a common and special problem for the dentist. The underlying medical problem, e.g. long-standing atrial fibrillation, deep vein thrombosis, prosthetic heart valve, or myocardial infarction, often prohibits discontinuing the anticoagulant. An acceptable, but uncommon, management strategy is to hospitalize the patient, discontinue the warfarin, and maintain the patient on a heparin bridge until the INR (international normalized ratio) returns to the normal range. An alternative option is to discontinue the warfarin 3 days preoperatively.

Care should be taken in considering the type of dentoalveolar surgery being performed. Many minor oral surgical procedures (such as single tooth extraction) can be done while the patient is anticoagulated, based on the coagulation profile. In general, for patients on warfarin, an INR <2.5 is generally acceptable if extraction of multiple (more than four) teeth is required. For extraction of one to three teeth, with no posterior teeth or surgical extractions, an INR of <3.0 is acceptable. Keeping this in mind for the patient who may need multiple extractions, staged visits may be most appropriate so discontinuation of the anticoagulants can be avoided.

Newer anticoagulants such as the oral factor Xa inhibitors (rivaroxaban and apixaban) and the oral thrombin inhibitor (dabigatran etexilate) have more rapid onset than warfarin, have fixed dosing, are not affected by food, have fewer interactions, and do not require monitoring. Despite the cost differential, they are therefore rapidly becoming the anticoagulants of choice for patients requiring anticoagulation and

Essentials of Oral and Maxillofacial Surgery, First Edition. Edited by M. Anthony Pogrel, Karl-Erik Kahnberg and Lars Andersson.
© 2014 John Wiley & Sons, Ltd. Published 2014 by John Wiley & Sons, Ltd.
Companion website: www.wiley.com/go/pogrel/oms

generally do not require any adjustment for routine dental extractions.

Treatment

Excessive postoperative bleeding can be prevented intraoperatively by appropriate tissue management and local measures. In general, careful removal of granulated/infected tissue, minimal manipulation of surgical flaps to avoid tearing, use of local anesthetic with vasoconstrictor, primary wound closure, and the application of topical agents, such as absorbable gelatin sponge, oxidized regenerated cellulose fabric, or chitosan bandage, can limit most postoperative bleeding. Direct pressure with gauze in the immediate postoperative setting is an important method of limiting bleeding as the initial clot forms. Patients should be instructed to continue to apply pressure to the wound until bleeding has stopped.

Bleeding that persists after the initial phase of clot formation should be treated first with local measures, starting with direct pressure to the surgical site. Careful examination of the operative site with illumination and magnification and good suction can be invaluable to identify the source of bleeding. It is not uncommon to identify an incompletely formed clot, a "liver clot", that is mobile and continues to aggravate the site. Careful removal of the clot is critical to control the bleeding successfully. Use of local vasoconstricting agents, such as local anesthetics with a vasoconstrictor such as epinephrine, is appropriate once the source of bleeding has been identified. If the vasoconstrictor is applied to the area prior to identification of the bleeding vessel, identification will be complicated. The wound may need to be repacked with a local hemostatic agent and sutured. Arterial bleeds that cannot be controlled with local measures should be treated with ligation or electrocautery. If bleeding persists, embolization, proximal vessel ligation, or other endovascular procedures may be required.

Pain

Etiology and prevalence

As with bleeding, postoperative pain is a side-effect of operative intervention. Pain associated with routine dentoalveolar procedures usually begins with the resolution of local anesthesia (6–12 hours) and typically peaks between 24 and 48 hours postoperatively.

Risk factors and prevention

Prevention of pain via intraoperative measures and adequate postoperative pain control measures is essential. Intraoperatively, minimizing tissue trauma and careful tissue manipulation will decrease inflammation and thus decrease pain. There is evidence that the administration of preoperative non-steroidal anti-inflammatory medications (salicylates, cyclooxygenase (COX)-2 inhibitors) can reduce the severity of postoperative pain. Postoperatively, the use of nonsteroidal medications, as well as narcotic preparations with acetaminophen (APAP) (hydrocodone, oxycodone, tramadol) are useful for treatment of moderate to severe postoperative pain. In addition, the use of long-acting local anesthetics, e.g. 0.5% bupivacaine with 1:200 000 epinephrine, can be beneficial in delaying the onset of pain, which may allow the patient to start postoperative analgesics prior to the onset of pain.

Swelling

Etiology and prevalence

Edema following the surgical removal of teeth and other routine dentoalveolar procedures is an expected finding during the postoperative course. The onset of swelling is typically between 12 and 24 hours following the procedure, with a peak swelling noted 48–72 hours postoperatively. Swelling typically begins to subside at 4 days postoperatively, with most patients experiencing resolution of surgical edema within 1 week postoperatively.

Prevention and treatment

It is important to inform patients of this time course and that swelling is an anticipated postoperative finding. In the early postoperative period, the use of ice may help with the management of swelling. In addition, patients should be told to sleep with the head of their bed elevated and not to sleep on their side, so as to avoid dependent swelling. Finally, perioperative steroids may be used to prevent swelling in patients undergoing significantly invasive procedures (e.g. third molar extraction). While the use of perioperative steroids may produce moderate decreases in swelling, these medications are typically short in action.

Surgical site infection

Etiology and prevalence

Because the oral cavity is home to a wide variety of bacterial flora, any intraoral wound will be exposed to a broad spectrum of aerobic, anaerobic, and facultative organisms with pathogenic potential. As such, postoperative infections should be primary among concerns for the practitioner when performing oral surgical procedures. Though the routine use of antibiotics for prevention of postoperative infections is still debated, there are several measures that can be implemented to reduce the likelihood of postoperative wound infection.

Prevention

Prevention of postoperative infection begins with identification of the patient at risk. A number of studies have demonstrated that the incidence of postoperative inflammatory complications increases with age, smoking, pre-existing infection/pathology in the surgical area, oral contraceptive use, and lack of surgical experience. When dealing with impacted teeth, mandibular third molars have been shown to have a higher rate of postoperative infections than maxillary teeth.

As with other common complications, careful tissue management, debridement/curettage of necrotic/ infected tissue, and thorough irrigation of the wound site will help to reduce the bacterial inocula within the wound site and reduce the possibility of infection.

Treatment

Patients presenting with infections will typically complain of persistent pain and swelling that is not improving with time, a foul taste, drainage from the wound, and limitation of jaw motion (trismus). Fever is variable and depends on the magnitude of the infection. Early recognition of an infectious process, typically a cellulitis, requires prompt treatment with an empiric course of antibiotics with broad-spectrum coverage for Gram-positive and anaerobic organisms. If the symptoms have persisted for more than 48–72 hours after the procedure, an abscess, or pus pocket, may have formed, in which case incision and drainage may be indicated, with collection of exudate for culture and sensitivity testing to guide antibiotic therapy. Prompt recognition and treatment are necessary to prevent the spread of infection into the submandibular, sublingual, submental, retropharyngeal spaces and spaces of the deep neck, which can result in airway compromise and the necessity for emergency airway management.

Alveolar osteitis

Prevalence and etiology

Among the most common complications associated with oral surgical procedures, specifically the removal of impacted teeth, is alveolar osteitis (AO), or "dry socket". The reported incidence is as high as 30% in some studies, though there exists a wide variation in reported incidence due to inconsistent diagnostic criteria. This condition, which was classically thought to be infectious in nature, is now understood to be associated with malformation, disruption, or other loss of a newly formed blood clot from an extraction socket. Patients presenting with AO will usually complain of a severe throbbing, radiating pain, often associated with a malodor from the surgical site. Trismus is an associated sign, related more to pain than swelling. Recognition of AO is based on the presence of new-onset severe pain, typically 3–5 days

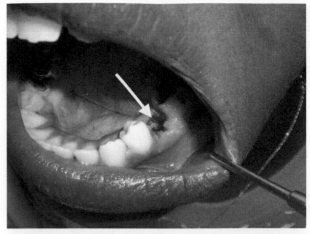

Fig. 7.1 Alveolar osteitis. This patient, a 30-year-old smoker, who was also on oral contraceptives, presented with severe pain of sudden onset 4 days after extraction of tooth 20. The clot is absent and exposed bone can be seen (arrow).

postoperatively, at which point pain and swelling associated with the operation should be beginning to subside. The lack of constitutional symptoms (fever), significant swelling, or intraoral discharge may help to distinguish AO from a surgical site infection. This distinction is important, since antibiotic treatment will not resolve AO. Physical exam findings may include a crypt-like socket with exposed bone and erythematous soft-tissue margins, food debris, or other detritus in the socket and extreme tenderness to palpation (Fig. 7.1). Radiographic examination should also be obtained to rule out the presence of a retained tooth structure or other surgical site complication, such as alveolar fracture.

Prevention

Preoperatively, there are a number of risk factors that have been identified that should alert the vigilant practitioner of the patient at risk. As with postoperative infections, age, oral contraceptive use, surgical experience, smoking, and mandibular surgery have been associated with AO. In addition, poor oral hygiene and pre-existing infections have been shown to increase the risk for AO. Intraoperatively, thorough lavage of the surgical site is associated with a decreased incidence of AO. The use of topical medicaments and antibiotics, clot stabilizers (Gelfoam®), platelet-rich plasma, and medicated mouthrinses have also been suggested for prevention of AO.

Treatment

As the condition is self-limiting, the treatment is supportive, with pain control being the primary goal. Treatment typically consists of gentle irrigation of the wound area with warm saline and application of medicated packing to the area, e.g. eugenol dressings, and aggressive use of oral analgesics. The packing should be changed every 24 hours until symptoms subside.

Fractures

Prevalence and etiology

While rare, fractures of the dentoalveolar process or mandible should be considered in the differential diagnosis of persistent pain or swelling after dentoalveolar procedures. Fractures are the result of using excessive force during tooth extraction (Fig. 7.2). If unrecognized and untreated, such fractures can lead to malocclusion, malunion, infection, and paresthesia.

Prevention

Preoperatively, there are few risk factors for fracture that have been identified. There is some evidence to suggest that age is a risk factor for fractures, presumably because of the loss of bone density, elasticity, and strength which are common findings in elderly patients. Atrophic mandibles or mandibles with large intrabony lesions are at risk for fracture.

Treatment

Recognition of the fracture is the most important management. Intraoperatively, recognition of an alveolar process or mandibular fracture can result from observing a mobile alveolar or mandibular segment or malocclusion. Postoperatively, any patient complaining of malocclusion, pain and swelling disproportionate to the procedure, tooth displacement or mobility, or persistent numbness should be evaluated for a possible fracture.

Once a fracture is identified, typically with the aid of imaging studies, e.g. periapical or panoramic radiographs or computed tomography (CT), treatment is guided by the nature of the fracture and functional limitation. Treatment ranges from dietary modifications (blenderized diet) and early immobilization to reduction and fixation of the fracture.

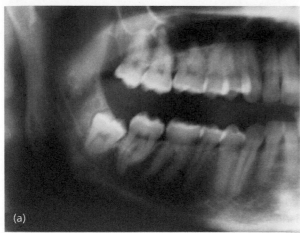
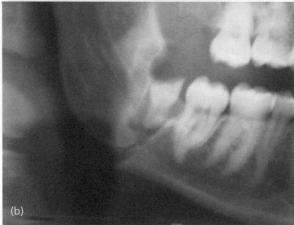
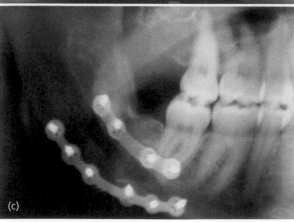

Fig. 7.2 Mandibular angle fracture upon attempted extraction of mandibular third molar. (a) Preoperative radiograph showing vertically impacted tooth 32. (b) The tooth has been partially extracted, with the roots remaining; there is a fracture of the mandibular angle. (c) After reduction of right mandibular angle fracture. (Photos provided courtesy of Leonard B. Kaban, DMD, MD.)

Root fracture

Prevalence and etiology

Root tip fractures are common after tooth extraction, especially in posterior, multirooted teeth. Fracture of the roots, or root tips, is typically due to excessive forces applied during extraction with inadequate separation of the roots from the extraction socket and is commonly unavoidable due to the root anatomy and bone quality. When such forces are applied, the torque generated will typically cause a fracture at the junction between that portion of the root still attached to the socket and that portion already freed from the alveolar wall.

Prevention

The prevention of root fractures is primarily based on use of proper surgical technique, minimizing excessive forces, and carefully ensuring that teeth are adequately elevated and mobilized prior to luxation. Recognition of teeth at risk for root fracture is also an important preventative measure. Multirooted posterior teeth, roots that are curved, canines or other anterior teeth that have root dilacerations, or teeth with widely spaced thin roots, all have an increased risk for fracture. Inadvertent root fractures can be avoided by operative planning and prudent sectioning of a tooth prior to elevation and removal.

Treatment

The most important step in treating a fractured root or retained root tip is recognition that such an incident has occurred. Once the tooth has been removed, it should be carefully inspected to confirm that the roots were removed completely. Reconstitute the fragments of a sectioned tooth to confirm complete removal.

If a root fracture is noted, the socket should be irrigated thoroughly and an attempt should be made to directly visualize the retained root/root tip. For teeth without preoperative evidence of periapical pathology or infection, small root tips (<3 mm) can be left in place without adverse effects. In fact, for posterior teeth, the risk of causing damage to the maxillary sinus or inferior alveolar nerve may often outweigh the risk of leaving the fragment in place, and sometimes this is carried out deliberately in the technique known as coronectomy.

If there is associated pathology with the tooth preoperatively, the root fragment should be removed. Once the fragment is directly visualized, root tip picks/elevators should be used to carefully separate the fragment from the alveolar socket, with special care taken not to apply apical pressure to the fragment. This gentle manipulation should be done until the root is mobilized, at which point it can be removed.

Root or tooth displacement

Prevalence and etiology

Displacement of root tips or tooth fragments is an uncommon but distressing complication nonetheless. Given the proximity of various fascial spaces to max-

illary and mandibular third molars, displacement of tooth fragments can occur into the infratemporal fossa and maxillary sinus or submandibular space and inferior alveolar canal, respectively.

Prevention

Displacement of tooth fragments into these fascial spaces can often be prevented by using careful surgical technique. For example, when elevating an impacted maxillary third molar, the use of a periosteal elevator posterior to the distal aspect of the crown can serve as a barrier to displacement into the infratemporal fossa. In the event of displacement into the infratemporal fossa, a minimal attempt should be made to visualize the fragment and remove it. If this attempt is unsuccessful, the wound should be closed and the patient should be given a course of antibiotics. Future exploration of the region should be anticipated and CT, plain film imaging or both should be obtained to aid in localization and surgical treatment planning.

Careful examination of preoperative radiographs can be useful in evaluating the association between the roots of impacted maxillary third molars and the maxillary sinus. In older patients, or those with significant periodontal disease, pneumatization of the maxillary alveolus can increase the likelihood of an association between the roots of the teeth and the maxillary sinus. In these cases, careful attention must be directed to avoiding excessive apical pressure to the teeth during the process of extracting teeth.

Treatment

In the event that a root fragment or tooth is displaced into the maxillary sinus (Fig. 7.3), the first step in treatment is localization of the fragment and prevention of further displacement. Typically this can be achieved by seating the patient in the upright

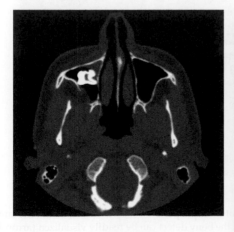
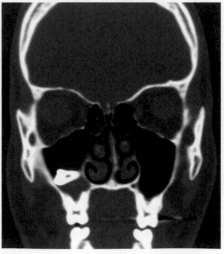

Fig. 7.3 Tooth displaced into maxillary sinus.

position and obtaining periapical radiographs of the region of interest. In the event that a root or fragment is visualized, various methods can be used for retrieval. The simplest method is forcing positive pressure through the sinus to displace the root – this can be accomplished by closing the nostrils and having the patient attempt to exhale through the nose. Alternative methods include attempting to remove the fragment using a thin suction tip or packing the socket with iodoform gauze and removing the gauze in a smooth stroke, hoping that the fragment will be caught in the gauze. In the event that such measures prove unsuccessful, the maxillary sinus can be explored to directly visualize and remove the fragment, either endoscopically or with open surgery involving a Caldwell–Luc incision. This can be done as a simultaneous procedure or at a future visit. If done at a future visit, the patient should be placed on sinus precautions, antibiotics and nasal decongestants.

Displacement of mandibular teeth into either the submandibular space or inferior alveolar canal is a rare occurrence. However, given the vital structures in these regions, any suspicion of displacement must be evaluated fully. Visualizing any fragments is best accomplished immediately using periapical and Panorex-type films, with occlusal films in addition for submandibular space invasion. These will be supplemented by cone-beam CT scans as time allows. Once the fragment is identified, a gentle attempt should be made to remove the fragment from the inferior alveolar nerve (IAN) canal or the submandibular space, but care should be taken not to compromise the spaces and further displace the tooth. In the event that the fragment cannot be easily removed, delayed removal may be indicated and the patient should be placed on antibiotics. For fragments in the IAN canal, if the patient does not demonstrate any signs of infection or paresthesia in the postoperative course, the fragment may be left without concern. For fragments in the submandibular space, exploration of the region with lingual dissection and separation of the mylohyoid muscle from the mandible is indicated approximately 6 weeks after the initial operation. This delay allows for tissue fibrosis to occur around the displaced fragment, thereby stabilizing its position. This procedure can be carried out intra-orally or extra-orally, depending on the position of the retained fragment.

Oroantral communication

Prevalence and etiology

Following extraction of maxillary posterior teeth, oroantral (sinus) communications are common, commonly unrecognized, and do not need treatment. Persistent, symptomatic oroantral communications are uncommon with a frequency of <1%. Oroantral communications may result from excessive manipulation of the operative site or poor technique. It should be readily acknowledged that communications typically result from intimate anatomic associations between the roots of the teeth and the floor of the maxillary sinus and may be unavoidable (Fig. 7.4).

Prevention

As with displacement of teeth into the maxillary sinus, prevention of oroantral communications starts

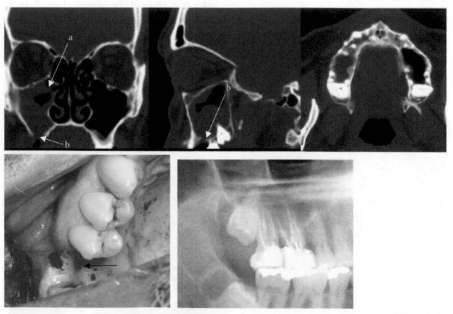

Fig. 7.4 Persistent oroantral communication following extraction of multiple periodontally involved teeth. The sinus on the right side is partially obliterated with inflammatory tissue (arrow a) and the bony defect can be readily visualized (arrow b) and is much larger than the apparent size of the lesion based on clinical examination (arrow in clinical photograph). Preoperative panoramic radiograph demonstrates close proximity of the roots to the maxillary sinus and a poorly defined margin of sinus floor around the apices of the dental roots.

with identification of the patient at risk. Evaluation of preoperative radiographs for any evidence of encroachment of the roots upon the floor of the sinus should alert the surgeon to the likelihood of this complication. Upon removal of the tooth, the socket should be curetted gently, avoiding the apical areas. If the tooth is not removed completely, judicious exploration should be undertaken, so as not to: (1) displace the remnant into the sinus; or (2) perforate the sinus floor while attempting to remove the fragment. A self-limiting oroantral communication may be an unavoidable side-effect of tooth removal due to the anatomic relationship between the roots and the sinus. Informing the patient of a likelihood of an oro-antral communication prior to tooth removal is preferable to explaining it after tooth removal.

Treatment

Diagnosis of a sinus communication is often made by having the patient force air through the nasal cavity while the nares are closed. If a large communication exists, air bubbles should be visible within the socket. This method may prove ineffective for small communications.

In the event that a communication is discovered, either by tactile sensation or forced air maneuver, the size of the defect and patient complaint guide treatment. As a general principle, any patient with a communication should be placed on sinus precautions, antibiotics, and nasal decongestants.

Most oroantral communications heal spontaneously with little intervention. At the time of the procedure, primary closure of the extraction socket is not indicated. The patient should be placed on broad-spectrum antibiotics, e.g. amoxycillin or clindamycin, and sinus precautions. Monitor the patient closely over the postoperative period to confirm closure of the oroantral communication. If an oroantal fistula develops, standard procedures to produce a layered closure of the wound and management of the sinus are indicated. Clinicians should remember that the size of the visible fistula is much smaller than the actual bony defect (Fig. 7.4).

Recommended reading

Susarla SM, Smart RJ, Dodson TB. (2010) Complications associated with dentoalveolar surgery. In: *Oral and Maxillofacial Surgery* (eds, Andersson L, Kahnberg K-E, Pogrel MA). Oxford, Wiley-Blackwell.

Part 2: Dentoalveolar Surgery

(Section Editor: Lars Andersson)

Chapter 8

Extraction of Teeth

Extraction of teeth is one of the most common surgical procedures worldwide. It has a psychological impact on the patient, because the patient will be losing a tooth, and the associations the patient will have with such a procedure. The patient will also face another problem in that the loss of a tooth often requires a later replacement of the missing tooth. For this reason patient information and consent is very important. Moreover, extraction of teeth incorporates basic principles from physics, mechanics, and surgery, and the clinician should therefore fully understand and master the techniques of extraction.

Indications for extraction

Although teeth in principle should be treated and maintained in the oral cavity as long as possible, provided they fulfill functional and esthetic criteria, it is sometimes inevitable that teeth have to be removed for various reasons. General indications for extractions, as listed in Box 8.1, are discussed under their respective headings; however, the decision to extract has to be made individually for each case.

Caries

When the tooth is subjected to severe caries with extensive loss of tooth substance that will not permit restorative procedures, it may sometimes be necessary to extract the tooth.

Periodontal disease

Periodontal disease should be treated as first alternative, but there are situations where severe periodontal disease can be an indication for extraction, especially when the prognosis is poor for periodontal treatment. Severe bone and attachment loss and irreversible tooth hypermobility may be an indication for extraction (Fig. 8.1). Long-standing, progressive periodontitis will result in alveolar bone loss. If implant treatment is going to be performed after extraction it is important not to wait too long before severely periodontally affected teeth are extracted. The severity of periodontal disease, long-term prognosis, and even cost/benefit aspects should be considered before making the decision.

Pulp disease when endodontic treatment is not possible or has failed

Irreversible pulpitis, pulp necrosis or internal resorption of the root canal where endodontic procedures are not possible or have failed are sometimes other indications for tooth extraction. This could be because of obliterated root canals, canals that are not accessible due to root anatomy, or when a patient chooses not to undergo such treatment.

Pathologic lesions in relation to teeth

Pathologic lesions associated with teeth, i.e. apical or juxtaradicular periodontitis, can usually be solved by endodontic treatment. If endodontic procedures are not possible, then extraction can be considered. If teeth compromise the surgical treatment of other pathologic lesions found in the tissues surrounding them, then extraction may be considered, e.g. in the treatment of osteomyelitis, or benign and malignant tumors of the jaw.

Essentials of Oral and Maxillofacial Surgery, First Edition. Edited by M. Anthony Pogrel, Karl-Erik Kahnberg and Lars Andersson.
© 2014 John Wiley & Sons, Ltd. Published 2014 by John Wiley & Sons, Ltd.
Companion website: www.wiley.com/go/pogrel/oms

Box 8.1 Indications for extraction of teeth

Caries

Periodontal disease

Pulp disease when endodontic treatment is not possible or has failed

Pathologic lesions surrounding teeth

Crown and root fractures

Malposition of teeth

Impacted teeth

Supernumerary teeth

Orthodontic indications

Teeth in bone fracture lines

Before prosthetic procedures

Before other surgical procedures

Before radiation therapy

Before bisphosphonate therapy

Other reasons for extraction

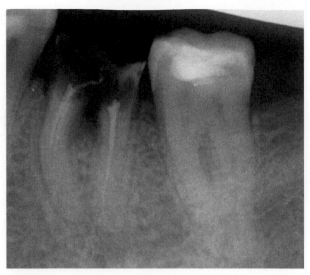

Fig. 8.2 Crown fracture of 36 leaving two delicate roots. These roots could be fragile and likely to fracture when extraction is attempted. Surgical removal of these roots should be considered.

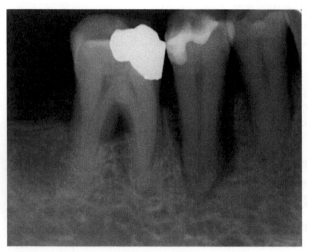

Fig. 8.1 Severe periodontal disease has led to extensive bone loss around 45 which is hypermobile and due to be extracted. Extraction in this case is easy.

Crown and root fractures

Crown, crown-root, and root fractures after trauma can most often be successfully treated and extraction avoided. However, there are other situations where fractures of the crown and root do not allow successful restorative therapy and extraction is the only alternative (Fig. 8.2).

Malposition of teeth

Although malposition of teeth is not an indication for extraction, there are situations where malposition is associated with other conditions such as trauma to soft tissue or blockage of eruption of adjacent teeth (Fig. 8.3). Another situation is when there is elongation of teeth due to the missing antagonist and where prosthetic rehabilitation is considered in the opposing jaw. The elongated tooth may then be considered for extraction.

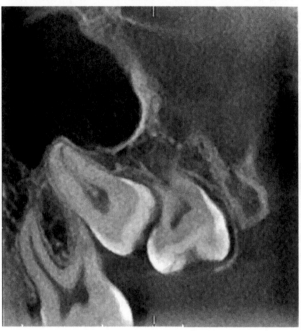

Fig. 8.3 Cone-beam computed tomography (CT) scan showing malposition of the upper left third molar blocking the eruption of the second maxillary molar.

Impacted teeth

Impacted teeth do not always reach functional occlusion, often because of lack of space. These teeth should be investigated and considered for extraction if they present a potential for the development of pathology in the future. These could include the risk for root resorption of adjacent teeth, loss of bone around adjacent roots or development of other pathologic conditions such as cysts. Impacted third molars are the most common teeth considered for extraction. However, there must always be an indication if third molars are going to be removed and prophylactic removal of impacted third molars without pathology or symptom is not justified today. For more details

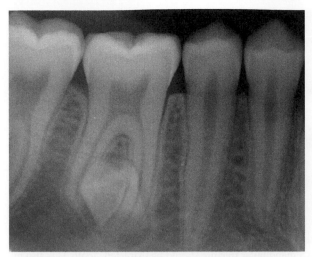

Fig. 8.4 Supernumerary tooth in the first molar region. This tooth will have to be followed radiologically and should be removed if any signs of pathology, such as progressive root resorption of the first molar, is suspected.

regarding strategies for third molar extraction see Chapter 9.

Supernumerary teeth

Supernumerary teeth that are potential sources for future pathology should sometimes be removed. However, supernumerary teeth without pathology do not have to be routinely removed (Fig. 8.4).

Orthodontic indications

Extraction of teeth is sometimes required to create space in order to carry out planned orthodontic treatment. The most common teeth for extraction on orthodontic indications are premolars. The decision on which tooth/teeth are to be extracted is made by the orthodontist.

Before prosthetic procedures

Before prosthetic reconstructions is carried out it is sometimes necessary to extract teeth. Teeth could interfere with the proper placement of a fixed or removable prosthetic appliance and may then be extracted. For example, in the case of rehabilitation of a jaw with implants where there are only one or two incisors remaining that have a dubious prognosis, in some situations it may be better to be radical and extract the remaining teeth and perform a full arch implant-supported reconstruction.

Before other surgical procedures

Sometimes teeth have to be removed prior to other surgical procedures. The most common indication in this regard is the removal of impacted molars prior to LeFort-I and sagittal split osteotomies. This is done if the teeth lie in the line of the planned osteotomies

or increase the risk for other complications such as undesired fractures.

Before radiation therapy

Careful consideration should be given to patients who are to undergo radiation therapy due to tumors in the head and neck region. These extractions should preferably be carried out before radiation treatment is starting. Teeth associated with pathologic conditions such as periapical periodontitis should be considered either for swift endodontic procedures or extraction. A radical approach by extracting rather than choosing doubtful restorative treatment with less chance of successful outcome is recommended to avoid later complications in the irradiated bone. There is a high risk of osteoradionecrosis if extractions have to be carried out after radiation therapy, especially with high doses of radiation (>60 Gray). This risk persists throughout the life of the patient.

Before bisphosphonate therapy

Patients treated with bisphosphonates, especially those treated for malignancies with intravenous administration of bisphosphonates, run a high risk of osteonecrosis if extraction is carried out after bisphosphonate treatment has started. Like in irradiated patients, this risk persists throughout the life of the patient. For this reason dental examination and appropriate treatment shall always be taken into consideration when such bisphosphonate treatment is planned. Extractions should be carried out before bisphosphonate therapy is started. Teeth associated with pathologic conditions such as periapical periodontitis should be considered either for swift endodontic procedures or extraction. A radical approach by extracting rather than choosing doubtful restorative treatment with less chance of successful outcome is recommended to avoid later complications. There is a high risk of osteonecrosis if extractions have to be carried out after intravenous bisphosphonate therapy is started. Patients on oral bisphosphonates, usually osteoporosis patients, are not subjected to the same high risk of osteonecrosis.

Teeth in bone fracture lines

Sometimes teeth in the line of a jaw fracture should be considered for extraction in order to prevent infection. Tooth luxation can almost always be treated by repositioning and fixation, but where there is severe luxation of teeth associated with complex jaw fractures, where teeth are in the line of the fractures and interfering with the repositioning, these teeth should be extracted (Fig. 8.5).

Other reasons for extraction

There are other situations where extraction may be chosen, even when the extraction may be on doubtful

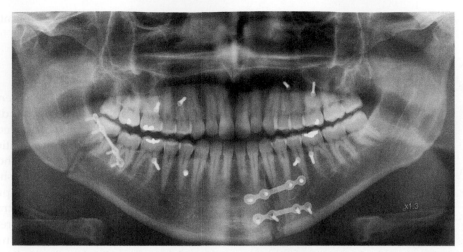

Fig. 8.5 Tooth 48 which is root fractured and is located in the line of a mandibular fracture should be extracted. Tooth 33 is also in the line of a fracture but can be preserved if it does not interfere with repositioning of the bone fragment.

indications. In these situations it is especially important to discuss alternative treatment and inform the patient preoperatively so the surgeon and patient agree on the choice of treatment. Extractions can sometimes be performed due to economic reasons. Patients might choose to extract a tooth rather than incur the costs of, for example, having endodontic treatment or a more expensive restorative procedure. Extractions can sometimes also be performed due to esthetic reasons. For example, the patient could choose to extract an upper malformed lateral incisor and have it replaced with an implant. Furthermore, a patient could choose to extract protrusive teeth in the upper front and have them replaced by an implant-supported prosthesis as an alternative to undergoing orthodontic or orthognathic surgical correction. Malformed or severely discolored teeth could also be considered for extraction due to esthetic reasons where the patients choose extraction and prosthetic reconstruction over other procedures such as veneers and crowns. Teeth could sometimes also be extracted due to difficulty in maintaining adequate oral hygiene. Most commonly, the third molars are extracted due the recurrence of pericoronitis and difficulties in maintaining oral hygiene.

Contraindications for extraction

The surgeon should also consider the contraindications for extracting the tooth, for example with consideration to the patient's general health or local conditions in the region of extraction. Contraindications for extractions are often relative and can be changed after treating or adjusting the underlying reason for the contraindication.

Systemic contraindications

These constitute all general health factors and mental factors which have influence on the patient's ability to withstand the surgical procedure. Severe dental anxiety is a relative contraindication to extraction in local anesthesia and in some cases patients can be treated in general anesthesia. One should pay extra attention to patients on medication such as anticoagulant drugs, cancer medication, glucocorticoids, immunosuppressants and bisphosphonates.

Patients with hemophilia or other coagulopathies should first have their disorders controlled before extraction. In general, most uncontrolled metabolic diseases, such as diabetes, constitute a relative contraindication until they are brought under control. Similarly, patients with severe uncontrolled hypertension and cardiac diseases should ideally be treated for these conditions first before extractions are carried out. Ongoing radio- and/or chemotherapy is also a relative contraindication. In all cases, one should be aware of the medications, especially those drugs that affect the immune system, delay or impair the healing process, or could interact with medication administered to manage an extraction. Some cancer medications, e.g. bisphosphonates, can also cause necrosis of the jaws after extractions.

Local contraindications

The most common local contraindication is an ongoing acute inflammatory or infectious process. The acute infection/inflammation should first be treated before proceeding with the extraction, depending on the location of the acute process. Extraction of a third lower molar during an ongoing acute pericoronitis could lead to a life-threatening postoperative infection. Local treatment of the pericoronitis is preferred and extraction may be carried out later.

However, there are also situations where an acute abscess is best drained by extraction of the tooth even in an acute phase. Therefore, an acute infectious and inflammatory process should not be considered as an absolute contraindication for extraction. The surgeon should, however, bear in mind that there could be other problems, such as severe pain, swelling, reduced mouth opening, and anxiety, which could make extractions associated with other acute conditions suboptimal. In such cases extractions should be deferred until the acute symptoms have subsided.

One of the most important contraindications to extraction is radiation therapy, past and present, involving the jaws. Delayed healing, dehiscence, and necrosis of the bone are often complications due to extractions performed in irradiated bone. Finally, teeth within the area of a malignant tumor should not be removed before the planning of tumor treatment has been performed.

Clinical evaluation of the tooth before extraction

Before starting extraction it is important to evaluate the condition of the crown. Deep caries or a large restoration may indicate a high risk for fracture of the crown during extraction, which would complicate the procedure. A tooth with missing crown will require a special approach. Other factors to consider

are tooth/root mobility. Ankylosis, which is often seen with infrapositioned primary teeth or teeth subjected to earlier trauma, often indicates a surgical approach for removal of the primary tooth or, with ankylotic infrapositioned permanent teeth in the anterior region, decoronation to preserve the alveolar bone crest in the anterior region should be chosen. It is also important to assess the status of the adjacent teeth to avoid damage to fragile teeth or teeth with large restorations. The clinical evaluation of the tooth to be removed is done in conjunction with a radiographic assessment.

Preoperative radiographic examination

Radiographic examination must always be carried out prior to extraction of teeth to evaluate the degree of difficulty of extraction. Root anatomy, presence of pathology in the root or surrounding bone, vital structures and relation to other roots, neighboring teeth and other factors such as ankylosis with replacement resorption or hypercementosis of the root are taken into consideration (Fig. 8.6). The

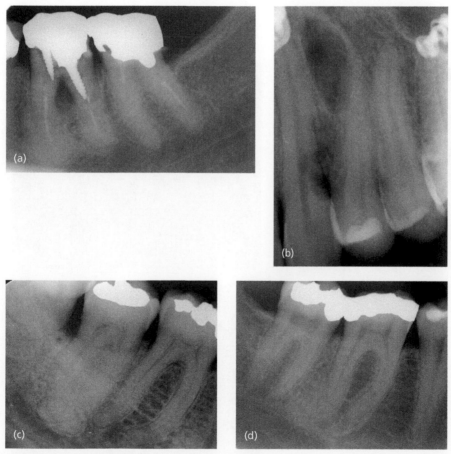

Fig. 8.6 (a) Hypercementosis of the mesial root of the first lower left molar would prompt surgical extraction of this tooth. Closed extraction in this case is impossible. The second molar has a large restoration, and the tooth could be fragile leading to fracture. The option of surgical extraction should be considered. (b) The extent of external root resorption makes extraction of the canine almost impossible due to the risk for fracture. Surgical extraction should be considered. (c) The root configuration of the second lower right molar makes it impossible to remove this tooth without a surgical procedure. (d) The lower first right molar has slender roots that taper towards each other apically. Besides, the cervical portion of the mesial root is narrower than the apical part. This will make extraction difficult and surgical extraction will have to be considered.

most common radiograph is a good quality intraoral periapical radiograph. Other techniques, such as panoramic radiographs, scanograms, and cone-beam computer tomography, are more valuable to evaluate the tooth in relation to vital structures such as inferior alveolar nerve and maxillary sinus.

In the mandible, the position of the mandibular canal should be noted, especially in relation to third molars (Fig. 8.7). The position of the mental foramen should be noted in cases where a flap has to be raised in order to remove the premolars (Fig. 8.8). In the maxilla, the proximity of the roots of the molars to the sinus should be assessed (Fig. 8.9). In some cases the sinus membrane can rupture during extraction of maxillary molars causing an oroantral communication.

Control of anxiety and pain

For a successful dental extraction, control of the patient's anxiety and pain is essential. Most patients have anxiety when undergoing an extraction procedure. Local anesthesia must be sufficient to eliminate pain and sensation from the involved tissues.

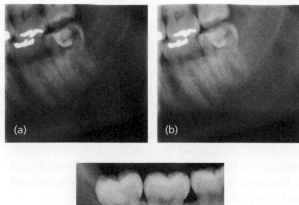
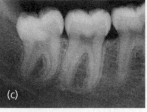

Fig. 8.7 (a) Scanogram showing the relation of the mandibular canal with respect to the apices of 37 and 38. Root anatomy makes it highly likely that the third molar would require a surgical extraction. The position of the mandibular canal must be determined before surgical extraction. (b, c) The distally angulated third molar and configuration of the root make an extraction avoiding a root fracture very difficult. Note the position of the mandibular canal in close proximity to the roots.

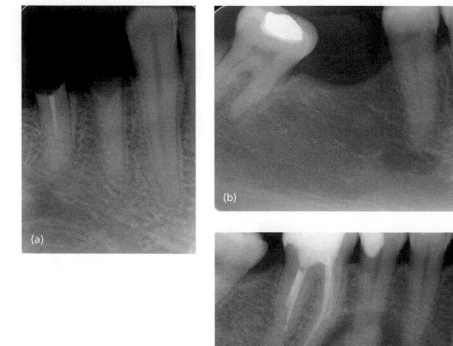

Fig. 8.8 (a) The mental foramen is just inferior to the roots of 45 with the anterior loop of the mental nerve visible. (b) The mental foramen is projected in contact with the apex of 45. The lamina dura of the root can be distinctly followed throughout, and this excludes apical pathology. (c) It is difficult to identify the position of the mental foramen from this single radiograph. Before surgical removal of the second premolar additional radiographs are needed to determine the relation to the mental foramen.

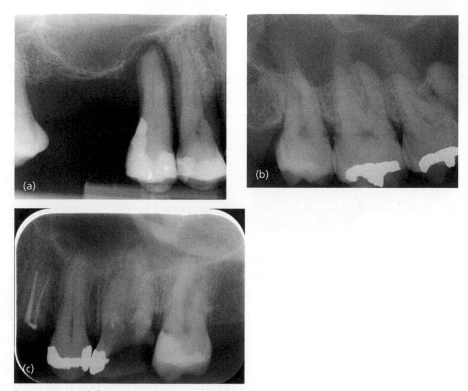

Fig. 8.9 (a) Note the proximity of the sinus membrane to 15. The infection around the apex of 15 can lead to destruction of the lower sinus wall and cause an oroantral communication when 15 is extracted. (b) Large maxillary sinus that extends over the apices of the molars with a risk for oroantral communication during extraction of these teeth. (c) Severe caries and loss of tooth substance will make extraction of 26 difficult. The maxillary sinus is in close relation to the apices which have apical periodontitis. This increases the risk for a rupture of the sinus membrane when extraction is attempted.

Sedation

Although pain associated with extractions is managed effectively through the administration of local anesthesia, patients are anxious because of the fear of pain. Anxiety control may vary from the surgeon simply showing concern and empathy for the anxious patient to the use of oral or parenteral drugs for sedation of the very anxious patients. In some patients general anesthesia has to be used to enable treatment.

Local anesthesia

A prerequisite for extraction is that the surgeon has knowledge of anatomy, innervation of teeth and surrounding soft and hard tissue and is familiar with the techniques of local anesthesia. Profound local anesthesia results in loss of all pain, temperature, and touch sensations, but it does not anesthetize the proprioceptive fibers. The patient still may therefore feel sensations of pressure which must be explained to the patient prior to local anesthesia and extraction. There are various local anesthetics in use. They can be used with or without vasoconstrictor. They differ in their concentration, and duration of anesthesia. Each local anesthetic has a recommended maximum dose to ensure safety of the patient and this must always be considered, especially when administering in very old or young patients.

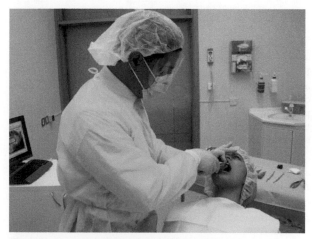

Fig. 8.10 Surgeon with proper clinical attire: gloves, mask, cap, and protective eye shield. Patient with sterile drape across the chest and a cap. The surgeon is in a standing position for extracting maxillary anterior teeth.

Preparation for extraction

To prevent injury or transmission of disease to their patients, themselves, and their assisting staff the surgeons should wear surgical gloves, surgical masks, gowns, surgical caps, and glasses or eye screens with side shields even for simple extractions (Figs 8.10, 8.11 and 8.12). For the patient, a sterile draping over the neck and chest is recommended. Preoperative

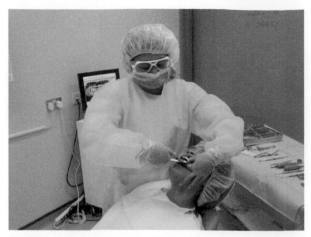

Fig. 8.11 Surgeon with proper clinical attire: gloves, mask, cap, and protective eye glasses. Patient with sterile drape across the chest and a cap. The surgeon is in a standing position for an extraction from the maxilla.

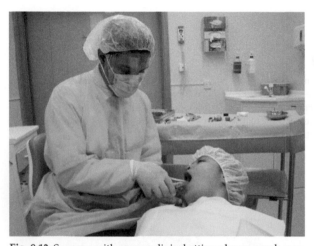

Fig. 8.12 Surgeon with proper clinical attire: gloves, mask, cap, and protective eye shield. Patient with sterile drape across the chest and a cap. The surgeon is in a sitting position with the patient lowered as low as possible so the mouth is level with the surgeon's elbow. The surgeon is in a sitting position for an extraction from the mandible.

mouthrinse with antiseptic, such as chlorhexidine, can be used to reduce the number of microorganisms at the surgical site.

Surgeon's position

The optimal position is when both patient and surgeon are comfortable (Figs 8.10, 8.11 and 8.12). Dental extraction can be performed with the surgeon sitting or standing. Most surgeons prefer the standing position. Regardless of whether the surgeon is sitting or standing, the correct positioning of the surgeon should allow him/her to deliver a controlled force to the patient's tooth through the forceps and elevators used. The patient's chair should be tilted backwards. The correct position allows the surgeon to provide stability and support and to enable a controlled force on the extraction forceps delivered from the arm and shoulder without engaging the wrist.

When extracting teeth in the maxilla, the surgeon should stand in front or by the side of the patient. The head can be supported by the surgeon's opposite hand or by the help of an assistant. For extraction of the mandibular teeth, the surgeon should approach the patient from behind during extraction of anterior and right posterior teeth. The approach from behind gives the surgeon a better visibility of the extraction site and it also allows the surgeon to be in a comfortable and stable position. When extracting left posterior mandibular teeth, the surgeon should approach the patient from the front. The mandible shall always be supported by the surgeon's opposite hand or by the help of an assistant to avoid unnecessary high load and injury to the temporomandibular joint.

Principles of simple (closed, non-surgical) extraction

The mechanical principles applied from physics where forces are transformed from long axes of the instruments and the surgeon's arms to deliver a force in an appropriate direction at the point of application on the teeth and roots. The principles of lever, wedge, and rotating wheel and axle are used for elevators and forceps.

Extraction of a tooth requires expansion of the alveolar socket and separation of the attachment of the periodontal and attaching gingival soft tissues. For this reason it is important to study the anatomy of the tooth and its root, its periodontal ligament, and oral soft tissue attachment prior to extraction.

Controlled force is delivered with dental elevators and forceps to expand and, in a controlled way, fracture the alveolar socket without fracturing the alveolar process, roots or crown of the tooth. The force delivered must be carefully applied to avoid excessive damage to the supporting structures and adjacent teeth.

The tooth has to follow a certain path upon delivery from its socket. Dental forceps and elevators have been designed to provide a mechanical advantage for the delivery by a controlled force. The instruments used to extract teeth should therefore be properly selected and handled in order to deliver a controlled force in appropriate directions.

To avoid fracture of the tooth the forceps should firmly engage the tooth as apical as possible without injuring the adjacent structures. The force delivered during removal while grasping the tooth as apical as possible can lower the center of rotation toward the apices of teeth, minimizing the risk of fracture of crowns or roots.

Some surgeons prefer to start with gentle reflection of the gingival tissue around the tooth neck with a periosteal elevator to prepare for the beaks of the forceps and minimize the soft tissue injury (Fig. 8.13).

The first step in extraction is gently expanding the alveolar bone. This is achieved by introducing a

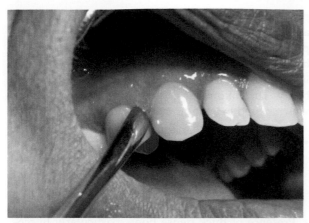

Fig. 8.13 The use of a periosteal elevator for releasing and expansion of gingival tissue before using elevators and forceps for extraction. This creates space for both instruments and minimizes soft tissue injury during extraction.

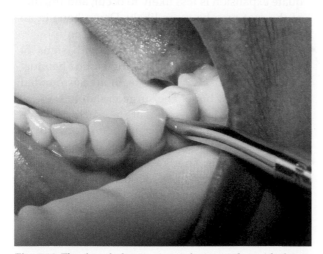

Fig. 8.14 The dental elevator is used as a wedge with the tip being forced into the periodontal space to expand the alveolar bone and force the tooth out of the socket.

dental elevator as a wedge as far apically as possible in the socket at the neck of the tooth to be extracted. The straight dental elevator is used for lever transmitting from a long lever arm with moderate force into a short lever arm with high force. It can be used as a wedge along the root in the periodontal space or according to the wheel and axis principle by inserting it into the interproximal space, perpendicular to the tooth long axis (Fig. 8.14) and rotating it toward the tooth to be extracted. This causes the alveolus to expand, loosen the periodontal ligaments, and forces the tooth in a coronal direction. The thumb and forefinger of the opposite hand should be used to hold the socket, with one finger on the buccal and the other finger on the lingual aspects; in this position, the surgeon can sense the force being applied and the degree of movement of the object tooth. This maneuver can also protect the surrounding soft tissue and adjacent teeth from inappropriately applied accidental forces. It is important not to deliver a high force by the elevator since this may result in fracture of the tooth.

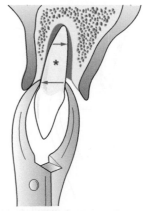

Fig. 8.15 The forceps is applied to the crown of a central maxillary incisor. The forceps is placed as far apically as possible so the center of rotation (star) is located as palatally as possible. Continued apical pressure is applied and the incisor is luxated buccally and lingually. Once some mobility is noted, the conical root allows rotational forces to be applied. Buccal, palatal, and rotational forces are used and finally the tooth is lifted out of its socket. The same technique can be used to extract maxillary lateral incisors and canines.

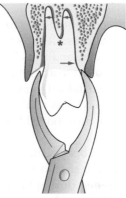

Fig. 8.16 The forceps is applied to a maxillary first premolar which has two thin roots. There is a high risk of fracture if careful technique is not applied. The forceps is placed as far apically as possible to move the center of rotation (star) as far apically as possible. The tooth is then luxated carefully buccally to expand the alveolus, and thereafter the tooth is luxated palatally. Rotational force should be avoided in teeth that have more than one root. After the tooth has been luxated it can be lifted out of its socket.

The appropriate dental forceps can then be applied with its beaks as far apically as possible and thereby acting as a wedge in the socket. The beaks must be parallel to the long axis of the tooth. A steady grip must be obtained and luxation pressure is then applied in lingual and buccal directions (Figs 8.15, 8.16 and 8.17), continuing with gently applied persistent force to expand the alveolus. It is important that the force is delivered with arm and shoulder and not with the hand only. The center of rotation should be kept as apical as possible. The luxations should be slow and the force must be held persistently for several seconds. One-rooted teeth can be rotated after initial luxation (Fig. 8.15), but teeth with more roots than one shall not be rotated. As the tooth gets more luxated and

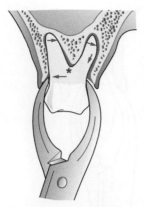

Fig. 8.17 Forceps is applied to a maxillary molar with two buccal and one palatal roots. Three-rooted teeth and root divergence will make the extraction difficult. The initial step is to seat the forceps firmly against the tooth and apply apical force to move the rotational center (star) as far apically as possible. Expansion of the sockets is achieved by careful buccal and palatal luxation. Large initial forces should be avoided and can result in uncontrolled fractures of the roots, buccal bone plate or tuberosity. Forces in buccal and palatal directions will enable bone expansion. After the tooth has been luxated the tooth is then carefully delivered out of the socket and mouth buccally.

loosened, the forceps should be repositioned more and more apically as possible; this will increase the efficiency of the forceps, and thus lessen the chance of fracture of the roots. Luxating the tooth buccally and lingually with sustained pressure over a long time will widen the alveolus so the tooth finally, as the very last step, can be removed from the socket by a slight traction.

After the tooth has been removed a compression of the alveolar process should be carried out since it has become expanded during the luxations. Sharp bone edges should be reduced by a rongeur or trimmed with a bone file so there is no sharp bone edge left.

Most erupted teeth can be extracted by simple extraction using the methods described. However, it takes some time and experience to get the right feeling for luxation without fracturing roots. As the surgeon gains experience, his or her efficiency will improve, and the surgeon will also develop a sense for teeth that may present problems in their removal. If the extraction is difficult, a decision should be made early to surgically remove the tooth rather than apply excessive force. This is important, in that excessive force increases discomfort and anxiety of the patient, the risk for root and crown fractures, and the time for extraction.

Surgical (open flap technique) extraction of teeth or roots

When teeth cannot be extracted simply, they are extracted by the use of an open, surgical flap technique. As a general rule, surgeons should consider performing an elective surgical extraction when they perceive a possible need for excessive force to extract a tooth. The term *excessive* means that the force will probably result in a fracture of bone, tooth root, or both. This will lead to an additional surgery and/or increase surgery time, which can cause undue morbidity. The following are examples of situations in which closed extraction may require excessive force:

- Failure to remove a tooth with forceps or closed extraction. Instead of applying a force that may be not controlled, the surgeon should simply reflect a soft tissue flap, remove some bone, section the tooth or roots, and extract the tooth in sections.
- Presence of thick dense bone, particularly bucco-cortical bone as assessed preoperatively. Surgical extraction should be considered. The extraction of most teeth depends on the expansion of the bucco-cortical plate. If this bone is thick and dense, adequate expansion is less likely to occur, and fracture of the root may be more likely. Dense bone in an older patient warrants even more caution.
- Presence of short clinical crowns with signs of severe attrition as a result of bruxism or habitual grinding. It is likely that the teeth are surrounded by dense heavy bone. The surgeon should exercise extreme caution if removal of such teeth is attempted with a closed technique. An open technique usually results in a quicker, easier extraction.
- Hypercementosis. This is a condition where cementum has continued to be deposited on the tooth and has formed a large bulbous root that is difficult to remove through the available tooth socket opening. Great force used to expand the bone may result in fracture of the tooth or bucco-cortical bone and in a more difficult extraction procedure.
- Teeth with long and divergent roots, especially the maxillary first molars or roots that have severe dilacerations or hooks, are also difficult to remove without fracturing one or more roots. By reflecting a soft tissue flap and sectioning the roots with a bur, a more controlled and planned extraction can be performed, with less morbidity (see Fig. 8.6c,d). Presence of large pneumatized maxillary sinus with the roots of maxillary molars extending into the sinus especially in the case of isolated molars (see Fig. 8.9b). Extraction may result in removal of a portion of sinus floor with the tooth leading to an annoying complication known as oroantral communication. If the roots are divergent, such a situation is even more likely to occur.
- Teeth with extensive caries, root caries, or that have large amalgam restorations are candidates for surgical extraction (Figs 8.9c and 8.18). Although the tooth is grasped primarily by the root, a portion of the force is applied to the crown. Such pressures can crush and shatter the crowns of teeth with extensive caries or large restorations. Planned open extraction will result in quicker and easier extraction. Teeth with crowns already lost secondary to extensive caries, and present in the mouth

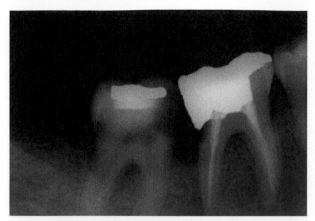

Fig. 8.18 Preoperative periapical radiograph showing severe caries in a second mandibular molar to be extracted. There is also evidence of a large amalgam filling on the first molar. Because of the high risk of fracture of crowns and filling a surgical extraction may be preferred.

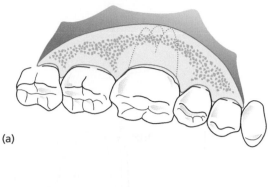

(a)

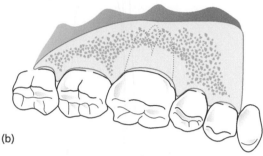

(b)

Fig. 8.19 (a) Envelope flap with incision along the gingival margin. (b) Envelope flap with incision along gingival margin and a vertical releasing incision.

as retained roots, can be considered candidates for surgical extraction.

- Primary (deciduous) teeth occasionally present problems for the surgeon and should not be underestimated. The prime consideration in the removal of deciduous teeth is to avoid injury to the developing permanent dentition. The enamel of the deciduous crowns is more brittle, and the roots are much flatter and more convex. Because the deciduous roots have already undergone resorption, seating the forceps far apically beneath the deciduous tooth may accidentally damage the developing permanent tooth. Primary teeth, especially the mandibular molars, may be submerged or ankylosed, so they should be percussed before extraction. If ankylosis is suspected, the tooth's removal should be reassessed. Radiographic changes include loss of evidence of a periodontal ligament space and apparent fusion of the bone and the tooth structure. Clinically, there is absence of mobility and a characteristic solid tone on percussion with a metal dental mirror handle. If extraction is necessary owing to infection or obstruction of an erupting permanent tooth, it is best done by a surgical procedure.

- Erupted mandibular third molars for which there is limited access, a forceps extraction is difficult to do due to difficulty of using the forceps properly and the presence of thick alveolar bone. Planned surgical extraction is performed by raising a soft tissue flap, and judicious removal of the buccal bone using fissure bur and surgical handpiece with copious saline irrigation to create a buccal trough to provide access for efficient instrumentation and atraumatic removal of the tooth. Surgical removal of third molars is covered in Chapter 9.

- Teeth previously treated with endodontic therapy are more prone to root fractures during extractions, especially when posts are anchored in the root and a surgical approach may be preferable.

Technique for surgical extraction

Surgical extractions should be carried out under high-standard aseptic conditions with the surgeon and assistant scrubbing in, wearing sterile gloves, caps, and masks, and using sterile instruments. The patient should be draped. High-speed air turbines should be avoided because of the risk for development of emphysema once a flap has been raised. Irrigation by sterile saline should be carried out when bone and teeth are cut by bur.

The flaps used with tooth extractions are envelope flaps, which are developed along the cervical necks of the teeth. If extended along the gingival margin they usually provide sufficient access to perform the necessary extraction surgery (Fig. 8.19a). It is best to extend this type of flap at least a minimum of one to two teeth both mesially and distally of the object tooth. Another flap used is a modification of the envelope flap, which requires a releasing incision in either the mesial or distal end of the incision, forming a three-corner flap (Fig. 8.19b). Occasionally, both ends of the flap are released forming a four-corner flap.

Bone is removed by rongeur or by a surgical bur to provide access to the tooth which can be removed atraumatically in a more controlled manner. The buccal bone is usually removed and the tooth delivered from buccal aspect. Bone removal varies with the practitioner's personal experience and preference. Bone to be removed should be limited and minimized to preserve the alveolus. This has become important since the widespread use of dental implants requiring sufficient bone volume.

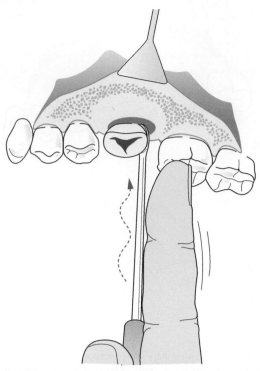

Fig. 8.20 The dental elevator is pushed apically along the root axis to expand the periodontal space and thus displacing the root out of its socket. Note the finger rest using the index finger to control the force delivered during removal of the tooth, preventing slipping with the instrument.

A straight dental elevator is used to expand the periodontal ligament space. The elevator is used as a wedge, pushing it apically to expand the periodontal space and thus displacing the tooth root out of the socket. It is important in this case to use the dental elevator carefully by applying a finger rest using the index finger to control the amount of force delivered during removal of the tooth and to prevent slipping of the elevator to avoid unnecessary trauma to soft tissues (Fig. 8.20).

Teeth with two roots, e.g. mandibular molars, can be sectioned into two halves and then removed similarly to two premolars. In situations where the crown is missing, it is easier to separate all roots and remove them individually (Figs 8.21, 8.22 and 8.23). Roots removal can be facilitated by drilling a hole in the root (purchase point) to facilitate leverage or use Cryer elevators (Fig. 8.23).

In cases where the tooth is surrounded by thick cortical bone, bone removal is essential and important for atraumatic surgical extraction. Again, a suitable surgical flap is reflected and a bone-cutting bur in a surgical handpiece is used with copious saline irrigation to remove at least one-half or two-thirds of the buccal bone covering the tooth root in the vertical dimension and about the whole mesio-distal dimension of the tooth in the horizontal dimension. The tooth can be then easily removed with an elevator or forceps in a buccal direction. Sometimes it might still be difficult to remove the tooth even after removal of bone. If the tooth is quite solid in the bone, a purchase

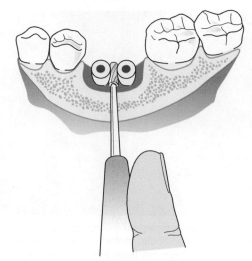

Fig. 8.21 Roots are separated by a bur and can then be more easily removed individually.

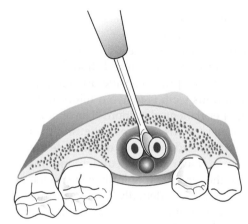

Fig. 8.22 Surgical removal of maxillary molar roots by elevator after root sectioning. The palatal root has been removed and the buccal roots are separated by an elevator before removal.

point can be cut in the tooth root and a suitable elevator, e.g. a Cryer elevator, is placed into the purchase point to elevate the tooth out of the socket.

A maxillary molar is removed by separating the crown from the roots and then the tooth is sectioned at the trifurcation area to separate the roots from each other and elevate them out individually. Care must be practiced when using the elevator not to use too much force to push the roots into the adjacent maxillary sinus and to prevent slippage of the elevator injuring the soft tissues.

It is good practice for a surgeon to inspect the extracted tooth or root and make sure it is removed entirely. This is very important when tooth sectioning is involved. All extracted pieces should be assembled at the end of the procedure and inspected to make sure that the whole tooth or root is removed successfully. A smooth tooth apex on digital palpation also confirms a complete tooth removal.

In all surgical extractions, the base of the flap should be thoroughly irrigated with saline solution and the extraction socket should also be irrigated,

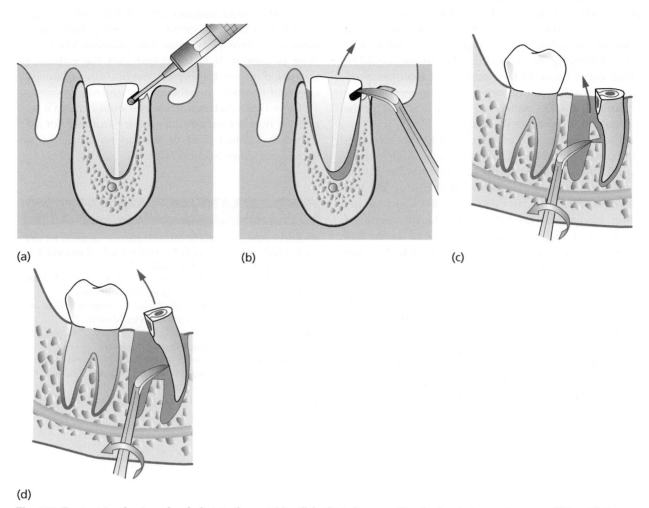

(a)

(b)

(c)

(d)

Fig. 8.23 Root retrieval using a bur hole into the root (a) will facilitate leverage. Standard technique using curved Warwick James or Cryer elevators (b) to remove interradicular bone and elevated retained root (c, d). Root tips can often be elevated using a Mitchell's trimmer.

especially when contaminated and when there are fragments of restorations or tooth present. Large sharp buccal bony edges should be removed with ronguers and then smoothened with a bone file. The flap is then adapted and sutured back.

Post extraction care and instructions

Regardless if a tooth is removed by a closed or open surgical method, the patient should receive postoperative instructions necessary to provide proper care. These instructions should be given verbally and in writing, allowing the patient to take them home. The patient and/or patient's guardian should be given the opportunity to ask any questions. After a tooth has been extracted, no debridement or curettage of the socket is necessary unless there is a pathologic process seen on a radiograph preoperatively. Obvious debris, such as tooth fragments, amalgam or calculus, may be present in the tooth socket after extraction and should be carefully removed with a curette or

suction. Too vigorous curettage of the socket may lead to additional injury and may delay healing.

Gentle digital pressure with the index finger and thumb should be applied to the bucco-lingual walls of the extraction socket to compress the usually expanded bucco-lingual plates after extraction to restore the original crest dimension. The overlying mucosa should then be palpated to check for any sharp bony edges or projections. If any are present, the mucosa and underlying periosteum should be reflected and sharp bony edges smoothened with a bone file.

Postoperative instructions should include a method of applying direct pressure for initial control of hemorrhage. A moist 2 × 2cm gauze should be applied directly over the extraction socket and the patient is instructed to bite down on the gauze for at least 30 minutes without interruption. It is important to place the gauze directly over the extraction site in the space occupied by the crown of the extracted tooth and not over the occlusal table of neighboring teeth to ensure that the pressure is correctly transmitted over the socket to achieve hemostasis. The patient should be informed that there may normally be slight postoperative bleeding during the first few hours; some oozing from the wound, which results in a red tinge of the saliva, can be expected for the first 24 hours following the extraction. The patient should be given extra gauze to take home and maintain pressure for another 30 minutes if bleeding resumes. If it is difficult for the patient to stop the bleeding, the patient should contact the surgeon.

The patient should be instructed to stay on a specific post extraction diet. A high-calorie, high-volume liquid diet is best for the first 12–24 hours. The patient must have adequate intake of fluid during the first 24 hours. The fluid can be juices, milk, water, or any other beverage. The patient should be instructed not to use a sucking straw; otherwise he or she will cause negative pressure that might lead to displacement of the coagulum and bleeding episodes. The diet should be soft and cool. Cool and cold foods help keep the local area comfortable. Hot and solid foods tend to cause local trauma and/or initiate bleeding episodes.

As with other surgeries, the postoperative course also varies with patients, depending on expectations and earlier experience. Mild to moderate postoperative pain is best managed by the use of over-the-counter analgesics, e.g. non-steroidal anti-inflammatory anal-gesics such as ibuprofen, aspirin, or acetaminophen. A combination of non-narcotics and narcotic analgesic drugs might be necessary for postoperative pain following extensive surgical manipulation. Whatever drug is chosen, it is important that the patient is instructed to start the pain medication before the effects of the local anesthetic have ended.

The written instruction sheet should contain a telephone number or any emergency number for the patient to contact if he or she has any question or should any complication arise.

Recommended reading

Al-Asfour A, Kanagaraja S. (2010) Extraction of teeth. In: *Oral and Maxillofacial Surgery* (eds, Andersson L, Kahnberg K-E, Pogrel MA). Oxford, Wiley-Blackwell.

Fonseca RJ, Frost DE, Hersh EV, Levin LM. (2000) *Oral and Maxillofacial Surgery*. Philadelphia, WB Saunders.

Hupp JR, Ellis EE, Tucker MR. (2013) *Contemporary Oral and Maxillofacial Surgery*. St Louis, Elsevier Mosby.

Lambrecht T. (2008) *Oral and Implant Surgery: Principles and Procedures*. Berlin, Quintessence Publishing.

Miloro M, Ghali GE, Larsen P, Waite P. (2012). *Peterson's Principles of Oral and Maxillofacial Surgery*, 3rd edn. Shelton, CT, People's Medical Publishing House.

Robinson PD. (2000) *Tooth Extraction. A Practical Guide*. Oxford, Wright.

Chapter 9

Management of Impacted Teeth

The management of impacted teeth is probably the most common problem in oral and maxillofacial surgery worldwide. Teeth that fail to erupt are usually the teeth which erupt last in a certain region where there is not enough space or because of crowding of teeth. The most common teeth which are impacted are mandibular and maxillary third molars followed by maxillary canines and mandibular premolars.

An impacted tooth is one which is prevented from completely erupting into a normal functional position. This may be due to lack of space, obstruction by another tooth, or an abnormal eruption path. The tooth may be soft tissue impacted or hard tissue impacted and may be unerupted or partially erupted. Impaction per itself is **not** an indication for removal, it is only a description of the position of the tooth.

However, impacted teeth may sometimes give rise to complications if they are left in place, and over several decades there have been recommendations that impacted teeth should be removed, even if they are asymptomatic. In the last 20 years, however, there has been much discussion and controversy regarding the need for prophylactic treatment of asymptomatic impacted teeth and there is now evidence that asymptomatic impacted teeth do not have to be removed. This discussion of prophylactic third molar surgery has been stimulated by research in medical decision-making, public health analysis, cost-effectiveness studies and by incorporating patient preferences in the decision-making process. It is well known in the practice of medicine that there is also a geographical and cultural variation in treatment indications and this variation can also be expected in the management of the third molar problem.

Since surgery is sometimes associated with complications, one must always balance the risk of complications caused by leaving the impacted tooth in place against the risk for complications and discomfort associated with surgery. The main complications related to third molar surgery are alveolar osteitis (fibrinolytic alveolitis, dry socket) infection and temporary or permanent nerve injury. Nerve injuries often cause temporary and permanent neuropathic pain or altered sensation in and around the mouth, resulting in significant difficulties for the patient with regard to eating, drinking, speaking, kissing, shaving, applying makeup etc. A nerve injury is one of the main causes of litigation in dentistry. Prevention of these injuries must therefore be taken into consideration before surgical removal of impacted teeth. The patient should always be advised of the risk of inferior alveolar nerve injury. It is probably easier for a patient to accept a permanent complication or disability of an intervention if it was properly based on a therapeutic indication than if surgery was performed on prevention and prophylaxis. Patient information about risks and complications is very important and the patient should always be part of the decision.

While many impacted third mandibular molars that cause problems are removed, impacted canines and premolars may often be guided to erupt spontaneously or by using orthodontic traction. Some impacted teeth, especially premolars, can be used as autotransplants to another region (see Chapter 11).

Management of impacted third molars

Indications for third molar removal

There should always be an appropriate indication for third molar removal. Indications can be local or for medical reasons.

Essentials of Oral and Maxillofacial Surgery, First Edition. Edited by M. Anthony Pogrel, Karl-Erik Kahnberg and Lars Andersson.
© 2014 John Wiley & Sons, Ltd. Published 2014 by John Wiley & Sons, Ltd.
Companion website: www.wiley.com/go/pogrel/oms

Local therapeutic indications

- Recurrent or severe pericoronitis;
- Periodontal disease with a pocket depth of 5 mm or more distal to the second molar;
- non-restorable caries in the third molar;
- Resorption of the third molar or adjacent tooth;
- Caries in the second molar where the third molar removal would render restoration possible or more simple;
- Apical periodontitis;
- Cysts or tumors associated with the third molar (or adjacent tooth);
- When required prior to orthognatic surgery;
- Removal of third molar in a fracture line;
- When a third molar may be considered for autogenous transplantation.

Medical conditions that require a serious consideration of prophylactic third molar removal

Prior to:

- radiation therapy for head and neck malignancies;
- organ transplantation;
- chemotherapy;
- bisphosphonate therapy.

Contraindications for third molar removal

There are situations when third molars should not be removed. Summarizing our current knowledge from the literature, published in reviews and guidelines, it is recommended that:

- third molar buds in young people should not be enucleated;
- asymptomatic pathology free third molars totally covered by bone should not be removed;
- routine removal of pathology free third molars totally or partially covered by soft tissue is not recommended but specific medical and local conditions may prove a prophylactic approach appropriate;
- third molar surgery is contraindicated in patients whose medical history or conditions expose the patient to an unacceptable risk to their health.

Presurgical assessment of third molars

In addition to a thorough history-taking, clinical and radiologic assessment should always be combined before considering removal of a third molar.

Clinical assessment

Clinical assessment should be carried out with the aim of assessing the status of the patient, the oral and maxillofacial region, the third molars and the adja-

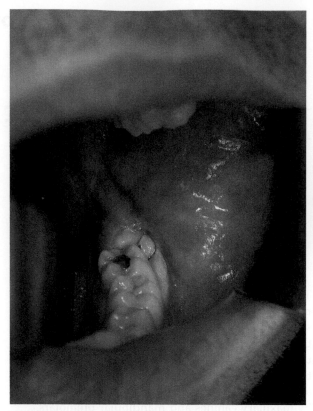

Fig. 9.1 Clinical photograph of partially erupted lower left molar with no local inflammation.

cent teeth (eruption status, caries, periodontal status, occlusion) (Figs 9.1 and 9.2).

Radiological assessment

Radiological examination is a complement to the clinical examination and is necessary in order to make decisions related to the procedure. A radiological evaluation will give information about anatomy of the impacted tooth, the region and the relation of structures. Usually a pair of periapical radiographs taken in different projections is enough and can be supplemented by a panoramic radiograph when more than one third molar requires assessment. If the initial radiographs suggest a close relationship between the roots of the lower third molar and the inferior alveolar nerve (IAN) canal, cone-beam computer tomography (CBCT) scanning can be used to give more detailed information of the anatomy in the region.

Important factors to consider

The following local factors are important to take into consideration when planning third molar surgery.

Application depth

The alveolar bone level and tooth position will dictate the application point depth (Fig. 9.3). The depth of application and the point of elevation will dictate the amount of bone removal that is required to gain access to the optimal application point. This factor is the most predictive of difficulty of surgery.

Another way to describe depth of impaction is Pell and Gregory classification, which assesses the relationship of the tooth to occlusal plane (classified as A, B, C) and relationship of the tooth to the anterior border of ramus (classified as 1, 2, 3) (Table 9.1). This classification may be used to describe the depth of impaction of the tooth but has been found to be less reliable in predicting difficulty than assessing the application point depth.

Angulation

The distinction between vertical, mesoangular, horizontal, and disto-angular orientation may affect the surgical approach, in particular with regard to the requirements for bone removal in order to gain access to point of application. The incidence and estimated degree of difficulty for the different angulations are:

- vertical impaction: 40% of all impacted mandibular third molars and usually the least difficult to remove.
- mesoangular impaction: 45% – can be of moderate difficulty;
- horizontal impaction: 10% – are generally of intermediate difficulty;
- distoangular: 5% – the most difficult to extract and frequently underestimated.

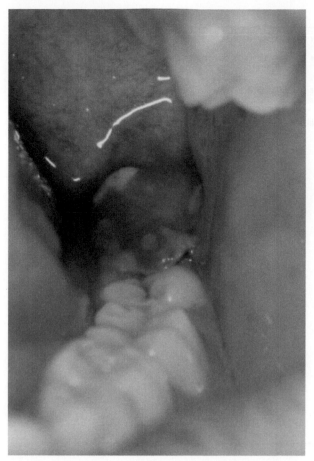

Fig. 9.2 Clinical photograph of partially erupted lower left with acute pericoronitis of 38. Notice the "imprint" of 28 occlusal surface.

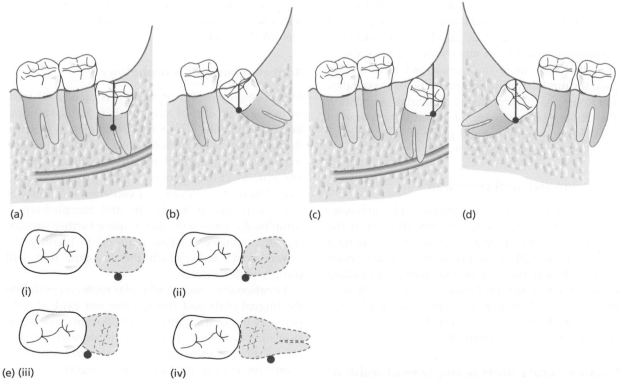

(a)　　　　(b)　　　　(c)　　　　(d)

(i)　　　　(ii)

(e) (iii)　　　　(iv)

Fig. 9.3 Diagram of application point depth. How is this measured? From the alveolar ridge to the point of application on the tooth. This will vary depending on the depth and angulation of the tooth. (a) Vertical; (b) mesoangular; (c) distoangular; (d) horizontal. Red line indicates application depth (mm); red dot indicates the application point. The length of the red line indicates the necessary vertical bone removal to reach the application point. (e) Key application points for each angulation: (i) vertical – mid-buccal; (ii) mesoangular – meso-buccal; (iii) distoangular – buccal/disto-buccal; (iv) horizontal – buccal.

Table 9.1 Pell and Gregory classification.

(1) Position A	The highest portion of the impacted mandibular third molar is on a level with or above the occlusal plane	
(2) Position B	The highest portion of the impacted mandibular third molar is below the occlusal plane but above the cervical line of the second mandibular molar	
(3) Position C	The highest portion of the impacted mandibular third molar is below the cervical line of the second mandibular molar	
(4) Position I	None of the crown is in the ramus of the mandible	
(5) Position II	Less than half of the crown is in the ramus	
(6) Position III	More than half of the crown is in the ramus	

The application point and necessary bone removal is not only dictated by the angulation of the tooth but also root morphology and proximity to adjacent structures (adjacent tooth, antrum and nerve). In association with identifying the tooth angulation, the potential space for application points must be identified. Often distoangular lower third molars are in close proximity to the adjacent second molar and have limited space for mesial application point. Several examples of radiographs of third molars illustrating angulation of teeth and a summary of potential application points for bone removal and planned sectioning are provided in Figures 9.3 and 9.4.

The crown size and condition

The crown width of the third molar can be an important factor in making surgery more difficult. If the tooth is impacted and the crown is wide, sectioning of the crown will be required to minimize bone removal thus reducing potential pain and swelling for the patient. If the third molar is carious or heavily restored, or indeed non-vital, this may render the tooth more brittle on elevation thus impacting on surgical difficulty. See Figure 9.5.

Distance across roots is larger than width of crown–root junction

If the root width is greater than the width of the tooth at the alveolar crest, the difficulty of surgery will increase and root sectioning will be indicated (Fig.

9.6). Multiple roots or hooked roots will also contribute to surgical difficulty and are more commonly seen in certain ethnic groups.

Hypercementosis or ankylosis of third molar roots will also increase surgical difficulty and must be identified on radiographic evaluation.

Root number and morphology

More complex root morphology is associated with increased difficulty of surgery (Fig. 9.7). Identification of such hooks is important, as they may fracture during removal of the tooth and a decision is then required as to whether to attempt their removal. Hooked, dancing or bent roots may provide a "challenge" to routine elevation. Even after sectioning of the crown and roots, if the root morphology is complex the roots will often require further sectioning and patience is often required to identify the "sweet spot" with which the resistant root will comply with elevation.

Occasionally lower third molar roots can perforate the lingual plate and this is often not evident until part way through surgery. Every effort must be made to ensure these roots do not get lost through the perforated lingual plate, one of the rare indications to raise a lingual flap for third molar surgery.

Root surface area

Assessment of the relative root surface area of the tooth to be extracted and the adjacent tooth must be

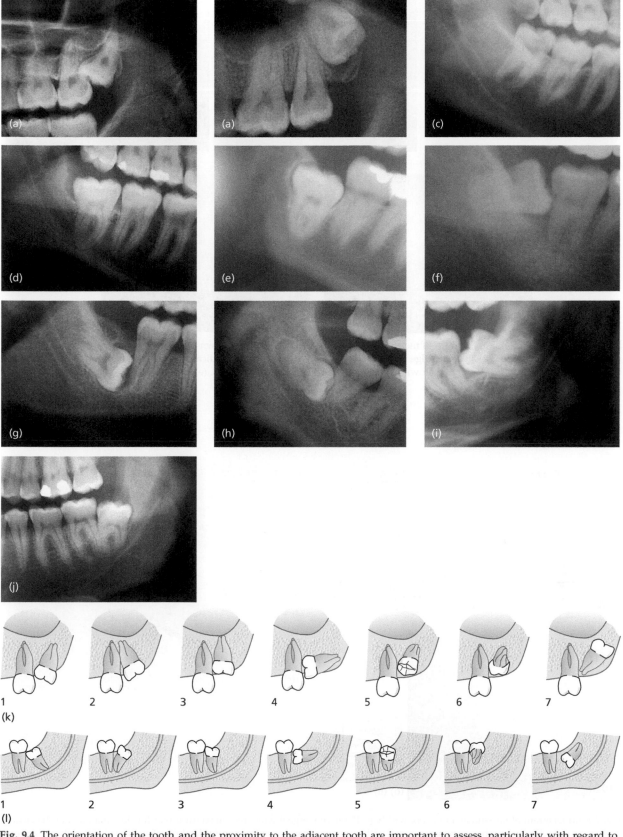

Fig. 9.4 The orientation of the tooth and the proximity to the adjacent tooth are important to assess, particularly with regard to distinction between vertical and distoangular orientation which may affect the requirements for bone removal. (a) Maxillary buccally erupted mesoangular 28 with no application space distal to 27. (b) Maxillary buccally partially erupted impacted distoangular 28. (c) Mandibular non-impacted erupted 48 in vertical position. (d) Vertical position, soft tissue impacted, partially erupted 48 with evidence of chronic inflammation with distal bone loss. (e) Vertical position, unerupted, bone impacted. (f) Horizontal position, partially erupted, tooth impacted. (g) Horizontal position, unerupted with oral communication. (h) Horizontal, unerupted below bone, no oral communication. (i) Mesoangular position, partially erupted, tooth impacted. (j) Distoangular, partially erupted, bone impacted. Diagrammatic summary of tooth angulation: classification of impaction of (k) maxillary third molars and (l) mandibular third molars: 1, mesoangular; 2, distoangular; 3, vertical; 4, horizontal; 5, bucco-angular; 6, linguo-angular; 7, inverted.

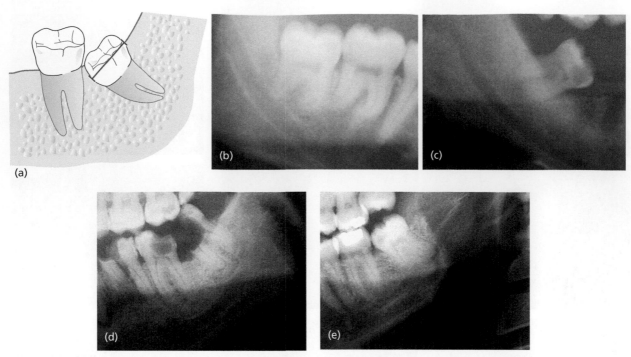

Fig. 9.5 Size of the crown. (a) Diagram of measurement of crown width. Red line drawn across maximum width of crown. If this is more than bony window in alveolar ridge (black line) then crown section will be indicated. (b) Crown wide. Wide crown width will increase surgical difficulty. (c) The crown condition – caries. (d) Gross caries of 38. (e) Crown heavily restored.

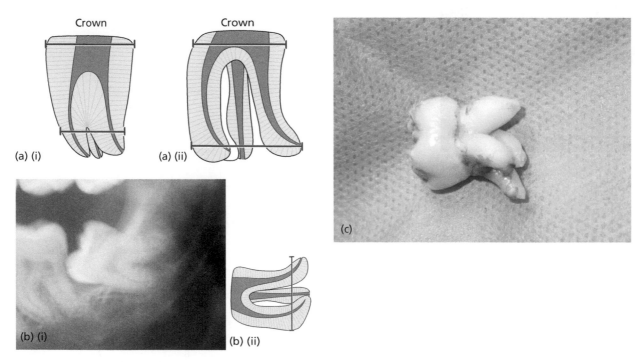

Fig. 9.6 (a) Diagram of measurement of root width. (i) Roots convergent when root maximum width is less than that of the crown base. (ii) Roots divergent when maximum root width is greater than base of crown (indication of increased difficulty of surgery and probable root section). (b) (i and ii) Splayed roots. Distance across roots is larger than width of crown root junction. (c) Lower third molar with four splayed roots.

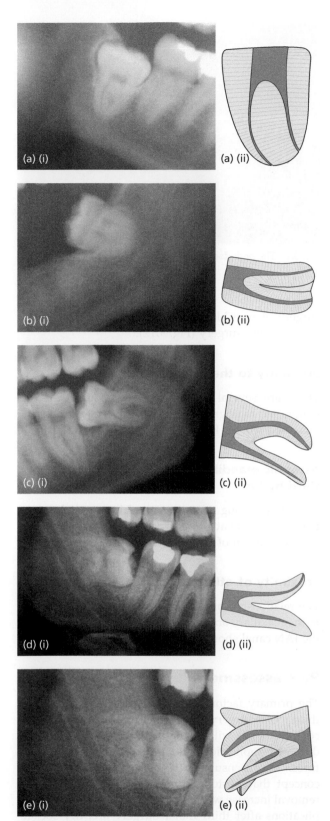

Fig. 9.7 (a) Conical/convergent roots. (b) Club-shaped roots. (c) Bifid roots. (d) Bifid divergent roots. (e) Multiple roots (may be penetrating lingual plate).

estimated (Fig. 9.8). If the third molar is multi-rooted adjacent to a second molar with conical roots, the adjacent tooth is more easily mobilized during elevation of the third molar. If the root surface area of the adjacent tooth is significantly less than that of the tooth to be extracted then the surgical approach must

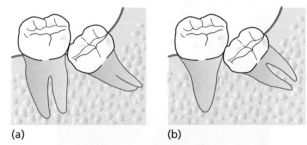

Fig. 9.8 Root surface area depends on length, width and number of roots. (a) Root surface area of 8 less than that of 7. (b) Root surface area of 8 greater than that of 7 (risk of displacing 7 on mesial application to 8).

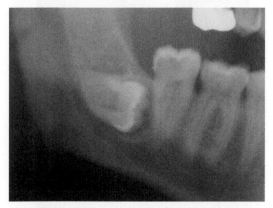

Fig. 9.9 Radiographic radiolucency adjacent to the crown of an impacted third molar may be due to enlarged follicle.

be adjusted accordingly to prevent any undue application of pressure near the adjacent tooth.

If the adjacent tooth is subluxated it should be immediately replaced and a figure-of-eight suture placed across the occlusal surface to "restrain" the tooth. Antibiotics and oral hygiene should be initiated, and, of course, the patient advised.

Follicular width

An enlarged follicle is usually considered to be non-cystic where the diameter is less than 1 cm. Radiographic radiolucency adjacent to the crown of a partially erupted third molar may be due to a previously enlarged follicle or chronic local infection (Fig. 9.9).

Pathology associated with third molars

Cystic lesions are the most common pathology associated with mandibular third molars. If the cystic lesion is associated with the crown of the tooth, the first differential diagnosis should be dentigerous cyst followed by odontogenic keratocystic tumor or ameloblastoma. Odontogenic keratocystic tumors are more likely to be associated with missing teeth. Surgical removal of third molars in association with pathology may be facilitated. However, the surgeon must ensure the pathology is correctly diagnosed and

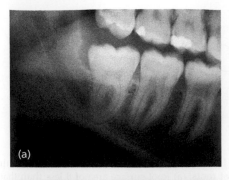

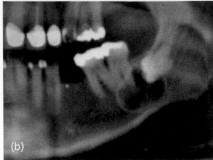

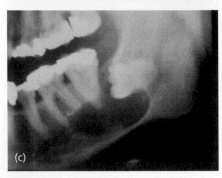

Fig. 9.10 Cystic lesions associated with third molar teeth. (a) Paradontal cyst associated with 38. (b) Monocystic lesions associated with crown of mandibular third molar likely to be a dentigerous cyst but could be mimicked by an odontogenic keratocystic tumor. (c) Multicystic lesion associated with impacted 38. This proved to be an ameloblastoma.

treated accordingly. Some examples of cysts associated with third molars are shown in Figure 9.10.

Periodontal status

The periodontal status of the adjacent tooth and that of the third molar (Fig. 9.11) will influence surgery. Bone loss due to periodontal disease will often facilitate the removal of the third molar tooth but care must be taken to prevent inadvertent removal of the periodontally involved adjacent second molar.

The restorative condition of the adjacent second molar

If the adjacent tooth to the third molar is carious or heavily restored, this may render the tooth more brittle and more at risk of damage on elevation of the third molar, thus impacting on surgical difficulty. It is important that the patient is warned prior to

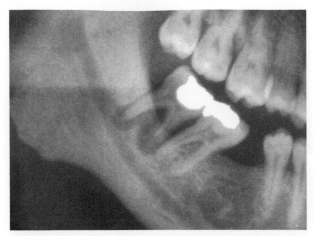

Fig. 9.11 The periodontal status of 48 is severe.

surgery of possible damage to the adjacent second molar during surgery (Fig. 9.12).

Proximity to the inferior alveolar canal

There are several radiographic signs assessed on panoramic radiographs that are associated with an increased risk for IAN injury (Figs 9.13 and 9.14).

Atrophic mandible or very long roots of third molar

Exceedingly long roots or atrophic mandible may place the patient at higher risk of mandibular fracture during removal of the lower third molar (Fig. 9.15).

Proximity of other structures

The relationship or proximity of upper third molars to the maxillary antrum and of lower third molars to the IAN canal should be assessed (Fig. 9.16).

Risk assessment

The primary factors that influence the difficulty of third molar surgery (length of procedure and related complications) will depend on patient factors, the depth of application, and proximity to vital structures. A consensus of the literature supports the concept that postoperative risks from third molar removal increase with age. The most important complications after third molar surgery are: dry socket (fibrinolytic alveolitis), postoperative infection, temporary or permanent nerve injury and marginal bone loss of the second molar. Patients must be informed of these risks before a decision of removal of the third molar is taken.

Assessment of difficulty of removal

Besides the tooth-related factors mentioned in Risk assessment, it is also important to take other factors

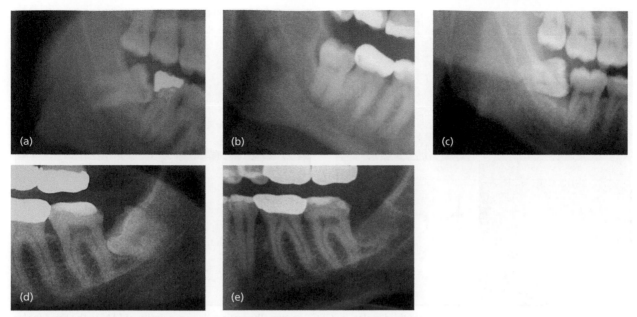

Fig. 9.12 (a) Restorative condition of adjacent 7 non-vital and crowned. (b) Heavily restored 47. (c) Caries distal surface of 47. (d) It is possible to excavate distal caries in the distocervical region of 37 whilst removing 48. (e) Restoration undertaken during removal of the mandibular third molar.

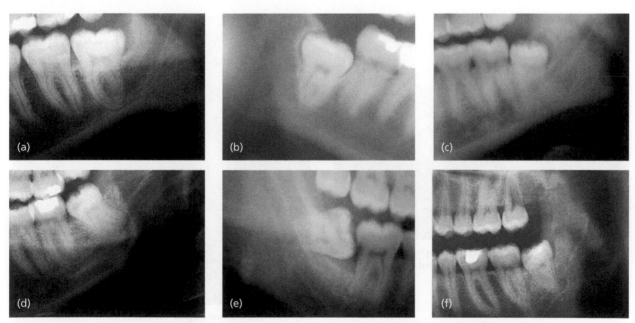

Fig. 9.13 (a) Superimposition of the IAN canal and third molar. (b) Diversion of the IAN canal. (c) Darkening of the root where it is crossed by the canal and widening of canal. (d) Interruption of the white lines of the canal. (e) Darkening of roots with associated widening of the canal. (f) Juxta-apical area. This apical area on a vital third molar may reflect a confluence of the periodontal membrane and the IAN canal; however, thus far neither CT nor MRI scan have been able to detect specific cavities. This radiographic feature was the main radiological risk factor for IAN injury.

into consideration in order to make a preoperative assessment of the degree of difficulty of removal. By doing this the dentist can decide if special resources will be required and if the case should be referred to a specialist.

The main factors that prolong operative time for third molar surgery, in order of importance, are:

- depth of impaction;
- density of bone;
- age of patient/ethnicity of patient;
- proximity to IAN canal;
- surgeon.

Surgical removal

Presurgical management

Pretreatment may be necessary for persistent local infection or a medical condition. If the patient is unable to cooperate or too anxious for care under

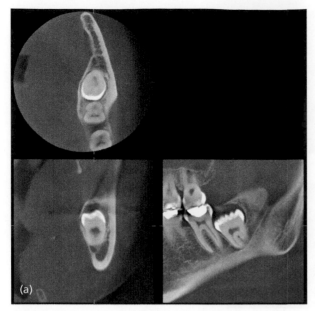

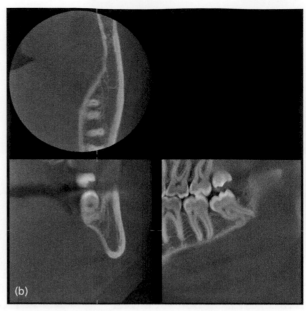

Fig. 9.14 Cone-beam CT (CBCT) scan of lower third molar. (a) CBCT section illustrating close proximity of IAN to the third molar tooth root on the lingual aspect. (b) CBCT section illustrating distant proximity of IAN to the third molar tooth root on the buccal aspect.

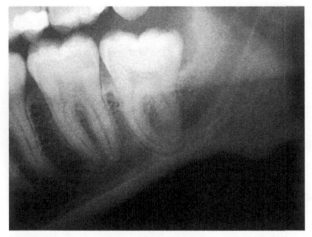

Fig. 9.15 Exceedingly long roots or atrophic mandible may place the patient at higher risk of mandibular fracture during removal of 38.

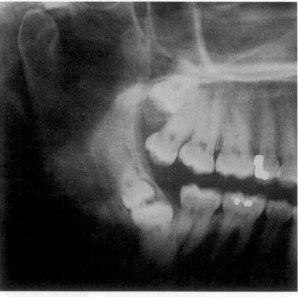

Fig. 9.16 The relationship or proximity of third molars to the adjacent unerupted teeth. Maxillary antrum to 18 and 48 and 49 to the inferior dental canal.

local analgesia, patient management will need to be modified accordingly. Although many third molars are removed in general practice, often the general practitioner may prefer to refer to a specialist because the removal is considered difficult or the case is complicated for other, often medical, reasons.

Patient information and consent

Good communication is central to the clinician–patient relationship and to good clinical care. Patients require information about the options available for management of their third molars, together with an explanation of the operation/procedure itself.

At the preoperative appointment, the potential outcome of any chosen course of action, adverse or otherwise, should be explained to the patient in terms that they can easily understand. Details should be noted in the patient's records and should include aspects relating to the patient's quality of life. In addition, care should be taken to explain to the patient the consequences of not having the tooth removed and other treatment options which may be required in this event. The information provided should be sufficient to enable the patient or their carer to make a valid informed decision and give consent. Valid consent must be obtained before starting treatment or physical investigation, or providing personal care, for a patient. This principle reflects the right of patients to determine what happens to their own bodies, and is a fundamental part of good practice. Patients have a right to choose whether or not to accept a dental professional's advice or treatment.

Removal without using a flap

In some cases, when the molar is erupted, a third molar can be removed using forceps or elevator without raising a flap using techniques described in Chapter 8.

Surgical flaps

Impacted third molars are extracted by first raising buccal triangular or envelope flap to gain access to the tooth (Figs 9.17 and 9.18). The flap should be a full thickness mucoperiosteal flap and, as pointed out in other another chapter, consideration must always be taken to the anatomy and sensitive structures in the region of the flap.

Bone removal

In the maxilla the overlying bone is thin and the maxillary bone is cancellous and elastic so extraction is usually accomplished by removing additional bone rather than by sectioning the tooth. For maxillary third molars, bone removal is done primarily on the lateral aspect of the tooth down to the cervical line to expose the crown (Fig. 9.17).

In the mandible an air-driven or electric hand piece with round or fissure burs is used. A fissure bur is be used to get clean sections for tooth splitting for elevation. For mandibular teeth, bone on the occlusal and buccal aspects of the impacted tooth is removed beyond the cervical line down to the roots of the tooth. It is advisable **not** to remove bone on the lingual and distal aspects due to the likelihood of damage to the lingual nerve. Figs 9.18, 9.19, 9.20, 9.21 and 9.22 illustrate surgical extraction of third molars.

Sectioning the tooth

Tooth sectioning is important and saves operative time. When sectioning the crown from the root a

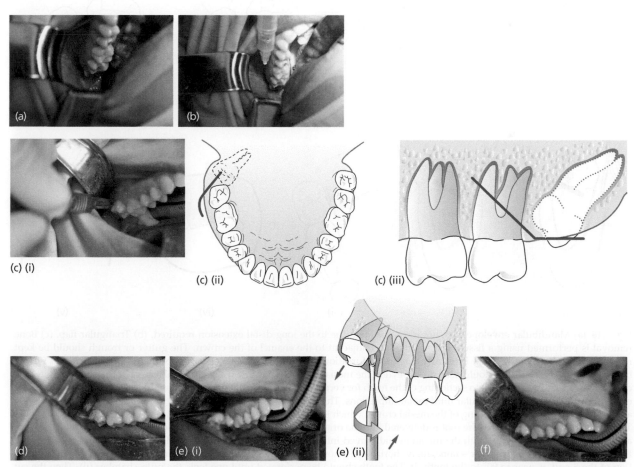

Fig. 9.17 Flap design for removal of maxillary third molar. (a) Preoperative view of 18. (b) Local anesthesia – buccal infiltration. (c) Placement of Minnesota retractor and incision with #15 blade. (d) Elevation of buccal flap, 18 retracted with Minnesota retractor. (e) Elevation upper root 18 with right-curved Warwick James elevator. The tooth is delivered with curved elevators applied on the mesio-buccal with rotational and lever types of motions. The tooth is always delivered in a disto-buccal and occlusal direction. (f) Socket 48 after extraction. Irrigate socket and use gloved finger to ensure no bony spicules are present and that the buccal plate is not fractured. No suture is necessary as the buccal flap remains sealed by the pressure of the cheek.

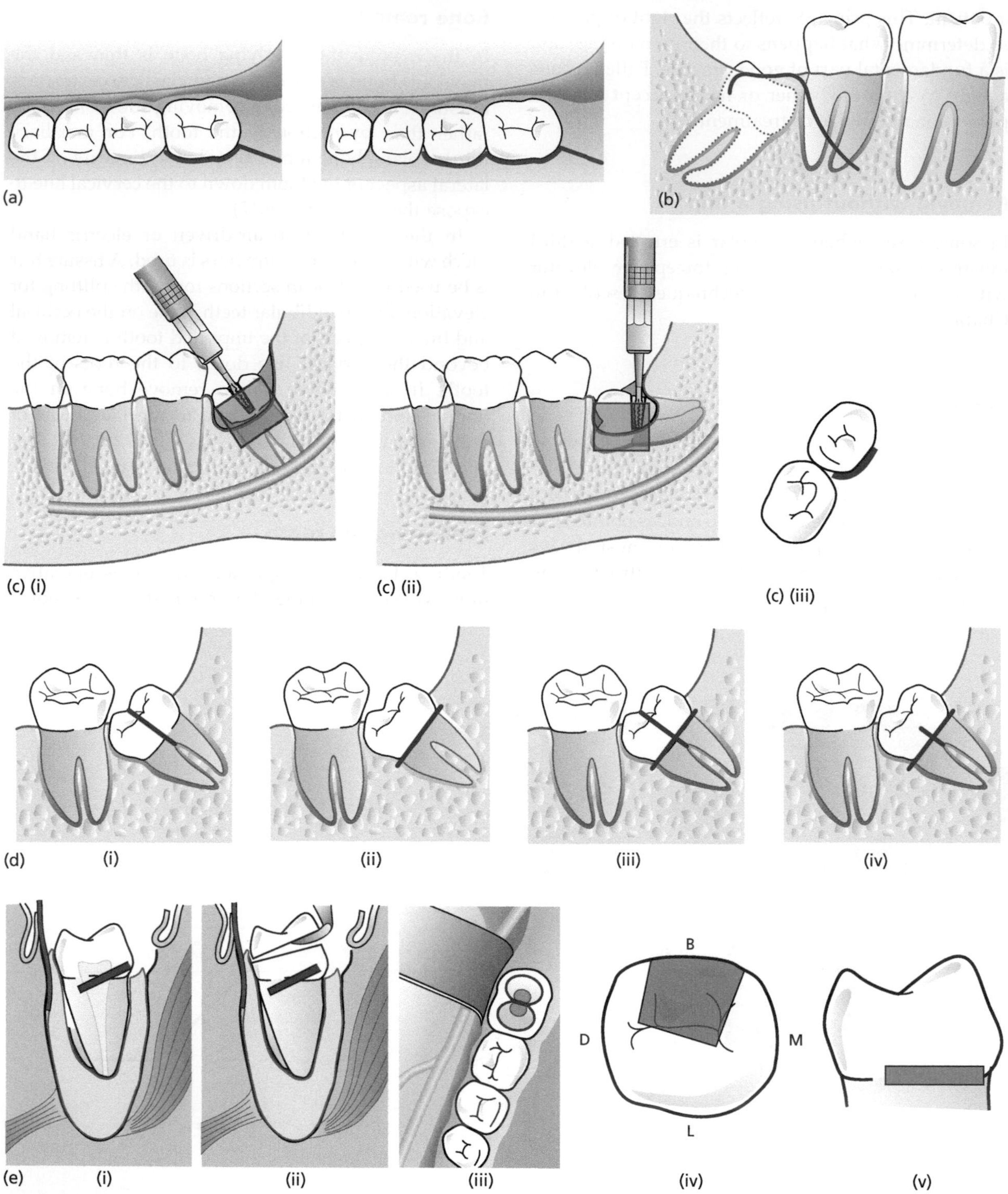

Fig. 9.18 (a) Mandibular envelope flap, not recommended due to the long distal extension required. (b) Triangular flap. (c) Bone removal is performed using a fissure bur at full speed adjacent to the enamel of the crown. The gutter or trough should be kept narrow (bur's width) and extend **inferiorly** *only* to the furcation of the tooth to allow elevation of the roots later without further bone removal. The bone cut should *not* extend beyond the mesial aspect of the crown *or* the buccal aspect of the tooth distally (see diagram). (d) Surgical approach to sectioning of the tooth for vertical, mesial, horizontal, and distoangular angulation. (i) Sectioning options for mandibular mesoangular third molar impactions. This view shows a cut longitudinally through the furcation. (ii) Same as (i), but with an additional cutting of the mesial crown, which is wedged under the second molar. (iii) Crown and root separation. The crown is removed and then the root is delivered into the original crown space. (iv) Crown removal as in (iii), but then the roots are divided longitudinally through the furcation and moved into the crown space for removal. Mesoangular – no section, i, ii, iii, iv; vertical – none, i; distoangular – none, iii, iv; horizontal – none, ii, iii, iv. (e) Using a fissure bur as near to the crown root junction of the 8 and as near to 90° to the tooth (i). The tooth should be perforated until one feels the pulp chamber (ii). Then the cut should be lateralized or verticalized depending on whether you intend to decoronate the tooth or vertically section it. Using a straight Warwick James elevator the crown should be "fractured off" (iii). If the roots require sectioning the fissure bur cut should *not* extend outside tooth material (iv) and the ideal underside of the sectioned crown should be cut only from the buccal aspect covering about 40% of the split surface (v). From the buccal aspect the crown section cut should be confined to the buccal surface and *not* extend through distal, mesial or lingual surfaces of the tooth.

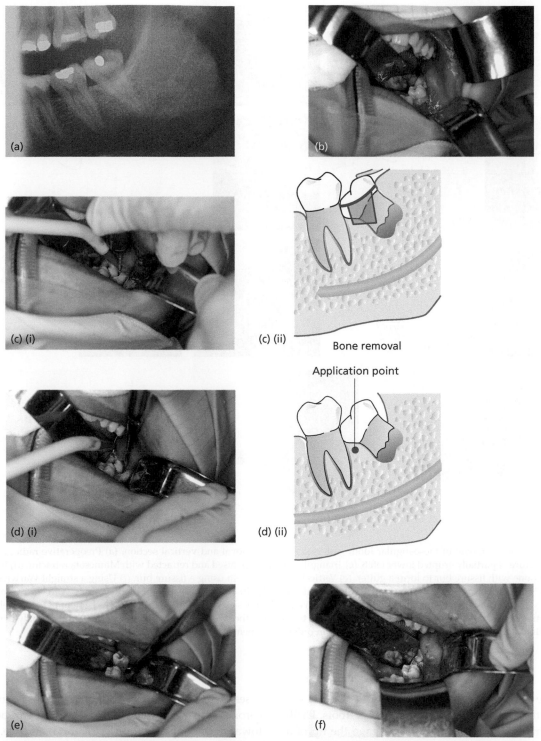

Fig. 9.19 Buccal flap with buccal bone removal for partially erupted third molar with deeper depth of impaction. (a) Preoperative film, 38 erupted non-impacted. (b) Clinical picture, 38 erupted, non-impacted. (c) Buccal bone removal with fissure bur to achieve narrow gutter. (d, e) Tooth elevated with contralateral (right) Warwick James elevator at mesial application point. This elevates the conical rooted tooth in a vertical and buccal direction. As the tooth moves superiorly the same Warwick James can be placed in the now exposed furcation of the tooth and final delivery is controlled. (f) After irrigation of the socket the buccal triangular flap is secured with a single 4/0 Vicryl™ Rapide suture.

fissure bur allows the surgeon to get a narrow clean section into the dental pulp then extend the slot within the confines of the tooth. At no point should the bur breach the mesial, distal or lingual surfaces of the tooth. Thus one achieves a "partial" section of the tooth covering about 40% of the split surface (Fig.

9.18e). After this section has been made the crown can be fractured with the help of an elevator in the slot.

Depending on the depth of application point and the angulation, the crown or root will need to be sectioned. When sectioning the roots the surgeon can use the dental pulp chambers to estimate where to

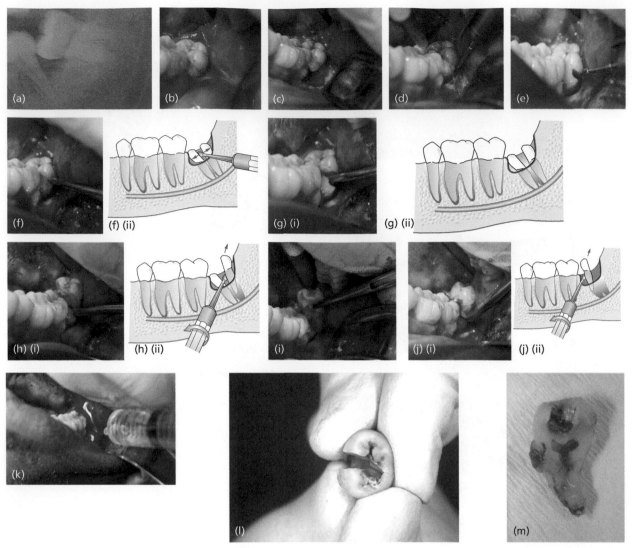

Fig. 9.20 Surgical removal of mesoangular tooth with buccal bone removal and vertical section. (a) Preoperative radiograph. (b) Clinical picture of partially erupted lower left 8. (c) Triangular buccal flap raised and retracted with Minnesota retractor. (d) Removal of buccal bone with fissure bur to form a gutter. (e) Vertical section of tooth using a fissure bur. (f) Using a straight Warwick James to "crack" the tooth into vertical sections. (g) Tooth cracked vertically. (h) The distal section of tooth elevated with No 1 Couplands. (i) The distal segment is elevated. (j) Using a contralateral Warwick James elevator mesially the mesial segment of tooth is elevated. (k) Irrigation of socket with saline. (l) Reapproximation of tooth out of the mouth to demonstrate that the tooth cut only penetrates into the dental pulp (m) not through the whole tooth in order not to penetrate the lingual aspect of the tooth.

split the roots. Again at no point should the drill cut extend through the lingual aspect of the roots. Drilling a small hole large enough to engage the tip of a curved Warwick James elevator is useful in gaining a "purchase point" to elevate the roots.

Coronectomy

Coronectomy (also known as partial tooth removal, partial odontectomy or intentional root retention) is a technique of partial root removal which should be considered when radiographic imaging suggests an intimate relationship between the roots of the lower third molar and the IAN and there is a high risk of nerve injury if too much bone has to be removed. In such cases only the crown is removed and the root is retained. The clinical procedure and two radiographic

cases are illustrated in Figure 9.23. In the years after coronectomy subsequent root migration can be seen towards the superior border of the mandible. Later root removal may be required but only in 2–6% of cases. Roots may require removal when they erupt later and become infected but sometimes the roots have then migrated away from the IAN thus minimizing potential injury to the nerve.

Post-surgical considerations

Antibiotics

The use of prophylactic antibiotic therapy following third molar surgery is common but there is very little evidence to support its routine use and there is, however, a growing body of data to suggest that this

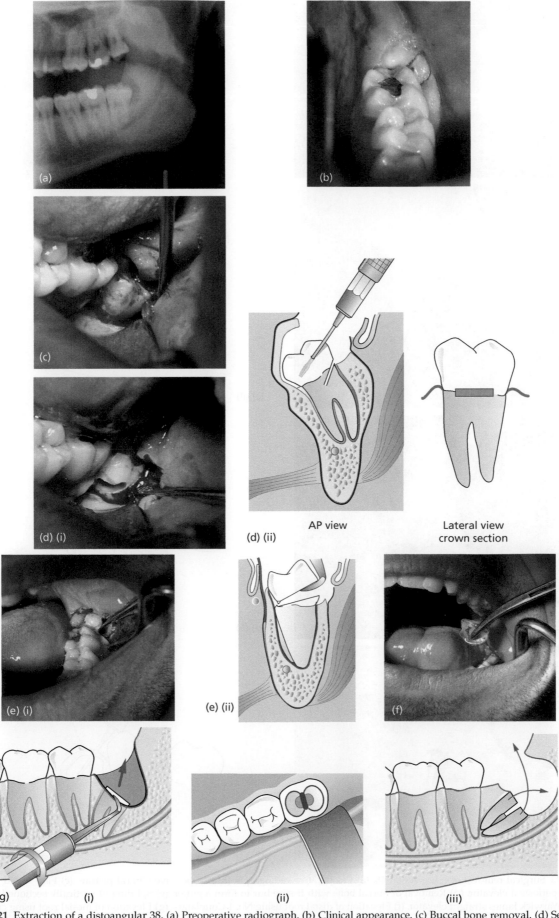

Fig. 9.21 Extraction of a distoangular 38. (a) Preoperative radiograph. (b) Clinical appearance. (c) Buccal bone removal. (d) Section of crown. (e) Elevation of crown. (f) Elevation of the crown, then elevation of the roots with curved Warwick James elevator. (e) Elevation of crown. (f) Elevation of the crown, then elevation of the roots with curved Warwick James elevator. (g) (i) Use Warwick James elevator to elevate roots together. If roots are immobile, section with fissure bur (ii) then elevate roots separately (iii).

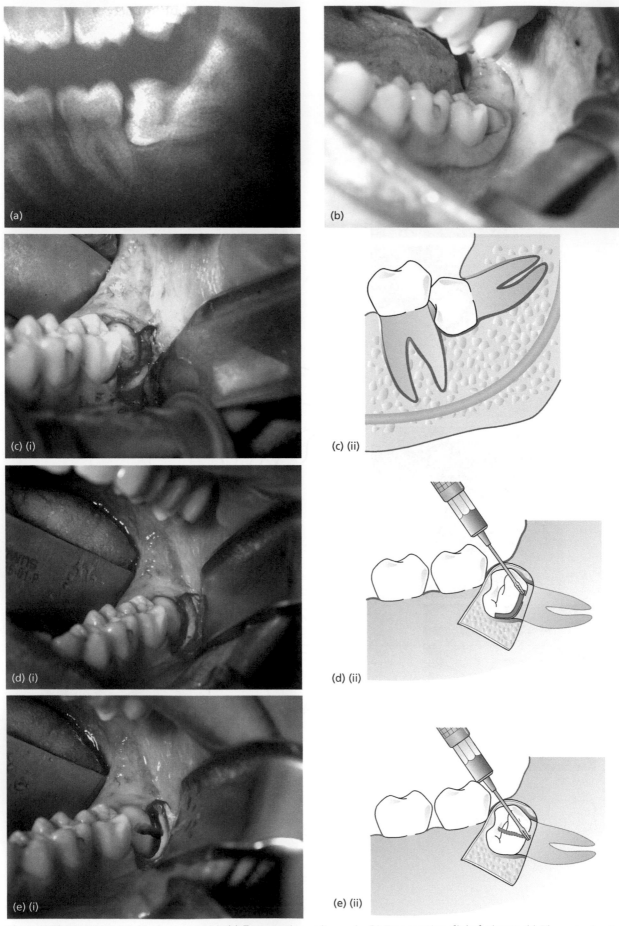

Fig. 9.22 Surgical removal of a horizontal 48. (a) Preoperative radiograph. (b) Preoperative clinical picture. (c) Flap raised using Wards periosteal elevator. (d) Removal of buccal bone with fissure bur to form a gutter. (e) Splitting of vertically sectioned tooth using Warwick James straight elevator. (f) Elevation of distal root using No. 1 Couplands. (g) Elevation of mesial root using curved left Warwick James elevator. (h) Approximation of wound prior to suture. (i) Alternative sectioning of a horizontal tooth may require decoronation (notice the angulation of the crown–root junction cut with narrowing of section inferiorly to maximize the ability to elevate the crown in one piece (i). If the crown is too impacted then section the crown into two pieces and then elevate the crown. This leaves the roots *in situ* (ii). Using the pulp chambers as "guide" one can section the roots with a fissure bur and then elevate the roots individually. The order will depend on root curvature. Drilling a small notch into the root surface will often facilitate root elevation (iii).

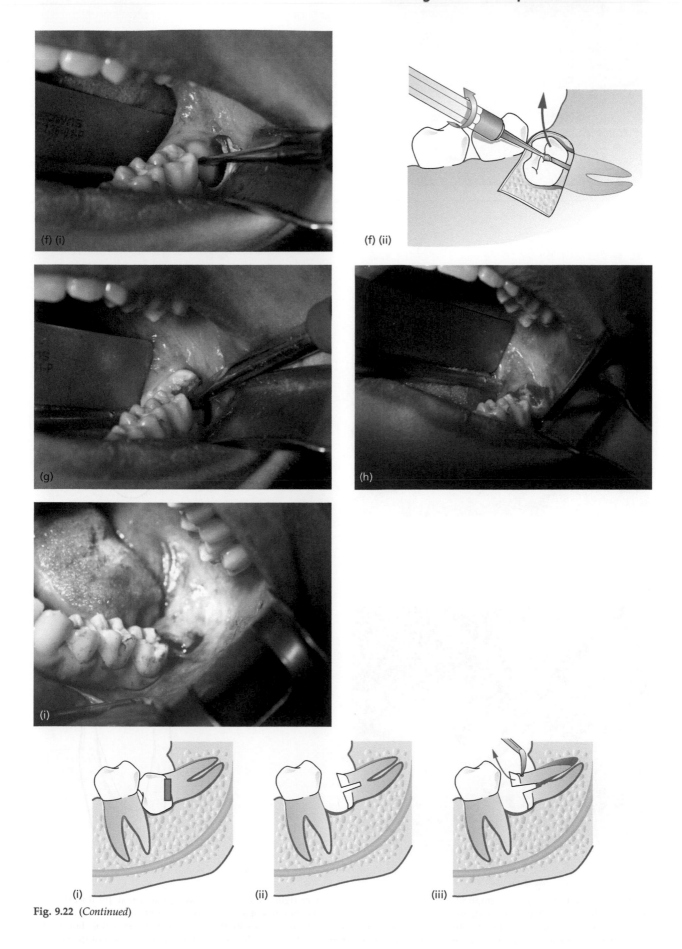

Fig. 9.22 (*Continued*)

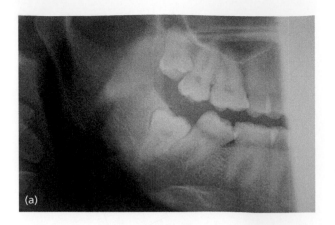

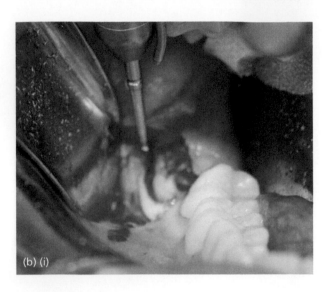

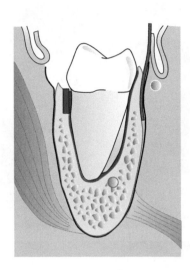

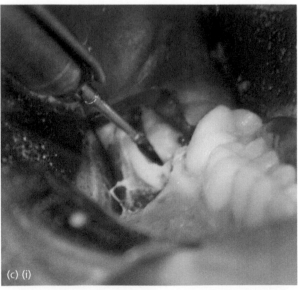

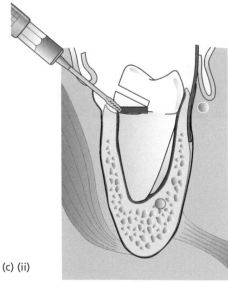

Fig. 9.23 Coronectomy. (a) Radiograph of vital vertically positioned lower right 8 with roots crossing IAN canal. (b) Buccal bone removal with fissure bur. (c) Sectioning of crown from roots level with the crown root junction subsequent to buccal bone removal with fissure bur. (d) Elevation of crown from roots with straight Warwick James. Usually the crown will elevate whole but if it is still impacted (too wide for space) then, using a fissure bur, the crown can be vertically sectioned to allow elevation of the crown. (e) Cracking crown apart into two segments using straight Warwick James. (f) Crown fragments extraorally. (g) Coronectomized roots *in situ*. The pulp chamber and live pulp can be seen. No dressing is necessary but you must ensure no enamel is left behind and trimming with a rose head bur may be necessary. (h) Closure of "socket" with single 4/0 Vicryl™ suture. (i) (i) preoperative radiograph of high-risk third molar. (ii) Postoperative radiograph of coronectomized third molar. (j) (i) Preoperative radiograph of high-risk third molar and second molar with dentigerous cyst. (ii) Postoperative (6 weeks) radiograph of coronectomized third molar and second molar with enucleation with good clinical healing.

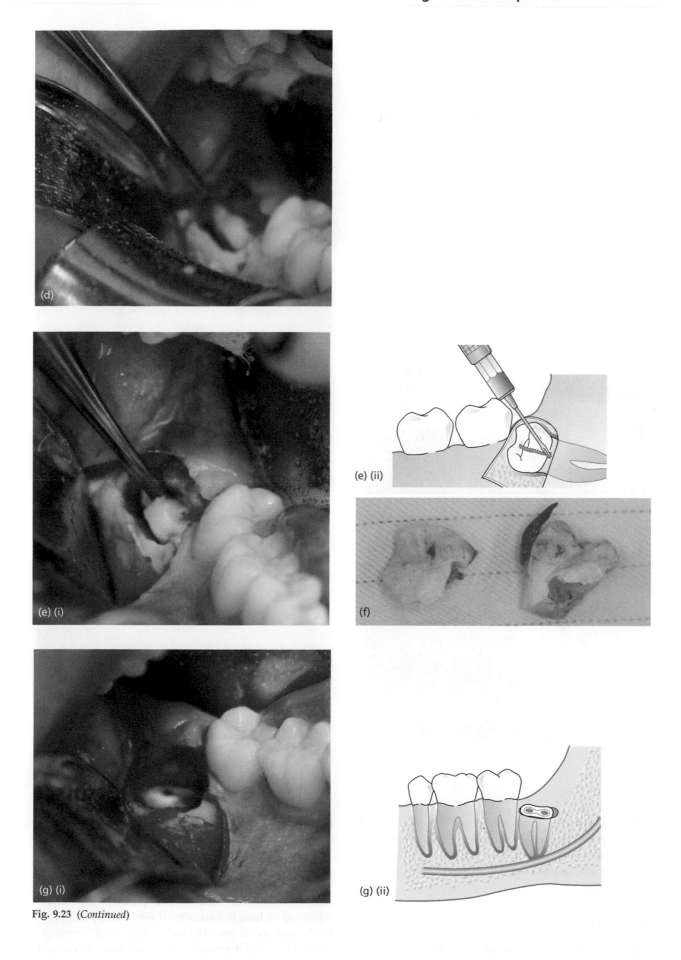

Fig. 9.23 (*Continued*)

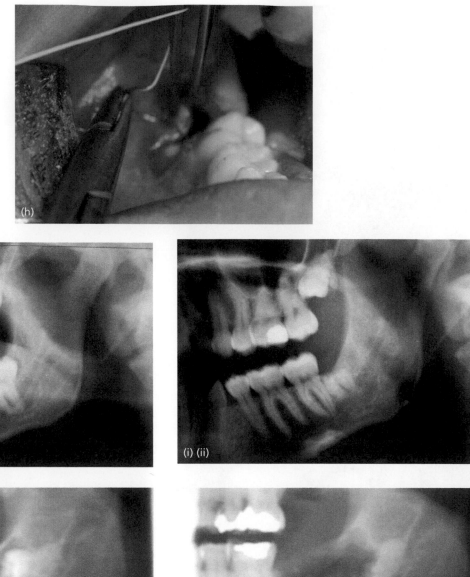

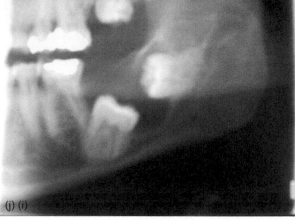

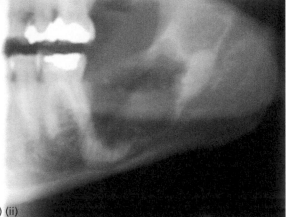

Fig. 9.23 (*Continued*)

practice wastes resources with very little prospect of health gain. However, in severe cases, where there is acute infection at the time of operation, significant bone removal, or prolonged operation, antibiotics can be considered.

Analgesia

Peak pain levels lasts for up to 12 hours. Normal practice is to prescribe or advise oral analgesics such as paracetamol (acetaminophen) or ibuprofen for outpatients.

Patient information

After third molar surgery the patients should be informed on how to look after their mouth postoperatively and about possible side-effects and complications. The patient should also know how to contact the surgeon in case of advice or emergency.

Management of impacted canines and premolars

Canines and premolars are, after the third molars, the next most commonly impacted teeth. These teeth can often be guided to erupt spontaneously or by using orthodontic traction. Some impacted teeth, especially premolars, can also be used as autotransplants to other regions. However, if these alternatives are not suitable extraction is often carried out.

Clinical and radiographic evaluation is important to determine the location of the impacted tooth, its relation to adjacent teeth and structures, and identification of potential pathologic findings in that area.

Periapical radiographs, occlusal radiograph, and panoramic radiograph are most commonly used as a first option to identify the location of the impacted tooth and its relationship to the adjacent teeth and relevant anatomic structures. Cone-beam CT is a very useful resource to identify the exact location and position of the impacted tooth in three dimensions and relation to anatomic structures, presence of pathologic findings, all of which can be valuable in treatment planning, assigning risk factors, and evaluating prognosis.

Treatment planning

Once the indications have been identified, the benefits and risks of the treatment should be communicated to the patient. A number of treatment options may be considered. These include observation, extraction, spontaneous eruption or guided eruption. Firstly, one must assess if the unerupted tooth possesses spontaneous eruption potential. This can be demonstrated by an incomplete root development with open apex. Guided eruption is achieved by widening the space by orthodontic treatment or with the help of traction of the impacted tooth. Guided eruption must be considered in all patients. Guided eruption is time consuming and often requires involvement of several specialists. This should be balanced against the patient's expectations and willingness to embark on a complex treatment. Extraction of the impacted tooth often appears to be a justified possibility; however, in reality it should be an option of last resort.

Orthodontic considerations and prognostic markers

The most important factors for the successful management of impacted maxillary canines are angulation of canine to the midline, age of the patient, vertical height, and bucco-palatal position. These factors can also affect the duration of the treatment.

Surgical management

For guided eruption of an impacted tooth, it is generally expected that the patient will undergo an initial phase of orthodontic treatment. The primary purpose of presurgical orthodontic treatment is to create adequate arch space to facilitate the eruption of the impacted tooth and sometimes leveling and alignment of the dental arches. In certain cases, with the proper alignment of the teeth and creation of adequate arch space, an unerupted tooth may only require surgical exposure to relieve the effect of the soft tissue on the delayed eruption. However, in many cases the surgical objective is indeed to surgically expose and bond an attachment to facilitate guided eruption with traction of the impacted tooth. Presence of a retained primary tooth may be an important factor to the patient, especially from the esthetic point of view. However, patients are often quite satisfied with bonding of a denture tooth to their orthodontic wires. This simple and small step can significantly impact the patient's esthetic needs, acceptance, and satisfaction with their treatment.

Exposure and bonding for guided eruption

Different approaches may be considered – one of the most important factors in surgical planning is related to the position of the tooth, palatal or buccal, the width of attached gingiva/mucosa and the depth of impaction. If the tooth is positioned palatally, the development of a soft tissue flap is quite straightforward. Once the flap is reflected, the bone overlying the impacted tooth may be removed with a hand instrument, such as a periosteal elevator or with round bur. Care must be taken to not remove bone in a manner that might compromise the tissues of the impacted tooth or the adjacent teeth.

If the tooth is positioned buccally, great care must be taken to maintain adequate keratinized and attached mucosa over the tooth. The presence of attached mucosa cervically is critical to the health and prognosis of the soft tissue around the erupted tooth.

An apically positioned soft tissue flap is one appropriate flap design when planning to expose and bond a buccally-positioned impacted tooth. An apically-positioned flap is designed as a full-thickness mucoperiosteal flap. A zone of keratinized gingiva must be included in the flap. The flap is mobilized by creating vertical releasing incisions on each side allowing it to be shifted later to the level of cemento-enamel junction of the erupted tooth, leaving the exposed crown open to the mouth. In such cases bonding of bracket can be performed 1–2 weeks after surgery.

When bonding is carried out under surgery, bone overlying the unerupted tooth is removed to facilitate bonding of a bracket (Figs 9.24 and 9.25). The ideal location of the bonded bracket is the most incisal portion of the crown. This position provides the most favorable application of orthodontic forces and best mechanical advantage needed to move the impacted

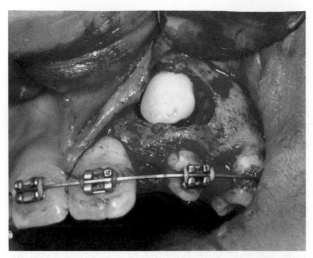

Fig. 9.24 Exposed crown of an unerupted maxillary canine. Bony defect around the crown of the impacted tooth is due to the dental follicle.

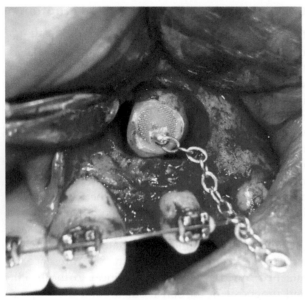

Fig. 9.25 A bracket and gold chain have been attached to the buccal surface of the impacted tooth. The excess bonding material should be cleansed from the tooth to reduce tissue irritation.

tooth into the desired position. Bleeding can hinder visualization of the tooth and bonding of the bracket. The oozing is best controlled by infiltration of local anesthesia containing a vasoconstrictor or packing with gauze, or cotton pellets soaked in local anesthesia or an epinephrine solution, before bonding. Upon completion of the bonding the flap may be repositioned in its original place and the traction carried out closed, with the traction chain or wire submerged. In cases with superficial positions of the crown and plenty of attached tissue on the alveolar crest, the flap may be positioned apically at the cemento-enamel junction of the impacted tooth and the traction and guided eruption performed with the crown exposed. Soon after recovery patients may continue orthodontic treatment.

Surgical removal

If removal of the impacted tooth is necessary, a full-thickness mucoperiosteal flap should be planned. This will allow adequate retraction of the flap and proper visualization. Upon dissection of the flap and exposure of the impacted tooth, adequate bony removal must be carried out to expose the coronal part of the tooth. Well-planned sectioning of the impacted tooth is often needed. Once the impacted tooth is removed, whole or in sections, the surgical site can be closed primarily by sutures.

Postoperative management and complications

The postoperative events and complications associated with surgical exposure of impacted teeth are generally similar to those of other dentoalveolar surgical procedures. The complication most specifically associated with exposure of impacted teeth is the failure of the initial bond or debonding of the bracket from the exposed tooth. This has been reported to range from 1% to 5% and has been attributed to failing to obtain a dry field during the bonding process.

Recommended reading

American Association of Oral and Maxillofacial Surgeons. (2007). White Paper. http://www.aaoms.org/docs/third_molar_white_paper.pdf.

Flick WG. (1999) The third molar controversy: framing the controversy as a public health policy issue. *Journal of Oral and Maxillofacial Surgery*, **57**, 438–45.

Friedman JW. (2003) Containing the cost of third-molar extractions is a dilemma for health insurance. *The Journal of the American Dental Association*, **134**, 450–5.

Hossaini M. (2010) Surgical treatment of impacted teeth other than third molars. In: *Oral and Maxillofacial Surgery*. (eds, Andersson L, Kahnberg K-E, Pogrel MA). Oxford, Wiley-Blackwell.

Hupp JR, Ellis EE, Tucker MR. (2013) *Contemporary Oral and Maxillofacial Surgery*. St Louis, Elsevier Mosby.

Knutsson K, Brehmer B, Lysell L, Rohlin M. (1996) Pathoses associated with mandibular third molars subjected to removal. *Oral Surgery, Oral Medicine, Oral Pathology, Oral Radiology, and Endodontology*, **82**, 10.

Long H, Zhou Y, Liao L, Pyakurel U, Wang Y, Lai W. (2012) Coronectomy vs. total removal for third molar extraction: a systematic review. *Journal of Dental Research*, **91**, 659–65.

Lysell L. (2010) Current concepts and strategies for third molar removal. In: *Oral and Maxillofacial Surgery*. (eds, Andersson L, Kahnberg K-E, Pogrel MA). Oxford, Wiley-Blackwell.

Management of unerupted and impacted third molar teeth. (2007). SIGN Publication, 43. http://www.sign.ac.uk/guidelines/fulltext/43/.

Miloro M, Ghali GE, Larsen P, Waite P. (2012) *Peterson's Principles of Oral and Maxillofacial Surgery*. Shelton, CT, People's Medical Publishing House.

NHS Centre for Reviews and Dissemination, University of York. (1998) Prophylactic removal of impacted third molars: is it justified? *Effectiveness Matters*, **3**, 2.

National Institute for Clinical Excellence. (2000) Guidance on the extraction of wisdom teeth. http://guidance.nice.org.uk/TA1.

Trigeminal Foundation. Nerve injuries. http://trigeminalnerve .org.uk/.

Renton T. (2010) Surgical management of third molars. In: *Oral and Maxillofacial Surgery.* (eds, Andersson L, Kahnberg K-E, Pogrel MA). Oxford, Wiley-Blackwell.

Renton T, Adey-Viscuso D, Meechan JG, Yilmaz Z. (2010) Trigeminal nerve injuries in relation to the local anaesthesia in mandibular injections. *British Dental Journal* **209**(9), E15.

Royal College of Surgeons of England, Faculty of Dental Surgery. The Management of Patients with Third Molar Teeth. Report of a working party convened by the Faculty of Dental Surgery, The Royal College of Surgeons of England. London: Faculty of Dental Surgery RCS (Eng), 1997.

Song F, O'Meara S, Wilson P, Golder S, Kleijnen J. (2000) The effectiveness and cost-effectiveness of prophylactic removal of wisdom teeth. *Health Technology Assessment*, **4**, 1–55.

Tegsjö U, Valerius-Olsson H, Andersson L. (1984) Periodontal conditions following surgical exposure of unerupted maxillary canines – a long term follow up study of two surgical techniques. *Swedish Dental Journal*, **8**, 257–63.

Vanarsdall RL, Corn H. (2003) Soft-tissue management of labially positioned unerupted teeth. *American Journal of Orthodontics* and *Dentofacial Orthopedics*, **125**, 284–93.

Chapter 10

Nerve Involvement in Oral and Maxillofacial Surgery

Nerves can be injured when surgery is performed in the maxillofacial region. Knowledge of anatomy is important to avoid and prevent nerve injuries. The possibility of nerve injuries must always be explained to patients prior to surgery so the patient understands the risks and be part of the decision to carry out surgery when there is risk for nerve injuries.

Trigeminal nerve

Injury to the terminal sensory branches of the trigeminal nerve (the lingual nerve, the inferior alveolar nerve, and the long buccal nerve) is relatively frequent and can occur as a result of many different forms of dental treatment.

Nerve injuries as a result of inferior alveolar nerve block

It is known that both temporary, and occasionally permanent, nerve damage can occur as the result of an inferior alveolar nerve block. The nerve predominantly affected appears to be the lingual nerve, which is affected approximately twice as often as the inferior alveolar nerve. The exact cause of injury with an inferior alveolar nerve block is unknown, but suggestions have included direct trauma from the needle in some way, hematoma to the nerve, or a neurotoxic effect from the local anesthetic itself. The incidence is unknown with estimates of *permanent* nerve damage resulting from inferior alveolar blocks varying from 1 in 20 000 inferior alveolar nerve blocks to 1 in 850 000 inferior alveolar nerve blocks. *Transient* damage from inferior alveolar nerve block probably occurs five or six times as frequently. Most cases recover within an 8–10 week-period, and a smaller number recover over a 9-month period. About 10% of cases prove to be permanent, with occasional disabling dysesthesia.

Inferior alveolar nerve damage from root canal treatment

Root canal therapy carried out on lower molars and premolars may damage the inferior alveolar nerve either from direct trauma from over instrumentation, from a hydrostatic pressure phenomenon or neurotoxicity from extruded root canal sealant (Fig. 10.1). Surgical removal of the material may be necessary in such cases.

Nerve damage from dental implants

The insertion of osseointegrated implants into the mandible has the potential to damage the inferior alveolar nerve and mental nerves due to overextension (Fig. 10.2). Today, with cone-beam computer tomography (CBCT), the distance to the nerve can be measured and installation depth and direction better planned prior to surgery (Fig. 10.3). Cases can also occur from implants inserted anterior to the mental foramen if consideration is not given to forward looping of the inferior alveolar nerve before it exits the mental foramen.

If there is anesthesia or paresthesia of the inferior alveolar nerve following implant insertion, once the local anesthetic has dissipated, consideration should be given to obtaining a cone-beam CT scan to accurately relate the position of the implant to the nerve, and early consideration should be given to removing the implant. This can be successful in the early stages when the involvement is due to pressure alone from the implants or hydrostatic pressure. However, many cases do not recover, presumably since the damage is more profound or was caused by the twist drill.

Essentials of Oral and Maxillofacial Surgery, First Edition. Edited by M. Anthony Pogrel, Karl-Erik Kahnberg and Lars Andersson.
© 2014 John Wiley & Sons, Ltd. Published 2014 by John Wiley & Sons, Ltd.
Companion website: www.wiley.com/go/pogrel/oms

Periodontal surgery

Periodontal surgery in the form of the distal wedge procedure and extensive surgery or deep root planing on the lingual side in the lower molar region can cause damage to the lingual nerve, particularly when the nerve lies in an aberrantly superior position as is known to occur in between 15 and 20% of cases (Fig. 10.4). In these cases the nerve can lie at the level of the crest of the lingual alveolar bone or even slightly above it. If periodontal surgery is to be performed in these areas, the surgeon must have knowledge of the possible aberrant positions of the lingual nerve and take this into account when performing the surgery. If the nerve is damaged with a sharp instrument such as a scalpel, early surgical nerve repair may give satisfactory results.

Dentoalveolar surgery and nerves

Dentoalveolar surgery carried out on the posterior mandible can cause damage to the lingual nerve, the inferior alveolar nerve, the long buccal nerve, and even the mylohyoid nerve. The commonest dentoalveolar procedure carried out in this area is third molar removal, but other surgical procedures in this area have also the potential to cause damage.

Inferior alveolar nerve

The incidence of inferior alveolar nerve damage from the removal of third molars varies in the literature from 0.5–5%. The cause is directly related to the anatomical relationship between the inferior alveolar nerve and the roots of the third molar. In many cases, this can be determined from panoramic radiograph,

and criteria have been developed to determine more exactly from a panoramic radiograph the relationship of the inferior alveolar nerve to the tooth. This is shown in Figure 10.5. When the image of the inferior alveolar canal is superimposed over the tooth with no loss of lamina dura of the canal and no narrowing

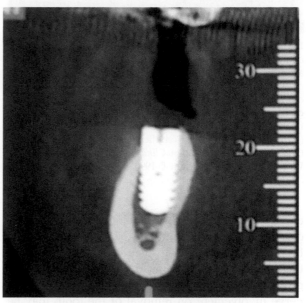

Fig. 10.3 CBCT scan showing implant and relation to inferior alveolar nerve canal and cortical bone walls.

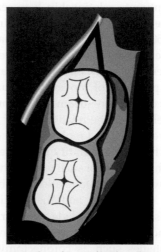

Fig. 10.4 Diagram to show how a distal wedge-type procedure can damage the lingual nerve if it lies in an aberrantly high position.

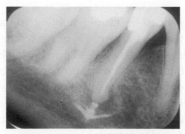

Fig. 10.1 Extruded root canal sealant in the inferior alveolar canal.

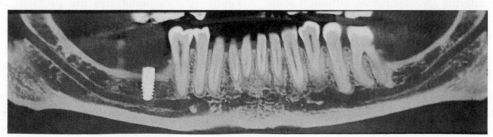

Fig. 10.2 Overextended implant into the inferior alveolar nerve canal.

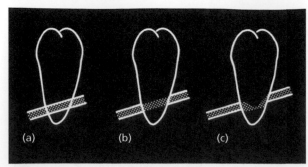

Fig. 10.5 Diagram to show the relationship of the inferior alveolar nerve to the roots of a mandibular third molar as seen on a panorex radiograph. (a) Superimposition only with no loss of cortical outline, narrowing or deviation. (b) Loss of cortical outline denotes grooving of the roots by the nerve. (c) Loss of cortical outline, narrowing, and deviation denote an intimate relationship between the nerve and roots of the third molar. (From Pogrel MA. (1990) Complications of third molar surgery. *Oral and Maxillofacial Surgery Clinics of North America*, 2: 441–51. With permission. Copyright © 1990 Elsevier.)

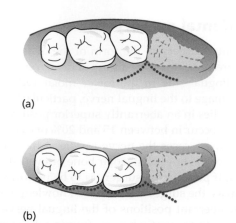

Fig. 10.6 Recommended incisions for removal of a lower third molar. (a) Triangular flap with buccal release. (b) Gingival margin envelope flap. Note that both incisions are buccally placed.

or change of direction, the relationship is probably one of superimposition with a low risk of nerve involvement as shown in Figure 10.5a. If, however, the nerve loses its lamina dura it may in fact be grooving the tooth, and the risk of inferior alveolar nerve involvement on removal of the tooth may be higher, as shown in Figure 10.5b. Figure 10.5c shows loss of the lamina dura, narrowing, and possible deviation of the path of the inferior alveolar canal and denotes an intimate relationship between the tooth and the nerve with a high risk of nerve involvement that may be 50% or higher. A pair of periapical films, taken at different angulations, may reveal relationships between the roots and nerves, by applying the parallax principle of movement ("same lingual, opposite buccal"). Cone-beam CT technology can now accurately show the relationship of the inferior alveolar nerve to the third molar in three dimensions and this has helped to quantify the issue of the risk involved in the removal of such teeth. Where suitable imaging shows an intimate relationship between the roots of the third molar and the inferior alveolar nerve, a decision must be made whether to proceed with the removal or not, or possibly consider intermediate strategies such as coronectomy or partial tooth removal whereby the portion of the root intimately related to the inferior alveolar nerve is left behind. Studies show that this is a safe and predictable technique with a high success rate in avoiding injury to the inferior alveolar nerve, although some of the roots may later move and some may even require subsequent removal.

Lingual nerve

Lingual nerve injuries in relation to dentoalveolar surgery are less frequent than inferior alveolar nerve injuries. Frequencies have been quoted as occurring in 0.2–2% of all lower third molar removals, although

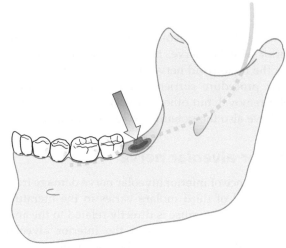

Fig. 10.7 Diagram to show how an aberrantly positioned lingual nerve can be attached to remnants of the dental follicle, which should be removed with caution.

they do appear to be more troubling to patients. In most cases the lingual nerve is protected beneath the lingual plate of bone, as it lies approximately 6–8 mm inferior to the lingual crest and some 2 mm medial; studies have shown, however, that in between 15 and 20% of cases the lingual nerve may lie at or above the level of the lingual plate and is therefore at risk during third molar removal.

Figure 10.6 denotes recommended incisions from a buccal approach for the removal of a lower left third molar, which should not endanger the lingual nerve. Figure 10.7 demonstrates the problem of retained dental follicle adjacent to an aberrantly placed lingual nerve, whilst Figure 10.8 demonstrates that sutures placed too deeply can damage the lingual nerve; sutures should be placed very superficially in this region. Lingual flap elevation and the placement of a subperiosteal lingual retractor is an acceptable technique in order to protect the lingual nerve during third molar removal if it is anticipated that bone will need to be removed in the distal or disto-lingual areas

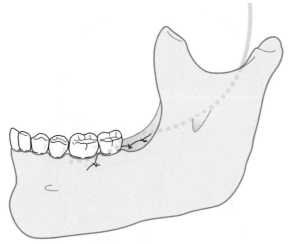

Fig. 10.8 Diagram to illustrate how deeply placed sutures following third molar removal can endanger an aberrantly placed lingual nerve. Sutures should be superficial only, or the sockets should be packed without suturing.

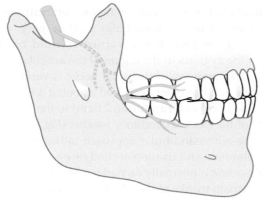

Fig. 10.9 Diagram to illustrate the usual position of the long buccal nerve, which is at risk with any extended incision for third molar removal.

or if the crown must be totally sectioned. It is accepted that there is a small risk of transient nerve involvement following the use of lingual retraction, but this virtually always recovers spontaneously in a few weeks.

Long buccal nerve

Considering the anatomy of the long buccal nerve (Fig. 10.9), it might be anticipated that this nerve would be involved in many cases during third molar removal. However, it is unusual for patients to be aware of damage to this nerve, partly because they are unaware of the altered sensation on the inner aspect of the cheek, and often because there is an overlapping nerve supply from surrounding nerves. Nevertheless, damage has been documented on a number of occasions and can occasionally be troublesome to patients. In practice, it is virtually impossible to find the long buccal nerve surgically, and equally impossible to repair it.

Mylohyoid nerve

Involvement of the mylohyoid nerve has been reported in up to 1.2% of third molar removals but is normally associated with lingual retraction, where the retractor has been placed too deeply. There is generally a localized area of paresthesia beneath the point of the chin on the affected side. It has been suggested that the mylohyoid nerve may provide part of the nerve supply to the tip of the tongue, possibly explaining different manifestations of nerve damage on the tip of the tongue versus other parts of the tongue. Involvement of the mylohyoid nerve is usually temporary and of little clinical significance.

Evaluation of trigeminal nerve damage

Most evaluation techniques for nerve involvement are semi-objective at best and do rely on the presence of a cooperative patient. The different testing techniques are used to evaluate the different types of nerve filaments that might be involved. In all cases the normal side is tested first and the abnormal side is compared to it. Patients should be referred to an oral and maxillofacial surgeon for such assessment. Various test can be used to test for sensation of touch, temperature, taste. The affected area is mapped and photographed to enable comparison of progress of recovery.

Facial nerve

The facial nerve, or VII cranial nerve, is the motor nerve which innervates the muscles of facial expression. It is at risk in a variety of oral and maxillofacial surgery procedures, mostly from procedures performed from an extraoral approach. The only time it is at risk from intraoral procedures is from an inferior alveolar nerve block, the local anesthetic injection technique commonly used to anesthetize the hemimandible, when the needle is incorrectly positioned and the local anesthetic is deposited posterior to the mandible in the parotid tissue where it can permeate to affect the branches of the facial nerve (Fig. 10.10). In this case, there will be a facial nerve weakness, which should be transitory and only last as long as the local anesthetic effects (Fig. 10.11). However, long-lasting, if not permanent, cases of facial nerve involvement have been described from this particular procedure, for which no active treatment is available.

The anatomy of the facial nerve is seen in Figure 10.12. On the face, the main trunk of the facial nerve emerges from the stylomastoid foramen and travels forward and laterally into the parotid gland, where it normally divides into an upper and lower trunk, which further subdivide into the five terminal branches, but there are many variations on this. The zygomaticotemporal, frontal, and buccal branches

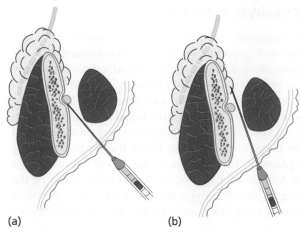

(a)   (b)

Fig. 10.10 Diagram to show how an inferior alveolar nerve block can affect the facial nerve if the local anesthetic is given too far posterior and the needle does not contact bone: (a) normal, (b) injection into parotid gland where facial nerve can be affected.

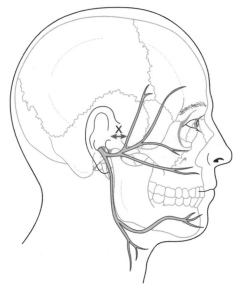

Fig. 10.12 Relationship of the branches of the facial nerve to the underlying bony structures. X = 0.8–3.5 cm.

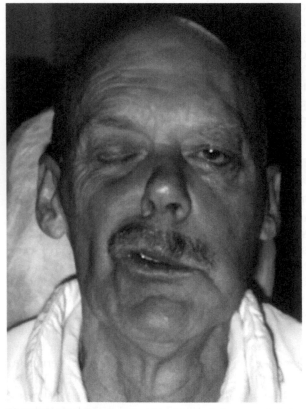

Fig. 10.11 Transient facial nerve weakness from an inferior alveolar nerve block.

arise from the upper trunk, while the mandibular and cervical branches emerge from the lower trunk. As they exit the parotid gland anteriorly, they lie in relation to the investing fascia of neck, deep to the platysma muscle. In this position they are at risk in many of the incisions and procedures carried out on the face. All of the branches are particularly at risk during parotid surgery, and this is described elsewhere in this textbook. Similarly, the upper branches

(particularly the zygomaticotemporal branch) are at risk during temporomandibular joint surgery, particularly if the dissection is carried forward on the arch of the zygoma in the region of the articular eminence. The anatomy of the facial nerve is variable in this area, and has been described as being anywhere from 0.8–3.5 cm anterior (mean 2.0 cm) to the anterior cavity of the external auditory meatus (Fig. 10.12).

In the retromandibular approach to the mandible for exploration and fixation of condyle neck fractures, the dissection is normally carried out bluntly between the two main trunks of the facial nerve, and although damage in this area is possible, it is actually quite unusual.

In the submandibular approach to the submandibular salivary gland and the mandible, both the mandibular and cervical branches of the facial nerve are at risk. The mandibular branch supplies the orbicularis oris, causing a weakness of the corner of the mouth, while the cervical branch supplies the platysma. An involvement of this nerve branch can also cause weakness of the corner of the mouth, though it is usually less severe than with mandibular branch involvement and is often transitory. An incision placed 2 cm, or one finger's breadth, below the angle of the mandible should avoid the mandibular branch of the facial nerve at all times. The cervical branch, however, runs progressively inferiorly as it progresses anteriorly, and in order to avoid contact with this nerve the incisions need to be placed 4 cm below the lower border of the mandible in the mandibular notch area, although 3 cm below the mandible at the angle is sufficient to avoid involvement of this branch. Both of these approaches are feasible for submandibular access surgery.

If these peripheral branches of the facial nerve are damaged during surgery, it is normally not possible to identify or repair them and spontaneous recovery is often incomplete. Surgical repair and reconstruc-

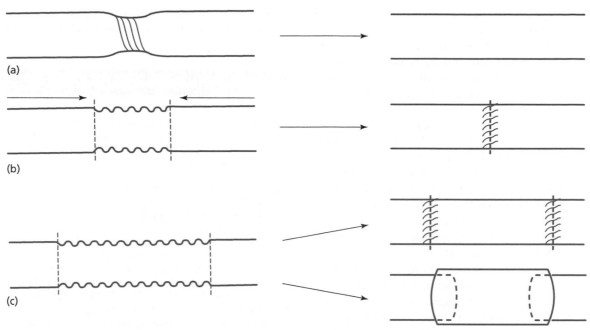

Fig. 10.13 Diagram to show the different types of microsurgical procedures possible. (a) Decompression for a localized compression from fibrosis, scarring or a bone fragment. (b) Direct anastomosis for a localized transection, or other injury. (c) A graft to repair a more extensive injury. (From Pogrel MA, Kaban LB. Injuries to the inferior alveolar and lingual nerves. *Cal Dent J* 1993; 21: 50–4. With permission. Copyright © 1997 California Dental Association.)

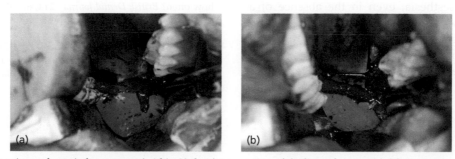

Fig. 10.14 Direct epineural repair for a recent (within 10 days) transection of the lingual nerve. (a) After exposure showing the two nerve ends. (b) After direct anastomosis with five 8/0 nylon sutures.

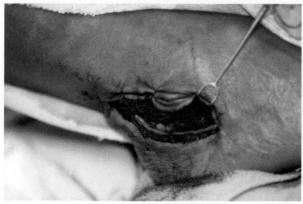

Fig. 10.15 Sural nerve graft taken from behind lateral malleolus of the right ankle.

tion of the main trunk and the upper and lower branches of the facial nerve may be possible on some occasions, but the results of surgery are generally less than satisfactory.

Microneurosurgery

Microneurosurgery has been attempted to repair injuries to the lingual and inferior alveolar nerve.

The type of nerve injuries that might be treated surgically would include compression injuries where decompression might result in a cure, and partial or complete severing of the nerve (Fig. 10.13). In these latter cases excision of the affected area of nerve is normally required, freshening up of the ends, and direct epineural repair when this is possible (Fig. 10.14). Undue stretching or devascularization of the nerve should be avoided, and in cases where direct apposition is not possible, a nerve graft or conduit must be used.

Donor sites for nerve grafting can come from the great auricular nerve in the neck or the sural nerve behind the lateral malleolus of the ankle (Fig. 10.15); the medial antebrachial nerve of the forearm has also been described as a donor. Rather than using nerve grafts, vein grafts are autogenous conduits which have met with some success.

Most authorities do feel that if surgery is to be successful, it should probably be carried out as soon as possible and certainly within a few months of injury. The longer one waits, the greater the chance can be of degeneration of the distal segment of the nerve and neuroma formation on the proximal segment, which would need excision and would complicate any repair procedure. Reports of results of microneurosurgery on the terminal branches of the third division of the trigeminal nerve are few, but do suggest that if surgery is carried out early on patients there can be some improvement in over 50% of cases, although virtually no cases return to normal. Repairs are normally performed under magnifying loupes or an operating microscope at magnifications of between 4 and 20 times, using 8/0 or 9/0 atraumatic nylon sutures.

Immediate microneurosurgical repair (within 3–7 days) can be recommended for a witnessed total transection, particularly of the lingual nerve, where the ends tend to retract and spontaneous recovery is rare, and also those cases with symptomatic endodontic paste within the inferior alveolar canal. Surgical exploration is also offered at 8–10 weeks postinjury, in those patients who are either totally anesthetic, or have severe dysesthesia, even in the absence of a witnessed transection. For longer times postinjury exploratory surgery may be offered but the results of surgery are poor.

Surgery appears to have little to offer for nerves injured by local anesthetic injections or by implant-related procedures; in the latter case the area of damage is often extensive and may require a graft.

Recommended reading

Fagin AP, Susarla SM, Donoff RB, Kaban LB, Dodson TB. (2012) What factors are associated with functional sensory recovery following lingual nerve repair? *Journal of Oral and Maxillofacial Surgery*, **70**, 2907–15.

Miloro M, Kolokythas A. (2011) Inferior alveolar and lingual nerve imaging. *Atlas of the Oral and Maxillofacial Surgery Clinics of North America*, **19**, 35–46.

Pogrel MA. (2007) Damage to the inferior alveolar nerve as the result of root canal therapy. *The Journal of the American Dental Association*, **138**, 65–99.

Pogrel MA. (2009) Coronectomy to prevent damage to the inferior alveolar nerve. *Alpha Omegan*, **102**, 61–7.

Pogrel MA. (2010) Nerve involvement in oral and maxillofacial surgery. In: *Oral and Maxillofacial Surgery*. (eds, Andersson L, Kahnberg K-E, Pogrel MA). Oxford, Wiley-Blackwell.

Pogrel MA. (2012) Permanent nerve damage from inferior alveolar nerve blocks: a current update. *Journal of The Californian Dental Association*, **40**, 795–7.

Renton T, Yilmaz Z. (2012) Managing iatrogenic trigeminal nerve injury; a case series and review of the literature. *International Journal of Oral and Maxillofacial Surgery*, **41**, 629–37.

Renton T, Janjua H, Gallagher JE, Dalgleich M, Yilmaz Z. (2013) UK dentists' experience of iatrogenic trigeminal nerve injuries in relation to routine dental procedures: why, when and how often? *British Dental Journal*, **214**, 633–42.

Trigeminal Foundation. Nerve injuries. http://trigeminalnerve .org.uk.

Umar G, Obiesan O, Bryant C, Rood JP. (2013) Elimination of permanent injuries to the inferior alveolar nerve following surgical intervention of the "high risk" molar. *British Journal of Oral and Maxillofacial Surgery*, **51**, 353–7.

Chapter 11

Autotransplantation of Teeth

Autotransplantation is a treatment alternative for replacing missing teeth, either those missing congenitally or those lost due to trauma or disease, by moving a tooth or a root to a more suitable position within the same individual.

Introduction

Teeth can be transplanted with good prognosis within the same individual. This is called autotransplantation and is defined as an organ or tissue moved from one location and placed in a different location within the same individual. Teeth can be transplanted from one place to another and a tooth or a root can also be transplanted to a more suitable position within the same socket.

Although replacement of lost or missing teeth in adults is nowadays more often carried out by implant treatment, there are a number of situations where autotransplantation seems to be a better alternative, especially in growing children and adolescents where implants should not be used due to the interference with growth of the alveolar process. A transplanted tooth with periodontal ligament (PDL) will follow and contribute to the development of the alveolar process and in many situations is therefore the first alternative for replacement in growing individuals. There are also some situations in adult patients where autotransplantation is a good alternative.

Donor teeth

Transplants can be taken by using teeth in crowded regions or by strategic extraction when equalizing the number of teeth between quadrants. Moreover, many premolars are extracted as part of the orthodontic treatment and can be used as transplants. Third molars can also be used. The transplanted tooth must have a suitable root length and shape.

Teeth with roots under development are easier to extract and have a better prognosis. Developing teeth can revascularize while teeth with fully developed roots do not revascularize and have to be endodontically treated. It is also important to take into consideration the development and growth status of the individual and an interdisciplinary approach is important when planning.

Indications

Congenitally missing teeth

Tooth aplasia is a suitable indication for autotransplantation (Fig. 11.1). Donor teeth can be other erupted or impacted teeth or strategically extracted, e.g. taken from a crowded area or when a tooth does not have an antagonist. Another indication can also be to equalize teeth between quadrants. If the space is too small, preoperative orthodontic widening may be necessary. An advantage with this type of transplantation is that a natural biological condition for bone and soft tissue development of the alveolar process in the young growing patient is achieved and normal eruption is promoted.

Unrestorable teeth

Autotransplantation may be indicated in situations with deep caries or where restoration or crown therapy is not feasible, or when endodontic treatment has failed (Fig. 11.2).

Crown–root and root fractures

Intra-alveolar transplantation, also called surgical extrusion, can be used to move a fractured root to a

Essentials of Oral and Maxillofacial Surgery, First Edition. Edited by M. Anthony Pogrel, Karl-Erik Kahnberg and Lars Andersson.
© 2014 John Wiley & Sons, Ltd. Published 2014 by John Wiley & Sons, Ltd.
Companion website: www.wiley.com/go/pogrel/oms

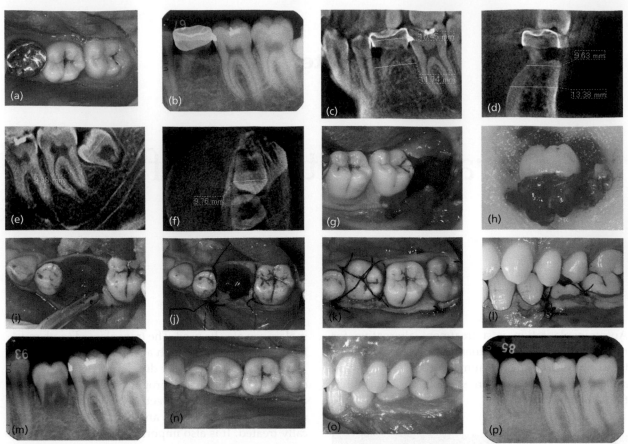

Fig. 11.1 Transplantation of immature impacted third molar to the site of congenitally missing second premolar. (a) The patient is a 20-year-old male with a congenitally missing premolar 35 and a remaining deciduous molar 75. The root has been resorbed. (b) Radiograph showing resorption of 75. (c, d) Cone-beam CT images of the recipient site. The measurement of the recipient space has shown it is wide enough to accommodate the donor mesio-distally and bucco-lingually. (e, f) Cone-beam CT images of the donor tooth. The measurement has revealed the tooth is small enough to be placed into the recipient site. The lower left impacted third molar 38 is considered to be a good donor tooth for transplantation. (g, h) Extraction of the donor tooth 38. Note the Hertwig's epithelial sheath is preserved at each apex. (i) Extraction of the tooth from the recipient site. (j) After careful try-in of the donor into the recipient site, suturing of the flap is performed without placing it in the socket. A knot is tied on the buccal aspect of the inter-proximal area and about 3 cm of one of the sutures is left. Another interrupted suture is tied across the vertical releasing incision on the mesial aspect. Again, 3 cm of one end is left. Next, a suture is placed through the interproximal area of the mesial aspect but in this procedure only one knot is tied loosely so that it allows space for the donor tooth to be placed into the socket. (k) Just after suture splinting. The loosely tied suture is tied tightly after placing the donor tooth. The tooth is tied into place by using a crisscross method. The remaining distal buccal end is tied with the mesio-lingual end and a knot is made on the center of the occlusal surface of the donor tooth. A horizontal mattress suture is tied on the disto-lingual aspect, and the remaining suture is tied to the remaining suture from the first crisscross knot. The remaining suture is then tied to the long remaining end of the suture from the vertical releasing portion. This allows the donor tooth to be seated in the correct position. Any excess suture is cut. (l) Occlusal adjustments are made on the antagonist so that articulating paper can freely slide through the contact. In this case, the opposing tooth was slightly extruded, so with the patient's permission, some adjustments were made to the opposing tooth in contact. (m) Radiograph immediately after transplantation. Note the apices are wide open. (n, o, p) Follow-up after 1 year, 8 months. The transplanted tooth has erupted and is in contact with the antagonist. Pulp healing and root development are seen.

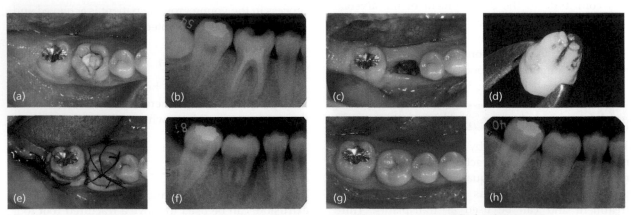

Fig. 11.2 Transplantation immature third molar 48 to replace an unrestorable first molar 46. (a) Occlusal view of the non-restorable 46. (b) Radiograph of 46. It was considered transplantation of an immature third molar would give a better prognosis than preserving 46 in this young patient. (c) 2 weeks after the extraction of 46. Transplantation was performed on the same day. (d) Extracted 48 as a donor. Note Hertwig's epithelial sheaths are preserved apically. (e, f) Immediately after transplantation. (g, h) 4 years' follow-up. The transplant shows a positive electric pulp test and normal healing is seen clinically and radiographically.

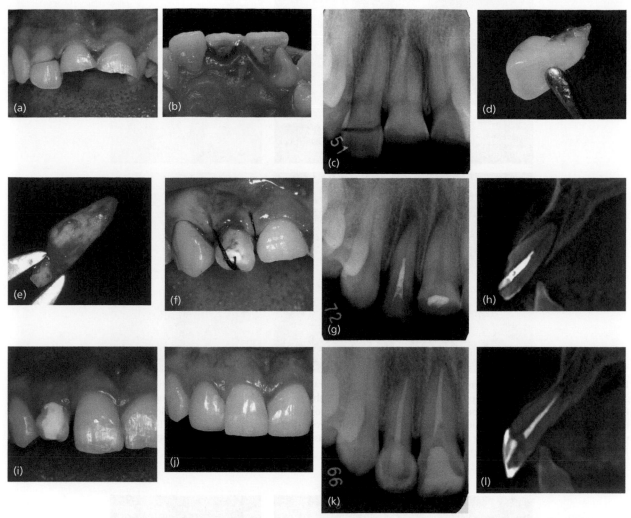

Fig. 11.3 Crown-root fracture and surgical extrusion. (a, b, c) A 32-year-old female has sustained dental trauma in the anterior area. Three incisors have been injured. Both central incisors were subjected to lateral luxation with crown fracture and the right lateral incisor suffered crown–root fracture. In this presentation, the treatment is focused on the lateral incisor. (d) Removal of the coronal fragment of 12. (e) The extracted crown root fragment 12 before transplantation. (f) The transplanted 12 immediately after surgical extrusion. The tooth was rotated 180°, so that the palatal aspect is now facing buccally, and transplanted to an extruded position. A suture has been placed to hold the tooth in the correct position. (g) Radiograph immediately after surgical extrusion and rotation of root fragment through 180°. The endodontic treatment was performed before surgery and the canal was filled temporarily with radiopaque calcium hydroxide. (h) Cone-beam CT image immediately after surgery. (i) 5 weeks postoperative appearance just before the restoration of the crown with composite. (j) 4 years' follow-up. The crowns of the three traumatized incisors 12, 11, and 21 have been restored with composite. (k) 4 years' radiographic follow-up. Normal healing is seen. (l) Cone-beam CT image of tooth 12 at 4 years' follow-up. Normal PDL space along the root surface is observed and the thin buccal bone plate is preserved.

more coronal position in the alveolar socket so crown therapy will be enabled (Fig. 11.3). The root can be extracted either directly with forceps or via an open flap approach if the root is submerged. If the remaining root is long enough to carry a crown the root can be transplanted to a more suitable position in the socket. In some cases it may be suitable to rotate the root to 180°, to achieve a larger area of the root within the alveolar bone. By doing this, the root is secured in its new position and does not slide back. Endodontic treatment should be performed within the first weeks after transplantation and crown therapy can usually be finished within 3 months after the transplantation. This method is a first choice of treatment in growing individuals where implant treatment is contraindicated, but can also be performed in adult patients as an alternative to implant treatment.

Lost teeth in young growing patients

Incisors are sometimes lost because of tooth avulsion or cannot be restored after complex trauma. In adults such lost teeth are often replaced by implants; however, when the patient is young and still growing implant treatment is contraindicated because implants will not follow the growth and development of the alveolar process. In such a case it can be difficult to achieve a good esthetic final result because the tissues do not develop normally in an esthetically sensitive area. Tooth transplant will enable continuing growth and development of the bone and soft tissues of the alveolar process while an individual is growing, and is therefore often a first choice when replacing teeth in young patients who are still growing (Figs 11.4 and 11.5).

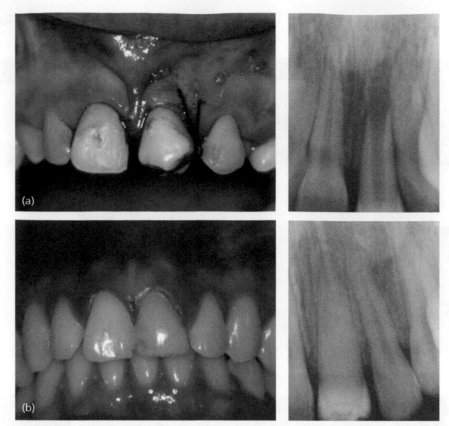

Fig. 11.4 Autotransplantation of mandibular premolar to the central incisor area with a closed technique. (a) Transplanted premolar sutured into position. The postoperative immediate radiograph shows incomplete root development. (b). Follow-up 9 years after transplantation. The crown has been built up by composite. Radiograph shows that full root development has been achieved and the usual obliteration is seen indicating the pulp has survived. (From Andreasen JO, Andersson L, Tsukiboshi M. (2007) Autotransplantation of teeth to the anterior region. In: *Textbook and Color Atlas of Traumatic Injuries to the Teeth*, 4th edn. Ch. 27. (eds, Andreasen JO, Andreasen FM, Andersson L). Blackwell Publishing, Oxford.)

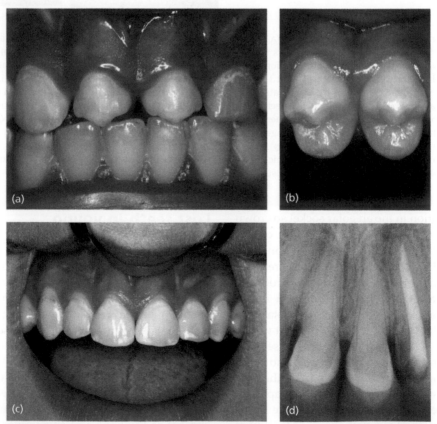

Fig. 11.5 (a, b) Autotransplanted premolars. (c) The transplants were later restored with porcelain laminate veneers. (d) Radiograph after restoration. (From Andreasen JO, Andersson L, Tsukiboshi M. (2007) Autotransplantation of teeth to the anterior region. In: *Textbook and Color Atlas of Traumatic Injuries to the Teeth*, 4th edn. Ch. 27. (eds, Andreasen JO, Andreasen FM, Andersson L). Blackwell Publishing, Oxford.)

Lost teeth in adults

Teeth lost in individuals who have finished growing are usually replaced by implants. However, autotransplantation can also be performed in adult patients after tooth loss; but, since these teeth have fully developed roots, they will not revascularize and must therefore be root canal-treated.

Autotransplants vs implants

Since the introduction of implants, many surgeons today prefer implants to replace lost teeth in *adult patients* who have finished growing. However, autotransplantation of teeth can, in principle, also be performed in adult patients. Third molars may still be undergoing root development in young adults; these can be excellent transplants and revascularization can occur. Teeth with fully formed roots can be transplanted provided root canal treatment is performed. Implant treatment cannot be afforded by all patients and autotransplantation may be an alternative.

In *young growing patients* implant treatment is contraindicated in the anterior maxillary region because it stops the vertical growth of the alveolar process and it can be difficult to achieve a good esthetic final result if an implant is placed before growth is completed. To support the development of normal tissue in the trauma area, and to secure growth and development of the alveolar process in an individual who is still growing, transplantation of the tooth is an excellent form of treatment.

Principles of healing after autotransplantation

Two tissues are of main importance for an autotransplantation to be successful: the pulp and the periodontal ligament. When a tooth is transplanted the vascular supply is immediately lost. Revascularization is therefore of utmost importance if the pulp is going to survive. Studies of transplanted teeth have shown that young teeth with ongoing root development and open apex can revascularize. Successful healing is related to the stage of root development. In order to optimize conditions for revascularization, transplantation should ideally be carried out before the root reaches full root length and when the root apex is still open (Fig. 11.6). Teeth with fully developed roots and a closed apex cannot be expected to revascularize but can still be transplanted provided root canal treatment is performed (Fig. 11.7).

Principles of surgery

Possible transplants can be strategically extracted teeth, e.g. premolars from areas with crowded teeth or areas where the number of teeth in a quadrant is going to be reduced and equalized to an adjacent quadrant. The treatment should therefore ideally be planned in a multi-disciplinary approach with, in addition to the surgeon, orthodontists, pediatric dentists, endodontists etc. The orthodontist has a central

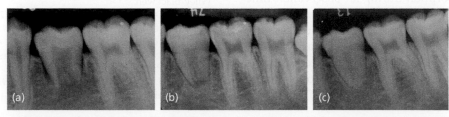

Fig. 11.6 Transplanted molar with optimal root length. The patient is a 17-year-old female. (a) Immediately after transplantation. (b) 8 months later. The root of the transplant is developing. (c) 6 years later. The root development is completed to full root length.

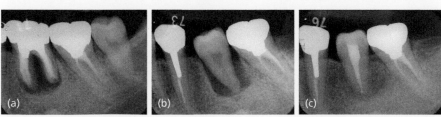

Fig. 11.7 Case illustrating bone healing capacity of PDL after transplantation. (a) Before transplantation. Tooth 36 is going to be replaced by 38, which is not in occlusion and lacks an antagonist. (b) Just after transplantation. Note the wide space between the donor and the socket walls. (c) 2 years postoperatively. New bone has been formed and a normal PDL space is seen around the transplanted tooth.

role to advise on a suitable transplant and perform preoperative and postoperative orthodontic treatment when required. It is important to have a thorough preoperative radiographic examination with panoramic radiographs and periapical dental films of both the donor and recipient areas to estimate root anatomy, root development, and space conditions. Cone-beam computed tomography is a helpful preoperative tool (see Fig. 11.1). Estimation of the degree of root development is the key factor in order to time the transplantation. A root development of 70–80% seems to be optimal.

Surgical techniques

A prerequisite for a successful result of transplantation is that the capacity of the tissues for healing and regeneration is preserved. For this reason there are special requirements regarding the surgical techniques. It is important that the surgeon has a full understanding of the highly sensitive tissues (PDL and pulp) involved. These are cases which should be referred to surgeons specially trained in this methodology. For more information about the surgical technique we recommend special textbooks (see Recommended reading).

Long-term prognosis

There are some studies reporting tooth survival after tooth transplantation in almost 100% of cases. However, evaluating with more strict criteria, i.e. not only survival but healing without any signs of progressive root resorption during an observation time of several years, achieves a more relevant success rate. Using such evaluation criteria, the success for a transplanted molar is 72–90%, for premolars, 89–98%, and for canines, 25–81%. The higher success figures are for studies with teeth with developing roots with open apices and revascularization. Transplant-

ing teeth with fully developed roots has a lower success rate due to a higher risk for damage of the PDL with resulting root resorption. For intraalveolar transplantation (surgical extrusion) a success rate of 88–90% has been reported. Numerous clinical and experimental studies of autotransplantation and replantation have resulted in today's understanding of the healing process and how to avoid or reduce the risk of complications after autotransplantation. In recent decades, in centers where multidisciplinary teams have been formed to perform autotransplantation, there is an increasing demand for this treatment in young growing patients.

Summary

Transplantation of teeth is a well-documented treatment method that should always be taken into consideration as a first treatment alternative in young growing patients with congenitally missing teeth and in situations of tooth loss after trauma in growing patients. A multidisciplinary approach is recommended for these cases. A transplanted tooth can contribute to normal development of the alveolar process when the patient is still growing. In adult patients there are also situations where autotransplantation sometimes can be a preferable alternative to other treatment although implant treatment is today more common for adult patients.

Recommended reading

Andersson L, Tsukiboshi M, Andreasen JO. (2010) Autotransplantation of teeth. In: *Oral and Maxillofacial Surgery* (eds, Andersson L, Kahnberg K-E, Pogrel MA). Oxford, Wiley-Blackwell.

Andreasen JO, Andersson L, Tsukiboshi M. (2007) Autotransplantation of teeth to the anterior region. In: *Textbook and Color Atlas of Traumatic Injuries to the Teeth*, 4th edn. Ch. 27. (eds, Andreasen JO, Andreasen FM, Andersson L). Oxford, Blackwell Publishing.

Tsukiboshi M. (2001) *Autotransplantation of teeth*. Illinois: Quintessence Publishing.

Chapter 12

Endodontic Surgery

Periradicular surgical procedures (PRS) are used to treat diseases and conditions of the tooth root that cannot be treated with orthograde root canal treatment. The majority of these surgical procedures will involve resection of the root apex (apicectomy) and retrograde obturation of the root canal to address persistent disease that has not resolved following an acceptable root canal treatment.

Indications for periapical surgery

An apicectomy is indicated when conventional non-surgical root canal treatment with orthograde root canal filling has failed or cannot be performed, and the tooth is associated with clinical symptoms or signs of continuing periradicular disease. A surgical approach cannot substitute non-surgical orthograde root canal treatment and should not be considered as the primary option to treat teeth with associated apical pathology, but seen as a supplement to endodontic treatment. Indications and contraindications for undertaking PRS are outlined in Table 12.1.

The surgical procedure aims to remove the necrotic and infected dental root apex, curettage and removal of the periradicular lesion, and seal off the apical aspect of the root canal. The apical seal of the root canal with a retrograde root filling has been demonstrated as being a major factor towards the successful outcome of PRS. There have been several significant advances in endodontic surgical procedures over the past decade. These include the development of improved root-end filling materials such as mineral trioxide aggregate (MTA), the introduction of magnification, and the use of ultrasonics in root-end preparation.

Preoperative imaging

Conventional radiology has been the principle technique for assessing periradicular anatomy prior to performing endodontic surgery. This facilitates the assessment of the number, length and shape of the roots, the presence of a sclerosed canal, and type of restoration present. However, these two-dimensional (2D) images of three-dimensional (3D) structures have their limitations. As a consequence, the use of 3D cone-beam computed tomography (CBCT) imaging is now becoming established in preoperative assessment for PRS. The detail provided by 3D CBCT imaging in diagnosing the precise size and location of resorption defects or periradicular pathology is greatly beneficial over conventional radiography. Such enhanced preoperative information allows improved precision in performing PRS procedures, thereby preventing complications arising through trauma to adjacent anatomic structures.

Magnification

The modern approach to PRS is through magnification, illumination, and microsurgery. The literature is now reporting greatly improved prognosis when these techniques are employed. Surgical operating microscope (SOM) and endoscopy are the methods used today. Microsurgical instruments are used (Figs 12.1, 12.2 and 12.3). Far more detailed examination of the root apex is possible, allowing anatomic features such as isthmuses, accessory canals, fracture cracks, and crazing to be identified. Angled ultrasonic instruments can be used to prepare the retrograde cavity with the aid of micromirrors.

Essentials of Oral and Maxillofacial Surgery, First Edition. Edited by M. Anthony Pogrel, Karl-Erik Kahnberg and Lars Andersson.
© 2014 John Wiley & Sons, Ltd. Published 2014 by John Wiley & Sons, Ltd.
Companion website: www.wiley.com/go/pogrel/oms

Table 12.1 Indications and contraindications for surgical endodontics. (Adapted from ESE guidelines 2006.)

Indications for surgical endodontics	Contraindications for surgical endodontics
Radiological findings of periradicular periodontitis and/or symptoms associated with a canal where an obstruction cannot be removed or will result in damage	Local anatomic factors, such as an inaccessible root end
Extruded material with clinical or radiological findings of apical periodontitis and/or symptoms over a prolonged period	Tooth with inadequate periodontal support
Persisting or emerging disease following root canal treatment where retreatment is inappropriate	Uncooperative patient
Perforation of the root or pulp chamber floor which cannot be treated from within the pulp cavity	Patients with a severely compromised medical history
Biopsy of persisting periradicular lesion is required	Tooth is unrestorable
If patient considerations preclude prolonged non-surgical root canal retreatment	Inexperienced operator with no training

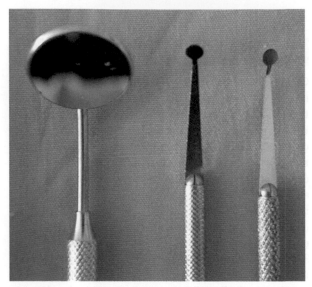

Fig. 12.1 Comparison of microsurgical mirrors to facilitate visualization of the root canal anatomy with a conventional dental mirror (left).

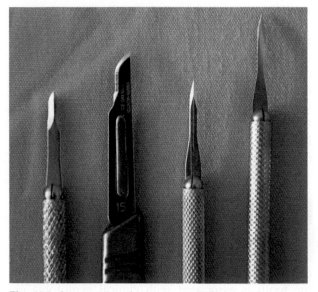

Fig. 12.2 Comparison of microsurgical blades with conventional surgical blade.

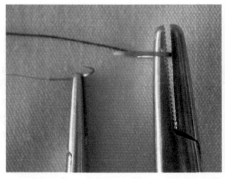
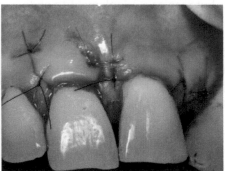

Fig. 12.3 (a) Microsurgical suture forceps and 5/0 suture in comparison to standard suture forceps and 4/0 suture. (b) Microsurgical suturing with papillae preservation.

Surgical procedures

Flap design

The rectangular flap (Fig. 12.4) is the most commonly used flap and comprises two vertical relieving incisions with a horizontal marginal incision. The natural retraction of the gingival tissues following surgery with a full-thickness sulcular flap may expose previously placed subgingival restoration margins. The patient should therefore be informed of this possibility in advance of the surgical procedure. If this is an unacceptable esthetic risk then an alternative flap design will be required and may involve papillae preservation.

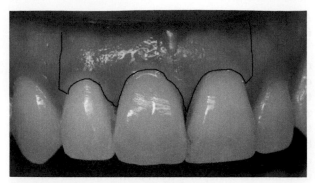

Fig. 12.4 Outline of rectangular flap.

Microsurgical approaches

The surgical operating microscope has facilitated the use of microsurgical scalpel blades and other microsurgical techniques. The potential for micro-suturing has permitted procedures designed to preserve the integrity of the interdental papilla with resultant improved postsurgical esthetics. Microsurgical sutures, size 5-0, will result in an excellent esthetic result if the procedures are followed precisely and the tissues kept moist during the surgery, especially if hemostatic agents are used. There is early clinical evidence that such papilla-based flaps achieve the best postoperative esthetic result (Fig. 12.3).

Careful assessment of the root length from preoperative radiographs prior to bone removal will help in locating the root apex. Extreme care must be taken when removing bone to identify the root apex, and when extending an exposed crypt so as not to generate heat which may rapidly cause irreversible damage to the bone. With the improved vision afforded by the microscope, the use of micromirrors and fine ultrasonic tips, bone removal can be kept to a minimum.

A thorough and detailed knowledge of the local anatomy is essential. PRS on maxillary anterior teeth may be relatively straightforward but on mandibular anterior teeth may be far more difficult due to the shallow labial sulcus and lingual inclination of the roots. Maxillary posterior teeth present additional problems in their proximity to the floor of the sinus, although the buccal roots usually lie very close to the cortical plate and frequently perforate this. Access to palatal roots will necessitate a significantly larger osteotomy. In addition, the mandibular posterior teeth are generally covered with a thick cortical plate making access very difficult.

Periradicular curettage

Periapical periodontitis is the body's natural immune response to the inflammatory mediators and infective agents within and around the root apex. Thus, no matter how thoroughly the granulation tissue that forms the periradicular disease lesion is removed from the surgical site, unless the actual source of infection within the root canal is addressed by root

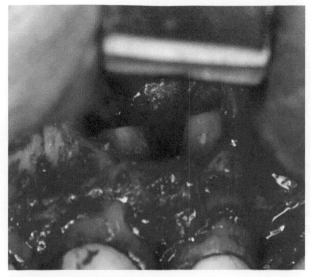

Fig. 12.5 Large apical lesion with root apices resected at 90°. Preparation of root canal with ultrasonic tips and use of micromirror prior to placement of retrograde root canal filling.

resection and retrograde restoration, the surgery will likely fail. Every effort should be made to dissect out the granulation tissue cleanly and without damage so that it may be placed immediately in a container of formalin and sent for a pathological report.

Root-end resection

The main reason for a surgical approach to an endodontic problem is to remove extraradicular bacteria and other contaminants causing clinical symptoms. However, the anatomy of the root apex is complicated, with multiple portals of exit and accessory canals.

It is therefore generally accepted that an apical resection of 3 mm will remove the majority, if not all, of these potential problem areas. This resection will additionally permit thorough inspection of the root canal, preparation of a cavity to encompass the canal shape and placement of a retrograde seal. The angle of resection should be as close to horizontal as possible (i.e. at right angles to the long axis of the tooth) (Fig. 12.5). This exposes a minimal number of dentine tubules, thereby reducing apical leakage and providing the best potential for healing.

Root-end preparation

The preparation of the retrograde cavity has two primary objectives. Firstly, it must thoroughly remove all traces of the previous failed and contaminated root canal filling material. Secondly, it must shape the apical aspect of the root canal system in order to permit placement of a hermetic seal. This will help to prevent the exit of further microbial contaminants. Once again, good visual inspection of the root apex using the SOM, good illumination, and the use of surgical micromirrors is essential. Traditionally a

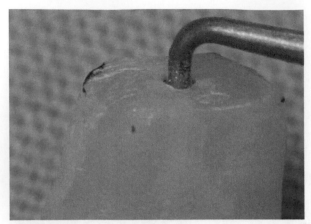

Fig. 12.6 Ultrasonic cavity preparation of 3–5 mm of the root canal for placement of the retrograde root canal filling.

micro-handpiece with a round bur was used to undertake root-end preparation. The currently preferred method involves the use of specially designed ultrasonic tips in a piezoelectric ultrasonic handpiece. Ultrasonic preparation of the root end produces cleaner, well-centered, and more conservative root-end cavities than conventional rotary instrumentation (Fig. 12.6). The use of ultrasonics for root-end preparation has been demonstrated to improve surgical outcomes in comparison to traditional techniques.

Restoration of the retrograde cavity

Before restoring the root-end preparation, there must be adequate hemostasis within the surgical site. This can be achieved by placing a gauze pack or a hemostatic material. These agents also help to act as a barrier to prevent the accumulation of excess retrograde filling material around the root apex tissues. The root-end preparation can then be dried with either paper points or the use of a micro-irrigating syringe.

The restorative material selected for the root-end filling must be radiopaque, easy to manipulate, and exhibit two principal characteristics. Firstly, it must provide an effective permanent seal to prevent leakage from the root canal system of any microorganisms or their by-products. As such, it must be stable and insoluble. Secondly, the material should be biocompatible, ideally promoting regeneration of the surrounding cementum and bone directly on to its surface. Although many materials have been advocated for this purpose in the past, only two are now recommended as retrograde filling materials. These are MTA or reinforced zinc oxide–eugenol cements.

Amalgam is no longer recommended as a material for root-end filling.

Mineral trioxide aggregate (MTA) is now recognized to have significantly better properties than any other material for this purpose. Unlike all of the other traditionally used root-end filling materials (amalgam, zinc oxide–eugenol cements, glass ionomer cements) the set of the freshly placed material is not affected by the presence of moisture, including blood. It is less cytotoxic and more tissue compatible than previously used materials. Reports from animal studies demonstrate less inflammation and greater cementum deposition over set MTA compared with other materials within days of surgery. Furthermore, scanning electron microscopy (SEM) images reveal cementoblasts adhering to the material. The only reported disadvantage of MTA is the slight difficulty in handling and placement.

Wound closure

Once the site has been inspected and any remaining foreign bodies removed, gentle bleeding may be encouraged by simple curettage to ensure a blood clot is present in the wound. A postoperative radiograph should be exposed at the suture removal appointment. Good clinical governance would involve exposing a further radiograph after 1 year to confirm healing and facilitate audit of clinical outcomes. The tooth should be monitored radiographically for up to 4 years.

Periradicular surgery outcomes

It has been demonstrated that periradicular microsurgical techniques can achieve success rates of 92.5% over a 3-year observation period. It is also established that the use of modern materials, magnification, improved surgical techniques, and better postgraduate training results in improved surgical success rates over traditional PRS techniques.

Recommended reading

Carotte P, Murray C. (2010) Endodontic Surgery. In: *Oral & Maxillofacial Surgery*. (eds, Andersson L, Kahnberg K-E, Pogrel MA). Oxford, Wiley-Blackwell.

European Society of Endodontology, quality guidelines for endodontic treatment: consensus report of the European Society of Endodontology. (2006) *International Endodontic Journal*, **39**, 921–30.

Chapter 13

Preprosthetic and Oral Soft Tissue Surgery

Preprosthetic surgery is the surgery that aims to improve tissue conditions for later prosthetic treatment. Earlier in the history of dentistry this meant surgery aiming at increasing the base for stability and retention of removable dentures. However, today the scope of preprosthetic surgery has changed to include also the improvement of the conditions for implant treatment. Nowadays, implant treatment is an increasingly chosen option. For these reasons, this chapter aims to cover both preprosthetic surgery prior to removable dentures and conditions improving the tissue around implants. Moreover, some other simple soft tissue surgical procedures aiming at improving functions and esthetics are covered. However, crestal preparation by bone augmentation prior to implant treatment is covered in Chapters 15–18.

crest for later implant placement. Decoronation of the ankylosed root is a good alternative, which will leave the root for osseous replacement, thereby saving the alveolar process.

When multiple extractions are carried out, there may be postextraction irregularities of the alveolar sockets. The irregular surface may be trimmed with a bur, a rongeur, a fine osteotome or a bone file. Whenever possible, it is better to use a file or rongeur in minor discrepancies to prevent decrease of alveolar height. Various methods for preparation of the crest prior to implant treatment are ridge splitting, filling the extraction socket with biomaterials, membrane techniques and distraction osteogenesis, some of which will be covered in Chapters 15–18.

Surgical methods for alveolar crest preservation

Already during extraction the clinician should be aware of the importance to preserve the alveolar bone crest. Conventional extraction methods may sometimes be traumatic and cause alveolar bone destruction during the healing period. In order to avoid postextraction bone and soft tissue loss, tooth removal may be performed by tissue preserving techniques such as the use of periotome (Fig. 13.1). Bone removal should be avoided or limited, especially the marginal bone to enable later implant installation. Removal of diverging roots can be carried out by first separating them by burs instead of sacrificing bone. Another method of preserving the bone is to remove the roots following drilling them from inside, starting from the pulp chamber. Teeth that have become ankylosed after replantation shall not be removed but left for osseous replacement by bone to preserve the bone

Surgical management of peri-implant soft tissue

Implant-related indications

Preservation of healthy peri-implant soft tissue is an important and challenging part of dental implant treatment. The keratinized attached gingiva seems to be an important factor to avoid inflammation and peri-implantitis and for achieving the best esthetics, especially important in the anterior region. This can be achieved during surgery by planning incisions and by tight adaptation of the soft tissue to the marginal section of a dental implant, forming a natural soft tissue barrier. In an edentulous area a crestal incision is widely used to facilitate soft tissue adaptation around necks of non-submerged implants (Figs 13.2 and 13.3). The incisions should be placed at the crestal level in order to leave adequate amounts of keratinized and well-perfused mucosa at both buccal and lingual sites.

Essentials of Oral and Maxillofacial Surgery, First Edition. Edited by M. Anthony Pogrel, Karl-Erik Kahnberg and Lars Andersson.
© 2014 John Wiley & Sons, Ltd. Published 2014 by John Wiley & Sons, Ltd.
Companion website: www.wiley.com/go/pogrel/oms

Regeneration

The papilla regeneration technique is a simple and innovative method to form a new papilla between implants or teeth. A small palatal or lingual crestal incision is made to uncover the implant and, immediately after a healing cap is inserted, a semilunar incision is performed in the keratinized gingiva and the tissue rotated interproximally to form a new papilla (Fig. 13.4).

Oral soft tissue grafting

Sometimes it may be advantageous to graft keratinized gingiva to increase the width of the attached gingiva of the implant site. The host region should provide proper vascularization properties for graft integration. Grafts can be taken from the palatal

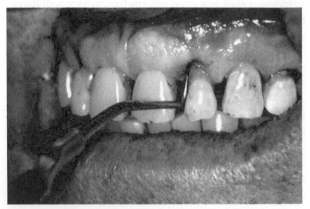

Fig. 13.1 Socket preservation. Removal of the maxillary lateral incisor by periotome.

mucosa and subepithelial connective tissue can be used to augment concavities.

Palatal mucosa grafting

Mucosal palatal grafts has been used successfully for years in periodontal practice to cover denuded roots. A similar philosophy can be applied to the soft tissue around dental implants in situations with loose alveolar mucosa. Attached keratinized gingiva can be grafted from the palate. Restoration of a wide band of attached gingiva around dental implants can be seen in Figures 13.5 and 13.6.

Subepithelial connective tissue grafting

Concavities in the crest (Fig. 13.7a) can be built up for enhancement of esthetics. Subepithelial connective tissue grafts harvested from the palate can be used. These grafts are inserted in a split thickness pocket. Healing is facilitated by the graft being interposed between split-thickness upper layer and the periosteum so it receives its perfusion from both sites (Fig. 13.7).

Recontouring of bone tissue

Treatment of bone exostoses, tori and genial tubercles

Exostosis of alveolar bone is a benign osseous hypertrophic formation of unknown etiology. Palatal and lingual exostoses, known as "tori" are observed

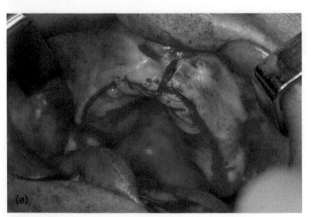

(a)

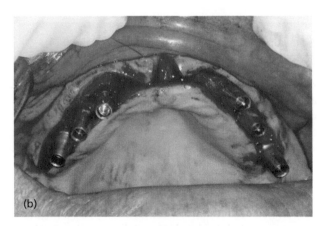

(b)

Fig. 13.2 Flap design for edentulous maxillary arch.

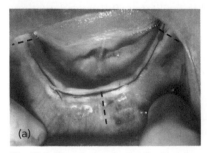

(a)

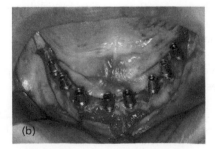

(b)

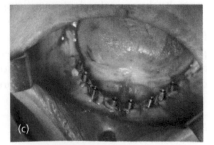

(c)

Fig. 13.3 Flap design for total edentulous mandibular arch. The dotted lines indicates the vertical releasing incisions if needed.

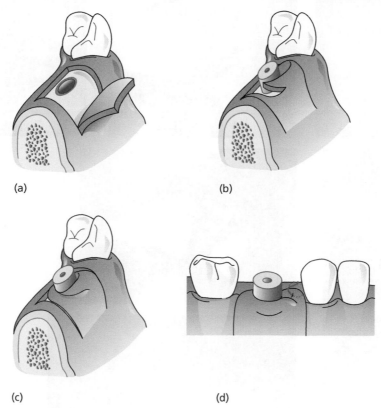

(a)

(b)

(c)

(d)

Fig. 13.4 The papilla regeneration technique.

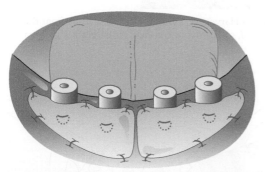

Fig. 13.5 Schematic representation of onlay palatal mucosa grafting to form peri-implant attached mucosa at the neck level of implants.

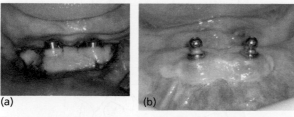

(a)

(b)

Fig. 13.6 (a) Palatal mucosal graft adapted to the host site. (b) Free palatal graft increased the width of labial attached gingiva.

mostly in the middle of the palatal vault. Palatal tori can be broad, lobulated, or nodular. If a patient's function is compromised, e.g. speaking, they may be removed, otherwise there is no indication for removal.

In edentulous patients, however, removal is recommended to facilitate denture retention and stability. To remove them, the principle is to raise a mucoperiosteal flap, resect the bone and smoothen the bone with an osteotome or a bur. Large tori are sectioned first with a fissure bur and then removed with an osteotome or a big round bur (Fig. 13.8). Extra care is taken to avoid extensive removal of palatal bone and subsequent perforation of the nasal floor. The flaps are sutured after irrigation with saline. A surgical stent, made prior to surgery, is inserted containing a tissue conditioner to avoid formation of a hematoma and dead space under the stent.

Lingual tori are generally bilateral and can be singular, lobulated or multiple. The lingual tori are accessed with horizontal crestal incision. Vertical incision must be avoided. Lingual tori can be removed with a bur or an osteotome.

The genioglossal muscle attaches to the genial tubercle located at the lingual aspect of mandible. As the mandible resorbs, the genial tubercle becomes prominent and the mouth floor ascends simultaneously with the resorption process. The activity of the genioglossal muscle and protuberance of the genial tubercle complicates wear of dentures by causing dislocation during function. A crestal incision is performed with scalpel along the anterior ridge. Subperiosteal dissection is continued under the lingual mucoperiosteum until the genial tubercles and muscles become evident. The genial tubercle is resected with a fissure or round bur.

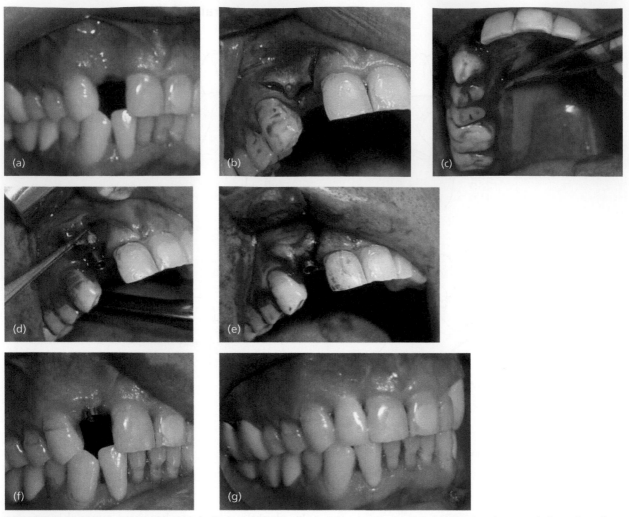

Fig. 13.7 (a) Mucosal cavity in the buccal gingiva. (b) Design of incision. (c) Harvest of a connective tissue graft from the palate. (d, e) Insertion of the graft and slight roll-up of the flap over the abutment. (f, g) Postoperative view of the grafted gingiva during and after prosthetic treatment.

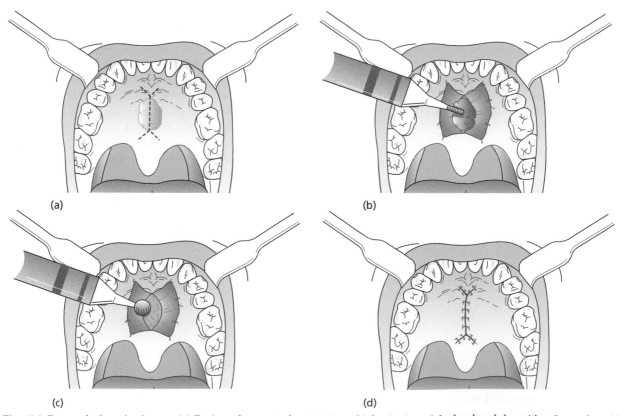

Fig. 13.8 Removal of a palatal torus. (a) Design of an open-door incision. (b) Sectioning of the hard nodules with a fissure bur. (c) Smoothing the palatal bone with an egg-shaped bur. (d) Final closure.

Recontouring of soft tissue

Maxillary tuberosity reduction

Fibrous enlargement of the maxillary tuberosity may increase vertical dimension at the posterior ridge and limit the intermaxillary space required for dentures and the fibrous tissue may also reduce the stability of the denture. To reduce the fibrous tissue, a wedge-shaped resection of excessive tuberosities is carried out (Fig. 13.9). Excessive fibrous

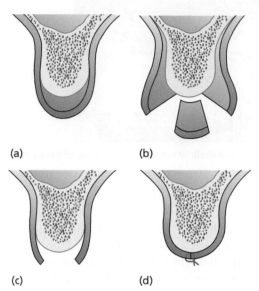

(a)   (b)

(c)   (d)

Fig. 13.9 Reduction of maxillary tuberosity. (a) Redundant soft tissues of the maxillary tuber. (b) The wedge excision. (c) Undermining the submucous tissues. (d) Final closure.

soft tissue is removed from the inside of the buccal and palatal flaps.

Frenectomy

Various techniques have been described for removal of active and strong frenum attachments.

The diamond-shaped excision is usually used and provides optimal results. Eversion of the upper lip also helps to identify borders of a frenum. Two hemostatic clamps are applied to the superior and inferior section of the maxillary midline diastema. The clamped tissue is resected immediately from the mucosa. The upper vertical incision is closed with simple sutures and the inferior part, localized at the attached gingiva, is left to heal secondarily (Fig. 13.10).

The Z-plasty technique may produce less scarring than the diamond-shaped excision. Z-plasty is usually indicated for a frenum with a wide crestal part and shorter alveolar height because it increases alveolar height. An incision is made directly along the length of a frenum. Superior and inferior incisions are placed to form triangles. After supraperiosteal undermining, the apex of the inferior triangle is rotated upwards and conversely the apex of the superior triangle is rotated downwards (Fig. 13.11).

Lingual frenectomy

In edentulous older patients, the lingual frenum may attach high at the crestal level. This attachment may cause speech difficulties and denture instability. Fibrotic tissue starting from alveolar ridge to the base of tongue is resected.

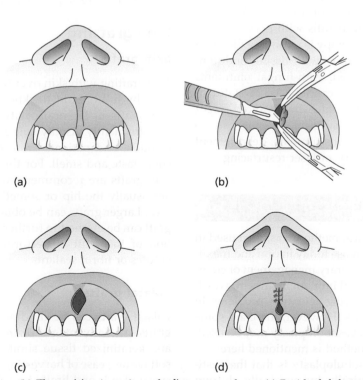

(a)   (b)

(c)   (d)

Fig. 13.10 (a) A labial frenum. (b) The excision is performed adjacent to a clamp. (c) Residual defect after excision. (d) Suturing upper end of the wound, the lower raw surface is left for secondary epithelialization.

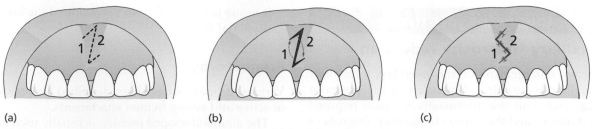

Fig. 13.11 The Z-plasty frenectomy technique. (a) Outlining of the Z flaps. (b) Creating the small triangular flaps. (c) Rotation of the flaps and final closure.

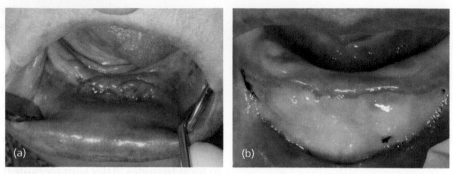

Fig. 13.12 (a) Preoperative intraoral view of a patient with a wide hyperplasia and shallow vestibular sulcus. (b) 10 days postoperatively. The healing occurs by secondary epithelialization.

Removal of palatal papillary hyperplasia

Papillary hyperplasia of palatal mucosa is a pathologic condition associated with suboptimally fitting dentures. Papillary hyperplasia is presented with reddish small nodular inflammation and edema of palatal mucosa. Mechanical irritation seems to be an initial factor; however, isolated cultures from lesions demonstrate predominance of *Candida albicans*, a species that increases in mouths with poor levels of oral hygiene. An initial therapy is removing ill-fitting dentures or relining dentures with tissue conditioners over a 6-month period. Anti-fungal ointments may be used to eliminate candidiasis. Nystatin or clotrimazole are drugs of choice. In advanced stages of papillary hyperplasia, surgical excision can be accomplished with rotary instruments, debridement with scalpel, electrocautery, or laser resurfacing.

Vestibuloplasty

This preprosthetic surgical method was often used in the past, but is seldom in use today in oral and maxillofacial surgery. Contemporary management of edentulous patients is by dental implant treatment, which is more effective for solving retention problems in extensively resorbed jaws. However, there are some special situations when vestibuloplasty may be used, so for this reason the method is mentioned here.

The principle of vestibuloplasty is that the vestibulum is extended apically by surgically shifting

tissue apically and the denuded open exposed soft tissue area is left for secondary epithelialization (Fig. 13.12). The thought behind this is that the denture-bearing area can be extended. However, the extension of the vestibulum results in rapid relapse due to scar contraction. To avoid this, attempts have been made to cover the denuded area by a graft, which can be either a free graft or by the use of a flap moved in from nearby areas (pedicled flap).

Free grafting

Skin grafts

Free grafting with skin over the denuded area can be used by full or split thickness grafts. Full-thickness skin grafts in the oral cavity are not ideal because they frequently display hair growth and thick keratinization, and patients are often disturbed by their color, taste and smell. For this reason split thickness skin grafts are recommended. The skin donor sites are usually the hip or sometimes the retroauricular area. Larger grafts can be obtained from the hip. The graft can be meshed to further increase the area. Fixation of the graft is performed by surgical stents, sutures or fibrin sealants.

Palatal grafts

Palatal grafts can be used as an alternative to skin grafts. The advantages of intraoral palatal grafting are: keratinized tissue similar to adjacent intraoral soft tissues; ease of harvesting; lack of hair follicles or sweat glands and limited morbidity (Fig. 13.13).

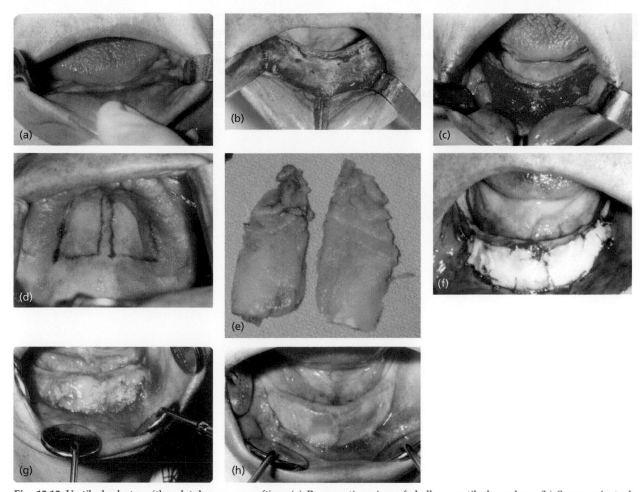

Fig. 13.13 Vestibuloplasty with palatal mucosa grafting. (a) Preoperative view of shallow vestibular sulcus. (b) Supraperiosteal dissection. (c) Suturing mucosal flap to the deepest level at the newly formed sulcus. (d) Marking the palatal mucosa prior to harvest. (e) The harvested palatal mucosa. (f) Healing after 1 week. (g) Complete healing of the palatal grafts. (h) The newly formed vestibular sulcus.

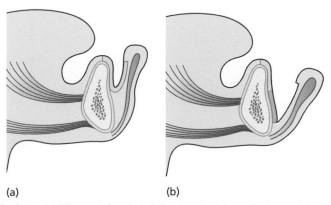

Fig. 13.14 Kazanjian's vestibuloplasty. (a) The crestal pedicled flap is raised from the inner side of the lip. (b) The flap is sutured over the periosteum to the deepest point of dissection.

Pedicled flaps

Coverage of the denuded crestal area can also be carried out with a pedicled flap from nearby tissue areas. An example of this is the vestubuloplasty where a transvestibular horizontal mucosal incision is made in the lower lip between the right and left premolars. The mucosa is dissected supraperiosteally to the alveolar crest, which is followed by supraperio-steal dissection of the mental muscles to the vestibular depth. The pedicled flap is sutured to the periosteum to the depth of the vestibular sulcus. The open wound in the vestibular sulcus and inner lip is left to heal by secondary epithelialization (Fig. 13.14). Variation of the method has been described but, as mentioned earlier, few of the preprosthetic vestibuloplasty methods are in use today due to the development of implant dentistry.

Recommended reading

Basa S, Uckan S, Kisnisci R. (2010) Preprosthetic and Oral Soft tissue Surgery. In: *Oral and Maxillofacial Surgery* (eds, Andersson L, Kahnberg K-E, Pogrel MA). Oxford, Wiley-Blackwell.

Fonseca RJ, Frost DE, Hersh EV, Levin LM. (2000) *Oral and Maxillofacial Surgery*. Philadelphia, WB Saunders.

Hupp JR, Ellis EE, Tucker MR. (2013) *Contemporary Oral and Maxillofacial Surgery*. St Louis, Elsevier Mosby.

Palacci P, Ericsson I, Engstrand P, Rangert B. (1995) Peri-implant soft tissue management: papilla regeneration technique. In: *Optimal Implant Positioning and Soft Tissue Management for the Brånemark System.* pp. 59–70. Chicago, Quintessence Publishing.

Part 3: Implant Surgery

(Section Editor: Karl-Erik Kahnberg)

Chapter 14

Implantology

Evidence-based oral implant therapy was presented to the dental community in the early 1980s. Foreign materials have, however, long been used to replace missing teeth. For example, subperiosteal and blade implants had been used for some decades when pure titanium screw-shaped implants were introduced by the experimental and clinical work of P-I Brånemark. Today, the use of osseointegrated oral implants is considered to be standard procedure for the treatment of total and partial edentulism. Long-term clinical data on modern implant systems on the market today have, in general, shown high survival rates and minimal marginal bone loss around the implants. However, critical reviews of the scientific literature have concluded that some, often low-price systems, are not yet sufficiently documented in long-term clinical trials.

One prerequisite for successful anchorage and long-term function of titanium implants is that a sufficient volume of healthy bone is available in order to house adequate numbers and sizes of implants. The density of the bone is also a determinant of implant success, since failure is more common in bone with low mineral content.

Biological principles behind osseointegration

Implant stability and loading considerations

In the early days of implant dentistry, the use of osseointegrated implants always included a healing period of typically 3–6 months from placement to prosthetic treatment. The formation of direct bone–implant contacts was considered a prerequisite before loading could be commenced (Fig. 14.1).

Today, immediate/early loading of dental implants is a clinical reality and numerous clinical studies have demonstrated as good results as those previously reported for two-stage implants. This has changed the understanding of what factors are important for a successful clinical outcome. In the early days, focus was mainly paid to the osseointegration process *per se*, whilst today a general stability concept is discussed where bone healing is one of several important factors.

The clinical manifestation of a successful dental implant is the absence of mobility. Thus, achievement and maintenance of implant stability are prerequisites for a successful clinical outcome with dental implants. The main determinants of implant stability are: (1) the mechanical properties of the bone tissue at the implant site and (2) how well the implant is engaged with that bone tissue. The first factor is determined by the composition of the bone at the implant site and is influenced by stage of healing, since soft trabecular bone seems to be transformed to dense cortical bone near the implant surface. The second factor is influenced by the surgical technique, the design of the implant, and the osseointegration process. Successful healing results in bone formation that reinforces the interface zone and forms bridges and a direct contact between the implant surface and the surrounding bone (Fig. 14.2). Unsuccessful healing results in formation of an interface fibrous scar tissue (Fig. 14.3), which can be caused by infection or mobility of the implant after installation.

However, a clinically stable and successful implant also shows a certain degree of mobility on the microscale when a load is applied. For instance, if applying a lateral load (bending) to an implant in bone, the implant will be displaced but will return to its original position as soon as the load is removed (Fig. 14.4). Thus, a stable implant can display different degrees of stability, i.e. different degrees of displacement or

Essentials of Oral and Maxillofacial Surgery, First Edition. Edited by M. Anthony Pogrel, Karl-Erik Kahnberg and Lars Andersson.
© 2014 John Wiley & Sons, Ltd. Published 2014 by John Wiley & Sons, Ltd.
Companion website: www.wiley.com/go/pogrel/oms

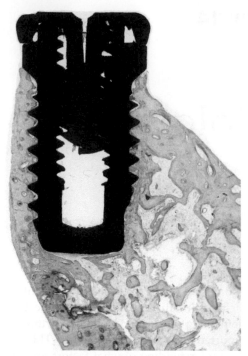

Fig. 14.1 Light micrograph of an osseointegrated implant, retrieved from the posterior mandible of a patient 6 months after placement. The implant is surrounded by cortical and trabecular bone.

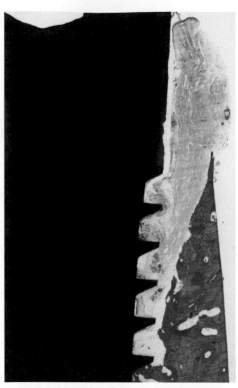

Fig. 14.3 Light micrograph of a clinically failed and retrieved implant. The implant is separated from the bone by a layer of fibrous scar tissue.

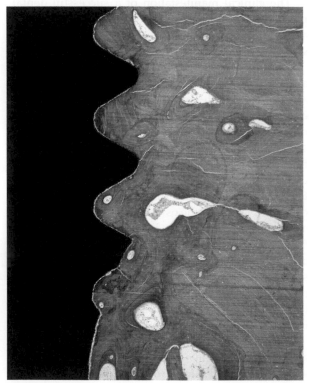

Fig. 14.2 Light micrograph of a clinically retrieved implant showing dense cortical bone in contact with the implant surface and with signs of ongoing remodeling.

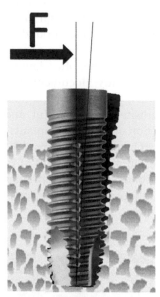

Fig. 14.4 Schematic showing displacement of an osseointegrated implant in the bone bed due to application of a lateral load.

resistance to load, depending on factors relating to the bone, the surgical technique, and the implant design. During clinical function, loading will be applied in axial, lateral, and rotational directions (Fig. 14.5). Furthermore, axial loads can be in push-in or

pull-out directions. Lateral loads can principally be applied from any direction 360° around the implant. Rotational loading can either be clockwise or anti-clockwise. Thus, the outcome of implant stability analysis depends greatly on the type of test used and in which direction the load is applied. In essence, stability measurements in bending give information about the stiffness of the implant–bone system, while application of shear forces, with for instance a reverse torque test, measures the strength of the interface. This means that a newly placed implant can show a high degree of lateral stability but is easily removed when applying reverse torque since bone has not been formed and interlocked with the implant surface. With time, bone formation will lead to an increased interlocking with the implant surface and an increased strength of the interface, whilst the lateral stability may be unaffected. Since most implants will be connected with a framework, reverse torque tests are probably less relevant than measurements of lateral stability.

Primary stability

Implant stability is the result of contact between the implant surface and surrounding bone tissue. The degree of primary stability after installation depends

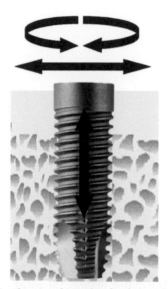

Fig. 14.5 An implant is subjected to loads in axial, lateral, and rotational directions.

on factors related to the bone, surgical technique, and implant design. The biomechanical properties of bone are determined by the ratio of cortical and trabecular bone at an implant site. Cortical bone is built up of densely packed mineralized lamellae, whilst trabecular bone is porous in structure and contains more soft tissue components than mineralized tissue (Fig. 14.6). For this reason cortical bone is 10–20 times stiffer than trabecular bone and provides a better support for an implant. The surgical technique can influence implant stability depending on the choice of drill diameters, depth of preparation, and whether pretapping is used or not. The implant itself also has impact on stability depending on its geometrical features. In a human cadaver study, it was demonstrated that bone density and implant design are important factors that influence primary stability as measured by resonance frequency analysis. They also found that 1° tapering of an implant dramatically increased the primary stability in poor bone. In continuing work, it was shown that primary stability also is influenced by drill diameter and whether pretapping is used or not. In essence, thinner drill diameters, omitting pretapping, and the use of a tapered implant will result in higher primary stability.

Secondary stability

After implant placement the bone tissue will respond to the surgical trauma, which with time results in: (1) a change of the cortical/trabecular bone ratio and (2) an increasing degree of bone–implant contact. The time needed for completion of bone formation and remodeling is in the range of 12–18 months. The impact of the degree of bone–implant contact for secondary implant stability is not known in detail, although it is generally anticipated that more bone contact means better implant stability. However, the change of the trabecular network into a more cortical

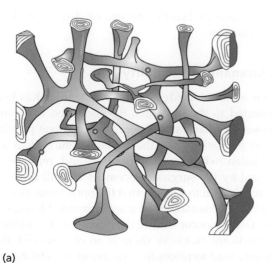

(a)

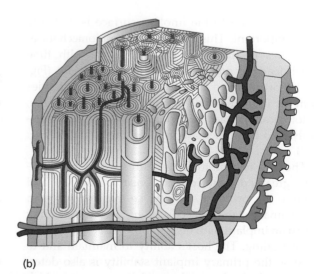

(b)

Fig. 14.6 (a) Schematic of trabecular bone. One unit of trabecular bone tissue is mineralized to 40–60%. (b) Schematic showing cortical bone. One unit of cortical bone tissue is mineralized to 90–95%.

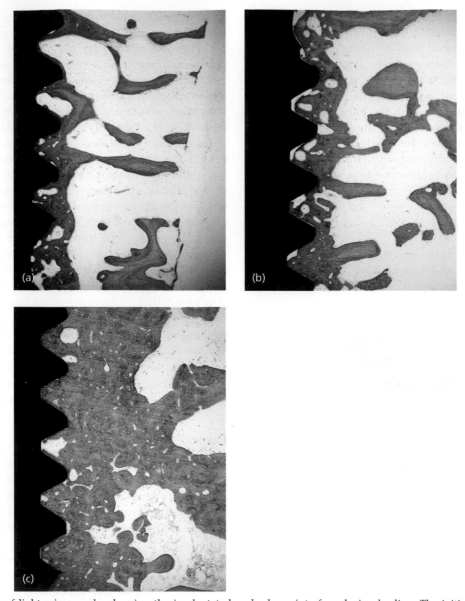

Fig. 14.7 Series of light micrographs showing the implant–trabecular bone interface during healing. The initially slender bone trabeculae forms direct contacts with the implant surface. Continuous apposition of bone results in an increased density of the peri-implant bone.

bone in relation to the implant surface is probably more important. This means that the biomechanical properties of trabecular bone improve with time which leads to greater stability of the implant (Fig. 14.7). Cortical bone already has favorable properties from an implant stability point of view. Therefore, histological changes of cortical bone will not necessarily lead to an increase in secondary stability (Fig. 14.8).

The time needed to achieve sufficient implant stability greatly depends on the density of the bone and thereby the primary stability, i.e. an implant with low primary stability needs a long period of healing whilst an implant with high stability needs only short or no healing. The host's ability to maintain and to increase the primary implant stability is also determined by the healing and remodeling capacity, which in turn is influenced by endogenous and exogenous factors such as health, the use of drugs, smoking, irradiation, etc.

Maintenance of stability

When a crown/bridge or an overdenture has been connected to the implants, the conveyed loads and stresses will have an influence on the bone physiology. In the early phase, the implant–bone system will be loaded while bone formation and remodeling induced by the surgical placement are still ongoing. It is reasonable to suggest that the bone tissue is more sensitive at this stage than after completed healing as most failures occur during the first year of loading. If the loads are excessive there is an obvious risk that this may lead to resorption, decrease of stability, and eventual loss of the implant. If the loads are within physiological limits it is probable that loading may

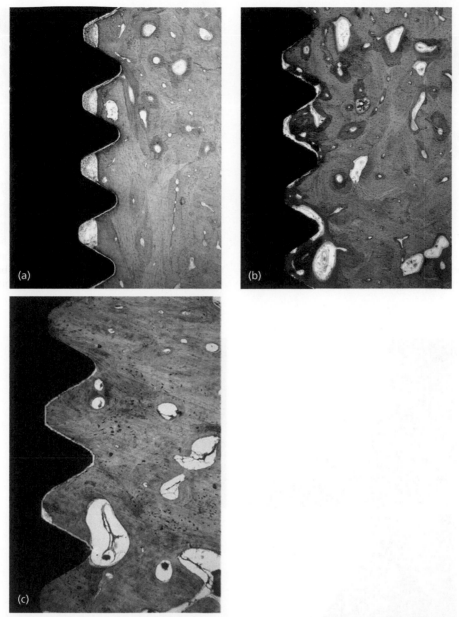

Fig. 14.8 Series of light micrographs showing the implant–cortical bone interface during healing. Apart from bone formation and fill of the voids at the interface, no major changes of the peri-implant bone density can be seen.

stimulate further remodeling and adaptation of the bone to the present load situation. Overload has to be looked upon as a relative parameter since this describes an imbalance between loads and the degree of implant stability. In other words, for a given load the overload threshold is lower for an implant with low stability than for one with high stability.

Bone tissue responses to implants

The bone healing process around a dental implant resembles that of normal bone healing. The surgical trauma created during the insertion of an implant initiates an immediate and preprogrammed healing response at the bone–implant interface. This process involves the formation of a blood clot containing erythrocytes and biologically potent cells such as leukocytes and thrombocytes. Cytokines and factors

from these cells, the coagulation process, and injured tissues act as chemotactic stimuli on leukocytes and other cell types. The fibrin network within the blood clot provides an important scaffold for migrating cells involved in the formation of new tissues, such as vessels, extracellular matrix, and bone. Mesenchymal cells in the granulation tissue will differentiate to preosteoblasts and subsequently osteoblasts and start to produce immature woven bone (Fig. 14.9). If a certain surface topography is present, new bone formation will occur directly at the implant surface (Fig. 14.10). Bone formation is also seen at the pre-existing bone surfaces facing the implant, probably as a result of activation of so-called resting cells and by populations of newly differentiated stem cells (Fig. 14.11). With time the new bone from adjacent bone surfaces will reach the implant surface and create bone–implant contacts and fuse with the bone initially

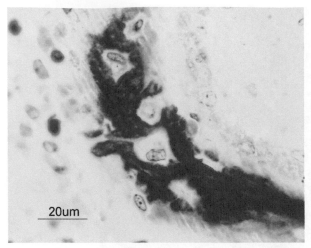

Fig. 14.9 Light micrograph showing osteoblasts producing woven bone in a loose connective tissue near an implant surface 7 days after surgery in the rabbit tibia.

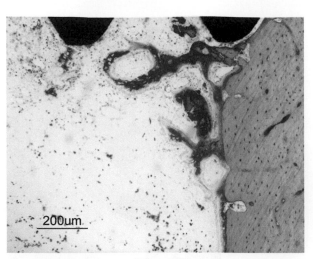

Fig. 14.11 Light micrograph showing formation of woven bone from the endosteal surface from the cortical bone towards an implant 7 days after insertion in the rabbit tibia.

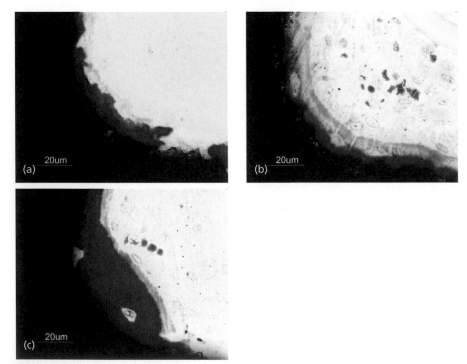

Fig. 14.10 Series of light micrographs showing bone formation directly on an implant surface in the rabbit tibia. (a) An acellular dark stained matrix is seen on the surface (7 days). (b) Osteoblasts producing osteoid are now visible (7 days). (c) Ongoing bone formation from the surface towards the adjacent tissues. Some osteocytes are seen near the surface (14 days).

formed in the granulation tissue near or at the implant surface. A rapid increase of new bone area and degree of bone–implant contact is seen during the early healing period (Fig. 14.12). Bone regeneration occurs in two stages and this is also the case around dental implants. The immature woven bone is replaced by mature lamellar bone through a remodeling process. This is done by bone metabolizing units (BMUs), which contain osteoclasts, which resorb the woven bone, followed by a seam of osteoblasts, which lay down new layers of bone (Fig. 14.13). It is anticipated that the early bone formation takes about 3–4 months,

whilst the remodeling process of the repair may take another 9–12 months in humans. However, physiological remodeling is a continuous process since it is part of the calcium metabolism system (Fig. 14.14).

The majority of early studies on implant integration used machined, minimally rough implants. Today, it is well known that implants with increased surface roughness can result in more rapid integration, with more bone contacts at an earlier stage as a result. Moreover, it seems likely the pathways of implant integration may be different for different surfaces and terms like "contact" and "distance" osteo-

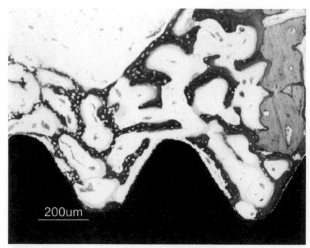

Fig. 14.12 Light micrograph showing extensive bone formation near and at the implant surface 14 days after insertion in the rabbit tibia.

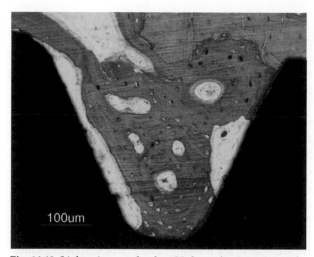

Fig. 14.13 Light micrograph taken 28 days after insertion in the rabbit tibia. Most of the thread is filled with new bone which is undergoing remodeling as indicated by the presence of secondary osteons.

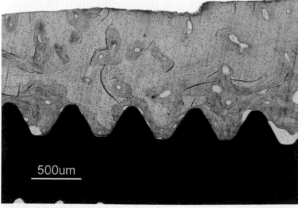

Fig. 14.14 Light micrograph of an implant that had been in clinical function for 9 months. Note the formation of secondary osteons indicating ongoing remodeling.

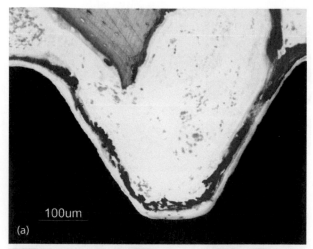

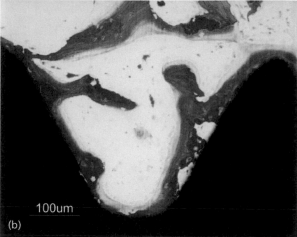

Fig. 14.15 Light micrographs demonstrating differences between a minimally rough and a moderately rough implant surface after 7 days of healing in the rabbit tibia. (a) Bone is formed at a distance from the turned and smoother surface. (b) Bone is formed at and along the surface of a moderately rough implant.

genesis have been coined to distinguish between the two modes of implant integration. Contact osteogenesis means that the implant is integrated by formation of bone directly to the implant surface and distance osteogenesis means that bone is formed from pre-existing bone surfaces towards the implant surface. The differences between contact and distance osteogenesis were demonstrated in a kinetic study comparing oxidized and machined implant surfaces in a rabbit model after 7, 14, and 28 days. The surface-modified implants showed bone formation by osteoblasts directly on the surface, whilst bone formation occurred in the granulation tissue at a distance from the machined implant surfaces (Fig. 14.15). This may be because the initial blood clot retains better to the rough implant surface. The clot can then serve as a scaffold/matrix for migration of mesenchymal cells to the interface. At a smooth implant surface, shrinkage of the blood clot, which occurs after some time, will result in a gap at the implant interface (Fig. 14.16a), whereas the interface is maintained at a

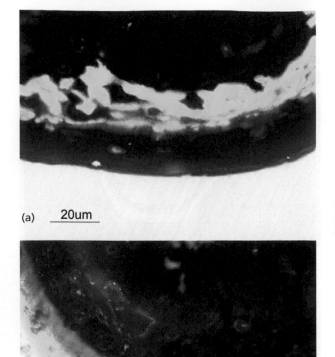

(a)   20um

(b)   20um

Fig. 14.16 Close-up of Fig. 14.15a, b. (a) Distance osteogenesis near a turned implant. (b) Contact osteogenesis at a moderately rough surface.

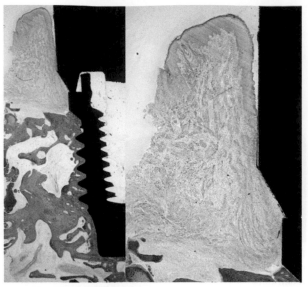

Fig. 14.17 Light micrograph of a clinically retrieved implant with mucosa penetrating abutment. The morphology of the implant–soft tissue interface resembles that of teeth.

rough surface (Fig. 14.16b). Using the microimplant technique, Ivanoff and co-workers demonstrated more bone–implant contacts as well as more bone in the threads of implants modified by blasting or by anodic oxidation compared with machined controls. They observed bone formation at and along the surface of the modified implants whilst the machined implants seemed to be integrated by bone formed from the surrounding pre-existing bone walls. However, in spite of the biological benefits with surface-modified implants, randomized clinical studies with up to 5 years of follow-up have demonstrated no differences in normal patient populations. Having said this, the experiences with surface-modified implants in more challenging situations, such as bone grafting and immediate loading, indicate superior outcomes with surface-modified implants. The failure rate with machined implants in reconstructive cases was reported to be around 8%. The same research group's experiences from the first 200 surface-modified implants, including varying reconstruction techniques, showed a failure rate of 0.5%. The results indicate that in biologically challenging situations surface modification may make a difference. Similar experiences have been noted when applying an immediate loading

protocol, which is another example of a biologically challenging situation. Glauser and co-workers reported a failure rate of 17.3% for immediately loaded machined implants and only 3% for oxidized implants. The histology of clinical oxidized implants, retrieved after 5–9 months of immediate or early (2 months of healing prior to loading) loading showed high degrees of integration. Formation of bone directly at the implant surface (i.e. contact osteogenesis) could be demonstrated.

The contact osteogenesis properties may have a significant impact on clinical results in terms of the integration of implants in situations where primary bone contacts are missing. The placement of implants in extraction sockets is one example of such a clinical situation. A study in dogs comparing the integration of machined and oxidized implants in bone defects demonstrated a more marked and rapid increase in stability for the latter as measured with resonance frequency analysis (RFA) after 4 and 12 weeks of healing. The histological evaluation also revealed differences in favor of the surface-modified implants, since more bone was in contact with the oxidized titanium after 4 and 12 weeks.

The marginal tissues

The soft tissue barrier around an implant or abutment is important for maintenance of implant stability and long-term clinical function, since it protects the integrity of the bone–implant interface (Fig. 14.17). The morphology of the barrier resembles that of gingiva around teeth and contains a sulcus epithelium, a contact epithelium followed by a zone of connective tissue down to the marginal bone. The presence of capillaries and postcapillary venules suggests that an effective defense mechanism is at hand as inflammatory cells can migrate into the interface for phagocytosis of bacteria and other foreign bodies. One major difference compared with gingiva is the direction of the collagen fibers which seem to run parallel with the implant/abutment surface, while perpendicular fibers are also present at teeth.

Some loss of marginal bone is expected during the lifetime of an implant. Studies have shown that the major changes, about 0.5–1.5 mm bone loss, occur during healing and the first year of loading. The reasons are not well understood, but the initial bone loss is probably related to healing and remodeling of the marginal bone following implant and abutment surgery as well as a response to loading. Mainly based on experimental dog studies, it has been proposed that a submucosal implant–abutment junction results in a micro-gap where microorganisms may be trapped and induce an inflammatory reaction and bone loss. However, follow-up studies have reported similar amounts of marginal bone loss around one-piece and two-piece implant systems, and thus do not support the earlier findings. Moreover, it is generally anticipated that surface roughness and geometric features such as micro-threads at the neck of the implant may minimize marginal bone loss. However, at present the results from clinical follow-up studies are not conclusive on this point. In general, well documented implant systems show minimal average bone loss over time. Having said this, some implants can show extensive marginal bone loss, with or without signs of infection. The incidence and causes of peri-implant bone loss are not well known and are under debate.

Implant components

Implant components are illustrated in Figure 14.18:

- implant fixture;
- cover screw;
- abutments.

Indications for implant treatment

The indications for bone-anchored fixed or removable prostheses are edentulism, partial edentulism, and single tooth loss. In other words, any type of tooth loss is an indication for implant treatment, but it is certainly not the only or even the best solution for all patients. The clinician should always consider the individual situation for each patient and present different prosthetic alternatives together with treatment plans and estimations of costs. The overall goal with implant treatment is to achieve a long-term successfully stable construction. Criteria for successful outcomes with implant-supported prostheses have been proposed. Implant therapy is prescribed to resolve prosthetic problems and such prostheses should meet the clinically evolved standards of func-

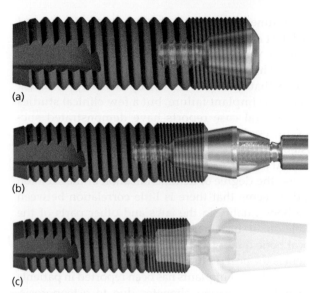

Fig. 14.18 (a) Cross-section of fixture and cover screw. (b) Cross-section of fixture and abutment + bridge screw for screw-retained construction. (c) Abutment in zirconium for a cement-retained crown.

tion, comfort, and esthetics. The prostheses should also allow for routine maintenance and should permit planned or unplanned revisions of the existing design. Treatment outcome success criteria for implant-supported prostheses should also be assessed in context of time-dependent considerations for any required retreatment. The success criteria comprise the following determinants:

1. The resultant implant support does not preclude the placement of a planned functional and esthetic prostheses that is satisfactory to both patient and clinician.
2. There is no pain, discomfort, altered sensation or infection attributable to the implants.
3. Individual unattached implants are immobile when tested clinically.
4. The mean vertical bone loss is less than 0.2 mm annually following the first year of function.

Contraindications

Medical contraindications

The absolute contraindications to implant treatment are few but similar to those for all other types of surgeries. As with any surgical intervention, the implant patient should be assessed preoperatively to evaluate his or her ability to tolerate the treatment. Absolute contraindications to implant surgery are limited to acute illness, terminal illness, uncontrolled metabolic disease, and severe bleeding disorders.

Systemic risk factors

Systemic or general risk factors such as age, smoking, and osteoporosis have been suspected to influence the treatment outcome. Follow-up studies have failed to detect any differences between patients under and over 60 years. Even the age group over 80 years showed high implant survival rates. It has been anticipated that osteoporosis/osteopenia may be a risk factor for implant failure, but a few clinical studies and several case reports have demonstrated successful clinical results in patients with diagnosed osteoporosis. So-called dual energy X-ray absorptiometry (DEXA) measurements have been used to assess the degree of demineralization of the skeleton and it seems that there is little correlation between the bone quality in the jaws and other parts of the skeleton. It has therefore been suggested that the local bone quality as classified during implant placement is the best predictor for implant failure. Interestingly, failure of implants has been reported in patients treated with bisphosphonates due to osteoporosis. There is, however, little evidence yet that oral bisphosphonate medication in relatively low doses increases the risk for implant failure. On the other hand, intravenous administration of bisphosphonates in high doses due to skeletal malignancies may increase the risk of jaw bone osteomyelitis/necrosis. Additionally, the combination of bisphosphonate treatment and corticosteroids may increase the risk for jaw bone disease.

Patients with metabolic diseases are known to have an impaired bone-healing capacity but well balanced diabetic patients have shown a failure rate similar to that of healthy patients.

Studies have indicated that tobacco smoking is associated with poor peri-implant soft tissue health, marginal bone loss, and implant failure. Even though other clinical investigations have demonstrated little or no negative influence on the peri-implant soft tissues and marginal bone level, in general, implant failure is about twice as common in smokers as in non-smokers. It is known that smoking has a negative influence on peripheral microcirculation and wound healing and it has been suggested that smoking influences bone quality, which in turn may lead to higher failure rate.

It has been suggested that ongoing chemotherapy could increase the risk for implant failure. Recent studies have not confirmed that, but of course ongoing treatment with chemotherapy should be considered as a risk factor.

Local contraindications

The primary local contraindication is irradiation to the head–neck region, ongoing and 1–2 years post treatment. There is a high risk of failure if implants are installed in irradiated bone tissue and there is risk of inducing osteoradionecrosis. Other local contraindications are untreated periodontal disease in residual dentition, periapical lesions at adjacent teeth, other untreated jaw bone infections or cysts, and diseases in the oral mucosa.

Treatment of children and adolescents with oral implants

There are situations when prosthetic rehabilitation of children is needed. Trauma or congenital lack of teeth, such as in cleft patient or children with syndromes, may call for prosthetic treatment. The mouth is important for appearance and self-esteem in the growing individual. Missing teeth should primarily be replaced by orthodontic spaces closure, composite retained onlay bridges or autotransplantation of teeth. Anchoring elements do not follow skeletal growth in space in the same way as biological teeth and therefore placement of osseointegrated implants is usually not indicated in children. During facial growth, the facial bones are displaced relative to each other and to the cranial base, while their surfaces undergo extensive remodeling. The midface grows generally in a downward and forward direction in relation to the cranial base. The mandible has a V-shaped growth pattern which implies a drift of the lingual and buccal cortical plates. Vertical growth is, to a considerable degree, a result of the development of the alveolar process, which in turn is essentially dependent on the presence of the erupting teeth. In experimental and clinical studies it has been shown that osseointegrated implants are stationary during growth and do not erupt with adjacent teeth, which subsequently leads to infra-occlusion for the implant-supported crown or bridge. Additionally, a fixed prosthesis may impede normal skeletal growth. There are, however, situations when the demands for fixed prosthetic rehabilitation with oral or maxillofacial implants are high. The goal in such cases is not to aim initially at lifelong function of the implants and superstructure in the growing patient but to temporarily rehabilitate and accept sequential installation of implants over time, as the maxillofacial anatomy matures.

A more common type of temporary anchorage element in children is the temporary orthodontic implant, which is used as an anchorage for orthodontic forces. This type of implant is pointed, does not require preparation and is inserted without raising a flap. It is inserted in alveolar bone or the palate and is usually not in place more than 12 months. It is simple to remove and local anesthesia is seldom needed at removal.

Treatment planning

Clinical examination

General medical evaluation

As with any surgical intervention, preoperative assessment should be carried out to evaluate the patient's ability to tolerate the procedure. Implant surgery may be associated with certain risks but since it is a relatively atraumatic procedure there are few immediate surgical risks. Absolute contraindications are, as described in Medical contraindications, acute and terminal illness, uncontrolled metabolic disease, and severe bleeding disorders.

Oral health status

A thorough clinical examination is mandatory. Visual inspection and palpation of soft tissues and underlying bone will usually detect excess tissue and give preliminary information of bone shape and width. Time since tooth extraction and status of any remaining dentition should be taken into consideration. Signs of infection or ongoing periodontal disease are contraindications to implant placement. If immediate installation of an implant is planned, the status of the tooth that is to be extracted should be evaluated. Additionally, prosthetic aspects such as loading conditions, interocclusal distance, extension of the superstructure, and any need for cantilevers should be addressed at this stage. Esthetic demands are usually high in the anterior region and therefore the smile line, lip support, mucosal biotype, intercanine distance, and buccal corridors should be clinically evaluated if implant-supported crowns or bridges are planned in the anterior region. Additionally, a facial analysis should be carried out so that any asymmetry or disharmony of the face is noted.

Jaw relations

The sagittal relation between the jaws changes over time in edentulous patients since bone resorption leads to posterior drift of the maxillary alveolar bone and anterior drift of the crest of the mandible. Subsequently, a class III relation will arise. This is, of course, unfavorable both from a loading point of view and maybe also from esthetic aspects. Bone resorption also tends to make the crests narrower, which is why a transversal registration is also of importance. Correct placement of the implants can, at least to a certain degree, compensate for this. In severe cases of resorption, bone augmentation will be needed prior to or in conjunction with implant placement.

Radiographic examination

A comprehensive clinical examination, as described in Oral health status, should always precede the radiographic examination, which should be done with techniques resulting in the lowest dose but still presenting all clinically necessary information. Failure to diagnose and treat pathologic conditions around remaining teeth and/or residual jaw bone can seriously compromise the results of implant therapy. Intraoral radiographs are still most common in dental practice and can be recommended if a paralleling technique is used. This way, a preliminary estimate of the vertical dimension of the implant site can be obtained. Panoramic radiographs are often used in the preliminary planning. Pathology in the jaws can usually be detected and available bone height can be assessed in both anterior and posterior regions. The best estimate of height and width, however, is obtained with cross-sectional tomography. This technique gives a higher radiation dose to the patient and should not be performed without a clear indication. There are some guidelines where indications for cross-sectional imaging in implantology have been presented. These are:

• when minimizing the risk of damage to important anatomical structures;
• to provide more information in cases where there is limited amount of bone height and/or width;
• to improve implant positioning that will optimize biomechanical functional and esthetic results.

Computed tomography (CT) and cone-beam computed tomography (CBCT)

Traditional medical CT scanners are big and expensive and have mostly been used for craniomaxillofacial trauma surgery and for planning of treatment of malignancies in the head and neck region. CBCT scanners have been available for craniofacial imaging since 1999 in Europe and since 2001 in the USA. These scanners use a cone-shaped X-ray beam rather than a conventional linear fan beam to provide images of the structures of the skull and maxillofacial bones. Conventional CT scanners use a single row of solid state detectors paired with a fan-shaped beam to capture the attenuated X-ray. CBCT scanners use a square two-dimensional array of detectors to capture the cone-shaped beam. This means that traditional CT provides a set of consecutive slices of the patient while the CBCT provides a volume of data. Both techniques make it possible to get a three-dimensional (3D) image of the anatomy when software is added to the equipment.

The CBCT scanner is smaller than a traditional CT scanner and the radiation dose is relatively lower, which makes it more popular in dental practice.

Radiographic classification of bone quality

Traditionally, classification of bone quality and sometimes also bone quantity has been registered during implant installation. A scale from 1 to 4 has been used, where 4 is the most demineralized type of bone and gives least mechanical support of the fixture at installation. Today, when tomography is getting more common, this rather subjective system can be replaced by the Hounsfield scale. The bone quality can be shown for each individual implant site (Fig. 14.19).

Hounsfield units:

• D1: >1250 HU;
• D2: 850–1250 HU;

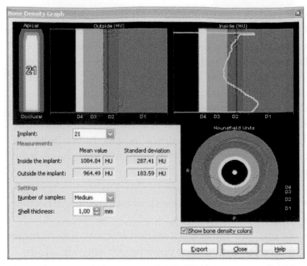

Fig. 14.19 Bone quality, Hounsfield scale.

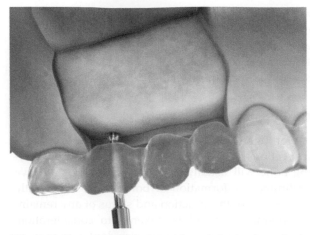

Fig. 14.20 First, the planned position of the implant site is marked with a guide drill. This will provide information about the quality of the marginal bone and is also a start point for the first twist drill.

- D3: 350–850 HU;
- D4: 150–350 HU;
- D5: <150 HU.

Model analyses

Model analyses are typically done on plaster casts and can be used for anatomic registration and for evaluation of occlusion and articulation. Implant fixture position can also be planned on the model. Modern software and the use of 3D planning will, however, most likely put the plaster cast in the history books fairly soon.

Surgical procedure

Regardless of the preoperative planning and choice of surgical protocol, treatment includes site preparation and installation of the implant, aiming at good primary stability. Figures 14.20, 14.21, 14.22, 14.23, 14.24, 14.25 and 14.26 provide a general overview of a standard implant site preparation with raised mucoperiosteal flaps.

If teeth have to be removed because they are impossible to use for prosthetic reconstruction, prepare for implant placement using an atraumatic extraction technique. The aim is to reduce unfavorable postextraction ridge remodeling. Bone grafts and/or resorbable membranes may be used to preserve the ridge during healing, especially in the esthetic zone. Immediate installation of implants after extraction is an alternative to a staged treatment protocol but there are some prerequisites that have to be fulfilled:

- absence of active infection;
- adequate residual ridge;
- possibility for primary stability;

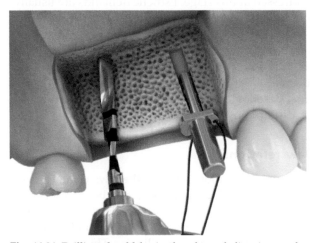

Fig. 14.21 Drilling should be in the planned direction to the appropriate depth under profuse irrigation. A secured indicator can be used to facilitate the direction of the subsequent drilling.

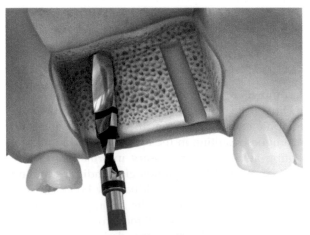

Fig. 14.22 Drilling is done stepwise to the planned diameter. Mesial–distal distance minimum 2mm to adjacent roots and 3–4mm between implants.

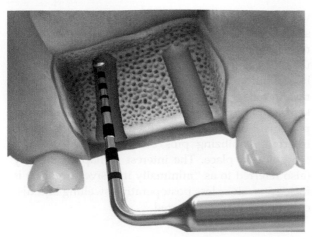

Fig. 14.23 Drilling depth is verified before the implant is inserted.

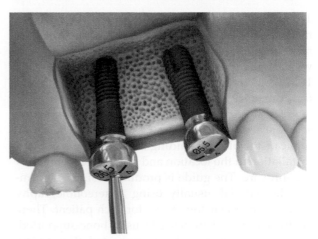

Fig. 14.26 One-stage procedure. Here, the flaps are sutured around the abutments.

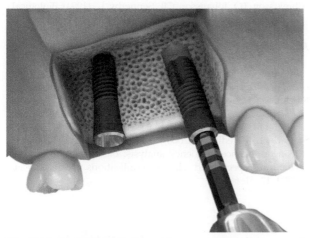

Fig. 14.24 Implant installation with a contra angle at low speed (25 rpm) and maximum torque 35 Ncm.

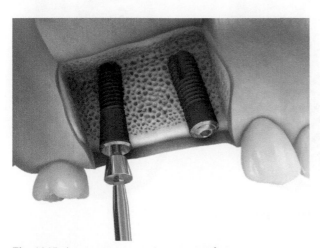

Fig. 14.25 A two-stage procedure means that cover screws are installed and the flaps are repositioned tightly. This method is used when healing period without loading is needed, e.g. in soft bone or when the primary implant stability is poor.

- adjunctive use of bone grafting techniques to correct residual defects may be used, especially if there is a gap of >2 mm between the implant fixture and extraction socket.

Maintenance

Postoperative check-ups are mandatory and the intraoral radiograph is still the gold standard for evaluation of marginal bone level. The requirements for radiographic check-up have changed recently and today an individualized follow-up regimen is advised, which depends on factors such as patient cooperation and marginal bone level changes during the first year post-treatment. Annual radiographs are not recommended if stable marginal levels have been established during the first 1–2 years of function. As a rule of thumb, radiographic evaluation of implants and surrounding bone should be carried out at delivery of the superstructure and then after 1, 3, 5, and 10 years in function. Clinical examination, including registration of plaque and bleeding at probing around the abutments, should be carried out 3 months after delivery of the superstructure and, if without remarks, annually. Good oral hygiene is mandatory after implant treatment, especially if the patient has a history of periodontitis.

Computer-guided implant treatment

When a patient is considered suitable for implant treatment, computer-guided planning and treatment can be used. Computer-guided implant treatment implies that the patient has to go through a CT scan (or CBCT), preferably with a radiopaque scan prosthesis in place, before the data can be imported into a software planning program. There are several different software programs available on the market.

To take full advantage of the concept it is recommended to define from the outset, the type of final restoration, the need for provisional restoration, and what surgical protocol to use. The software (Fig. 14.27) can either be used alone or as a base for manufacturing a surgical guide. If a surgical guide is used, it will be the link between the planning done with the software and the actual surgery. Cylinders in the guide replicate the plan by guiding the drilling and implant installation in the location and orientation defined by the software. The guide is produced using a biocompatible material, usually using a stereolithography process, and is custom-made for each patient. There are three different guides to be used: bone-supported, mucosa-supported or tooth-supported (Fig. 14.28). The bone-supported guide means that a flap has to be raised and the guide should be relatively stable when placed on the alveolar crest. The tooth-supported guide is also fixed and stabilized by the residual dentition and a flapless technique can be used. The so-called mucosa-supported guide means by definition that the surgery is performed without raising a flap. This type of guide will be difficult to keep stable in position during the preparation and placement of implants, so three to four horizontally inserted, stabilizing pins/screw are used to keep the guide in place. The interest in flapless surgery (also referred to as "minimally invasive surgery") is increasing, since less postoperative swelling and discomfort have been reported.

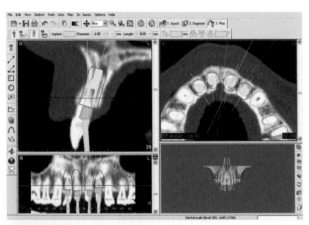

Fig. 14.27 Software for computer-guided implant planning.

Recommended reading

Adell R, Lekholm U, Rockler B, Brånemark P-I. (1981) A 15-year study of osseointegrated implants in the treatment of the edentulous jaw. *International Journal of Oral Surgery*, **10**, 387–416.

Albrektsson TO, Johansson CB, Sennerby L. (1994) Biological aspects of implant dentistry: osseointegration. *Periodontology 2000*, **4**, 58–73.

Albrektsson T, Zarb G, Worthington P, Eriksson AR. (1986) The long-term efficacy of currently used dental implants: a review and proposed criteria of success. *International Journal of Oral and Maxillofacial Implants*, **1**, 11–25.

Rasmussen L, Sennerby L. (2010) Implantology. In: *Oral and Maxillofacial Surgery* (eds, Andersson L, Kahnberg K-E, Pogrel MA). Oxford, Wiley-Blackwell.

Sennerby L, Meredith N. (2008) Implant stability measurements using resonance frequency analysis: biological and biomechanical aspects and clinical implications. *Periodontology 2000*, **47**, 51–66.

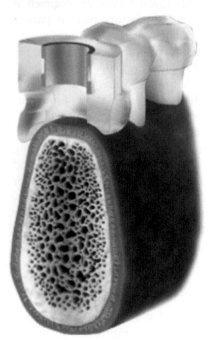
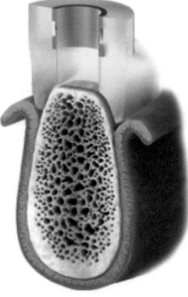
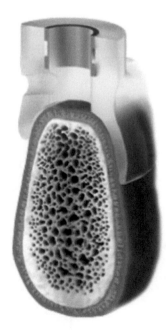

Fig. 14.28 Surgical guides: bone-supported, tooth-supported, and mucosa-support.

Chapter 15

Optimal Implant Placement in the Esthetic Zone by the Use of Guided Bone Regeneration

Biological factors influencing the reconstruction of alveolar bone

An absolute prerequisite for implant treatment is the availability of sufficient alveolar bone to support and retain the endosseous implant. Factors such as infection, cystic lesions, tooth/alveolar trauma or congenital tooth agenesis cause a reduction of the alveolar ridge dimensions to a varying degree. With the increasing drive for optimal esthetic outcome of implant treatment, restoring both the hard and soft tissue levels is essential (Fig. 15.1).

Tooth replacement in the anterior maxilla is a demanding treatment, since the absence of, or poor, preoperative planning, or the choice of an inappropriate treatment approach, can lead to everything from esthetic shortcomings to real disasters.

Esthetic complications can be related to malpositioned implants and the choice of inappropriate prosthetic components. The most critical factors, however, are the anatomic causes that include bone deficiencies in the horizontal or vertical dimensions, and often a combination of the two. This is not infrequently associated with soft tissue defects of the alveolar ridge. Alveolar atrophy and anatomic alterations will have a negative influence on the proper buccal–palatal position of the implant. Malposition of the implant may have effects on the shape, emergence profile, and interproximal contour.

It is important for the clinician to understand that the anatomic contour of the ridge comprises the soft tissue and the underlying supporting bone tissue in all directions. Hence, the soft tissue contour is heavily influenced by the bone anatomy present.

The concept of the so-called biological width has increased the knowledge and understanding of the interaction between the different tissue types and different biomaterial surfaces. In brief, the soft tissue demonstrates relatively constant dimensions in thickness; the peri-implant soft tissue thickness is about 3–4 mm. It is slightly thinner on the buccal aspect and more pronounced at the interproximal areas. The soft tissue is also slightly thicker in the anterior maxillary area in contrast to the posterior region of the mandible, which demonstrates the thinnest portion in the oral cavity.

Due to the relatively constant dimensions of the soft tissue, it is inevitable that the underlying bone structure of the alveolar process plays a key role in the overall esthetic appearance. This is particularly pronounced in the anterior region of the maxilla. This area is also defined as the esthetic zone.

The resorption pattern of the alveolar process following single or multiple tooth loss has been studied in detail and this knowledge is important in the treatment planning of esthetic implant dentistry. Frequently, loss of the buccal bone plate (horizontal resorption) is seen in trauma patients (Fig. 15.1a). This is most pronounced during the first 6 months following the injury. Another important anatomic structure to consider is the interproximal crest height since it plays a significant role in maintaining the peri-implant papillae. Today it is well accepted that vertical resorption of more than 5 mm from the top of the bony crest to the contact point reduces the probability of an intact papilla by approximately 75%. This is particularly the case in situations with multiple tooth loss.

Today's state-of-the-art esthetic treatment not only involves optimally designed crown and bridge solutions. It also involves restoration of the adjacent tissues (Fig. 15.1). Based on the discussion at the beginning of this chapter, a solid base needs to be created. Thus, reconstruction and correction of bone defects are needed. Numerous methods have been

Essentials of Oral and Maxillofacial Surgery, First Edition. Edited by M. Anthony Pogrel, Karl-Erik Kahnberg and Lars Andersson.
© 2014 John Wiley & Sons, Ltd. Published 2014 by John Wiley & Sons, Ltd.
Companion website: www.wiley.com/go/pogrel/oms

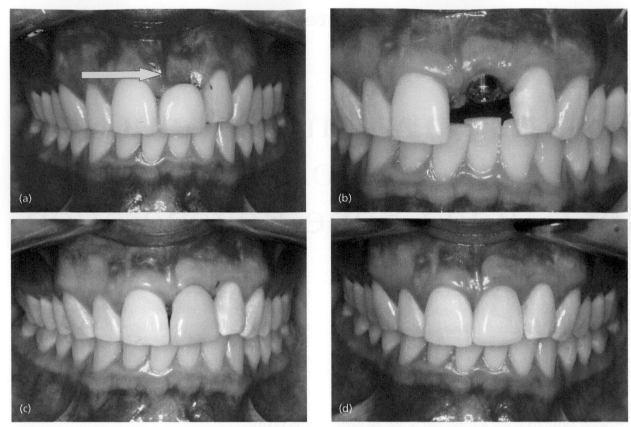

Fig. 15.1 (a) Clinical case demonstrating a trauma at young age and subsequent tooth loss (21). Note the buccal atrophy and concavity (arrow) of the hard and soft tissue. Due to the loss of tissue optimal restoration is not possible from an esthetic point of view. The patient has been temporarily restored with a Maryland bridge while waiting for skeletal growth to be completed. (b) Healing following implant placement and simultaneous GBR procedure. The buccal bone has been augmented with BioOss® and a Bio-Gide® membrane. Note the regained harmony of the contour of the keratinized gingiva of the soft tissue. (c) Ample time should be provided for the soft tissue to mature and stabilize prior to the finalization of the tooth. A combination of a permanent abutment in a biocompatible material and a high-quality temporary crown is provided for at least 2 months. (d) Final restoration of tooth 21 with optimal esthetic result. Note the harmony of the hard and soft tissue in the region providing an ideal emergence profile for the final crown.

used in an attempt to overcome this problem. Previously, one of the most common methods involved the harvesting and implantation of fresh autogenous bone grafts. However, this involves an extra surgical site, and the morbidity for the patient following such an event should not be ignored. Numerous different types of bone substitute materials have been developed and recent advances are of great interest.

The materials can be divided into three categories:

- *Allografts.* This group of materials is derived from an individual of the same species and contains no viable cells. The principles for incorporation of allografts follows the same principles as for fresh autogenous bone grafts but the incorporation process probably proceeds more slowly due to the absence of living cells which are both osteoinductive and responsible for triggering the inflammatory process. Frozen or freeze-dried, mineralized or demineralized bone, demineralized dentin, and antigen-extracted allogenic bone (AAA) are all examples of allograft materials.
- *Alloplastic grafts.* These are developed and derived synthetically and follow the same principles as for allografts, except that the materials contain no proteins and have osteoconductive properties only. Hydroxyapatite (HA) is probably the best known material in this family. Bioactive glass ceramic is another member of this family that has been tested and demonstrates active bone formation. Calcium sulfate (plaster of Paris) has also been evaluated as a grafting material. Recently great interest has been shown in tricalciumphosphate (TCP) materials. This material is osteoconductive and has the capability to be slowly resorbed and eventually replaced by new bone.
- *Xenografts.* A xenogeneic graft is derived from bone tissue originating from various species. In order to avoid an immunologic response and subsequent rejection after implantation, the proteins have to be eliminated. The osteoinductive capacity of the material therefore disappears and this type of graft material only acts as an osteoinductive scaffold. During the last decade a bovine hydroxyapatite (BHA) (Bio-Oss®, Geistlich, Wolhusen, CH) has been developed and widely used in conjunction with implant treatment. It is by far the best documented material available on the market at

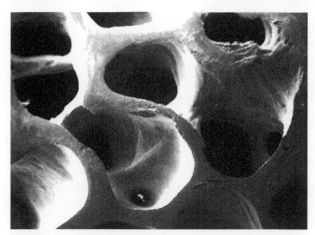

Fig. 15.2 Scanning electron microscopy image of the bovine hydroxyapatite (BHA) structure of BioOss® after deproteinization. The crystalline structure of BHA is very similar to that of human bone.

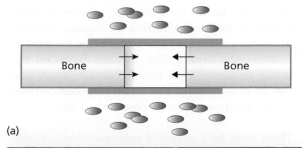

(a)

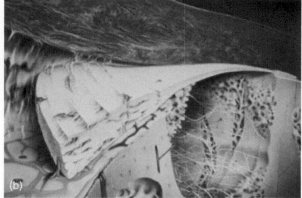

(b)

Fig. 15.3 (a) Schematic drawing illustrating the principle of guided bone regeneration. Barrier membranes are placed in direct contact with the bone surface thereby protecting the defect from interfering soft tissue cells. A secluded environment is created into which only cells from the adjacent bone can migrate. (b) Illustration showing the principle of an e-PTFE barrier membrane. Note the more open portion in the periphery of the barrier, designed to allow more rapid ingrowth of the soft tissue. This will stabilize the membrane and minimize micromovements. Also note the more cell-occlusive portion placed over the defect.

present. The material is quite similar to human bone in its configuration and is considered to be osteoconductive (Fig. 15.2).

However, there is a discussion about whether BHA is resorbable, or is slowly degraded, or is phagocytable or non-resorbable. Recent findings claim that virtually no resorption occurs even after several years. The biological impact of these findings remains to be fully understood. The fact that BHA particles are incorporated into newly regenerated bone could actually be of an advantage in esthetic situations where the material will act as "reinforcement" of the newly formed bone tissue and thereby prevent early resorption of the regenerated bone.

The biological principles of guided bone regeneration

Over the last two decades, the development of the technique of guided bone regeneration (GBR) has had a significant impact on esthetic reconstruction in conjunction with implant therapy. This technique involves the use of physical barrier membranes during the healing phase in order to avoid ingrowth of undesired tissue types into a wound area.

During the 1980s the principle of guided tissue regeneration (GTR) was developed for regenerating periodontal tissues lost as a result of inflammatory periodontal disease. A series of studies documented the possibility of excluding undesirable cells from populating the wound area by means of membrane barriers. This favors the proliferation of defined tissue cells to produce a desired type of tissue (Fig. 15.3).

The principle of physical sealing of an anatomic site for improved healing of certain tissue types is by no means new. During the mid-1950s attempts were made for neural regeneration by the use of cellulose acetate filters.

GBR refers more precisely to the goal of the membrane application than GTR. This concept promotes bone formation by protection against an invasion of competing, non-osteogenic tissues. To this end, bone defects are tightly covered by a barrier membrane of defined permeability and excellent biocompatibility.

Experimental studies have proven that certain tissues within the body possess the biologic potential for regeneration if the proper environment is provided during healing. The ultimate goal of GBR is to use a temporary device to provide the necessary environment so the body can use its natural healing potential and regenerate lost and absent tissues.

The efficacy of barrier membranes in conjunction with bone healing and reconstructive therapy is probably the result of a combination of different mechanisms – mechanical, cellular, and molecular. Examples of these are:

- prevention of fibroblast mass action;
- prevention of contact inhibition by heterotopic cell interaction;
- exclusion of cell-derived soluble inhibitory factors;
- local concentration of growth stimulatory factors;
- stimulatory properties of the membrane itself.

The basic studies on GBR have shown that the sequence of healing occurring in regular fracture repair follows the same basic pattern that is found in osseous lesions during GBR therapy. Based on the scientific evidence available, it can be stated that certain conditions must be met for new bone formation to be predictably accomplished by GBR:

1. There must be a source of osteogenic cells. Viable bone must be present adjacent to the defect where regeneration is desired.
2. An adequate source of vascularity is essential. This supply originates mostly from the adjacent bone surface (Volkmann's canals and marrow compartment).
3. The wound site must remain mechanically stable during healing.
4. An appropriate space must be created and maintained between the membrane and the parent bone surface.
5. Soft connective tissue cells must be excluded from the space created by the membrane barrier. The structure of the material used must be able to accomplish this.

The general function of a membrane used for GBR therapy is to create an environment that will allow the normal healing process to form bone in a defined region (Fig. 15.3). Hence, the host tissue–biomaterial interaction should not interfere with bone formation and maintenance to a clinically significant degree. Biomaterial chemistry and structure should result in minimal foreign body response. Optimal bone–biomaterial interaction characteristics are also desirable. A GBR membrane that allows close adaptation of bone tissue will allow more complete fill of the space defined by the membrane and stabilization of the membrane within the overall system.

Tissue integration

The phenomena of ingrowth and surface bonding of tissue to a biomaterial are termed integration. Surface and microstructural characteristics are usually responsible for these events (Fig. 15.4). The clinical benefits of GBR membranes that have the capacity to integrate with surrounding tissues are a result of a more mechanically stable (and therefore predictable) wound healing environment. While tissue integration appears to be necessary for optimal performance of a GBR membrane, chemical and structural properties that encourage tissue integration must be balanced with the overall functional needs for alveolar ridge augmentation (Fig. 15.4).

Membrane design criteria and material selection

The acceptance of membrane-assisted regeneration of osseous lesions in the oral cavity has introduced

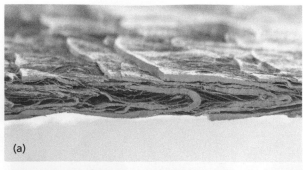

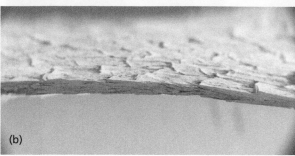

Fig. 15.4 (a) The outer surface of the GTAM (Gore-Tex Augmentation Material) is designed to create a barrier to passage of cells and to allow connective tissue attachment. The material is 50% air by volume and 25 μm between nodes. (Scanning electron microscopy image.) (b) The inner surface of the GTAM is designed for connective tissue attachment. It is 30% air by volume and less than 8 μm between nodes. (Scanning electron microscopy image.)

reconstructive dentistry to new therapeutic procedures and biomaterials. Clinicians are being exposed to an increasing number of membrane materials used, or proposed for use, in GBR. In order to select the best material for a specific clinical indication, it is imperative to understand the functional requirements demanded of membrane barriers for GBR procedures.

If the only requirement of a membrane material used in GBR were to provide a barrier to the proliferation of fibrous connective tissue, any suitable biocompatible material in the form of a cell-occlusive film could be used in clinical practice. However, a membrane that is used for alveolar ridge augmentation must meet a number of requirements in addition to acting as a passive physical barrier:

1. The membrane must be constructed of acceptable biocompatible material. The interaction between the material and the tissue should not adversely affect the surrounding tissue, the intended healing result, or the overall safety of the patient.
2. The membrane should exhibit suitable occlusive properties to prevent fibrous connective tissue (scar) invasion of the space adjacent to the bone and provide some degree of protection from bacterial invasion should the membrane become exposed to the oral environment (Fig. 15.4b).
3. The membrane must be able to provide a suitable space into which osseous regeneration can occur.

Spacemaking provides necessary volume with specific geometry for functional reconstruction.

4. The membrane should be capable of integrating with or attaching to the surrounding tissue. Tissue integration helps to stabilize the healing wound (Fig. 15.4a). It helps to create a "seal" between the bone and the material and prevent fibrous connective tissue leakage into the defect, and retards the migration of epithelium around the material should it become exposed.

5. The membrane must be clinically manageable.

Two different types of membrane are the most commonly used on the market. Non-resorbable, e-PTFE (expanded polytetrafluoroethylene) membrane was the first material to be successfully applied for GBR. The use of this material requires a removal procedure once the healing is completed. Although this material demonstrates superior biological response, the extra steps in clinical handling led to the development of biodegradable membranes such as collagen or synthetic polymers. Furthermore, attempts have also been made using other types of barrier membranes such as lyophilized dura, calvarial bone, and peritoneal tissue. However, the results regarding these latter materials are still somewhat limited in applications related to implant treatment.

Biocompatibility

When discussing the clinical outcome of membrane materials, biocompatibility is a fundamental requirement for acceptable function of any implantable medical device. Although this requirement is often taken for granted, tissue interactions involve many application-specific factors that are governed by complex mechanisms.

A classical definition of biocompatibility by Williams is, "the state of affairs when a biomaterial exists within a physiological environment, without the material adversely and significantly affecting the body". This should be interpreted with regard to biomaterial used, the indication, and the environment in which the material is placed and maintained. For example, degradable materials are clearly affected by the environment of the body; however, safe degradation is one of the primary intended functions of this class of biomaterials. Biocompatibility is a relative term. All implanted materials interact with the host tissue to some extent. Biomaterials with dissimilar chemical composition or biomaterials with the same chemical composition but with different macro- and microstructure will demonstrate different cellular or systemic responses.

Non-resorbable membranes

As previously described, non-resorbable membranes were the first materials successfully used in GBR. The best documented material is e-PTFE (expanded polytetrafluoroethylene) (Gore-Tex Augmentation Mate-

rial, W.L. Gore & Ass. Inc., Flagstaff, AZ, USA). Originally used in medical applications such as synthetic vascular graft and heart patches, the material has an extensive documentation with regard to tissue response and safety. In the 1990s, barrier membranes with special characteristics for GBR were developed and became commercially available (Fig. 15.4). Substantial experimental and clinical data are available for this type of membrane. The biological response is near to ideal and the e-PTFE membrane is still considered the "gold standard" in membrane technology. The material is made up of carbon and fluorine chains strongly bonded to each other. This creates a highly chemically stable and hydrophobic material which is ideal for biocompatible tissue interaction. The material has an open outer structure for early tissue integration and stabilization and an inner portion which is responsible for the occlusive properties of the device (Fig. 15.4).

Biodegradable barrier membranes

Collagen membranes are resorbed by enzymatic degradation, while synthetic polymers are resorbed via degradation into lactic acid and water.

Bio-Gide® was the first collagen barrier membrane designed for GBR and is by far the best documented product in the literature. It is made from native, non-cross-linked collagen types I and III and consists of two functional layers. The compact layer is cell occlusive and fulfills barrier function, whilst the porous layer allows tissue integration (Fig. 15.5). The membrane has hydrophilic properties, which enable self-adherence to the bone surface, thus providing easy clinical handling. Due to the lack of stiffness, collagen membranes are usually used in combination with bone chips or bone substitutes.

Pure synthetic biodegradable membranes are also available on the market. These materials usually

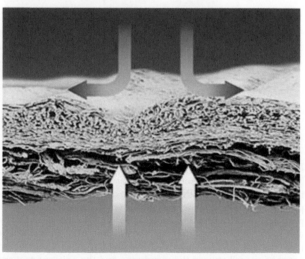

Fig. 15.5 Scanning electron microscopy image showing cross-section of a biodegradable Bio-Gide® collagen membrane. The double layer design is created in order to stabilize the material and prevent soft tissue penetration.

consist of a combination of PLA/PGA (polylactide and polyglycolide). An example of such membranes is RESOLUT (W.L. Gore & Ass. Inc., Flagstaff, AZ, USA). Although this demonstrates excellent biological behavior in experimental studies, the amount of clinical data is still somewhat limited.

Indications for GBR treatment

When a defect in the alveolar bone is present, three basic situations can require the use of a regenerative procedure:

- Bucco-palatal bone thickness is reduced, but still allows placement of the implant although with the result of either a dehiscence or fenestration-type defect (simultaneous approach) (Fig. 15.6a).
- Horizontal bone thickness is reduced in such a way that optimal implant placement with regard to prosthetic planning is not possible (simultaneous approach).

- Bone thickness is so reduced that implant placement is not possible with proper primary stability. In this situation, ridge augmentation is required prior to implant installation (staged approach).

Basic surgical technique of GBR

Preoperative antibiotics

The same antibiotic prophylaxis is recommended as in conjunction with implant placement according to standard protocol. Usually a 1-day regimen including 2g fenoxymethyl-Pc × 2 is enough. For advanced GBR cases, 1 week's antibiotic coverage postoperatively is recommended.

Flap design

A full-thickness crestal incision, slightly buccal but still within attached mucosa, is performed and extended mesially and distally to the adjacent teeth.

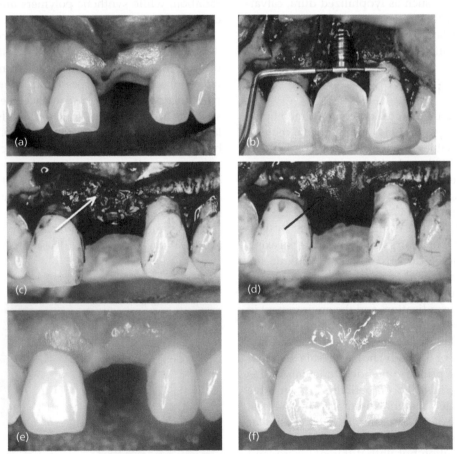

Fig. 15.6 (a) Buccal concavity in combination with minor vertical bone loss due to earlier trauma. The bone tissue is not sufficient either for optimal implant placement or support of the soft tissue. (b) Buccal mucoperiosteal flap raised. Note the design of the flap including one extra tooth on each side of the implant site. The implant is placed in optimal position according to the preoperative prosthetic planning using a surgical stent. Lack of buccal bone and several exposed threads of the implant are evident. (c) BioOss® particles mixed with autogenous bone particles harvested from preparation of the implant site are placed in the defect area and also used to cover the surface of the implant. (d) A Bio-Gide® membrane is trimmed and placed over the defect area. Note that the membrane is allowed to extend into the periphery from the graft material. Also note the trimming which leaves approximately 1 mm of space between the membrane and the adjacent root surfaces. (e) Clinical photograph showing uneventful healing after 6 months. Note the harmony of soft tissue contour compared to prior to treatment (see (a)). (f) Completion of the treatment. Final crown (Procera®) in place. The soft tissue contour including the height of the papillae is evident.

Diverging releasing incisions are then performed buccally (Fig. 15.6b). Full-thickness mucoperiosteal flaps are elevated.

Site preparation

Based on the available amount of host bone present, simultaneous implant placement can be performed. If optimal position and direction and satisfactory primary stability cannot be obtained, a two-stage procedure should be considered.

The bone surface in the augmentation area should be carefully debrided in order to remove all remnants of soft tissue. If implant placement is performed it should be performed according to the protocol of the implant system used, aiming at a prosthetic-driven position (Fig. 15.6c).

Prior to placement of graft material and the barrier membrane, the buccal bone plate in the defect area must be perforated to create access for multipotent cells and blood vessels emanating from the marrow cavity. This can be performed either with a spiral or a round bur with a dimension of approximately 1 mm. This surgical procedure is believed to stimulate osteogenesis by activating a cascade effect of growth factors. Furthermore it allows the formation of an appropriate coagulum which will act as a matrix for the initial bone formation.

Graft material

The use of spacemaking materials underneath the membrane has been proven to provide a more predictable regenerative result and is today considered state of the art. Many different materials, including autogenous bone chips, freeze-dried-dimeneralized, deproteinized bovine bone, and synthetic graft materials such as TCPs, have been tested with varying results. The best documented filling material with predictable outcome is a combination of deproteinized bovine bone (Bio-Oss, Geistlich, Switzerland) and autogenous bone chips mixed in a ratio of 1:1. The addition of Bio-Oss has been shown to minimize resorption of the newly regenerated bone (Fig. 15.6c).

Membrane selection and positioning

The anatomic shape of the defect to be regenerated dictates the choice of membrane material. The following protocols can be recommended.

Biodegradable membranes

Most defects can be treated with resorbable membranes together with autogenous bone chips alone or in combination with bone substitutes. Usually the autogenous bone chips are placed in contact with either the bone surface or the exposed parts of the implant and then covered with a layer of Bio-Oss. Alternatively the two filling materials are mixed together in a ratio of approximately 1:1.

The membrane must be cut and trimmed to adapt to the anatomy of the ridge and applied over the defect in order to cover the bone graft. Due to the hydrophilic properties of the Bio-Gide membrane, it will "stick" to the bone surface once wetted either with saline or blood. Hence, no fixation screws or tacks are needed for stabilization in most cases (Fig. 15.6d).

Non-resorbable membranes

When a large volume of bone (outside the bone envelope) must be regenerated, the use of non-resorbable e-PTFE membrane is indicated. The preparation of the augmentation site is identical to that described in Site preparation. However, extra attention must be paid to the membrane adaptation and fixation. The membrane must be cut to extend at least 4–5 mm beyond the filling material to avoid interference with the surrounding soft tissue. It is important to avoid creating sharp edges since they can increase the risk for membrane perforation during healing. A critical note is to trim the membrane so a distance of 1–2 mm is maintained from the root surface of the neighboring teeth. This is to avoid contamination due to bacterial downgrowth along the root and also to enhance periodontal reattachment.

Finally, the membrane should be fixated using either micro-screws or specially designed tacks. It is practical to start this procedure on the palatal side prior to the placement of the bone graft material (Fig. 15.7). A critical technique is the adjustment of the flaps prior to suturing. A completely tension-free environment must be created by performing periosteal releasing incisions at the base of the buccal flap.

Suturing

Suturing is recommended using non-resorbable sutures in a biocompatible material. A double suture layer should be created with a combination of horizontal mattress sutures (4/0) (on top of the crest) followed by single interrupted sutures (5/0 or 6/0) for mucosal closure.

Follow-up

Due to the compromised wound, the recommendation is to maintain the sutures in place for at least 14 days. The patient should receive systemic antibiotics (amoxicillin) for 5–10 days when they have undergone a more advanced GBR procedure. In addition, the patient should rinse with chlorhexidine solution for 3 weeks after placement of the GBR barrier. This could thereafter be switched to a 1% chlorhexidine gel which is gently applied in the wound area only once daily.

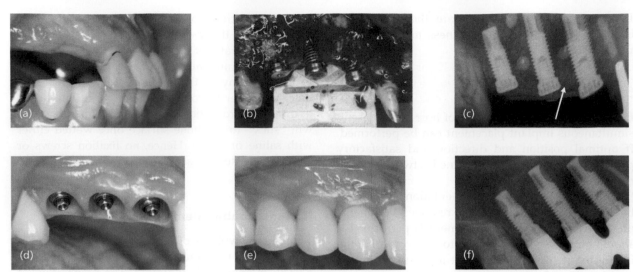

Fig. 15.7 (a) Edentulous area in the posterior maxilla. Both horizontal and vertical bone loss are present. Without bone augmentation in conjunction with implant treatment, a less than ideal esthetic outcome regarding the length of the clinical crowns would be evident. (b) Esthetic-driven implant placement. Implants are placed according to prosthetic planning transferred via a surgical stent. Note the level of the present bone in relation to the placement of the fixture heads. A titanium-reinforced GTAM has already been secured palatally by means of titanium fixation tacks. The defect area will subsequently be filled with a mixture of BioOss® and autogenous bone particles. Finally the membrane will be wrapped over the graft buccally and sealed with micro tacks. Suturing is according to the described protocol. (c) Radiograph showing the augmented area after 6 months of healing. Note the newly formed bone between the implants (compared to Fig. 15.7b). The tacks used for membrane fixation are also visible on the radiograph. (d) Clinical photograph after abutment connection and subsequent healing. (e) Final reconstruction: Procera® crowns placed. Note the optimal length of the clinical crowns that matches the neighboring teeth. (f) Radiological follow-up after 1 year in clinical function. Note the bone height is maintained in between the implants. The bony support allows a stable soft tissue level around the superstructure.

The e-PTFE membranes are removed after 6–8 months (either at the time of fixture installation or abutment connection). During this healing period, the patients are checked once a month for plaque removal and any complications.

Temporary dentures

Implant treatment and related bone augmentative procedures are usually associated with a situation where the patient needs a temporary solution during the respective healing phases. Clinical studies have demonstrated a clear correlation between membrane exposure and pressure from temporary dentures in the wound area. Hence, strict rules apply for the design of the temporary solution in conjunction with GBR. Ideally, fixed solutions such as Maryland bridges or conventional temporary bridges are the first choices if possible. If a temporary removable denture is necessary, it should be designed in such a way that no contact is present between the base of the denture and the soft tissue covering the GBR membrane. Furthermore, occlusal support of the denture is mandatory in order to prevent a pumping pressure when chewing.

Membrane removal

A non-resorbable barrier membrane is removed under local anesthesia. Technically the easiest way to approach the membrane is from the lateral aspect and

to dissect it free from the covering soft tissue layer. Following this procedure, it is usually easy to remove the barrier from the underlying bone tissue. Great care should be taken to remove the entire membrane material. This is usually performed in conjunction with either implant placement or abutment connection. Biodegradable barrier membranes do not usually require this procedure. Most biodegradable membranes on the market are designed with a resorption pattern of less than 6 months.

Clinical results of GBR

A variety of techniques and materials has been used to establish the structural base of osseous tissue for supporting dental implants. GBR is a surgical concept which has been in clinical use for well over two decades. It has undergone several developments and improvements and is nowadays considered a predictable treatment modality, once the previously described issues have been taken fully into account. Doubts have previously been raised regarding the quality and lasting capability of membrane-regenerated bone when being put into clinical function. Previous experimental studies have clearly shown the positive dynamics of this type of bone over time. Recently this has also been confirmed in several clinical studies. In a recent review study by Aghaloo and Moy, the GBR technique was compared to different types of grafting procedures such as autogenous onlay, veneer (OVG), interpositional inlay grafting (COG), distraction osteogenesis (DO), and ridge splitting (RS). The data originated from a database search which identified 526 articles. Finally, 335 articles met the criteria. Implant survival rate was 95.5% for GBR technique, 90.4% for OVG, 94.7% for DO, and 83.8% for COG. Hence, GBR technique performed better or equal to more advanced bone grafting procedures using autogenous bone.

Another interesting clinical finding is that it seems slightly easier to augment bone in the maxilla compared to the mandible. The use of provisional restoration during the healing period seems to improve the result. Early implant placement also seems to be preferable if possible, due to alveolar ridge preservation, more favorable defect morphologies, and probably a higher regenerative capacity of the adjacent bone.

Bone augmentation of atrophic jaw bone and, particularly, in the esthetic zone in the maxilla is a delicate and technique-sensitive procedure. The principle of GBR offers an alternative that is less resource demanding and also results in less morbidity for the patients. Predictable results can be obtained if a thorough understanding of the biological principles is applied in the clinical setting (Fig. 15.7).

Recommended reading

Araújo MG, Lindhe J. (2005) Dimensional ridge alterations following tooth extraction. An experimental study in the dog. *Journal of Clinical Periodontology*, **32**, 212–18.

Buser D, Martin W, Belser C. (2004) Optimizing esthetics for implant restorations in the anterior maxilla: anatomic and surgical considerations. *International Journal of Oral and Maxillofacial Implants*, **19** (Suppl), 43–61.

Dahlin C. (2010) Optimal implant placement in the esthetic zone by the use of guided bone regeneration. In: *Oral and Maxillofacial Surgery* (eds, Andersson L, Kahnberg K-E, Pogrel MA). Oxford, Wiley-Blackwell.

Dahlin C, Linde A, Gottlow J, Nyman S. (1988) Healing of bone defects by guided tissue regeneration. *Plastic and Reconstructive Surgery*, **81**, 672–6.

Zitzmann NU, Schärer P, Marinello CP. (2001) Long-term results of implants treated with guided bone regeneration: a 5-year prospective study. *International Journal of Oral Maxillofacial Implant*, **16**, 355–66.

Chapter 16

Implant Placement in the Posterior Mandible

Anatomy of the posterior edentulous mandible

Normal topography

The curvature of the alveolar process of the mandible is narrower than the body itself; the posterior parts of the alveolar process are positioned much more lingually than the mandibular body. In the second and third molar area the bony substance of the oblique line, running from the coronoid process, is superimposed on the outer alveolar plate because of this divergence of the alveolar process and mandibular body. This gives an impression of a thick alveolar plate. Lingually, the temporal crest from the medial part of the coronoid process follows the course of the oblique line. Behind the third molar these two lines form the retromolar triangle which continues anteriorly as the alveolar crest. To accommodate the comparatively thicker roots of the molars the alveolar crest is wider and the crest flatter in the posterior than in the anterior parts of the mandible. Lingual to the second and third molars the downwards sloping mylohyoid line adds to the thickness of the superior parts of the alveolar crest. Hence, a cross-section of this part of the mandible is angulated lingually.

In the first and second molar area there is a shallow concavity in the lingual surface, the submandibular fossa. Further anteriorly, in the area corresponding to the premolars, the more distinct sublingual fossa is found.

As the oblique line continues anteriorly and inferiorly it gets less pronounced which gives the impression of a thinner mandible. The orifice of the mental canal, the mental foramen, is found in the buccal cortex, between the roots of the first and second premolar, usually a couple of millimeters below the apices. As the curvature of the mandible increases in this region, the anterior rim of the orifice is sharper than the posterior.

The mandibular canal

The mandibular neurovascular bundle enters the mandibular canal through the mandibular foramen. This is a wide opening situated approximately in the center of the lingual surface of the mandibular ramus, hidden behind a thin, bony process, the lingula. During the first 8–10 mm the canal runs close to the lingual cortex. As it descends it moves to a more central position in the bone in a smooth curve downward and forward into the mandibular body some 6–8 mm from the mandibular base. The curvature of the canal is less pronounced as it continues in the mandibular body. This means that the canal runs continuously closer to the mandibular base until it reaches the area between the first and second molar from where it moves upwards to the mental foramen in an increasingly sharp curve. As the canal moves inferiorly it moves lingually and reaches its most lingual position at its most inferior position, between the first and second molar. From there it runs closer to the buccal cortex. When the mandibular canal forks into an incisor canal, containing the anterior plexus of the nerve, and a mental canal (usually called the mental foramen), containing the mental nerve, the canal is positioned approximately 3–4 mm from the buccal surface. What is known as the mental foramen is actually a canal through which the first 2–4 mm of the mental branch of the mandibular nerve run before it leaves the mandibular body apical to, and between, the first and second premolar. However, in a few cases its location may vary from the canine to the first molar. The mental canal usually runs perpendicular to the sagittal cardinal axis of the head. Thus it runs slightly posteriorly to the surface of the

Essentials of Oral and Maxillofacial Surgery, First Edition. Edited by M. Anthony Pogrel, Karl-Erik Kahnberg and Lars Andersson.
© 2014 John Wiley & Sons, Ltd. Published 2014 by John Wiley & Sons, Ltd.
Companion website: www.wiley.com/go/pogrel/oms

mandible after leaving the mandibular canal but the pattern of emergence seems to vary between population groups. The posterior direction may be readily seen in lateral radiographs and has been interpreted as a loop. The length of the loop has been measured at between 0 and 7.5 mm. However, others have shown that the loop is a radiographic artifact rather than an anatomic structure and that it should have no impact on implant surgery. The anterior and posterior walls of the mental canal are frequently not parallel, but converge towards the foramen, which may explain the difference in findings between radiographs and clinical findings.

As the upwards curve of the mandibular canal is accentuated close to its ramification, the mental canal reaches the mental foramen slightly from below. The incisor canal continues anteriorly after the furcation of the nerve. The size of the canal anterior to the furcation varies considerably; from being the same size as the main canal to a diminutive, almost invisible canal. However, even in cases where the canal is initially rather wide it soon narrows as it runs anteriorly.

The expression "mandibular canal" may give a false impression of a rather robust structure with thick cortical walls. In a few cases this may be true (Fig. 16.1a) but in most cases the walls are fairly thin, in some cases they seem almost non-existent (Fig. 16.1b). Normally the walls of the mandibular canal are perforated by small vessels and nerve fibers leaving the neurovascular bundle to the teeth. It is not known whether these perforations eventually disappear when the vessels and nerve fibers atrophy after teeth have been extracted. The mental canal seems to be usually surrounded by solid cortical walls, which are a continuation of the buccal cortex.

The periosteum that covers the exterior surface of the mandible continues into the mental canal and along the mandibular canal as an endosteum covering the surface of the walls of the canals.

Resorption patterns of the alveolar ridge

As the alveolar crest is wider in the premolar and molar area than in the anterior region, vertical resorption is slower in the posterior parts. On the other hand, molars and premolars are usually lost earlier than incisors. Thus when patients seek implant placement, the posterior regions are usually equally or more resorbed than the anterior.

In the posterior molar area resorption usually results in a wider arch and a wider crest as resorption reaches the oblique and mylohyoid lines. In the first molar and especially in the premolar area, two different resorption patterns are seen, although combinations of the two are common. Whether the resorption mode is due to the angulation of the alveolar crest or genetically determined is not known.

The usual pattern is vertical resorption. This results in a flat and rather wide crest. If the resorption is moderate, leaving more than 10 mm height of bone superior to the mandibular canal, implant placement is usually uncomplicated. However, as resorption continues, the height above the mandibular canal is reduced and in advanced cases, where resorption reaches the level of the mandibular canal, the foramen is found on the top of and even slightly lingual to the

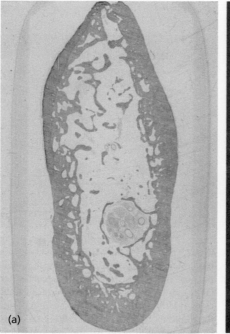
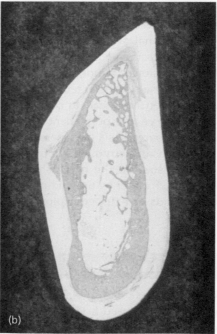

(a)   (b)

Fig. 16.1 (a) Cross-section of the mandible. Mandibular canal with a thick cortical wall. (b) Cross-section of the mandible. Mandibular canal with an extremely thin cortical wall.

top of the crest with part of the alveolar nerve positioned under a thin layer of bone or even directly under the alveolar mucosa.

The other, less frequent, resorption pattern is lateral resorption. This results in a narrow crest, in advanced cases in a very high, thin ridge made up of cortical bone which is totally unsuitable for implant placement.

Implant placement superior to the mandibular canal

Conventional implant placement in the posterior mandible may be associated with the risk of nerve damage. However, as long as the distance between the superior cortex and the mandibular canal is 13 mm or more, implant placement in the posterior mandible is little different from elsewhere if the difficulties mentioned in the preceding section are observed. The distance between the surface of the alveolar crest and the roof of the mandibular canal can relatively accurately be calculated by means of a panoramic radiograph once the position of the mental foramen has been clinically established. When the distance is less, more accurate measurement becomes imperative. Numerous methods to establish the location of the mandibular canal have been presented. When extreme accuracy is needed, a surgical guide based on a three-dimensional (3D) model should be made and used during surgery.

Nerve damage may occur even if the canal is not directly traumatized during implant surgery. The implant seat is usually drilled 0.5–1 mm deeper than the length of the corresponding implant. When working close to the canal it is tempting to be cautious and drill less deep. This may result in the implant being placed a little deeper than the seat allows, compressing the apical cancellous bone, and, indirectly, the roof of the canal, without the surgeon realizing. This results in pressure on the neurovascular bundle. If the compression is minor, only a part of the sensory area may lose sensation temporarily. A more severe compression may lead to compartment syndrome in the nerve and permanent nerve damage with anesthesia, paresthesia or hyperesthesia. Should the surgeon observe any such symptoms postoperatively, the pressure on the nerve should immediately be eliminated, either by unwinding the implant one or two rounds or by open exploration of the nerve.

The use of wider implants

To compensate for the reduced bone–implant contact area when shorter implants are used, wider implants may be considered. These also have an esthetic advantage in the posterior area; the wider neck of these implants mimics the size of the cervix of the molars. Both the esthetic and functional results may therefore be enhanced.

When using wider implants the surgeon should be aware that with increased diameter the speed at the periphery of the drill and implant are exponentially increased. Gentle drilling and placement of the implant are imperative to avoid failures due to overheating of the bone.

Placement of implants lingual to the neurovascular bundle

To allow the use of longer implants, placement lingual to the mandibular canal has sometimes been recommended. The impression that the implants are placed lingual to the neurovascular bundle and secured into the cortex at the base of the mandible may be given by illustrations such as Figure 16.2. However, as can be seen in Figure 16.3, the bone lingual to the mandibular canal is too thin to allow insertion of implants. To obtain a result as shown in Figure 16.2 the implants have to be angulated to perforate the lingual cortex immediately above or at the level of the canal and the implants are thus inserted into the floor of the mouth. This may have the advantage of double cortical anchorage but the method is highly dangerous and may even be life-threatening; fatal incidents have been reported after accidental perforations into the floor of the mouth. Due to the resilient tissues in the floor of the mouth, bleeding may pass unnoticed until it suddenly manifests itself as an airway obstruction. As the implant seat is drilled without visible or easily calculated reference points, laceration of the neurovascular bundle is also highly probable.

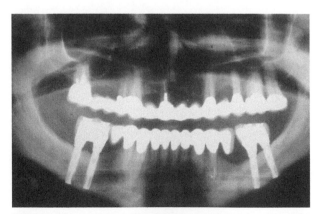

Fig. 16.2 Nerve transposition has been performed on the right side. As bone chips have been placed between and lateral to the implants the former alveolar canal can no longer be seen across the implants. As the buccal cortex has healed, a new "retromolar" foramen has been formed posterior to the implants on the right side. On the left side a so-called "lingual placement" of the implants has been performed. Note that the canal can still be seen across (buccal to) the implants. A false impression is given that the implants are secured into the base of the mandible but in reality are placed into the floor of the mouth.

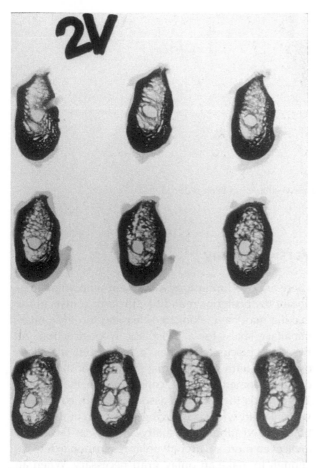

Fig. 16.3 Set of cross-sections of a mandible from the mental foramen (upper left) to the third molar area (lower right). The amount of bone available for implant placement lingual to the neurovascular trunk is insufficient.

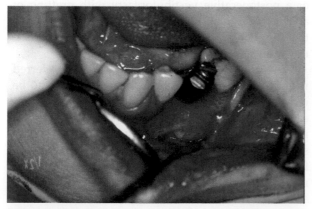

Fig. 16.4 Lingual placement of an implant. Note how the implant has been unfavorably angulated to avoid interference with the neurovascular bundle.

Of course, it may be argued that this technique allows for a bicortical anchorage of the implant, and in a few selected situations this technique may have its place. However, if the distance to the mandibular canal is short, the implants have to be angulated in a way that makes it difficult to achieve a satisfactory esthetic and functional prosthetic reconstruction (Fig. 16.4); in cases where the height above the canal is

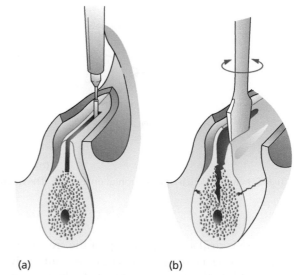

(a)   (b)

Fig. 16.5 Schematic sketch of a crestal split. A groove is made with a fissure bur along the crest into the cancellous bone, and a chisel is gently inserted and twisted until a space wide enough for insertion of the implants is created.

sufficient, a safer choice would be to choose to place a shorter and maybe wider implant above the canal rather than taking the risk of placing it lingual to the nerve bundle.

Crestal split

Sometimes an advanced lateral resorption pattern of the alveolar crest results in a high but very narrow crest unsuitable for implant placement, even if implant perforations both lingually and buccally are accepted. In such cases, the intermaxillary space permitting, a so-called crestal split may be considered. Typically the method is used in the anterior maxilla but it can be adopted for use in the posterior mandible as well. The crest has to have a wide base containing cancellous bone that runs well into the top of the crest and the cortex must not be too thick. In these cases success rates in the range 85–95% have been reported. However, in the posterior mandible very few cases qualify for this procedure. The bone has to be elastic to permit bending or a controlled breaking. Thus the patient has to be young. In most cases the thin crest is made up of a unified lingual and buccal cortex without any cancellous bone in between. This makes a split highly unpredictable or even impossible. In most cases other methods are to be preferred.

Surgical technique

After an incision has been made along the top of the crest, a lingually based flap is raised (Fig. 16.5). A buccal flap only about 2 mm wide is raised, to preserve the blood supply to the buccal cortical plate. A

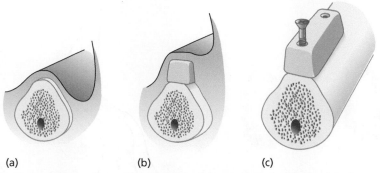

(a)   (b)   (c)

Fig. 16.6 Schematic sketch of a horizontal onlay graft. The depth of the vestibule has been reduced.

thin groove is drilled along the top of the crest until cancellous bone is reached. A chisel is cautiously driven well into the groove by a mallet while care is taken not to interfere with the neurovascular bundle. The chisel is then gently rotated until the gap widens and, in most cases, a green-stick fracture is produced at the base of the buccal cortex, which is nourished by the attached periosteum. If the cortex is thick or only a short length of the crest is involved in the operation, additional vertical cuts may have to be made at both ends. Vertical incisions for these cuts should be placed anterior and posterior to the bony cuts and narrow vertical flaps raised to expose the area planned for the cuts. The implants can then be inserted in the gap. In some cases it is not even necessary to prepare a seat. The gap between the implants may either be covered by a membrane and/or the space filled with a particulate bone graft. If the buccal bone has fractured it has to be secured by lag screws into the lingual cortex to provide initial stability for the implants. Soft tissue covering is produced by the lingual flap; this may sometimes be difficult. Second-stage surgery can be performed after 5–6 months.

Onlay augmentation in the posterior mandible

Indications for augmentation of the posterior mandible may be esthetic as well as functional. An esthetic problem is found in cases where the edentulous posterior part of the mandible is resorbed to a level well below the marginal level of the anterior, dentulous area. A residual crest thinner than 4 mm or with a residual height above the mandibular canal less than 7–8 mm presents a functional problem. In both cases, augmentation could be one of several possible solutions.

Onlay grafts and implant placement can be performed as a one-stage or a two-stage procedure, with autografts, allografts, xenografts, mixtures of these and various bone cements. Block grafts or particulate grafts may be used. At present, autogenous cancellous bone grafts seem to be the "gold standard" against which the merits of other grafts are measured.

Vertical onlay

There are two limitations associated with augmentation of the posterior mandible; the antagonists in the maxilla may have elongated, leaving too little intermaxillary space for a prosthetic reconstruction. As has been discussed earlier, a segmental maxillary osteotomy with superior displacement of the osteotomized segment may be considered in these cases. The other is the problem associated with covering a vertical graft while preserving the depth of the vestibule. The vestibule is usually shallow in the molar area, even more so after alveolar resorption extensive enough to make an onlay graft necessary. When an onlay graft is covered there is a tendency for the vestibule to be reduced even further; in extreme cases it can be totally lost leaving the augmented mandible lying in the buccal soft tissues (Fig. 16.6). A second procedure, either a preoperative tissue expansion or a postoperative vestibuloplasty with grafting of attached gingival, should thus be included in the therapy plan when augmentation is planned in the molar area.

A cortico-cancellous block is usually preferred when the height of the posterior mandible is to be reconstructed. Adequate volume of this material is easily available from the iliac crest and, in contrast to most autogenous and allogenic alternatives, it offers stability to implants during the time it acts as a scaffold for new bone formation. The drawback with this material is that the degree of resorption is unpredictable. It is imperative to carve the transplant to an exact fit and to secure the transplant firmly to the recipient. As the residual amount of bone is unpredictable a two-stage procedure is preferred where the implants are inserted about 4 months after the transplantation.

In a few selected cases another approach may be chosen; if adequate stability can be obtained by inserting the implants one third to two thirds of their lengths into the mandible, compressed cancellous bone mixed with 20–30% allogenic bone substitute may be added around the implants to form a crest of adequate size for the implants. In this case the allogenic bone is used as a temporary filler, to increase

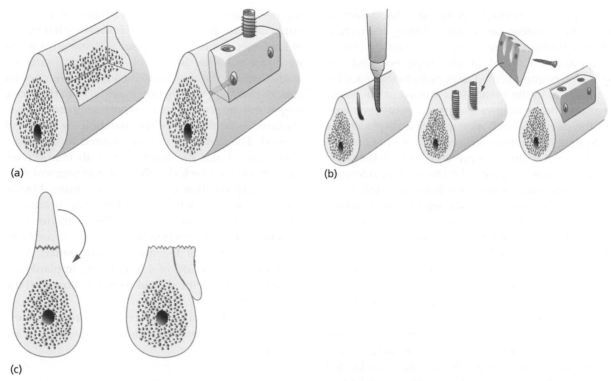

Fig. 16.7 (a) Schematic sketch of a buccal on-/inlay graft. A lateral box has been cut in the sloping buccal wall of the mandible and an onlay that has been adapted to fit this box tightly is secured to the recipient site. The implant seats are then drilled through the onlay/inlay into the mandible and the implants are placed. (b) Schematic sketch of a buccal onlay graft. Implant seats are drilled into the mandibular body and the implants placed. Due to the thin crest only the apices of the implants are secured into the mandibular body. An onlay graft is then cut/drilled to as good a fit to the mandible and implants as possible, gaps are filled with particulate bone, and the graft is secured to the recipient site. (c) Schematic sketch of a crestal downfracture.

the volume of the bone and, more importantly, to reduce the speed of resorption to allow adequate bone formation. The use of a contoured titanium mesh membrane to reduce the pressure on the graft is highly recommended in these cases. Alternatively, the implants themselves may reduce external pressure on the graft by acting as "tent poles".

Lateral onlay

There are three principle methods for widening a thin alveolar crest. Usually cortico-cancellous block grafts from the chin or lateral part of the corpus/ramus are used. Again, the graft should be contoured to a perfect fit to the recipient surface and secured by screws (Fig. 16.7a). If the cortical plate is thin, the vascularization offered by the recipient is usually less than when onlays are used to increase the vertical dimension. Hence, the risk for resorption may be higher and the "take" of the graft is usually slower and more unpredictable. The procedure is usually a two-stage procedure. When implants are placed 4–5 months after the transplantation there is still a risk of the graft loosening from the recipient crest.

In some cases vertical concavities with the diameter of the implants can be drilled into the buccal surface of the thin crest. The implants are then partly inserted into these concavities and secured apically in the cortex of the wider mandibular body. A par-

ticulate bone graft or particulate autogeneous bone mixed with hydroxyapatite could be packed between and buccal to the implants/crest and covered with a titanium membrane and left to heal for at least 6 months (Fig. 16.7b).

A third method is downfracture of the crest. After an incision 2–3mm buccal to the top of the crest a vestibularly-based buccal flap is raised and a horizontal cut is made along and almost through the crest, preferably with a thin fissure bur. The tip of the crest is then downfractured buccally to add to the width of base of the crest (Fig. 16.7c). The advantage of this method is that the blood supply to the "transplanted" bone is preserved by the soft tissue attachment. The drawbacks are that the height of the crest is reduced, the final width of the crest cannot be controlled, and attached gingiva is lost on top of the newly formed crest.

Distraction osteogenesis in the posterior mandible

Alveolar distraction was introduced by Chin and Toth in 1966. This procedure has advantages compared to onlay grafting; the result is usually more predictable and there is no soft tissue displacement. The latter is especially important in the posterior parts of the mandible as the vestibule and the attached gingiva can be preserved. On the other hand distraction implies patient compliance during distraction and consolidation, more visits, and the added cost of the appliance. Control of the appliance and the vectors can be complicated, especially as the space for the appliance in the vestibule is limited in the posterior mandible. It follows that mechanical problems with the device as well as unplanned displacement and tipping of the transport segment are not uncommon. Distraction involves pressure on both the reference and transport segment. Fractures of the reference segment, the basal bone, have been reported. Pressure on the superior, transport, segment may induce not only suture dehiscence but progressive surface resorption with eventual collapse or fracture of this segment if it is not thick enough. This means that distraction is increasingly more difficult to perform as the distance between the alveolar crest and the canal is reduced. To prevent fractures a bone height above the canal of at least 5–6 mm is recommended. The procedure seems to be well tolerated by most patients but a high incidence of complications including bleeding, transient nerve damage, unplanned displacement or fractures of bone segments, malfunctions or fractures of appliance may occur; incidences between 0 and 100% have been reported. This may indicate that thorough preoperative planning and gentle surgical technique is a prerequisite for success. Awareness of this together with the relative complexity of the procedure may limit the usefulness of the procedure to rather few, carefully selected cases.

Surgical technique

A horizontal incision is made in the vestibule corresponding to the area of the alveolar crest to be distracted (Fig. 16.8). Care should be taken not to damage the branches of the mental nerve at the anterior end of the incision. Superiorly directed relief incisions are made at both ends. At the posterior end this may be replaced by an elongation of the horizontal incision. The flap is raised to expose the lateral part of the mandible. However, the top of the crest should be exposed as little as possible. While the index finger is placed against the lingual side of the mandible a horizontal osteotomy is made almost through the mandible not closer than 3 mm to the anticipated level of

the neurovascular bundle. A medium-sized fissure bur is ideal for this purpose as it is readily felt by the index finger before the soft tissue is lacerated; a reciprocal saw is harder to control. Two vertical cuts are made through the crest at both ends of the horizontal cuts, slightly converging downwards. With the index finger still in place, the transport segment is then fractured from the rest of the mandible by means of a chisel. The distractor is then secured to the transport segment and the basal bone with mini-screws and activated to check that the transport segment may move freely and that the vectors are correct. Finally the distractor is inactivated and the flap resutured. After a latency period of 1 week the distractor may be activated for distraction by 0.5 up to 1.0 mm/day. An overcorrection of 1–2 mm is recommended. After a consolidation period of 4 months the implants are placed. The distractor should be in position until the implants are placed.

Penicillin V is administered: 2 g preoperatively and 2 × 2 g postoperatively until the suture lines are healed.

Nerve transposition

There is widespread confusion in the literature as to what this procedure should be called. The terms lateralization, transposition, and repositioning are frequently used interchangeably. In this text, *nerve lateralization* includes procedures where the nerve is manipulated laterally posterior to the mental foramen. *Nerve transposition* is defined as a procedure where the neurovascular bundle is manipulated laterally after the incisor branch has been cut. This procedure was originally used to facilitate orthognathic surgery of the anterior mandible. The area of the mental foramen is thus included. The expression *nerve repositioning* means "placed in the original position"; it is not applicable in this context and should be avoided.

The main advantage of nerve transposition and nerve lateralization is that both these methods permit installation of implants in cases where other methods would fail or be impossible to use. They may thus be regarded as "rescue operations". Both methods offer bicortical implant stability. The implant survival rate is high, around 93–95%. Marginal bone resorption

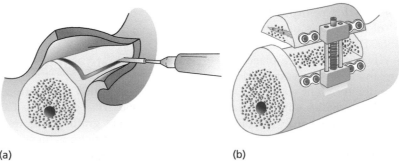

(a)   (b)

Fig. 16.8 Schematic sketch of the principles of distraction osteogenesis in the posterior mandible.

does not differ from what is found after conventional implant placement and less than after distraction. Once the surgeon is familiar with the procedure it is a quick procedure that can be made under local anesthesia. Nerve transposition may also be used to preserve neurosensory function in association with mandibular hemiectomies/reconstructions.

However, the procedure involves repeated trauma to the neurovascular bundle; the first trauma occurs when the incisor branch of the nerve is cut and a reactive swelling of the nerve follows. This swelling may induce a so-called compartment syndrome within the nerve trunk resulting in a "strangulation" of the vessels and hence lack of neurosensory function. The second trauma occurs as the nerve trunk is manipulated out of the mandibular canal. The alpha-fibers of the nerve are highly sensitive to traction. If the nerve is bent at any point up to approximately 5%, temporary neurosensory disturbances will occur. Normal sensation may be expected within 4–6 weeks although it may take considerably longer in some cases. However, if the traction is more than 5% the perineural vessels will rupture and permanent lack of neurosensory function or deficit function will result. Immediate postoperative loss of sensation or deficit nerve function can be expected in most cases but gradually normal neurosensory function is regained. Six to 12 months postoperatively only a few percent of the patients have persistent loss of sensation and some of these patients do not seem aware of this. In a study on 100 cases approximately 80% of the cases had no or deficient sensibility 1 week postoperatively, 25% 6 months postoperatively and 6% 18 months postoperatively. If corticosteroids are administered to reduce the peri- and postoperative swelling of the nerve, normal function seems to be regained a little earlier but the end result is approximately the same. Although these figures may seem encouraging, patients seem to find it harder to accept nerve disturbances following nerve lateralization/transposition than after, for example, sagittal split operations. It may be the implant patients are generally older and find it harder to adapt or there may be some quality factor in the nerve disturbance not registered by the method used. Some authors have advised against the use of this method as a routine procedure. Devitalization of the incisors after nerve transposition has not been reported, not even after bilateral procedures.

As the cancellous bone of the mandible is widely exposed during surgery and as the devitalized buccal cortex is reused in particulate form, the administration of antibiotics is imperative to avoid severe infections that have occasionally been reported. In extensively resorbed cases where the "buccal window" will cover most of the buccal surface there is a certain risk of mandibular fracture, especially if the seats are drilled deep into or through the cortex at the base of the mandible leaving only the lingual cortex to stabilize the mandible. The risk is most acute 1 week postoperatively when the decalcifica-tion phase of the remodeling coincides with the patient regaining full chewing force. However, it should be pointed out that fractures in conjunction with conventional implant placement in the posterior mandible have been reported.

Surgical technique

A subperiosteal flap is outlined by an incision along or slightly lingual to the top of the alveolar crest with a deep relieving incision into the vestibule anterior to the position of the mental foramen. To protect the anterior branches of the mental nerve, this should not be positioned too close to the mental foramen or made too vertical. Usually it is advantageous to add a posterior releasing incision. The flap is raised to expose the crest and buccal surface of the mandibular body, the mental foramen, and the base of the mandible. The subperiosteal dissection should continue into the mental canal to free the endosteum from the surrounding walls. A panoramic radiograph can usually provide information about the approximate level and course of the mandibular canal; the mental foramen indicates the highest point of the canal in the mandibular body. With a thin dissector between the roof and the nerve in the mental canal, a horizontal cut, parallel to the base of the mandible, is made from a point at least 6–8 mm anterior to the mental foramen and at the level of the roof of the mental canal, until a point some 8–10 mm posterior to the planned position of the most posterior implant seat. This horizontal cut should be made through the cortex and 1–2 mm into the cancellous bone. A second cut, as long as and parallel to the first, is made below the anticipated level of the mandibular canal. This cut involves two difficulties: access below the mental foramen and estimation of the level of the canal. To facilitate access to the area below the mental foramen a very shallow cut could be made through the periosteum/endosteum that covers the nerve branches as they leave the foramen. This will expose the neurovascular bundle, usually the two main branches, and allow the flap to be retracted a little further. A correct estimation of the level of the floor of the canal is crucial. If the cut is not made into the cancellous bone but into the cortex of the mandibular base, the subsequent steps of the procedure will be more difficult and there is a definitive risk for mandibular fracture. If the cut is made too high, the nerve will be damaged. All cuts are made by means of a thin fissure bur. When in doubt the cut could be prepared by using a thin round bur to localize the correct position of the cut. Once the two horizontal cuts are made, these are united at both ends, in front of the foramen into the cancellous bone and at the posterior end only just through the cortex to avoid accidental cutting of the nerve (Fig. 16.9a). The thin elevator is again inserted into the mental canal and the roof of the canal is cut with a fissure bur, starting from a position adjacent to the elevator and working upwards in a V-form to

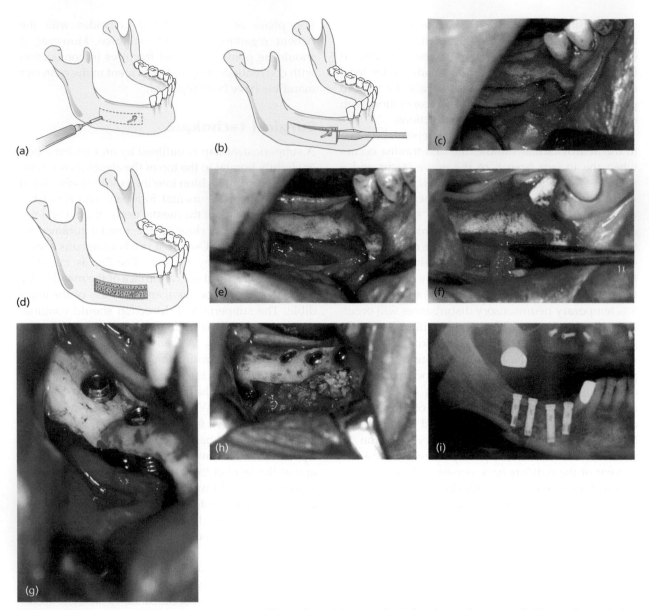

Fig. 16.9 (a) Schematic sketch of nerve transposition. The outline of the cortical window, later to be removed. The window includes the mental foramen. The superior, inferior, and anterior bone cuts are well into the cancellous bone; the posterior, however, is only almost through the cortex to avoid trauma to the neurovascular bundle. (b) The roof of the mental canal has been removed. The buccal window is gently being removed. (c) Clinical illustration of (b). (d) The buccal cortex has been removed. Schematic sketch. (e) Clinical view of (d). At the furcation the rather thick main trunk divides into a thinner mental branch and an even thinner incisor branch. Note that the nerve is situated more lingually in the posterior part of the mandible. (f) The incisor branch is transected and immediately starts to contract and swell as it is gently removed from the mandibular body. (g) The implants are placed. (h) The former buccal cortical window is cut into bone chips that are placed between and lateral to the implants. The neurovascular bundle now leaves the mandibular body posterior to the implants where eventually a "retromolar foramen" will be formed. (i) Radiographic view after implant placement.

remove the cortical roof of the mental canal. The buccal bone plate encircled by the cuts is then gently removed (Fig. 16.9b, c). The course of the mandibular neurovascular bundle in the mandible, the furcation at the mental foramen and the incisor branch are exposed (Fig. 16.9d, e). Usually small remnants of bone on top and below the bundle have to be removed with an elevator to free it completely. The incisor branch is cut some 7–8 mm anterior to the furcation and, starting from the mental foramen area, the neurovascular bundle is carefully lifted out of the mandible (Fig. 16.9f). It should be noted that the main

trunk will start to retract and swell as a response to the trauma when the incisor branch is cut (Fig. 16.9f).

When the nerve is dissected out of the mandibular body care should be taken not to bend the nerve as this will induce neurosensory disturbances. Usually the nerve is more easily removed and the bleeding less, the longer the patient has been edentulous, as the small nerve fibers and vessels that earlier ran to the teeth are vestigial. While the nerve trunk is gently protected the implant seats are drilled, making only small impressions in the basal cortex, and the implants are inserted. They should be lightly stabilized against the cortex in the base of the mandible but not necessary perforating it, as this may increase the risk for mandibular fracture. It has been shown that the nerve trunk may be repositioned into the mandibular body protected from the implant surfaces by a resorbable membrane or even without a membrane (Fig. 16.9g); however, the author prefers to avoid direct contact between the implant and the nerve trunk in case an infection develops around an implant or the implant has to be removed for other reasons.

The bone plate that was removed earlier is cut into 2–3 mm pieces that are packed between and buccal to the implants while the neurovascular bundle is allowed to leave the mandibular body distal to the most posterior implant (Fig. 16.9h). Eventually a new foramen will be formed in this area (Fig. 16.2). Cover screws are placed and the flap resutured. The patient is given penicillin V (2 g) and corticosteroids (4 mg) preoperatively. Later the same day the patient is given penicillin V tablets (2 g) and corticosteroids (3 × 4 mg). Penicillin V (2 g) is given for another 10 days postoperatively and corticosteroids are given, reducing the dose as follows: 4 × 3 mg the first, 4 × 2 mg the second and finally 4 × 1 mg the third postoperative day. Figure 16.9i shows the postoperative radiographic result.

In cases of extreme resorption where the neurovascular bundle is close to or on top of the crest, the superior cortex is removed to reach the nerve which should be transpositioned posteriorly and into the lateral wall of the mandible. In these cases the crest should be allowed to heal before the implants are placed and the procedure should thus be performed as a two-stage procedure where the implants are inserted approximately 6 months after the transposition of the nerve.

Nerve lateralization

Nerve lateralization is one of the procedures indicated when implants are to be inserted posterior to the mental foramen (preferable from the first molar)

and the height above the canal is inadequate. The method seems to offer both advantages and disadvantages compared to nerve transposition; as the area of the mental foramen is not involved, the procedure could be expected to be faster and easier to perform, and as the incisor branch of the nerve is not cut, one trauma less is inflicted on the nerve. On the other hand, localized traction has to be applied to the nerve when the implants are placed and postoperatively it may come to rest against the threads of the implant, which may constitute an additional long-term trauma. As the anterior cut through the cortex is placed in an area where the nerve runs close to or, in some cases, actually within the buccal cortex when nerve lateralization is performed, there is an increased risk of accidentally cutting the nerve in this area.

Due to better access, implant placement in the area of the second premolar seems to be facilitated by nerve transposition. Otherwise, the results of the two methods seem comparable; neither implant survival nor postoperative neurosensory function seem to differ significantly. Hence, the choice of method seems to be up to the personal preferences of the surgeon.

Surgical technique

The flap design is identical to that used in nerve transposition. It is important to expose the mental foramen to help localize the level of the canal but the dissection is not continued into the mental canal. In the area where implant placement is planned two horizontal cuts are drilled 1–2 mm into the cancellous bone, parallel to the base of the mandible, by means of a thin fissure bur, one about 2 mm superior to the anticipated level of the neurovascular bundle and the other below the mandibular canal. As in nerve transposition the level of the lower cut is the hardest to place correctly and any misjudgement involves the same risks. The horizontal cuts are then united by vertical cuts at both ends, at the posterior end only just through the cortex to avoid accidental cutting of the nerve (Fig. 16.10a). The anterior cut has to be

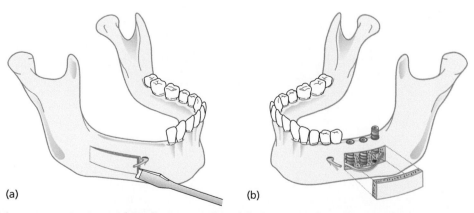

(a)   (b)

Fig. 16.10 (a) Schematic sketch of nerve lateralization. Outline of the buccal window. The mental foramen is not included in the window. (b) The cortical window has been removed, and the nerve trunk is gently pulled buccally as the implants are placed.

made through the cortex which involves a certain risk of cutting the nerve if this is close to or within the cortex. A more cautious cut that does not penetrate the cortex will make luxation of the buccal cortex and dissection of the nerve much more difficult, riskier and time consuming. To prevent accidental cutting of the nerve, preoperative tomograms are recommended.

When the buccal bone plate has been removed any small remnants of bone on top and below the nerve bundle are removed with an elevator to facilitate lateralization of the bundle. This has to be done more carefully than when transposition is performed as the medial part of the nerve bundle has to be accessible from a lateral approach. The neurovascular bundle is then gently pulled 2–3 mm (or as required) out of the operation field. The author uses a home-modified instrument; a small dissector with the tip bent 120°. As has been pointed out above it is extremely important to apply only gentle traction to the nerve to reduce the risk of nerve damage. As in nerve transposition the nerve may start to swell as the vessels within the trunk rupture, but the swelling is usually less than when transposition is performed. The implant seats are drilled only a couple of millimeters into the basal cortex. The implants are placed and the neurovascular bundle is allowed to slip back into the mandible (Fig. 16.10b). Frequently, the bundle contracts to lie against the treads of the implants. The long-term neurosensory impact of this is not known. To avoid a postoperative buccal concavity in the mandible the bone plate that was removed earlier can be cut into 2–3 mm pieces that are gently packed between and buccal to the implants and the neurovascular bundle. Any pressure should be avoided. Cover screws are placed and the flap resutured. The patient is given penicillin V 2 g preoperatively and 2 × 2 g postoperatively for 10 days, as well as corticosteroids 4 mg preoperatively and 3 × 4 mg postoperatively on the day of operation and 4 × 3 mg, 4 × 2 mg and 4 × 1 mg, respectively, the following postoperative days.

Ethical considerations

Before every single operation the surgeon should consider the balance between what the patient may gain and the risks involved. Implant surgery is an elective procedure; it does not save lives or prevent disablement. Hence, the surgical risk should be moderate. Unfortunately, it is not possible to give general recommendations on what level of risk is justifiable; that depends on each case and each patient. Some of the procedures discussed in this chapter are well proven and should be safe, others involve moderate risks and discomfort, while still others involve considerable risks for failure, pain, impairment, and may even prove fatal.

Recommended reading

Greenstein G, Tarnow D. (2006)The mental foramen and nerve: clinical and anatomical factors related to dental implant placement: a literature review. *Journal of Periodontology*, **77**, 1933–43.

Kahnberg KE, Ridell A. (1987)Transposition of the mental nerve in orthognathic surgery. *J Oral and Maxillofacial Surgery*, **45**, 315–18.

Klinge B, Petersson A, Maly P. (1989) Location of the mandibular canal: comparison of macroscopic findings, conventional radiography, and computed tomography. *International Journal of Oral and Maxillofacial Implants*, **4**, 327–32.

Rosenquist B. (1994) Implant placement in combination with nerve transpositioning: experiences with the first 100 cases. *International Journal of Oral and Maxillofacial Surgery*, **9**, 522–31.

Rosenquist B. (2010) Implant placement in the posterior mandible. In: *Oral and Maxillofacial Surgery* (eds, Andersson L, Kahnberg K-E, Pogrel MA). Oxford, Wiley-Blackwell.

Chapter 17

Use of Autogenous Bone Material for Implant Rehabilitation in the Bone Deficient Maxilla

Introduction

Surgical techniques today enable us to reconstruct bone-deficient regions equally well in the maxilla and the mandible. Bone grafting techniques, using autogenous bone from the iliac crest, mandibular symphyseal region, mandibular angle or cranium, can provide material for reconstruction purposes. Onlay grafting is especially indicated for defects, thin ridges and as a complement to inlay grafting. Inlay grafting, in combination with orthognathic surgery, has a predictable outcome. The sinus lifting technique is especially useful for reconstruction in the bone deficient posterior maxilla.

Background

Functional rehabilitation with dental implants has been in practical use for over 40 years with extremely good results. Early long-term studies over 15 years, in rehabilitation of edentulous mandibles, show success rates of over 90%. Edentulous, resorbed mandibles were the most problematic situations and these were also where fixed implant bridge solutions were most indicated. The long-term results have been remarkably good, which today means that it is possible to have immediate loading in most edentulous mandibles. The maxillary region is more problematic, especially with regard to the anatomic situation, where the maxillary sinus and nasal cavity occupy large areas. The cortical structure of the bone tissue in the maxilla is not the same as in the mandible, due to factors such as muscle influence on the mandible. The fact that the mandible is the mobile part of the chewing system explains some of the differences between the two jaws. The edentulous maxilla may require much more augmentation than the edentulous mandible, in order to be suitable for implant rehabilitation. There is a spectrum of surgical techniques available today which enable us to solve all kinds of bone-deficient situations, equally satisfactorily in the maxilla and the mandible.

Bone graft sources

The most frequently used regions for bone graft harvesting are the mandibular angle region and the chin region when there is only need for a limited amount of bone graft. For larger reconstructions the iliac bone is by far the most used source for autogenous bone graft.

Cortical bone graft can be harvested from the mandibular chin on the buccal side. By use of a Lindeman drill or a round burr, or an oscillating saw, a piece of bone can be taken with due consideration to the incisor roots and the mental foramina (Fig. 17.1). It is recommended not to perforate the lingual cortex in order to avoid bleedings from the floor of the mouth.

When harvesting bone graft from the angular region, the surgical approach is similar to the sagittal split approach. An incision is made outside the molar region extending up on the anterior ramus. The buccal part of the crest is exposed and a bone incision made outside the teeth into the marrow space. Vertical bone cuts are made on both sides of the horizontal and another one at the bottom of the planned graft area about one centimeter above the mandibular base.

The bone graft is splitted out with a chisel. With the right technique there should be no interference with the nerve canal (Fig. 17.1).

Essentials of Oral and Maxillofacial Surgery, First Edition. Edited by M. Anthony Pogrel, Karl-Erik Kahnberg and Lars Andersson.
© 2014 John Wiley & Sons, Ltd. Published 2014 by John Wiley & Sons, Ltd.
Companion website: www.wiley.com/go/pogrel/oms

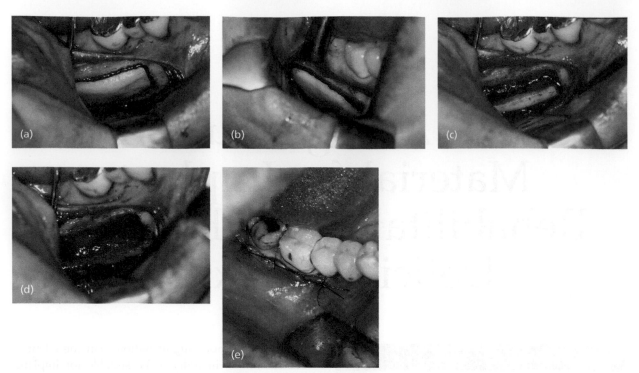

Fig. 17.1 (a) Bone incision in the mandibular angle. (b) Vertical bone incision posterior to the mental foramen. (c) The buccal cortical bone piece is split out buccally. (d) The bone graft site after removal of graft. (e) Closing of the graft site.

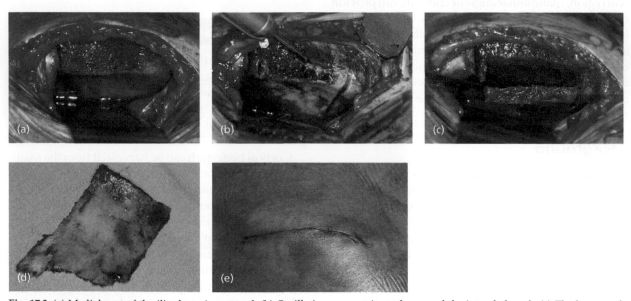

Fig. 17.2 (a) Medial part of the iliac bone is exposed. (b) Oscillating saw cut is made around the intended graft. (c) The bone graft is split out medially. (d) A large bone bloc is harvested. (e) The iliac crest after reconstructing and suturing.

When there is a need for larger amount of bone graft you have to harvest from the iliac bone (Fig. 17.2). While harvesting bone graft from the mandible is made in local anesthesia harvesting from the iliac bone has to be made in general anesthesia.

There are several different approaches to the iliac bone but it is an advantage for the patient to have an unchanged contour of the iliac crest after the surgical procedure.

In our experience the periosteum together with the upper part of the selected graft region (Fig. 17.2) is cut and bent aside and the medial surface of the iliac bone exposed. An oscillating saw can be used to take the desired amount of graft; bleedings are stopped eventually by use of bone wax and the wound closed. The upper loose bony part of the crest can now be fixated with plate screws and the skin incision sutured. A drain can be used for the first 24 hours.

Aspects of bone graft behavior

Autogenous bone graft material is the gold standard for reconstruction of bony defects in the facial skeleton, such as tumor resections, congenital defects or atrophy of the jaws. Fresh, immediately harvested bone graft is by far the most reliable. The bone graft may then be replaced by new bone by osteoconduction or by osteoinduction through surviving osteogenic cells. The microvascular system in the bone graft may also make minor anastomosis with the surrounding vital tissue and revascularize the graft material. The predictability of the graft volume has not always been certain. Postoperative resorption may radically reduce the volume by up to 50–70% of the graft when it is in a passive state. Several factors may be of importance in maintaining as much bone graft volume as possible. Recent literature reviews indicate that the embryonic origin is important for the graft survival. Membranous bone should be superior to endocondral bone with less resorption over time. The revascularization of the graft is extremely important for starting new bone formation. Another important factor in preserving bone graft volume is rigid fixation of the graft, probably because this creates an appositional phase earlier, and thereby promotes improved osteoconduction.

The recipient bed for the bone graft may also be of importance for graft survival and volumetric changes. The influence of the bone graft recipient site on the survival of onlay bone grafts has been studied in several publications. The degree of contact between bone graft and recipient site as well as the orientation of the bone graft may have a significant effect on remodeling of vascularized bone grafts. Cortical preparations of the recipient bone marrow site allow exposure of osteogenic stem cells to the graft and may improve bone healing. Several publications support the theory that perforated bone is superior to unperforated. The perforations may increase initial healing of the bone graft, but there is no evidence that they help to maintain bone graft volume. Osteopromotive membranes have been used to improve bone graft survival and stability; these allow free diffusion of tissue fluid and prevent cellular ingrowth from adjacent connective tissue.

Block or particulated bone

Bone block grafts are structurally stable and initially resistant to resorption. The autogenous bone block will be almost totally necrotic after the grafting procedure and needs revascularization to survive. Incorporation of the graft is initiated by an inflammatory reaction during the first weeks, which then turns into a granulation phase, followed by osteoclastic activity. The new bone in and around the bone block is formed by creeping substitution and development of lamellar bone. This process proceeds gradually and has not reached normal physiological strength until 1 year. Normal biological properties are not present for at least 2 years, and part of the block will still contain residual necrotic original bone. Mechanical strength will be reduced during the first year.

Particulated bone graft can be both cortical and cancellous. Particulation can be done with a bone mill or the bone can be cut into pieces with bone scissors. Cancellous particulated bone has a larger surface area exposed to the surrounding tissue and vascular ingrowth may proceed faster than in bone block grafts. Compared to cortical graft it regains biological properties faster but it is also more exposed to resorption activities. The cancellous bone graft gradually increases in mechanical strength and it takes 1–2 years to reach normal mechanical strength, much like the bone block graft.

Onlay grafting

Different methods for reconstruction of the atrophic maxilla can be used, depending on the actual situation. An atrophic alveolar ridge, with sufficient height but which is too thin, may be suitable for onlay grafting, where bone graft from either the hip or the mandible can be used for augmentation. Onlay grafting aims to widen the crest and make it possible for implant insertion. It is very important not to reduce the vertical height of the crest, since vertical augmentation may be very difficult to achieve.

The first attempts to treat severely resorbed maxillae were made in the 1980s with large horseshoe-shaped bone blocks grafted to the maxillary ridge (Fig. 17.3). Technical difficulties with the technique made it unpredictable and there was a relatively high morbidity rate.

The buccal onlay grafting technique is useful in the posterior mandible as well as in the maxillary alveolar process. To achieve as good a result as possible it is advisable to make small perforations in the buccal cortical bone before attaching the graft with plate screws. If there is a discrepancy between the graft and the host bed it is also advisable to put bone graft material in the space to optimize the contact between bone graft and crest. The bone graft may be harvested from the mandibular angle, chin region, iliac crest or cranial sites. The most important issues in this procedure are to achieve rigid fixation of the bone graft and to close the covering soft tissue in such a way as to prevent microorganisms from the oral cavity entering the grafted area. The flap covering the bone graft should have a relaxed position and not be forced into a position by use of a strong suture. If this is not achieved, the graft may be totally destroyed due to wound dehiscence and compromised vascular blood supply.

A large onlay graft was the initial method of choice for reconstruction of the resorbed edentulous maxilla. The bone graft was obtained from the iliac bone

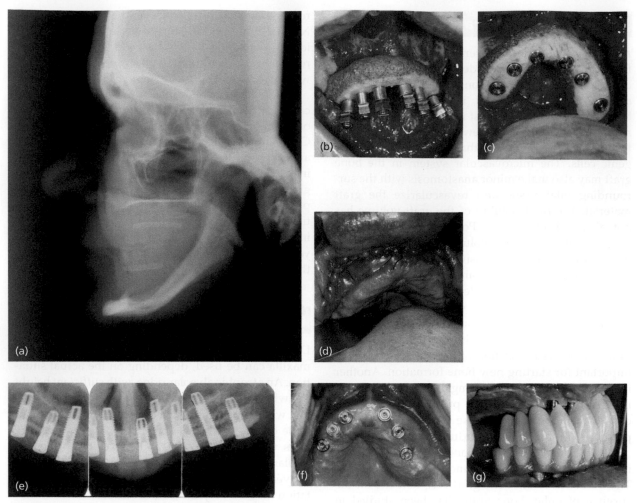

Fig. 17.3 (a) Lateral radiograph of edentulous maxilla and mandible. (b) Onlay grafting with block graft from the iliac bone and simultaneous implant insertion. (c) Implant and bone graft in place. (d) Soft tissue closure. (e) Radiograph of implant placement. (f) Abutment connection 6 months later. (g) Implant-supported bridge construction.

beneath the iliac crest not involving the arch of the crest (Fig. 17.3a, b). The horseshoe-shaped bone graft was modeled to fit on to the exposed upper jaw crest (Fig. 17.3b). The remaining, exposed crest of the upper jaw was ground to fit the graft better and the cortex was perforated with a small round drill to form a better vascular bed for the grafted bone. After modeling of the bone graft to fit on to the crest, implants could be inserted into the graft and retained in the residual crestal bone in a one-stage procedure; alternatively the graft could be attached to the crest with plate screws in a two-stage procedure, thus allowing the graft to become more vascularized before implant insertion. The choice of a one- or two-stage concept depends, of course, on the amount of available bone volume. More residual bone allows for a better and safer implant stability and is therefore more suited for one-stage procedures. Large onlay block grafts have been shown to achieve a good result in long-term follow-up with one-stage implant surgery and also with a two-stage surgical technique.

Long-term clinical and radiographic follow-up studies have shown very good success and survival rates with onlay grafts with only minor drawbacks.

With all autogenous bone grafts, healing follows the same principles, according to Wolf's law. The bone graft has to be functionally stimulated in order not to be resorbed. So a bone graft without functional stimulation by chewing through implants will resorb more or less completely. This functional stimulation is very well achieved by the implants. One should always allow for some remodeling resorption where excess bone graft material will disappear.

Bone graft will always adapt to functional load and stimulation. Thus in the horseshoe-shaped iliac bone grafts with excess volume outside the implants, functional remodeling, especially in a buccal–lingual direction was clearly evident. In patients with a retrognathic position at the upper jaw this resorption of 2–3 mm was negative since the retrognathic look of the maxilla was still noticeable even after implant surgery.

A technical problem of onlay grafting for small and larger surgical procedures is that the additional bone material has to be covered by a vital, vascularized flap, which must not be stretched or damaged. Careful closure of the incision without communication with the oral cavity is another important factor for a successful result. Big bone blocks for treatment of edentulous maxillae are especially vulnerable since there is so much foreign material to be incorporated within the tissue. Therefore it is of utmost importance to have as thick a flap as possible, with good vascularization to form a tension-free cover over the bone graft material (Fig. 17.3d).

The onlay bone graft can be attached to the residual crest with either the implants (one-stage procedure) or in a two-stage procedure with either plate screws or osteosutures. The choice of which technique to use depends on the clinical situation (Figs 17.4, 17.5).

Inlay grafting

In cases with an atrophic maxilla, bone grafting can be performed using orthognathic surgical proce-

dures. Maxillary osteotomy Le Fort I with down-fracturing of the maxilla is an excellent method for augmenting the alveolar process. After mobilization of the maxilla it can be manually repositioned with the fingers or carefully with Rowe and Killey's disimpaction forceps. The sinus membrane and the sinus recesses are carefully extirpated. The nasal mucosa should be intact or repaired to avoid contamination from the mouth or from the nose. Bone graft material is modeled to fit into the sinus recesses and nasal floor and secured with osteosutures. Normally five wire loops are sufficient to attach the bone graft of combined cortical plate and cancellous bone to the sinus recess and nasal floor. The maxilla is then held in its planned position with plates and screws. Anterior repositioning up to 10–15 mm is possible in most cases. Inferior repositioning can also be done to adjust the relationship between lip and upper jaw crest.

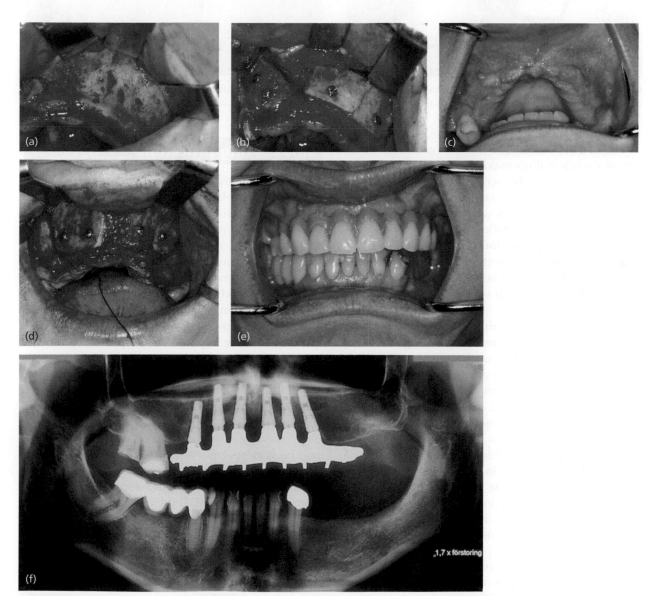

Fig. 17.4 (a) Clinical view of thin but high alveolar crest in the anterior region of the maxilla. (b) Onlay grafts positioned to increase the width of the alveolar crest. (c) Soft tissue healing. (d) Bone graft healing. (e) Implant-supported bridge in place. (f) Panoramic radiograph after bridge construction.

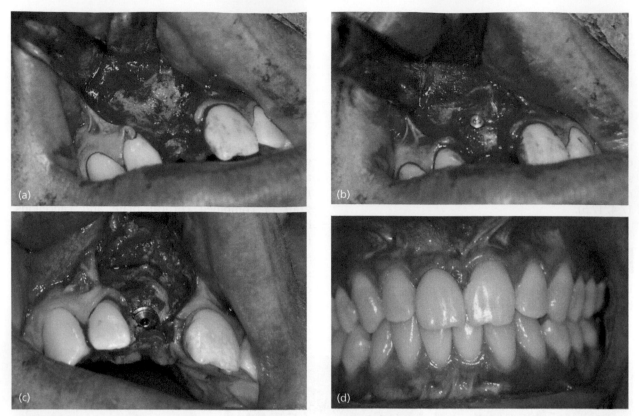

Fig. 17.5 (a) Single tooth loss in the anterior maxilla. Thin alveolar crest. (b) Onlay graft in place to increase bone volume of the crest. (c) Implant insertion in the reconstructed crest. (d) Implant-supported crown in place.

The Le Fort I technique for bone graft augmentation of the edentulous maxillae was originally introduced by Sailer who simultaneously performed grafting and implant installation. In the present model the bone graft is allowed to heal for 4–5 months before implants are installed. Implants can then be positioned as required for the prosthetic solution (Fig. 17.6). Slightly different approaches can be used for this procedure but the outcome with the treatment is usually very good with success and survival rates of 90–95%.

Preparation of the grafting site to optimize the healing process can be done by peforating the cortex of the recipient site with a small round bur. The cortical surface can also be roughened to stimulate bone formation. When pure cortical bone graft is placed against a cortical ridge the healing time should normally be extended 1 or 2 months to avoid the risk of inadequate healing between the two cortical surfaces.

The advantages with this method for treatment of deficient bone volume in the maxillary alveolar process are the predictable result and the possibility of correcting sagittal discrepancies between the jaws to some extent to improve the prosthetic possibilities. The problem with soft tissue closure which may arise in onlay grafting is not a problem in inlay grafting. The choice between one- or two-stage procedure as well as early loading is up to the surgeon. The author's own experience suggests a two-stage procedure with bone graft healing for 4–5 months and implant healing for at least 3–4 months (Fig. 17.4).

Sinus lifting procedure

For a long time the sinus lift procedure has been the solution for implant rehabilitation in the posterior maxilla with a limited amount of bone below the sinus cavity. Sinus lift involves opening a bone window to get access to the sinus cavity and gentle lifting of the sinus membrane, thereby creating a space for graft material. There are several surgical modifications and methods for the procedure but the aim of all of them is to increase the amount of bone for implant integration.

It is extremely important to keep the sinus membrane intact when it is elevated in connection with bone graft inlays. Since the drainage from the maxillary sinus is effected only through the osteum, a small canal leading out in the nose below the second nasal concha, there is a huge risk that infections established in the maxillary sinus cavity with minimal drainage will be very severe. As soon as bony fragments or salivary products gain access into the sinus cavity there is a risk for sinusitis development. A massive sinus infection will drastically reduce the chance of inlay grafts surviving and thus prevent anchoring of implants.

If the available amount of bone volume below the sinus cavity approximates 10–15 mm there may be no need for a sinus lift procedure. It is therefore important to have determined the bone volume preoperatively by tomographic measurements or computed tomography (CT) evaluation.

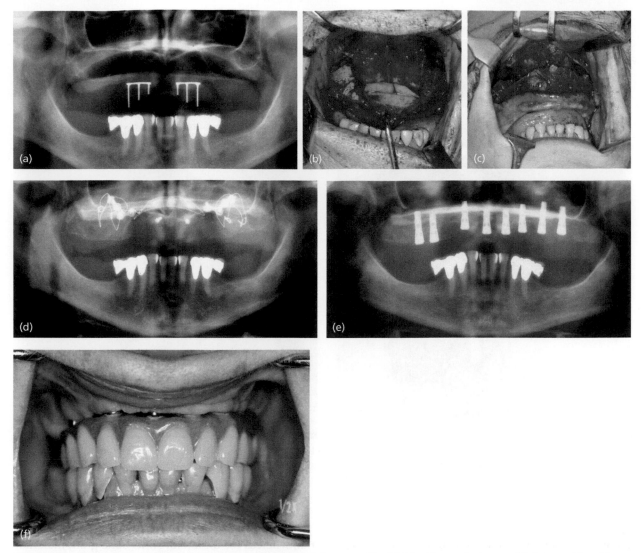

Fig. 17.6 (a) Panoramic radiograph of severely resorbed edentulous maxilla. (b) Maxillary osteotomy with interpositional bone graft. (c) Reconstructed maxilla with bone graft from the iliac bone. (d) Panoramic view of bone graft reconstruction. (e) Implant surgery at a second stage 4 months later. (f) Implant-supported bridge in place.

Morphologic aspects

The maxillary sinus in the adult can vary considerably in size and there is a continuous extension with increasing age. Expansion of the maxillary sinus into the alveolar process is especially observed in connection with extraction of molar teeth and also premolar teeth. Edentulism creates a situation where finally only a paper thin bony wall exists between the oral cavity and the sinus cavity. The maxillary sinus cavity is usually one big solitary cavity but it may also sometimes be divided into smaller chambers separated by septa. The origin of these septa may be a consequence of the sinus going deeper in the molar region and thereby forming septa towards the anterior part. The maxilla has a dense vascular network. The maxillary sinus is supplied by branches from the maxillary artery via the infraorbital artery and the greater palatal artery and the facial artery. Venous flow is via the sphenopalatine vein, the pterygoid plexus, and the facial vein. There seems to be a con-

nection between reduced vascularity and atrophy of the alveolar process. Loss of the maxillary teeth and increasing age result in marked reduction in the vascularization of the alveolar process.

Surgical technique

The lateral window technique is by far the most frequently used surgical procedure (Fig. 17.7). The lateral window gives access to the sinus cavity and enables positioning of graft material. The buccal windows are made by a round bur, diamond bur or piezoelectric surgery for gentle removal of bone over the sinus membrane. All possible precautions should be taken to avoid perforation of the sinus membrane. The smooth touch technique is recommended in approaching the sinus membrane. The window may be infracted, in which case the superior part of the bone incision is only part way through the buccal bone.

Alternative options are to loosen the window but still have it attached to the sinus membrane, or

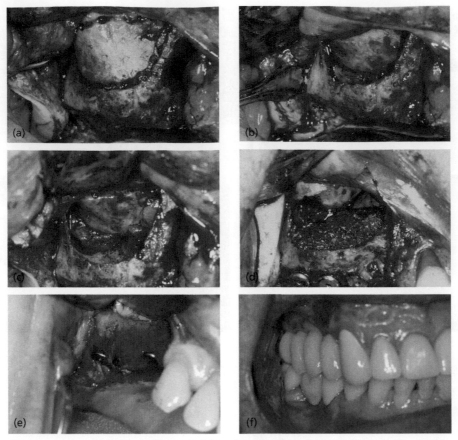

Fig. 17.7 (a) Sinus lift by use of the "window technique". A lateral bone "window" is created using a round bur. (b) Infraction of the buccal window. (c) Sinus membrane is lifted and a space is created below the window and the sinus membrane. (d) Bone graft is positioned in the lower part of the sinus cavity and kept in place by the implants (one-stage surgery). (e) Bone healing after 6 months. (f) Implant-supported bridge in place.

remove the window completely and use it as a free graft (Figs 17.8, 17.9, 17.10). The sinus membrane is carefully elevated with a blunt instrument from the bottom of the sinus cavity. It can be difficult to elevate, especially if extractions have been performed recently, causing a tight connection with the sinus membrane (Figs 17.9, 17.10).

Another critical point is in the superior corner of the window when the infraction technique is used. The infraction may give rise to sharp contours which may easily cause perforation of the sinus membrane. If the perforation is very small a resorbable membrane (Bio-Gide®) can be used to cover the perforation. If the membrane is manipulated or wrinkled too much, trying to suture it, to cover the perforation, there is a clear risk that the perforation will be enlarged and destroy any chance of sinus lifting augmentation. Complications like sinusitis may occur if there are loose particles within the sinus cavity.

Bone graft material can be obtained from the iliac bone, cranial bone, tibial bone or mandibular bone. Small amounts of bone material can also be obtained by use of the bone collectors like Bone Trap® or safe scraper (Fig. 17.11). The amount of bone needed depends on the type of procedure. Bilateral sinus lifting for rehabilitation of the premolar and molar regions demands a large amount of bone graft mate-

rial, whereas for unilateral sinus bone graft, material from the mandibular angle or chin is enough. Sinus lift for single tooth replacement needs even less bone graft material.

The bone graft material from the mandible is mainly cortical, as is cranial bone graft, whereas bone graft from the iliac bone and tibial bone consists of cancellous bone material. Cortical bone graft is more resistant to resorption but normally a mixture of cortical and cancellous bone graft is used.

The bone graft material, either in cortical block or particulated bone, is placed below the sinus membrane in the inferior chamber of the sinus cavity. Depending on the clinical situation the graft material can be immobilized with wires, plate screws, or it can just be packed below the sinus membrane. It is important to ensure that the bone material is stable and not moving around. A piece of cortical bone can be used as a roof for the particulated bone which is collected in the sinus inferior recess. The bone can easily be immobilized with wire osteosutures or plate screws. The surgeon may choose to use a resorbable membrane to cover the bone graft. In a two-stage procedure the bone graft is normally left to heal for at least 4 months. Shorter healing time will risk failure of the bone graft; if the healing time is too long, resorption of the graft will begin. The question of whether to do

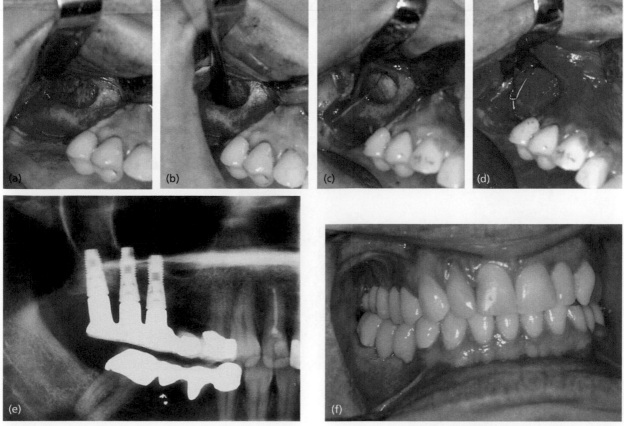

Fig. 17.8 (a) Sinus lift by use of a two-stage technique. Bone window is removed and sinus membrane is lifted. (b) Space for the bone graft is created in the basal part of the sinus cavity. (c) Cortical bone graft is positioned as a roof in the basal part of the sinus cavity. (d) Particulated bone graft is placed below the cortical "roof" and secured with wires. (e) Radiograph of implants in the sinus graft. (f) Implant-supported bridge.

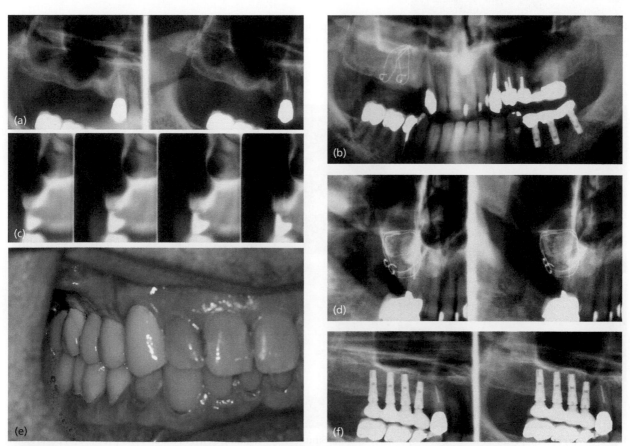

Fig. 17.9 (a) A case with a large sinus cavity and minimal residual bone volume. (b) The same case after sinus lift and bone grafting. (c) Tomograph in close section of the posterior maxilla before grafting. (d) Tomograph after sinus lift and bone grafting. (e) Clinical view of implant-supported bridge in place. (f) Radiograph after implant rehabilitation.

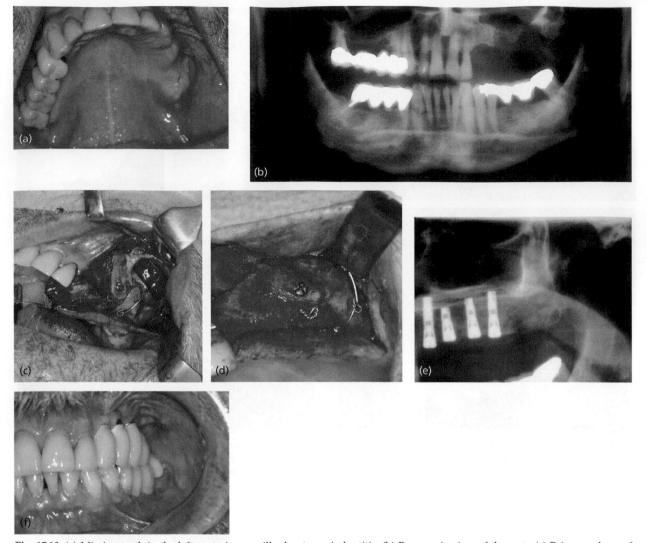

Fig. 17.10 (a) Missing teeth in the left posterior maxilla due to periodontitis. (b) Panoramic view of the case. (c) Primary phase of sinus lift and bone reconstruction. (d) Bone graft healing after 4 months. (e) Radiograph of implants in bone grafted posterior maxilla. (f) Implant-supported bridge construction.

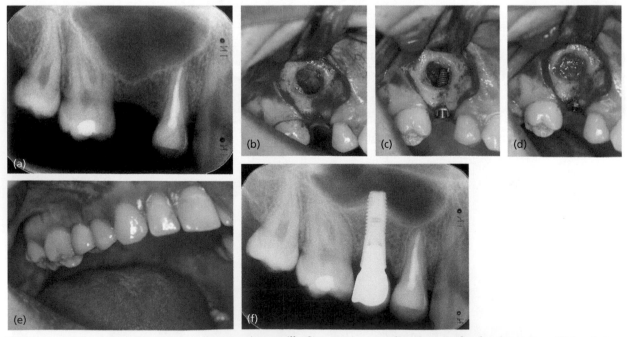

Fig. 17.11 (a) Second premolar missing in the posterior maxilla. Sinus cavity extending down in the alveolar process. (b) Local sinus lift by use of a circular bone window. (c) Implant insertion into the sinus cavity using the implant as a tent pole for the sinus membrane. (d) Particulate bone from Bone Trap® placed around the implant. (e) Crown restoration in place. (f) Two-year postoperative control showing a satisfactory bone filling around the implant.

the bone grafting and implant placement in one or two stages is still open to discussion and needs more clinical scientific follow-up and analysis.

It is extremely important to have enough bone volume below the sinus cavity when doing one-stage surgery, attaching the bone graft with implants. Bone graft and implants have to be stabilized rigidly and even resist some reduction of marginal bone level and the grafted bone in the postoperative remodeling phase. If the alveolar bone below the sinus cavity is too thin (<5–6 mm) there is a high risk that the implants, together with bone graft material (blocks or particulated), become mobile with subsequent failure of the implants and the bone graft. However, in cases with more bone volume available in the alveolar process the one-stage technique can be suitable. Primary stability should be enough for one-stage surgery when there is 5–10 mm of residual bone volume in the alveolar process.

There are many opinions on immediate or early loading of the implants placed in grafted bone. If the residual bone volume in the alveolar process below the maxillary sinus is qualitatively and quantitatively sufficient to stabilize the implants and give them an initial primary stability (Rf ≈ 6 0) it is possible to use early loading. The maxillary bones, however, are not often of good enough quality for immediate loading. Immediate or early loading can have a stimulating effect on bone healing and osseointegration, depending on the extent of loading and the primary stability of the implants. However, even with resonance frequency measurements (RFM), which give the surgeon an idea of primary stability, it is difficult to know whether immediate loading will be appropriate in individual cases.

Sinus lifting procedures using an impaction technique were originally presented by Summers. The purpose of this technique is to initiate a split of the alveolar crest between the inner cortical part towards the sinus cavity and the outer cortical part (towards the crest). The residual bone in the alveolar crest should be at least 6–7 mm and contain both cortical bone and marrow to be suitable for the impaction procedure. The intention with Summers' impaction technique is to fracture the cortical bone underlying the sinus cavity in such a way that the sinus floor can be elevated without rupturing the sinus membrane.

The procedure begins with flap elevation then preparation of implant sites with a round bur and spiral bur, but only through the cortical bone and slightly into the spongeous bone (2–3 mm). The subsequent surgery is done with osteotomes which normally have the same diameter as the implant surgery drills. By gradually enlarging the implant site with osteotomes up to the desired length and width the implants can be installed without perforating the membrane. Usually the best result is obtained with two to three implant sites in a row to be able to induce the sinus floor fracture. With only one implant site it is more difficult to achieve the same sinus floor eleva-

tion. The effect with only one impaction site may be very limited and the risk of sinus membrane perforation increases. In indicated cases, sinus impaction is a less demanding procedure for the patient, but still with predictable results. The choice of filling the space below the elevated sinus floor with bone graft or biomaterial is up to the surgeon. However, it is important to check for eventual perforations in the sinus membrane. Healing time after impaction and implant installation should be a little more extended than for conventional implant surgery.

In cases of single tooth replacement in the posterior maxilla where the available bone volume is too small to allow for conventional implants, a modified kind of sinus lift can be made. Where the sinus cavity has expanded down into the alveolar process after tooth extraction there is an ideal situation for a local sinus lift (Fig. 17.11). A crestal incision is made in the edentulous area and connected with diverging relaxation incisions in the vestibule. A circular area over the sinus cavity bone is removed to the sinus membrane and the bone material collected with a bone collector during the preparation. The sinus membrane is carefully lifted and the implant installed through the crestal bone by standardized technique. The implant is allowed to penetrate into the sinus cavity below the sinus membrane about two to three times the residual bone volume. The sinus membrane is thus held up by the implant which acts as a tent pole for the membrane. The bone material is placed around the exposed part of the implant but no attempt is made to completely fill the space around the implant. Recent results indicate a predictable outcome of the method.

Use of platelet-rich plasma

The use of platelet-rich plasma (PRP) in connection with bone grafting was been introduced by Robert Marx in 1948. He used a concentrate of platelets when doing cancer reconstruction cases. The theory of getting a concentrate of platelets into the wound area is to concentrate bone morphogenetic proteins, bone morphogenetic enzymes, and immunoglobulins as close as possible to the bone graft material in order to enhance and speed up the bone regeneration and bone integration processes.

Later studies with both animals and humans have not been able to confirm the effect on bone regeneration. However, a markedly noticeable effect on soft tissue postoperatively has been observed. Concentration of enzymes and immunoglobulins may reduce the initial inflammatory surgical response and therefore result in a less pronounced inflammatory postsurgical reaction. Human grafting studies by Thor and co-workers do, however, suggest that there may be a slight adjunctive effect of PRP on bone healing and bone regeneration, especially in conjunction with use of implants which have a moderately roughened implant surface. Further studies will be needed to verify the benefit of PRP in bone grafting cases.

The reason for the limited effect on bone graft healing could be that PRP releases enzymes and bone morphogenetic proteins with a very brief action time span, while bone regeneration is a slow process with a time span of weeks and months. Once it is possible to have slow-releasing adjuvants or surfaces on implants to allow for slow release of enzymatic substances, there may be a dramatic change in the effect of PRP and related substances. Until then it is advisable to reduce surgical time both in the bone graft harvesting and positioning and modeling of the bone graft, in order to maintain the graft's vitality. In a cortical bone graft block there will be a gradually "creeping substitution" of capillaries to vitalize and build up the new bone from inside and outside.

Staging of grafting procedures

Bone grafting by use of autogenous bone graft material can be done in one- or two-stage procedures. A one-stage procedure means that the implants are installed at the same time as the grafting procedure. A two-stage procedure means that one waits for healing of the bone graft before placing the implants. In a one-stage procedure the outcome of the implants depends on revascularization and vitalization of the bone graft before osseointegration can occur. Experimental studies have shown that there is a slow phase in bone-to-implant contact in the bone graft area compared to normal non-grafted bone tissue. The implants will depend on the residual bone tissue for primary stability and osseointegration before the bone graft gets enough microcirculation and living cell population for the osseointegration process. If the primary stability in the residual bone is too poor or the naturally occurring remodeling process due to the surgical trauma impairs the primary stability, there is a big risk of failure of the implant. The matter of immediate or early loading of the implants also depends on the initial stability and on the loading forces. Immediate or early loading can provide stimulation for the osseointegration process but may also be a disaster if the balance between stability and loading is negative.

Split crest surgery

An option already discussed for reconstruction of the alveolar crest which is too thin for implant placement is the buccal onlay graft, which will enlarge and thicken the crest thus enabling implant placement. However, if the anatomy is suitable for splitting of the crest, i.e. two cortical layers and an intermediate marrow space, it may be possible to split the crest in the middle and place bone graft in between the two plates. If the alveolar crest is composed of only corti-

cal bone there is a big risk of fracturing and destroying the crest. The incision should be made on the alveolar crest top, with minimal exposure of the bony surfaces on either the palatal side or the buccal side, so that the circulation to the two bony plates is not jeopardized. An osteotomy can be carried out with a chisel, oscillating saw or Lindemann drill to get the right direction. The two bony pieces are then separated with a chisel and the buccal bone segment with attached soft tissue fractured out of the base of the alveolar process. Particulated bone or Bio-Oss® can now be placed adjacent to the implant and the soft tissue closed. The procedure may be most successful in cases where there is a possibility of placing thinner implants without splitting the crest. However, in those cases where there is an indication for split crest surgery, the method has proven to be successful. If the crest is split in pieces a more complicated grafting procedure has to be done.

The zygoma implant

In certain cases it is possible to avoid bone grafting to improve the bone volume of the maxilla. Special made implants, so called zygoma implants, can be surgically anchored in the zygoma process and through the sinus cavity end up in the maxillary alveolar process. By use of two zygoma implants one on each side and combined with short implants in the anterior part of the upper jaw an implant supported prosthetic construction can be made.

Complications

Complications may arise due to inadequate coverage of the graft or flaps which are stretched too much, with compromised vascular circulation. Exposure of the graft may result in loss of part or all of the graft. Smoking may seriously affect graft healing since capillary sprouting is reduced by nicotine.

Wound dehiscence problems may be the most frequent complication, since healing contraction may disrupt the wound. That is why it is so important to have a flap which covers the surgical area without tension. Stretching of the flap to close the wound may impair healing due to strangulation of the small vessels and capillaries. Wound dehiscence in the early stage of healing is mostly located in the incision line; however, in later stages after several weeks of healing, dehiscence may appear where the vascular supply is inadequate to supply and revascularize the bone graft material.

In early dehiscences there is a big risk of losing the bone graft totally and contamination from the oral cavity will make a reclosure almost impossible since the bone graft has already been contaminated. When the dehiscence occurs at a later stage, when a major part of the bone graft has been incorporated by revascularization and regeneration of bone, the problem is more limited to the actual area of exposure. The part of the bone graft which has been exposed and devitalized can gradually be removed and secondary healing will close the dehiscences over vital bone tissue.

Inlay grafting is performed with extremely thin maxillae, so there is always a risk for fracturing of the palate or the sinus walls. It is possible to repair fractures by use of bone graft but it may be difficult to advance the maxilla once it has been fractured. Sinus infection can occur but is not a common complication.

The most frequent complication associated with sinus lifting procedures is perforation of the sinus membrane with maxillary sinus infections. Drainage from the sinus cavity is very limited with only the osteum as a natural canal, so there is a high risk for sinusitis after perforation with graft material moving around in the sinus cavity. Sinusitis must be treated with antibiotics and, often, the sinus must be reopened and cleaned, maybe removing part of the graft material. Dislocation of an implant into the sinus cavity may also occur which demands exploration and extirpation. Complications like lack of osseointegration, as in conventional implant surgery, may also occur. The complications in sinus impaction surgery are also connected with perforation of the sinus membrane and dislocation of graft material.

Recommended reading

Isaksson S. (1994) Evaluation of three grafting techniques for severely resorbed maxillae in conjunction with immediate endosseous implants. *International Journal of Oral and Maxillofacial Implants*, **9**, 679–88.

Kahnberg K-E. (2010) Treatment of bone-deficient ridges in implant rehabilitation. In: *Oral and Maxillofacial Surgery* (eds, Andersson L, Kahnberg K-E, Pogrel MA). Oxford, Wiley-Blackwell.

Kahnberg K-E. (2010) Implant rehabilitation in the posterior maxilla using autogenous bone material. In: *Oral and Maxillofacial Surgery* (eds, Andersson L, Kahnberg K-E, Pogrel MA). Oxford, Wiley-Blackwell.

Kahnberg K-E, Vannas-Löfqvist L. (2005) Maxillary osteotomy with an interpositional bone graft and implants for reconstruction of the severely resorbed maxilla: a clinical report. *International Journal of Oral and Maxillofacial Implants*, **6**, 938–45.

Kahnberg K-E, Vannas-Löfqvist L. (2008) Sinus lift procedure using a 2-stage surgical technique. I Clinical and radiographic report up to 5 years. *International Journal of Oral and Maxillofacial Implants*, **23**, 876–84.

Kahnberg K-E, Nyström E, Bartholdsson L. (1989) Combined use of bone grafts and Brånemark fixtures in the treatment of severely resorbed maxillae. *International Journal of Oral and Maxillofacial Implants*, **4**, 297–304.

Khoury F. (1999) Augmentation of the sinus floor with mandibular bone block and simultaneous implantation: a 6-year clinical investigation. *International Journal of Oral and Maxillofacial Implants*, **14**, 557–64.

Tatum H. (1986) Maxillary and sinus implant reconstruction. *Dental Clinics of North America*, **30**, 207–29.

Chapter 18

Biomaterials for Bone Replacement in Implant Surgery

Introduction

When bone reconstruction of the posterior atrophic maxilla is needed, different surgical procedures can be used. Following the loss of teeth, alveolar ridge resorption leads to a combined vertical and horizontal reduction of the bony support, at the same time increasing maxillary sinus pneumatization. Such a condition makes implant placement impossible, either because of insufficient vertical bone volume or an alteration of the intermaxillary relationship which is not compatible with prosthetically guided implantology. As for other areas, bone augmentation procedures can be performed prior to placement of the implant, concurrent with implant placement, or subsequent to it.

Up to 10 years ago, autogenous bone was considered to be the gold standard in the reconstruction of atrophic areas of the jaws, due to its osteoconductive, osteoinductive and regenerative properties; it should still be chosen as the most suitable material in severe atrophies (class V and VI according to Cawood and Howell). In the treatment of smaller defects (class III and IV), bone substitutes of synthetic and xenogenic origin have been playing an important role in implant surgery. All those materials, generally called "biomaterials", are able to favor the adherence of cells and tissue regeneration thanks to a variable degree of osteoconductive activity; after being tested for several years through randomized prospective or retrospective studies, they can be considered as a reliable way to rebuild bone.

Something fundamental is to remember that the difficulty in rebuilding a bone defect is more related to its extent than its depth. In other words, a very deep but localized defect is easier to treat than a superficial but extensive one. Careful preoperative analysis of the site to be regenerated is important instead of deciding at the time of surgery.

Biomaterials

The term biomaterial generally indicates any substance used to create a medical device destined for diagnosis, prevention, control, mitigation or therapy of a human disease, on condition that it persists in the body for at least 30 days after implantation. First of all, cytotoxicity, genotoxicity, and hemocompatibility of a biomaterial have to be evaluated. After that, attention has to be paid to its macrostructure and microstructure, by evaluating the isotropy. Finally, its mechanical, physical, and chemical properties should be taken into consideration. Which characteristics should a biomaterial have to be considered for implantation in the human body? They can be summarized as follows:

- non-carcinogenic;
- non-antigenic;
- hydrophilic;
- radiopaque;
- easy handling;
- versatile (usable in several clinical fields).

Biomaterials can be obtained from the patient (autogenous), from beings belonging to the same species (homologous), from beings belonging to different species (xenogenic) or from minerals (alloplasts). Apart from autogenous bone, which has osteoconductive, osteoinductive, and osteoproliferative properties, and homologous bone, whose properties are mainly osteoconductive and slightly inductive, all the biomaterials used for bone regeneration are only osteoconductive scaffolds. Bone substitutes were

Essentials of Oral and Maxillofacial Surgery, First Edition. Edited by M. Anthony Pogrel, Karl-Erik Kahnberg and Lars Andersson.
© 2014 John Wiley & Sons, Ltd. Published 2014 by John Wiley & Sons, Ltd.
Companion website: www.wiley.com/go/pogrel/oms

created in order to promote bone regeneration, avoiding the necessity of harvesting bone from the patient. The first materials on the market were represented by ceramic hydroxyapatite of different macrostructures (coral, bioglass, ceramic hydroxyapatite) and the osteoconductive potential, and the resorbability, were not excellent with regard to the implant field. A few years later, demineralized freeze dried bone allograft (DFDBA) from human donors was introduced in the US; osteoinductive properties were claimed for this, because the demineralization process was able to expose bone morphogenetic proteins (BMP). In addition, some publications confirmed an osteoconductive property for this material. Unfortunately, the properties of DFDBA were not confirmed by later histologic and clinical studies in sinus elevation and guided bone regeneration (GBR) procedures.

At the same time, xenogenic anorganic bone was obtained from cattle, followed by similar materials from equine or porcine sources. These mineral scaffolds, resulting from a treatment to eliminate any trace of organic material, promote colonization of bone tissue via osteoconduction. They are slowly replaced by newly formed bone; both the quality and the quantity of lamellar bone is well documented and, at the moment, they are considered a first-choice material in bony defect repair in implantology, with the exception of class V and VI atrophies (Cawood and Howell), where the use of autogenous bone, alone or in association with xenogenic materials, is mandatory to rebuild the bony architecture prior to implant placement.

Biomaterials currently used in osseointegration

Anorganic bovine bone

This is an osteoconductive and slow-resorbing material composed of an anorganic mineral matrix deprived of the organic scaffold in order to leave intercrystalline microtunnels and microcapillaries between the bovine apatite crystals. The high osteoconductivity is due to the natural microstrucure of the material, which demonstrates a large inner surface area and a system of intracrystalline spaces and microtunnels available for ingrowth of blood vessels and osteoblast migration. Long-term stability has been proved by many clinical studies. There must be no direct contact of the material with the implant surface for good implant osseointegration. The only early contact is between the clot and the matrix particles, and the angiogenesis and osteoblasts deposition occur from there. Integration is due to replacement of the bone substitute with newly formed bone. Histomorphometric analysis demonstrated that anorganic bovine bone increases the mineral portion in regenerated areas as compared to host bone areas. Some of the material remains in the bone tissue and

is slowly embedded in lamellar bone, resulting in denser bone, and this could explain the high survival rate of implants placed in areas augmented with it.

Calcium phosphate

Depending on the Ca/P ratio, the presence of water and impurities, this material crystallizes into two different shapes:

- calcium hydroxyphosphate or hydroxyapatite (HA);
- beta calciumtriphosphate (beta TCP).

Synthetic HA has the same chemical composition as human HA, but a slightly different structure. Its rate of metabolism by the human body depends on its structure, chemical composition, and interface surface area.

Beta TCP is also resorbable and is slowly converted to HA inside the human body; it supports early bone apposition (woven bone), although beta TCP's degradation products may provoke an inflammatory response that impairs and reverses bone apposition in the defect site. Histologic evaluations showed a solid host–bone connection at 9 months, but newly formed bone is confined to the periphery of the graft, the center being partially filled with connective tissue. This material can only be said to be basically resorbable, and no conversion process to trabecular, functional spongiosa occurs, since remodeling cannot take place. A recent report on sinus elevation showed no difference between a test site treated with beta TCP and a control site treated with autogenous bone in terms of quantity and rate of ossification in a significant sample of patients.

Calcium sulfate

This material has been used as a synthetic grafting material. Once the sulfate is embedded with water, an exothermic reaction results in crystallization and hardening of the granules. The host bone forms in concentric layers around the resorbing sulfate, which is different to the situation with other ceramics. Dense calcium sulfate does not seem to stimulate early bone apposition, but bone repair is more advanced at 12 weeks as compared with those treated with beta TCP, despite beta TCP's support for direct bone apposition at 1 week. Calcium sulfate appears to provide a more stable osteoconductive scaffold and seems to be a good material in sinus elevation. The osteoconductivity of calcium sulfate is documented, but the clinical experience remains limited.

Calcium carbonate

This material is derived from calcified coral polyp skeletons with an aragonite crystal structure and mineral trace elements. Histologic examinations showed absence of direct bony ingrowth of the carbonate in the bone, while connective tissue appeared to encapsulate the implant, isolating it from the autogenous bone and preventing osteoconduction. Bone remodeling looks incomplete due to an insufficient amount of newly formed bone.

Bioactive glass

This is a resorbable amorphous material composed of silicon dioxide, calcium oxide, and sodium oxide. The osteoconductive property is documented, but the most reliable clinical studies in sinus elevation were carried out using a mix of bioactive glass and autogenous bone in single-arm studies or comparing a mix with a control test represented by autogenous bone alone. Studies evaluating bone repair using bioglass alone are necessary to verify the properties of such a material.

Demineralized freeze-dried bone allograft

This material, from human donor bone, has been extensively used in the treatment of periodontal and periapical osseous defects. The material provides a source of type I collagen, which is the only organic component of bone. The processed bone results in lyophilized particles demineralized with hydrochloric acid. The particles are then recovered by centrifugation, frozen and freeze-dried again. Many reports confirm its ability to induce new bone formation thanks to the exposure of BMP, whose inductive properties are well known. Despite this property, DFDBA's osteoinductive action has never been demonstrated and it seems that the regenerated bone is insufficient either in quality or in quantity to allow predictable implant placement, particularly following sinus elevation procedures. Other clinical studies confirm the reliability of DFDBA in sinus elevations, but always in conjunction with other materials. Similar results are reported relating to the use of DFDBA in association with expanded polytetrafluoroethylene (e-PTFE) membranes.

Surgical techniques

The choice of procedure for reconstructing the posterior areas of the maxilla depends both on the depth and the extent of the defect. Starting from the postextraction defects up to the most severe atrophies, the classification according to Cawood and Howell clarifies, in a simple way, what kind of surgical technique is the most suitable for each specific bony defect. In accordance with that classification, the defects can be listed as follows:

* postextraction sites;
* horizontal defects (including dehiscences and fenestrations around implants);
* vertical defects;
* combined (vertical and horizontal defects);
* sinus elevation.

Postextraction sites

An alveolar bone loss of 23% in the first 6 months after tooth extraction and of 11% during the following 5 years was demonstrated by Carlsson. Alveolar bone loss not only reduces the amount of bone available for adequate support of the prosthetic load, but can also adversely affect the implant position, the peri-implant hard and soft tissue anatomy, and, consequently, the final esthetic and functional outcome. The immediate insertion of an implant in a postextraction site would therefore preserve a greater amount of alveolar bone and also reduce the treatment time. Whenever an immediate implant placement cannot be carried out due to the impossibility of obtaining primary stability for the fixture, physiological resorption due to the remodeling processes must be avoided. This goal can be easily achieved by filling the alveolus with bone substitutes and a free gingival graft, and implant placement surgery can be carried out about 6 months later.

Where there is an infection in the extraction area, immediate implant insertion should be avoided and the surgery postponed until 40–60 days after the extraction.

Immediate technique

When the gap between implant and alveolus is less than 1 mm, tissue regeneration is entrusted to the clot. For larger gaps, bone substitutes can be used to fill the defect and the area is covered with a collagen membrane and a free gingival graft, which improves the quantity and the quality of the soft tissues around the implant at the time of connection of the healing abutment (Fig. 18.1). The soft tissue graft is obviously useless in cases of immediate temporary crown placement.

Delayed technique

In this situation, 6–8 weeks are needed to rebuild the gingival tissue after extraction and implant placement is performed by means of a standard procedure.

Horizontal defects

These defects occur where there is adequate height but insufficient width of the ridge. They include implant dehiscences and fenestrations and can be treated with GBR procedures associated with autogenous bone chips and bone substitutes as well as ridge expansion techniques (at implant placement time) or autogenous bone blocks (prior to implant placement).

Dehiscences and fenestrations

Dehiscences are exposures of the implant at the level of its head, occurring when the thickness of the ridge

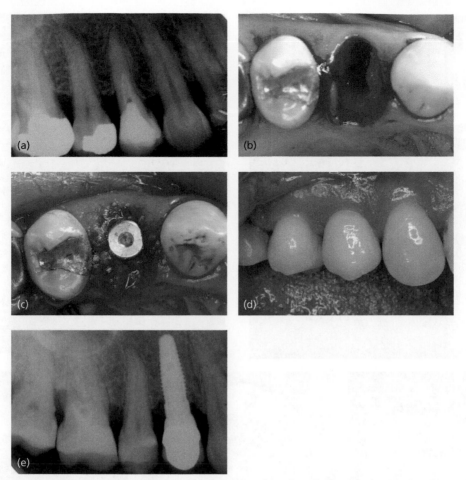

Fig. 18.1 Case 1. (a) Periapical radiographs: first premolar affected by external root resorption can be seen. (b) Tooth extraction: the socket can be seen. (c) A 4.3mm implant placed immediately after tooth extraction. Anorganic bovine bone is used to fill the gap between implant surface and bone structure. (d) Final intraoral view after gold ceramic crown placement. (e) Periapical radiograph: final control.

is insufficient in the most coronal area. Fenestrations are exposures of the middle third or the apical portion of the implant with or without involvement of the implant head.

A bone regeneration technique using autogenous chips, bone substitutes, and resorbable or non-resorbable membranes is a possible treatment. Most dehiscences and fenestrations can easily be treated with a resorbable membrane acting as a stabilizer of the underlying material (granules or chips). When the exposed surface of the implant exceeds 1 mm outside the bone envelope and a large volume of bone has to be regenerated, non-resorbable e-PTFE membranes are indicated. In both cases, membranes have to be stabilized with pins or mini-screws and periosteal releasing incisions of the buccal flap are mandatory to avoid tension at suturing. Vertical mattress and single sutures are required in all the techniques.

Autogenous intraoral or extraoral blocks

Harvesting bone blocks from inside the mouth (chin, mandibular body or ramus) is indicated in the correction of a class IV atrophic ridge, particularly in the case of an extended narrow ridge. When a larger amount of bone is necessary (such as a resorbed max-

illary ridge in edentulous patients) blocks can be harvested from the hip or the calvaria. In all these situations, attention must be paid to the block's resorption during the 4 months' healing. An average resorption of 20–30% can be observed at implant placement time, in blocks harvested from the chin or the hip, due to their cancellous component; and 15% resorption occurs in blocks harvested from the mandibular body and the ramus, which are basically made of cortical bone. An original technique to reduce the resorption of autogenous blocks was presented in 2005, involving a layer of anorganic bovine bone placed on the top of the block and covered by a collagen membrane. Using this procedure it is possible to maintain the original size of the block; it can be successfully used for either intraoral or extraoral grafts (Figs 18.2, 18.3).

Vertical defects

If the bone height is insufficient to guarantee long-term implant stability or the prosthetic rehabilitation would result in too long crowns, vertical ridge augmentation is mandatory. Vertical augmentation can be achieved by means of corticocancellous blocks harvested from the chin or the ramus or, alternatively,

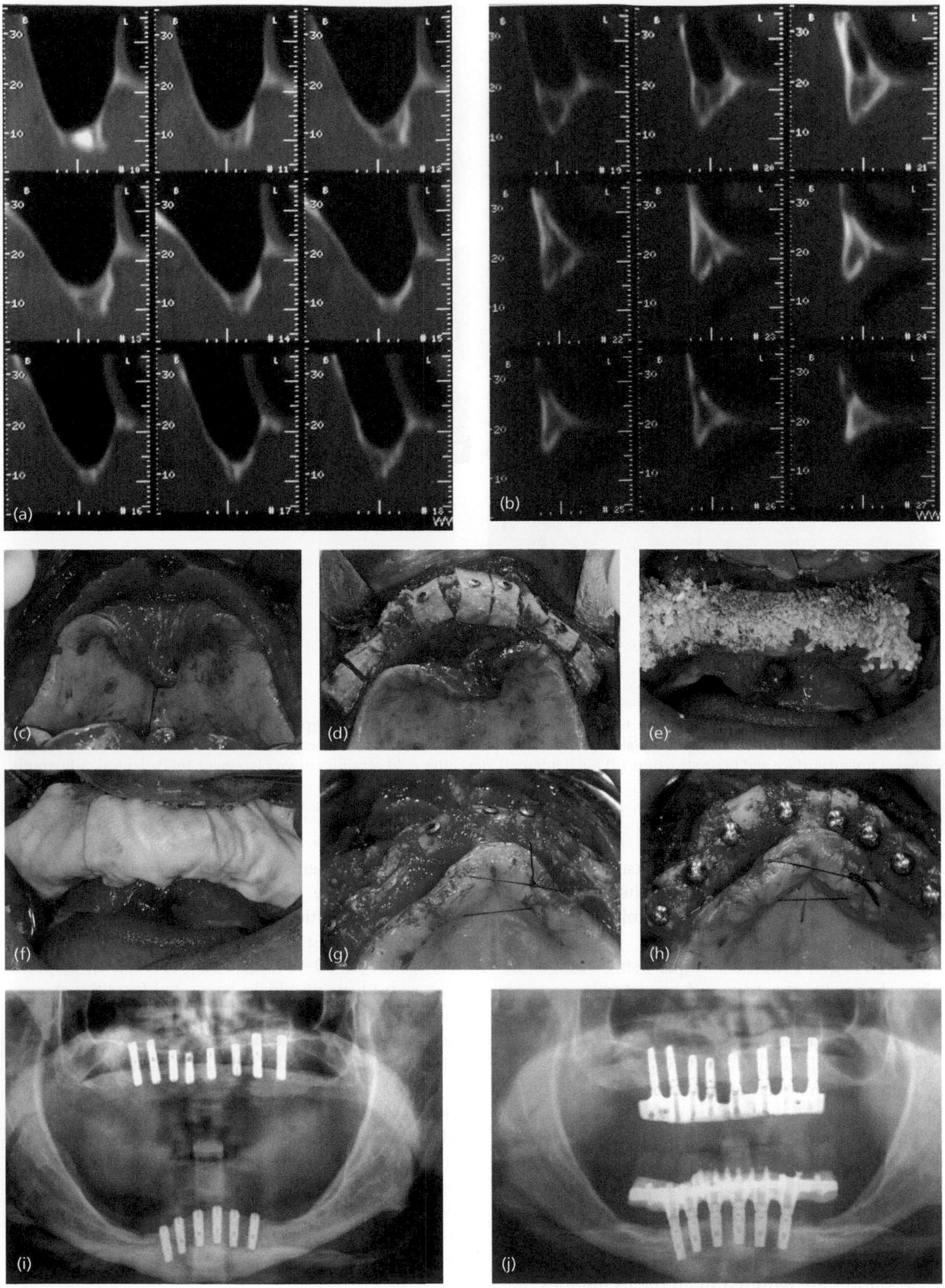

Fig. 18.2 Case 2. (a, b) CT scan view: sinus pneumatization and horizontal bone atrophy can be appreciated. (c) Intraoral view after bilateral sinus lift procedure: before grafting procedure. (d) Autogenous bone block harvested from the hip stabilized to the recipient site by means of cortical screws. (e) Anorganic bovine bone coverage to reduce bone block resorption. (f) Resorbable collagen membrane used to stabilize the anorganic bovine bone. (g) Intraoral view: the new ridge width can be appreciated after removal of cortical screws and before implant placement. (h) Eight implants placed in the newly formed bone. (i) Postoperative panoramic radiograph. (j) 1-year follow-up panoramic radiograph.

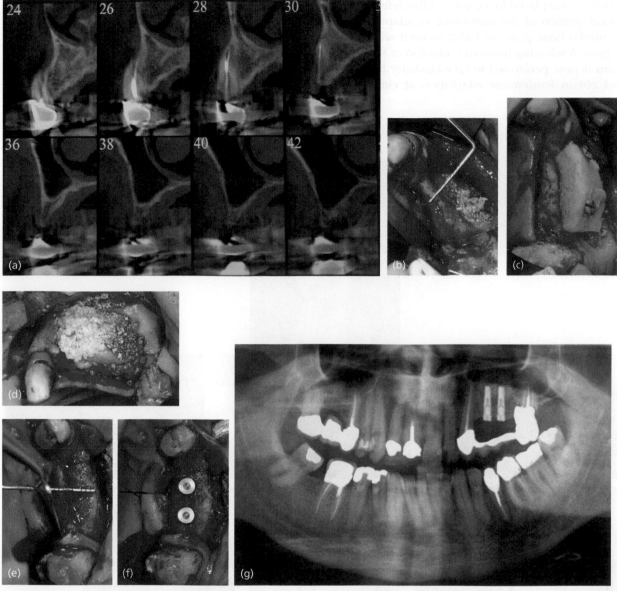

Fig. 18.3 Case 3. (a) CT scan view: sinus pneumatization and horizontal bone atrophy can be appreciated. (b) Intraoral view after sinus lift procedure: a 2 mm wide atrophic ridge can be noticed. (c) Corticocancellous bone block harvested from the chin stabilized by means of cortical screws. (d) Anorganic bovine bone coverage. (e) Intraoral view after 3 months' healing: the newly formed bone can be appreciated. (f) Two implants placed in the augmented edentulous ridge. (g) Postoperative panoramic radiograph.

with cancellous bone chips, bone substitutes, and a titanium-reinforced e-PTFE membrane.

Vertical GBR with membrane

This procedure is very predictable, but it has to be carried out strictly according to the surgical protocol, in order to limit the risks of the membrane exposure.

The most common flap design comprises a full-thickness mid-crestal incision within the keratinized mucosa of the edentulous ridge, extended mesially and distally to at least one adjacent tooth. Vertical releasing cuts are performed at the mesial and distal line angles of the incision. A proper preparation of the recipient site is crucial for new bone formation. The buccal and palatal flaps are reflected and gently

managed to avoid any perforation of the flap. Stainless steel mini-screws are used as "tent poles" to prevent collapse of the membrane and to predetermine either the width or the height of the future alveolar ridge. The mini-screws are placed and left to protrude out from the bone level to the expected height. The cortical plate is then drilled with a round bur to expose the cancellous bone and to provoke some bleeding. The titanium structure of the e-PTFE membrane is bent with pliers to adapt it to the ridge anatomy and it is trimmed with scissors to extend at least 4–5 mm beyond the margins of the defect. Once placed over the surgical recipient site, the membrane is secured to the lingual/palatal aspect of the bone crest with fixation mini-screws or pins. The cancellous autogenous chips mixed with the bone substitute are placed to reconstruct the defect and the buccal portion of the membrane is adapted to the vestibular bone plate, and also secured with screws or pins. A releasing horizontal incision of the periosteum is now performed to give elasticity to the flap and obtain tension-free adaptation at closure. The two margins of the flap can be considered sufficiently released when they overlap by at least 7–10 mm. Closure is done with horizontal mattress sutures first and with interrupted sutures later. The membrane is usually removed 6 months after surgery, at implant placement time (Fig. 18.4).

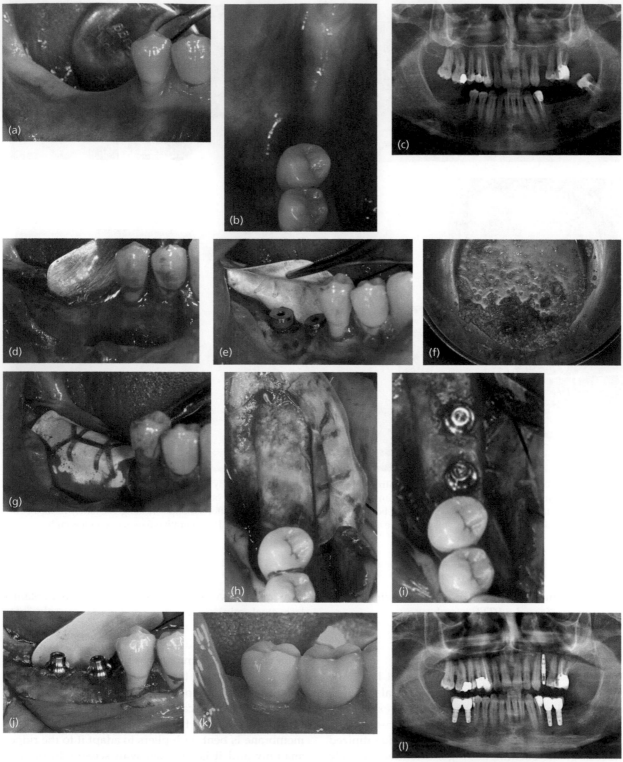

Fig. 18.4 Case 4. (a, b) Intraoral view: a horizontal and vertical defect can be appreciated. (c) Panoramic radiograph: vertical bone resorption can be seen in area 4.6–4.7. (d) Atrophic ridge after flap elevation: vertical bone resorption can be seen. (e) Two implants placed in the ideal position and non-resorbable membrane fixed to the lingual plate to perform vertical bone augmentation. (f) Anorganic bovine bone mixed in 1:1 ratio with autogenous bone harvested from the ramus. (g) Non-resorbable Gore-Tex membrane stabilized after grafting procedure. (h) Newly formed bone after 7 months' healing during membrane removal. (i, j) Healing abutment placed: the horizontal and vertical regeneration can be appreciated. (k) Final restoration. (l) 1-year follow-up panoramic radiograph.

Sinus elevation

When atrophy of the posterior maxilla reduces the amount of bone suitable for implant placement and a bone augmentation procedure is required, first of all one needs to evaluate if the sinus really has migrated from apical to coronal towards the margin of the alveolar ridge or if the sinus is in its previous position and the vertical height loss is due to vertical resorption. In the first case, a sinus elevation procedure is indicated, while in the second situation vertical ridge augmentation should be performed without any sinus involvement.

Once the necessity of performing a sinus elevation has been decided upon, the second step is the choice between a one- or a two-stage procedure. According to the recent literature, a residual alveolar ridge of 4 mm is the absolute minimum height for bone augmentation and simultaneous implant placement and a two-stage technique must be done where there is a residual height of 0–4 mm.

The surgical procedure is the well known Boyne and James technique and autogenous bone or bone substitutes have been used for a long time to fill up the subantral cavity. At present, long-term prospective and retrospective studies confirm that bone substitutes are able to regenerate new bone without harvesting autogenous bone and that the implant survival rate in augmented sinuses with biomaterials is significantly higher than that obtained using autogenous bone chips. In Cawood and Howell class VI defects only autogenous bone is recommended, since the severe atrophy needs all the power of an osteoproliferative material. This means that at least 80% of sinus elevation procedures can be done by using biomaterials alone.

What kind of bone substitute should be chosen to get the best result? All the bone substitutes currently used in the sinus elevation procedures, either xenogenic or alloplasts, offer osteoconductive properties only. The decision should be taken after considering the human hydroxyapatite structure: the more a granule of a biomaterial is similar to a human hydroxyapatite crystal, the more it is possible to get an osteoconductive effect. Another parameter to be taken into consideration is the biomaterial's resorption time. A material which is resorbed too quickly does not allow the osteoblasts and the new vessels to promote formation of woven bone. A material which is resorbed too slowly, by delaying its total substitution with newly formed bone, inhibits bone–implant contact, which is essential for osseointegration. A resorption time of 6–10 months can be considered reasonably ideal. In the author's experience, anorganic bovine bone has given excellent results in over 15 years of sinus elevation surgeries, giving a new bone quality close to a class 2 native bone and a very good osteoconductive property, as verified from many histomorphometric studies. Nevertheless, the author has been using other bone substitutes, such as beta TCP, calcium sulfate, and DFDBA, whose clinical efficacy has been demonstrated in some studies, although with a lower predictability in terms of bone quality and implant survival rate.

When the height of the residual ridge is 6–7 mm, the surgeon can decide whether to use short implants or elevate the sinus floor 2–3 mm with the Summer's osteotome technique. The procedure, wrongly named "minor sinus elevation" is a blind procedure and should be considered with care. In order to elevate the sinus membrane with this procedure, any of the biomaterials can be equally used, since the primary stability of the implant is guaranteed by the residual ridge. See Figures 18.5, 18.6.

Biomaterials in major advanced osseointegration

As described with regard to the intraoral autogenous blocks, biomaterials can be successfully used to reduce the iliac crest blocks with the same coverage technique. The author's clinical experience using anorganic bovine bone as an agent to limit autogenous bone resorption allows him to conclude that the coverage technique can be routinely used with absolute predictability even in cases of a whole maxillary or mandibular reconstruction.

Another way to use biomaterials in major reconstructions is the combination of bone substitutes and cancellous iliac bone as described by Boyne in his presentation of the titanium mesh technique for the upper jaw. The cancellous–anorganic bovine bone mix in a 1:1 ratio is used to fill up a titanium mesh model made in an individual tray (Fig. 18.7). The titanium mesh is secured to the palatal vault and kept in place for 5 months. The use of such a bone substitute helps to maintain the original volume of the graft during remodeling and contraction of the autogenous part, and so helps to determine increased firmness of the regenerated bone at implant placement time.

Developments: growth factors and BMP

A new field in implantology is developing with the aim of finding new ways to improve the osteoconductivity of bone substitutes and to study new molecules able to dictate cellular differentiation and improve bone regeneration. The so-called growth factors are biological mediators which promote cell proliferation. Some of these growth factors have been proved to have the ability to contribute to bone regeneration, PDGF (platelet-derived growth factor) in particular. PDGF is secreted by different cell types, such as platelets, osteoblasts, and activated macrophages, and is able to stimulate chemotaxis, cell proliferation, and protein synthesis. Some clinical studies are currently running on the use of different carriers

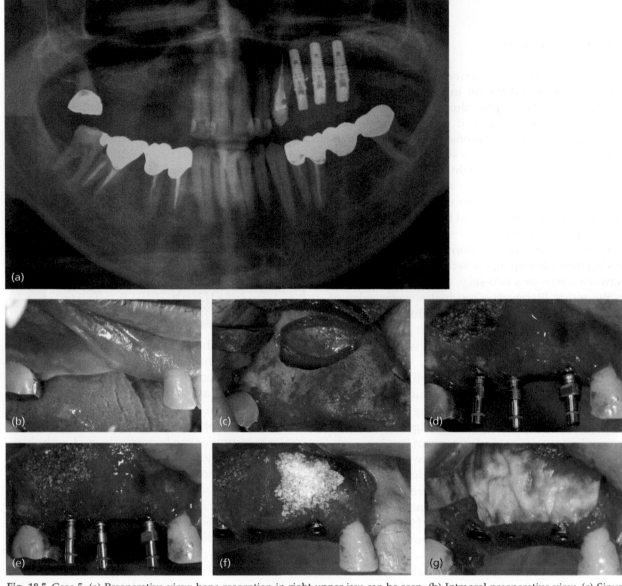

Fig. 18.5 Case 5. (a) Preoperative view: bone resorption in right upper jaw can be seen. (b) Intraoral preoperative view. (c) Sinus lift procedure: lateral approach to lift sinus floor. (d) Implant placement after grafting procedure in the medial portion of the subantral cavity by means of anorganic bovine bone. (e, f) Grafting procedure completed. (g) Resorbable membrane to stabilize the anorganic bovine bone.

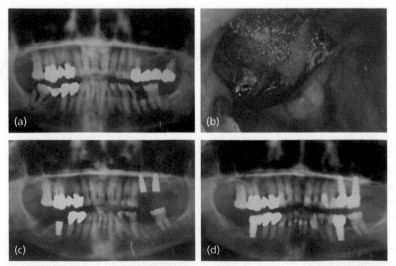

Fig. 18.6 Case 6. (a) Preoperative panoramic radiograph: before teeth extraction in the left upper jaw, 2 months before sinus lift procedure. (b) Sinus lift procedure and implant placement. Hydroxyapatite granules used to fill the subantral cavity can be seen. (c) Postoperative panoramic radiograph. (d) 1-year follow-up panoramic radiograph: no sign of graft resorption or peri-implant bone loss can be seen.

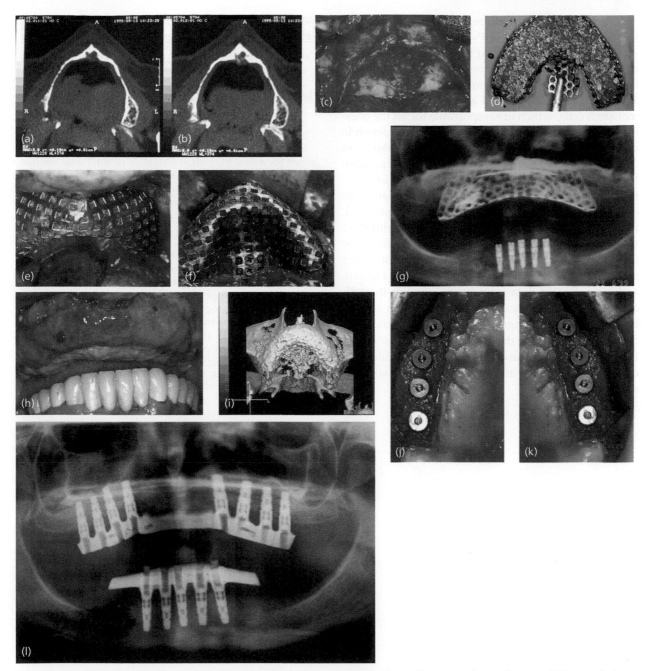

Fig. 18.7 Case 7. (a) Preoperative computed tomography (CT) scan: severe horizontal bone atrophy can be seen. (b) Intraoral view: extreme bone resorption can be appreciated. Bilateral sinus lift procedure performed before bone augmentation by means of titanium mesh. (c) Titanium mesh filled with a mixture of anorganic bovine bone and autogenous bone chips harvested from the hip. (d, e, f) Titanium mesh fixed to the palate by means of two cortical screws. (g) Postoperative panoramic radiograph. (h) Soft tissues healing after titanium mesh removal and fornix deepening procedures. (i) Three-dimensional reconstruction from CT scan: the newly formed bone and ridge dimensions can be seen. (j, k) Implant placement: 4.5 mm implants placed in the augmented alveolar ridge. (l) 5-year panoramic radiograph follow-up.

for PDGF in GBR. PDGF is also one of the factors contained in platelet-rich plasma (PRP), a platelet concentrate produced by plasmaphoresis using centrifugation; this is mixed with autogenous bone chips or bone substitutes in order to add osteoinductive properties to the graft. Different growth factors can be recognized within PRP: transforming growth factor (TGF-beta), insulin-like growth factor (IGF), fibroblast growth factors (FGF), and others. The initial technique was presented by Marx, starting from a large blood sample. Variations were applied in order to simplify the original procedure. After the first promising results using PRP in different ways, studies confirmed that the activity of PRP is significant only in the presence of autogenous bone, while disappointing results are reported in cases where PRP is used in association with bone substitutes. In fact, no significant differences in terms of vital bone production in sinus elevation with anorganic bovine bone or DFDBA are reported.

The real future in bone regeneration seems to be in connection with the BMPs, currently obtained by synthesis using recombinant DNA. BMPs are part of the TGF-beta family but, different to the other growth factors, they have an osteoinductive property. They are exogenic cytokines and act on adult mesenchymal stem cells, which are responsible for all the bone healing processes; their effect, however, depends upon the vector used to deliver the fluid BMP into the site to be regenerated. Different carriers have been studied, such as collagen, polylactic acid granules, anorganic bovine bone, corals, etc., and the ability of BMP-2 and BMP-7 has been investigated. In the first studies in humans by Boyne, rhBMP-2 was used in sinus elevation, showing trabecular bone formation after 16 weeks and similar results in terms of bone regeneration came from Cochran, Howell, and Jung. Recent data from Boyne confirm the reliability of rhBMP-2 in sinus elevation when carried by a resorbable collagen sponge. Further data are necessary to confirm the preliminary results, but in the near future the use of BMPs will considerably change the approach and the treatment of maxillary atrophy.

Recommended reading

Cawood JL, Howell RE. (1988) A classification of the edentulous jaws. *International Journal of Oral and Maxillofacial Surgery*, **17**, 232–36.

Hallman M, Sennerby L, Lundgren S. (2002) A clinical and histologic evaluation of implant integration in the posterior maxilla after sinus floor augmentation with autogenous bone, bovine hydrxyapatite, or a 20:80 mixture. *International Journal of Oral and Maxillofacial Implants*, **17**, 635–43.

Jensen SS, Aaboe M, Pinholt EM, *et al.* (1996) Tissue reaction and material characteristics of four bone substitutes. *International Journal of Oral and Maxillofacial Implants*, **11**, 55–66.

Maiorana C. (2010) Biomaterials for bone replacement in implant surgery. In: *Oral and Maxillofacial Surgery* (eds, Andersson L, Kahnberg K-E, Pogrel MA). Oxford, Wiley-Blackwell.

Maiorana C, Redemagni M, Rabagliati M, *et al.* (2000) Treatment of maxillary ridge resorption by sinus augmentation with iliac cancellous bone, anorganic bovine bone and implants: a clinical and histologic report. *International Journal of Oral and Maxillofacial Implants*, **15**, 873–8.

Maiorana C, Sommariva L, Brivio P, *et al.* (2003) Maxillary sinus augmentation with anorganic bovine bone and autologous platelet rich plasma: preliminary clinical and histologic evaluations. *International Journal of Periodontics and Restorative Dentistry*, **23**, 227–35.

Part 4: Oral Pathologic Lesions

(Section Editor: Tony Pogrel)

Chapter 19

Initial Evaluation and Management of the Oral and Maxillofacial Pathology Patient

The first step to approaching a patient with oral and maxillofacial pathology is to take a thorough history and perform a physical examination. Information gleaned from the history and physical examination will provide clues to the correct diagnosis and guide the clinician in selecting the appropriate tools to validate the diagnosis.

Obtaining the history

In taking the history of present illness, one should first establish a timeline for the disease. One should ask when the patient first noticed symptoms. Symptoms of interest include pain, paresthesia, dysphagia, dyspnea, otalgia, trismus, voice changes, weight loss, fevers, chills, and malaise. Although not necessarily present, pain is the most common presenting symptom for head and neck cancer. Paresthesia in the head and neck area is also highly concerning, and should be considered a sign of potential malignancy until proven otherwise. Either of these symptoms, when occurring without a likely explanation, should prompt a thorough investigation including a neurologic exam, imaging studies, and, potentially, tissue sampling.

The surgeon should inquire about any prior treatment or diagnostic tests. If biopsies have been performed in the past, it is essential to review both the pathology report and the pathology slides with a pathologist experienced in the diagnosis of oral pathology lesions. One should not take a prior pathologic diagnosis at face value, as errors can occur.

Other diseases, such as infectious diseases and autoimmune diseases, may present with oral lesions similar to oral cancer. Ask about symptoms that can rule in or out these other diseases if the initial history is suggestive of pathology other than cancer. The patient's history should be reviewed for exposures, constitutional symptoms, or systemic manifestations. An acute onset, presence of fever or chills, rapid swelling, and signs of acute inflammation are suggestive of an infectious process. A chronic process with dermatologic findings, arthralgias, or multiple organ system involvement is suspicious for an autoimmune disorder.

The clinician should take the time to take a thorough past medical history. The history may provide additional information helpful for stratifying a patient's risk for developing oral cancer. The past medical history may provide the etiology of the disease. Inquire about a history of dysplasia, immunocompromised states, other types of cancer, and a history of head and neck radiation.

A history of tobacco and alcohol use should be determined. Ask about cigarette usage in addition to other forms of tobacco use, such as snuff, cigar, or pipe tobacco. The quantity of tobacco and length of time used should be recorded. An accurate alcohol history is often difficult to gather, as most people underestimate their use. It is helpful to corroborate history with family and friends. It is also helpful to inquire about betel nut use, particularly in patients of Asian or South Asian descent. One should inquire about environmental exposures at work and home. A history of dental neglect should be recorded.

The focused physical examination

The focused examination of the oral and maxillofacial pathology patient should always include an examination of the neck, the face, the salivary glands, and the oral cavity. Examination of the eyes, ear, nose, pharynx, larynx, and cranial nerves should be performed as directed by the patient's presenting symptoms and the clinician's differential diagnosis.

Essentials of Oral and Maxillofacial Surgery, First Edition. Edited by M. Anthony Pogrel, Karl-Erik Kahnberg and Lars Andersson.
© 2014 John Wiley & Sons, Ltd. Published 2014 by John Wiley & Sons, Ltd.
Companion website: www.wiley.com/go/pogrel/oms

Imaging studies

Once the initial history and physical exam are completed, the next step in the clinical evaluation is often the ordering of imaging studies. There are a number of modalities available to the oral and maxillofacial surgeon, each with their own strengths, limitations, and varying degrees of invasiveness. As with any study, it is important for the surgeon requesting the imaging to have specific questions to be answered. When requesting imaging, the surgeon aims to: (1) better characterize the location, composition, and behavior of the lesion to assist in a diagnosis; (2) delineate the full extent of the lesion and its proximity to adjacent vital structures to aid in prognosticating as well as treatment planning; and (3) in the case of malignant disease, determine whether there is metastatic spread to the neck lymphatics.

Plain radiographs

Plain radiographs are two-dimensional images created by projecting X-rays through a patient on to a film or digital sensor. These include, dental panoramic tomograms, dental radiographs and chest radiographs.

A chest radiograph to screen for metastasis or synchronous lung primaries is part of the standard comprehensive evaluation of a patient diagnosed with head and neck cancer. Many of the risk factors that predispose a patient to developing oral cancer are also risk factors for other pathology. As many as 10% of oral cancer patients have chest metastases and 5% of patients have synchronous lung carcinomas that are detected on chest imaging.

Dental radiographs, such as periapical, bitewing, and occlusal films, are sometimes helpful in the evaluation of lesions of the dentate segments of the mandible and maxilla.

The dental panoramic tomogram (orthopantomogram or Panorex) is a film that is commonly used by dentists and oral and maxillofacial surgeons. Much like other dental radiographs, it is quick and inexpensive. It also has the advantage of being able to effectively image the maxilla and mandible. For these reasons, it is routinely part of the initial assessment of a patient presenting with pathology of the oral and maxillofacial region, and can be very helpful in diagnosing tumors and cysts of the jaws.

Computed tomography (CT)

CT allows the surgeon to appreciate a tumor's location and size in three dimensions, thus accurately defining a tumor's relationship to important vital structures, such as the great vessels, skull base, and orbit. In addition, CT is far superior in appreciating differences in soft tissue planes and vasculature. Fat, muscle, and water can be differentiated fairly easily. This ability is further enhanced by contrast. This has also allowed surgeons to screen for nodal metastasis with reasonable sensitivity.

Although the cost of a CT scan is decreasing as accessibility increases, the study still remains expensive. The effective dose of radiation from a head and neck CT is relatively small when compared to annual exposure to natural radiation. But, at around 1000–4000 μSv, it is not insignificant. This is, however, still a greater effective dose than that of plain radiography, and may be of concern to some patients, especially when serial CT scans are required, or the patients are children. Another drawback of the use of CT in the maxillofacial region is the obscuring of the image from artifacts arising from high-density materials such as dental filling or surgical hardware.

Recently, the cone-beam CT is an iteration of the technology that has been increasingly adopted for use in the oral and maxillofacial region, in particular for use in prosthodontic and orthodontic treatment planning, but also for use in diagnosing pathology as well as surgical and radiotherapy treatment planning. Cone-beam CT uses an X-ray beam in the shape of a cone that rotates and scans the entire volume of interest, as opposed to a conventional fan-beam CT, which uses a fan-shaped X-ray that rotates around and advances along the volume of interest. Because of this, cone-beam CT decreases the effective dose to roughly around 23–52 μSv. In addition, cone-beam CT is less susceptible to dental artifacts. The spatial accuracy is comparable to conventional CT, with its relative geometric error measured in tenths of a millimeter. However, some of the drawbacks of the cone-beam CT are its inferior soft tissue visualization, which limits its use in diagnostics for oral and maxillofacial pathology and staging of the neck, and that it is limited in the total volume that can be visualized with a single scan.

Another advance in surgical planning has been the use of conventional CT to create stereolithic models and customized surgical reconstruction plates.

Magnetic resonance imaging

MRI is a technology that is based upon the science of nuclear magnetic resonance. The system works by placing a patient in a magnetic field that aligns the protons of hydrogen atoms (most commonly found in water) in the direction of the field. A second magnetic field is then momentarily introduced that causes protons to be deflected from this axis and, in the process, absorb some of its energy. Once this second field is released, the protons that were previously deflected return to the initial axis of the first magnetic field and release the absorbed energy as a radiofrequency. The radiofrequencies are then detected by the MRI scanner and are used to determine the position of the respective protons. Several of these additional fields are used along the volume of interest and the information is compiled into a three-dimensional image that can be viewed in sections. Gadolinium, a paramagnetic material, is used to enhance areas of inflammation or increased vascularity.

As with CT, the MRI creates spatial imaging that allows the surgeon to visualize a tumor in three dimensions and appreciate the tumor's relationship to adjacent structures. In addition, MRI has several advantages over CT. It has superior soft tissue resolution, and, as such, is the preferred imaging of choice of neurologic pathology. It is minimally affected by artifacts from high-density materials. MRI also does not use ionizing radiation and is considered non-invasive. In addition, the use of certain protocols, namely magnetic resonance angiography (MRA), allows for the imaging and detection of blood flow, which is useful in the preoperative assessment of vessels for microvascular reconstruction.

As the technology uses a strong magnetic field, implanted paramagnetic materials, such as pacemakers, cochlear implants, deep brain stimulators, or older vascular aneurysm clips, are an absolute contraindication for MRI. These can cause motion and thermal injury to surrounding tissues. MRI scanners are much slower than CT scanners, with scanning times up to 40 minutes on older machines. Because of this, motion artifacts are a problem and patients who are unable to lie still (such as children) may require anesthesia to have an MRI. Furthermore, patients who suffer from claustrophobia may also find undergoing an MRI difficult.

Positron emission tomography (PET) and PET/CT

PET is an imaging modality that highlights areas of the body with increased metabolic activity. Radionuclides are bound to molecules that are important to human metabolism. The most common tracer used in PET is F2-fluoro-2deoxy-D-glucose (FDG), which is a radioactively labeled glucose. FDG is administered intravenously and becomes sequestered in cells that are actively taking up glucose. Malignant cells that are more mitotically and metabolically active would then have relatively greater uptake than surrounding nonmalignant cells. Once sequestered in cells, the FDG undergoes radioactive decay to a more stable molecule, emitting positrons in the process. These positrons combine with electrons within the adjacent tissues and annihilate, resulting in a release of gamma rays 180° from each other. These gamma rays are then picked up by detectors within the PET scanner. PET is often combined with CT, or even MRI, to give enhanced localization.

Ultrasound

Ultrasound images are created from the recording of the amplitudes of reflected high-frequency sound waves. The primary advantage of this tool is that anatomy can be visualized dynamically in real time by the sonographer. Other advantages are that ultrasound is extremely safe and relatively inexpensive.

Ultrasound has several indications. It is useful in evaluating superficial nodules of the neck, salivary glands, and thyroid gland. Ultrasound is very effective in identifying cystic lesions, which appear as well defined hypoechoic (dark) masses. Benign tumors of the salivary and thyroid glands are similarly well defined, lobular, and hypoechoic. Lesions that are less well defined are suspicious for malignancy and should prompt the clinician to order additional studies.

Obtaining a tissue diagnosis

Much information can be gathered from taking the history, performing the physical exam, and acquiring the appropriate imaging studies. However, histologic analysis is absolutely essential for a definitive diagnosis of oral pathology. For suspicious lesions of the soft or hard tissues of the oral cavity, a tissue biopsy is the sole method to obtain this.

Once the decision is made to perform a biopsy, the surgeon must determine: (1) whether the biopsy should be excisional or incisional; (2) what is the setting that the biopsy should be performed under; (3) what type of instrumentation should be used; and (4) decide where the biopsy specimen should be taken from.

Excisional and incisional biopsy

For an excisional biopsy, the entire lesion is removed. This approach is indicated if the suspicious lesion is likely to be benign, likely to be cured by local excision, and small enough that local excision is feasible. For an incisional biopsy, only a sample of representative tissue is taken from the patient, leaving the rest of the lesion in situ. This is indicated if the lesion is suspicious for malignancy or the area involved is larger than can be excised simply.

Setting for performing the biopsy

Many lesions are amenable to biopsy in the clinic. These include lesions of the skin, lesions of the lip, and mucosal lesions of the oral cavity. However, large lesions of the oral cavity that extend into the oropharynx or oral lesions with an intraosseous component may be more efficiently sampled in the operating room under general anesthesia. Having the patient under general anesthesia affords the surgeon the opportunity to take the time to adequately expose and visualize the lesion and sample enough tissue in enough locations, without being limited by concern for keeping an awake patient comfortable. In addition, if the plan is to perform an excisional biopsy, frozen section analysis of incisional biopsy specimens can be performed initially to verify that a lesion is, in fact, benign and not in need of an oncologic resection.

Instrumentation for performing the biopsy

A biopsy should be done with a sharp cutting instrument. A scalpel, fine scissors, a biopsy punch, or a combination of these can be used. The punch biopsy is particularly useful in sampling friable lesions. In these lesions, it may be difficult to adequately grab the tissue, as it often crumbles under the pressure of the tissue forceps.

Deciding where to sample with the biopsy

When performing an incisional biopsy, much depends on selecting a representative sample of the lesion to be diagnosed. The portion of the lesion that yields the most information will vary depending on the nature of the lesion and what is suspected to be the most likely diagnosis.

In ulcerative lesions that are suspicious for malignancy, the biopsy should be performed on the ulcer itself, near the edge of the ulcer. Normal mucosa does not need to be removed, as it does not provide any meaningful information. Do not perform the biopsy in a necrotic area as one may miss the diagnosis and get necrosis only. The biopsy should have a minimum depth of 5 mm to enable the pathologist to view the depth of invasion.

If the ulcerative lesion more closely fits an autoimmune process, a biopsy of the normal tissue should be performed. In vesiculobullous diseases, such as pemphigus vulgaris or erythema multiforme, the tissue from the ulcer itself does not provide helpful information, The surgeon should take more than one biopsy specimen so that one can be processed and stained with the standard hematoxylin and eosin stains and the other can be processed for direct immunofluorescence.

The differential diagnosis for intraosseous lesions includes odontogenic cysts or tumors, non-odontogenic cysts or tumors, fibro-osseous diseases, epithelial neoplasms that have eroded bone, vascular lesions, infectious processes, and metastatic diseases. Before an intraosseous lesion is accessed, it is advisable to rule out a vascular lesion, as cutting into a high-flow vascular malformation could lead to catastrophic hemorrhaging. Exam findings, such as a pulsatile lesion, audible bruits, or palpable thrills would be suggestive of a vascular lesion. Often there are associated soft tissue changes. The overlying mucosa may appear expansile and blue in color. In high-flow lesions affecting the dentoalveolar segments, there is frequently gingival hypertrophy with bleeding from the gingiva sulci. The increased vascular flow may also cause ipsilateral maxillary or mandibular hypertrophy. A Doppler examination may also be helpful in making this determination.

Once the area involved is visualized, a window in the bone may be created if the lesion has not already perforated the bone cortex. This will allow the lesion to be seen grossly. If the lesion is cystic, take note of the nature of the cystic contents, documenting the consistency, color, and whether it is characteristic for certain pathology. Generously sample the cyst lining. If the lesion is solid or solid with cystic components, sample tissue from the most central part of the lesion.

It is a common practice, if the lesion is obviously cystic, to marsupialize the cyst and place a drain that starts within the deepest portion of the cystic space and exits through the soft tissue flap into the oral cavity. In this way, if the lesion ultimately is diagnosed as either a keratocystic odontogenic tumor (formerly known as odontogenic keratocyst) or a dentigerous cyst, it has also been simultaneously treated.

Fine-needle aspiration biopsy

Fine-needle aspiration biopsy (FNAB) is a technique in which a fine needle is passed into a mass, cells are aspirated, and these cells are then prepared on slides and analyzed by a cytopathologist. The use of aspiration biopsy has been practiced for well over a century. Initially, the technique involved the use of a largebore needle under local anesthesia, but it has since evolved to be used with fine-gauge needles. At most institutions, this is performed by specialized cytopathologists.

Indications

FNAB can be used as the method for initial diagnosis for almost any mass in the head and neck region, particularly in disease processes that are not clearly infectious. This technique is helpful in distinguishing neoplastic processes from those that are inflammatory or reactive. However, the most common indication for the use of FNAB is a mass located in the neck, thyroid gland, or salivary glands.

Adjunctive diagnostic tools

Many premalignant and malignant lesions are small and are difficult to appreciate. Even when they are visualized, providers who do not frequently deal with diagnosis of diseases of the oral and maxillofacial region are, understandably, reticent to aggressively biopsy all suspicious lesions. Both of these scenarios are especially true when the lesions are relatively innocuous appearing. As a result, it is common for the generalist to dismiss more serious diseases, such as oral cancer, from the differential diagnosis, because they are rare or the patient's demographics do not necessarily fit the disease. Unfortunately, this is a fallacy, as it has been demonstrated that innocuous lesions can indeed be cancer and that there is an increasing incidence of oral cancer in younger adults who have never used tobacco or abused alcohol.

Therefore, the ability to perform a minimally invasive test to detect inconspicuous lesions or determine

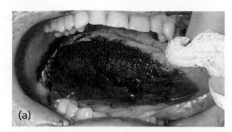 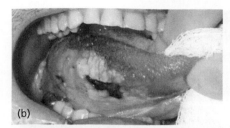

Fig. 19.1 (a) Staining of the oral tongue by toluidine blue prior to decolorization. (b) Tongue stained with toluidine blue after decolorization. The area of dysplasia retains the vital stain and remains dark blue. Note that the filiform papilla of the dorsal tongue stains a pale blue.

the malignant potential of borderline suspicious lesions would be a highly attractive tool. The most commonly available adjunctive diagnostic tools that have been used to fill this niche are discussed under their various headings.

Toluidine blue

Toluidine blue is a vital dye that stains nuclear material. As a consequence, it preferentially stains tissues with high rates of cellular turnover, namely neoplastic mucosa.

Technique

To perform the stain, have the patient first rinse his or her mouth with 1% acetic acid for 20–30 seconds. Following this, the patient should rinse with water twice, again for 20–30 seconds each time. Next, have the patient rinse with 1% toluidine blue solution. Follow this with 20–30 seconds of rinsing with 1% acetic acid and 20 seconds of rinsing with water.

Dark blue staining indicates a positive result, pictured in Figure 19.1, which represents the dye binding to nuclear material. Pale blue staining is more representative of benign lesions, which show no nuclear stains on histology. The papillae of the dorsal tongue also tend to retain toluidine blue.

Indications

Toluidine blue has been demonstrated to be an effective adjunctive screening tool in identifying premalignant lesions or oral cancer recurrences in high-risk populations, particularly those who have already been diagnosed with having oral dysplasia or oral cancer.

Tissue fluorescence

Autofluorescence is a property of cells whereby specific wavelengths of light are absorbed by molecules within cells, causing them to move into an excited state. As the molecules return back to their resting state, the energy from the excitation is released in the form of fluorescence emissions. There are several types of molecules that exhibit autofluorescence, but most commonly exist in the mitochondria and lyso-

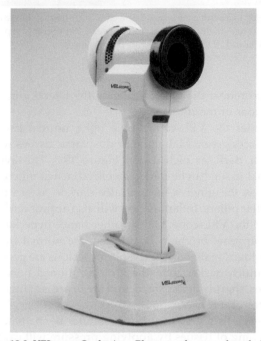

Fig. 19.2 VELscope® device. Photograph reproduced from LED Dental Inc. with permission.

somes of the cell. Porphyrins in erythrocytes also contribute to autofluorescence.

It has been observed that cancer cells have different autofluorescence emission patterns than normal tissues. This has led to the development of technologies that aim to highlight the differences in autofluorescence in order to aid in detection of pathologic oral lesions.

VELscope® (Fig. 19.2) is an example of an adaptation of this technology that uses a handheld device that shines high-intensity blue excitation light (400–460 nm wavelengths) into the oral cavity while the provider can visualize the different fluorescence patterns.

Technique

After performing a thorough history and physical exam under normal incandescent lighting, repeat the intraoral examination while shining the VELscope light into the oral cavity. Keep the light approximately 5 cm away from the entrance of the oral cavity to maximize the area to be illuminated. While shining the light, examine the entire oral cavity through the filter that is attached to the handheld light, taking

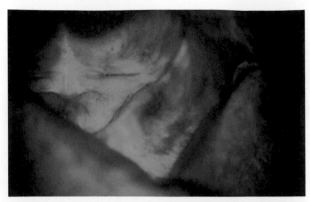

Fig. 19.3 Darkening of oral tongue due to difference in tissue fluorescence highlighted by VELscope®. Photograph reproduced from LED Dental Inc. with permission.

care to retract the tongue to view the lateral tongue and floor of mouth.

Under the VELscope's blue light, normal tissue fluoresces green. Malignant or dysplastic tissues will appear dark, as pictured in Figure 19.3. However, normal tissue can be dark as well. Attached mucosa, such as the gingiva, is typically darker, as are the tonsillar pillars. Inflammation will also appear darker under the VELscope. On the other hand, hyperkeratosis appears brighter. To differentiate normal from pathologic, malignant or dysplastic lesions are generally much darker than the aforementioned normal tissues, sharply demarcated, and are in areas at higher risk for oral cancer.

Areas that are suspicious should be palpated. Blanching of tissues by applying pressure will cause areas of inflammation that appear dark to fluoresce more like normal tissue.

It is important to correlate what is seen under the VELscope with the conventional oral examination. If, after considering all the information gathered the lesion remains suspicious, then the area should be biopsied.

Indications

The VELscope, as recommended by the manufacturer, is meant to be an adjunctive screening tool, to aid in the detection of suspicious oral lesions that may require a surgical biopsy when performing a conventional oral examination. In addition, the manufacturer suggests that it may also be used to delineate the full extent of a lesion when determining margins of resection.

Certainly, one study of 44 patients reported that the VELscope has a sensitivity and specificity of 98 and 100% for identifying dysplasia or carcinoma verified by surgical biopsy. It is important to point out that all of these lesions were visible with standard incandescent lighting and the majority of them were clinically suspicious. Unfortunately, whether the VELscope is useful in detecting suspicious lesions that are not visible, or for highlighting areas of concern within larger innocuous lesions, has not been determined.

Furthermore, it cannot be overemphasized that the VELscope was designed only to serve as an adjunctive diagnostic aid, and is not intended to replace the surgical biopsy for diagnosing oral lesions. Therefore, it should not be used to rule out malignancy in visible lesions.

Tissue reflectance

Tissue reflectance, or chemiluminescence, is an adjunctive screening tool that has been used for detection of premalignant or malignant lesions of the cervical mucosa. Recently, this method has been applied to the identification of suspicious oral lesions as well. Two such systems are currently available, ViziLite® Plus and MicroLux™ DL, pictured in Figures 19.4a and 19.4b, respectively. Tissue reflectance is a tool meant to enhance the visibility of pathologic lesions, as shown in Figures 19.4c, 19.4d, and 19.4e. Theoretically, the increased nuclear to cytoplasmic ratio of squamous neoplasms causes increased light reflectance relative to normal epithelium, an observation of which these tools attempt to take advantage.

Technique

After performing a thorough history and head and neck examination, have the patient rinse with a 1% acetic acid solution for 30 seconds as a mucolytic agent. Next, use the light source of the available system to inspect the mucosa of the oral cavity, taking special care to examine areas at higher risk for oral malignancy such as the floor of mouth and tongue. The ViziLite Plus system uses a chemiluminescent light that is disposable, whereas the MicroLux DL is battery operated. In either case, the manufacturer recommends that the light be kept about 0.5 cm from the area of epithelium being inspected. Suspicious lesions will appear "acetowhite". Surgical biopsy is necessary to confirm a diagnosis of dysplasia or cancer.

Indications

Tissue reflectance technology is intended to be an adjunctive screening tool to the conventional oral examination and requires confirmation by surgical biopsy. However, it is debatable whether or not the use of these instruments provides any added benefit over the conventional oral examination under standard incandescent lighting. Although the sensitivity for highlighting potentially pathologic lesions is high, it has been observed that many obviously benign lesions, such as leukoedema and traumatic ulcers, test positive. In the majority of the studies evaluating its efficacy, lesions detected by tissue reflectance were also visible under incandescent lighting. Furthermore, actual sensitivity and specificity are difficult to report, as surgical biopsies were not used to diagnose all detected lesions in any of the available studies. One study by Oh and Laskin

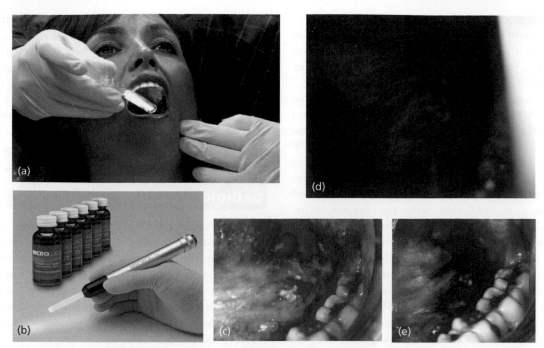

Fig. 19.4 (a) ViziLite device. Photo reproduced from Zila Pharmaceuticals, Inc. with permission. (b) Microlux/DL device. Photograph reproduced from AdDent, Inc. with permission. (c) Tongue with carcinoma in situ, viewed under standard incandescent lighting. (d) The same lesion viewed with ViziLite chemiluminescent lighting. (e) The same lesion viewed after staining with toluidine blue.

reported that the use of ViziLite actually made visualizing lesions more difficult due to the distracting highlights it created.

Brush cytology

The brush biopsy (Oral CDx® from CDx Laboratories) is a technique developed as a bridge to the surgical biopsy. It is intended for oral lesions that appear innocuous and would normally not be subject to a surgical biopsy. In these situations, rather than wrestle with the pitfalls of taking the "watch and wait" approach in a high-volume practice not specialized in following oral and maxillofacial pathology, the provider can perform a brush biopsy to assess the malignant potential of the lesion.

Indications

The brush biopsy is intended to be an adjunct diagnostic tool, as opposed to a screening tool. In other words, in lesions that have been detected, the brush biopsy is meant to assist in establishing a diagnosis.

Because the brush biopsy is targeted towards those lesions that clinicians might not necessarily biopsy, it must be highly sensitive for detecting malignancy in lesions that are clinically innocuous.

Management of premalignant disease

In oncology, it is a commonly held tenet that cancers that are detected early can be treated more effectively

and with less morbidity, thus increasing a patient's chances for survival. It has been theorized that cells that ultimately become malignant must go through a succession of genetic changes that allow them to be derailed from the usual growth restrictions of normal cells in tissues, a process described as multistep carcinogenesis. Thus, if a cancer can be detected early, before it has acquired all of the mutations necessary for invasion and metastasis it may be possible to successfully treat the disease locally. Certainly, this has been shown to be true in several cancers including colorectal cancer and cervical cancer.

Natural history of premalignant disease

Several lesions within the oral cavity have been said to be premalignant. They include leukoplakia, erythroplakia, lichen planus, and submucous fibrosis, among others. However, only leukoplakia and erythroplakia contribute significantly to the incidence of premalignant lesions and oral cancer.

Silverman *et al.* have described a unique form of leukoplakia that has very high rates of malignant transformation called proliferative verrucous leukoplakia (PVL). These lesions tend to appear initially as hyperkeratosis. However, they aggressively spread to include large areas of the oral cavity and often are multifocal. Although slow growing, they are persistent, and invariably recur after being excised. Over time, they can become exophytic and verrucous in appearance. Even as these lesions become progressively malignant in behavior, the histopathology can often remain as benign hyperplasia. Therefore, these lesions should be evaluated by their clinical behavior and not their pathology. Malignant transformation is expected if patients are followed for enough time, with rates of transformation at 60–100%.

It has been suggested that the human papilloma virus (HPV) may also play a role in leukoplakia and premalignant disease in the oral cavity, as is the case with oropharyngeal cancer. Whether certain HPV subtypes increase the risk of developing oral cancer remains a contentious issue. One of the difficulties with establishing a relationship between HPV and oral cancer is confusion with the nomenclature. The distinction between oral cancer, oropharyngeal cancer, and head and neck cancer is often not made explicit or is simply disregarded. In addition, PCR assays for HPV in oral cancer are not nearly as sensitive as they are for cervical cancer. At the present time, the general consensus is that HPV is not strongly associated with the development of oral cancer.

On histopathologic analysis, leukoplakias are also heterogeneous in presentation. Biopsy findings can be variable, demonstrating hyperkeratosis, varying grades of dysplasia, carcinoma in situ, or invasive squamous cell carcinoma. The discovery of dysplasia may provide some diagnostic benefit, as patients with biopsy-proven dysplasia are at higher risk for malignant transformation.

Surgical management of dysplasia

The most common method for managing biopsy-proven dysplasia of the oral cavity is local surgical excision. However, it is important to recognize that there is currently no evidence that surgical excision is effective in removing all premalignant cells. Nor is there any evidence that suggests excision prevents recurrence of the dysplasia, prevents transformation, or reduces mortality. In actuality, nearly 30% of dysplasias recur in the same location after excision.

Medical management of dysplasia

Given that surgery is probably ineffective in treating dysplasia, especially in the setting of field cancerization, the use of systemic or topical chemopreventive measures is particularly attractive. Several agents have been studied for this purpose, including vitamin A and retinoic acid, taken systemically or applied topically, systemic beta-carotene, systemic lycopene, topical ketorolac, and topical bleomycin. Although

beta-carotene, lycopene, vitamin A, and retinoids showed a small amount of benefit, they were associated with adverse effects and had high recurrence rates with cessation of the therapy. At the present time it is not felt that any chemopreventative measures are of any benefit for treating premalignant disease or preventing malignant transformation.

Summary of the approach to the oral and maxillofacial pathology patient

The evaluation of the oral and maxillofacial pathology patient begins with a focused history and physical examination. An experienced clinician will develop a differential diagnosis early on and will test and refine his or her hypotheses as they interview and examine the patient. Imaging studies are selected and ordered to answer specific questions and based upon specific indications, as each type of study has its strengths and weaknesses. If a neoplastic process is suspected, it should be confirmed with a tissue diagnosis. FNAB is extremely helpful as a first-line evaluation tool for neck or salivary gland masses. For most diseases, a surgical biopsy is necessary for a definitive diagnosis. If a neoplastic disease is suspected, the clinician should not hesitate to perform a biopsy or refer to an appropriate specialist.

Recommended reading

Cheng A, Schmidt BL. (2010) Initial evaluation and management of the oral and maxillofacial pathology patient. In: *Oral and Maxillofacial Surgery* (eds, Andersson L, Kahnberg K-E, Pogrel MA). Oxford, Wiley-Blackwell.

Hansen LS, Olson JA, Silverman S, Jr. (1985) Proliferative verrucous leukoplakia. A long-term study of thirty patients. *Oral Surgery, Oral Medicine, Oral Pathology*, **60**, 285–98.

Lane PM, Gilhuly T, Whitehead P, *et al.* (2006) Simple device for the direct visualization of oral-cavity tissue fluorescence. *Journal of Biomedical Optics*, **11**, 024006.

Oh ES, Laskin DM. (2007) Efficacy of the ViziLite system in the identification of oral lesions. *Journal of Oral and Maxillofacial Surgery*, **65**, 424–6.

Reiner B, Siegel E, Sawyer R, Brocato RM, Maroney M, Hooper F. (1997) The impact of routine CT of the chest on the diagnosis and management of newly diagnosed squamous cell carcinoma of the head and neck. *American Journal of Roentgenology*, **169**, 667–71.

Shiboski CH, Schmidt BL, Jordan RC. (2005) Tongue and tonsil carcinoma: increasing trends in the US population ages 20–44 years. *Cancer*, **103**, 1843–9.

Chapter 20

Cystic Lesions of the Jaws

Cystic lesions of the jaws are common pathologic lesions. This group of lesions comprises a number of different conditions, either odontogenic or non-odontogenic in origin.

Odontogenic cysts are the most frequent, and of these the radicular cyst is seen most often. Odontogenic cysts arise from the epithelial remnants of tooth formation, and consequently they are epithelially lined and develop in the tooth-bearing areas of the jaws. These lesions are benign, but very rare instances of associated malignancy or malignant change in the cyst wall have been reported.

Non-odontogenic cysts were classically thought to arise from epithelial remnants from the fusion of the maxillary and frontonasal processes and mandibular processes in the embryo. Aneurysmal and solitary bone cysts, on the other hand, are non-epithelial lined non-odontogenic cysts. These theories have, however, been challenged and most are now felt to be odontogenic or respiratory in origin.

Many of these lesions are slow growing and asymptomatic, often found as incidental findings at dental check-ups or with the use of panoramic radiographs for dental assessment. Accurate diagnosis and appropriate treatment are required, as these lesions will generally continue to grow and may affect adjacent teeth and other structures and even result in pathologic fracture.

The small group of developmental soft tissue cysts will be considered at the end of this chapter.

Odontogenic cysts

Apical or radicular cysts

Radicular cysts are the commonest jaw cysts, comprising half to two-thirds of all such lesions. The cyst is most commonly found associated with the apex of a tooth, but lateral periodontal cysts may be found associated with lateral canals, and residual cysts persist and enlarge following extraction of the causative tooth leaving cystic remnants behind. The cyst usually arises following the development of periapical granuloma from the necrotic remnants of the dental pulp. Chronic inflammation of this tissue initially stimulates the cell rests of Malassez, resulting in epithelial proliferation. This initiation phase is then followed by a phase of cyst development, followed by cyst growth. Radicular cysts are fluid-filled lesions that expand in the jaw by osmotic pressure and cytokines cause local resorption of bone.

Radicular cysts are uncommon in children, and become more frequent in adolescents but are most often seen in adults of all age groups. They are reported to be more prevalent in men than women, although this may be due to women taking greater care of their teeth and visiting the dentist more often than men. The maxilla is more commonly involved than the mandible. Most radicular cysts present as slow-growing, painless swellings associated with a non-vital or root-treated tooth or as incidental findings on panoramic radiographs. Less frequently, radicular cysts become infected and present as a facial abscess or cellulitis.

At presentation the oral soft tissues are often normal, but careful examination may reveal a firm, hard, smooth swelling at the apex of the tooth. As the cyst enlarges the overlying bone may become resorbed leaving a soft swelling or even a thin layer of bone that may be felt to give way on palpation (egg shell crackling). As the cyst is palpated the patient may report pain. The causative tooth will be found to be non-vital and other teeth involved as the cyst enlarges may also become devitalized.

Investigation is by vitality testing of the associated teeth and periapical or panoramic radiographs. The

Essentials of Oral and Maxillofacial Surgery, First Edition. Edited by M. Anthony Pogrel, Karl-Erik Kahnberg and Lars Andersson.
© 2014 John Wiley & Sons, Ltd. Published 2014 by John Wiley & Sons, Ltd.
Companion website: www.wiley.com/go/pogrel/oms

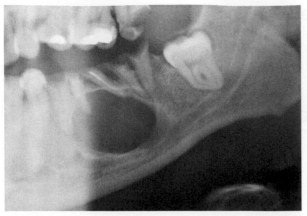

Fig. 20.1 Radicular cyst arising from non-vital roots of lower left first molar tooth. Note displacement of inferior dental canal by cyst posteriorly.

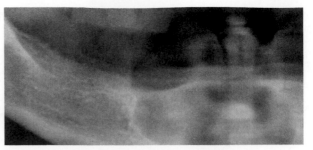

Fig. 20.2 Residual cyst from lower second premolar.

radiographic features are of a smooth, rounded, unilocular radiolucency with a radiopaque outline associated with the apex of a non-vital tooth. Adjacent structures may be displaced by the expanding cyst (Fig. 20.1).

Treatment is by removal of the cause of the inflammation either by root canal treatment, or by extraction of the causative tooth. Small cysts are reported to regress; however, larger lesions will require enucleation. In teeth previously root treated with a good periapical seal, or those restored with a post crown where the post is large and threatens root fracture if an attempt is made to remove it, apicectomy can be performed if the tooth is not extracted.

Following enucleation, the soft tissue overlying the bony cavity is closed and the resulting hematoma ossifies. Some surgeons prefer to fill large cavities with corticocancellous bone chips to accelerate bone regeneration, but there are no studies to show that this practice has benefit. More recently the use of bone morphogenic protein has been described to improve rates of bone regeneration. In mandibular lesions where removal of the cyst threatens to cause a postoperative pathologic fracture, miniplates can be placed prior to closure to strengthen the weakened area of jaw. Patients with very large lesions and those who are severely medically compromised and unable to withstand a prolonged oral surgical procedure may be best treated by marsupialization (decompression) of the cyst allowing bony regeneration. The cyst is decompressed and the lining sutured to the oral mucosa.

Residual cysts

Residual cysts develop from residual periapical infection or from cyst fragments left following extraction of a non-vital tooth. They present with similar features to the radicular cyst and radiographically are found as isolated, circumscribed, unilocular radiolucent lesions in the alveolar process but without an obvious causative tooth (Fig. 20.2). They require enu-

cleation or marsupialization as described in Apical or radicular cysts.

Lateral periodontal cysts

These lesions are usually asymptomatic and identified radiographically between the roots of teeth, often in the mandibular canine and premolar area. The adjacent teeth are vital and the cysts are thought to arise from the cell rests within the periodontal ligament. The botyroid odontogenic cyst and glandular odontogenic cyst are variants of the lateral periodontal cyst and are both uncommon. Botyroid odontogenic cyst is found in adults of 50 years and older, and involves the bicuspid area of the mandible. The glandular odontogenic cyst may be multilocular and is reported to be prone to recurrence. Treatment is usually by enucleation, although on occasion extraction of the involved tooth may be required.

Dentigerous cysts

Dentigerous or follicular cysts account for approximately one sixth of dental cysts. They are a fluid-filled expansion of the dental follicle and are attached to the crown of the tooth at the cemento-enamel junction. As the cyst expands it prevents the eruption of the tooth and may even displace the tooth into the jaw. The most commonly involved teeth are the mandibular third molar and maxillary canine.

Dentigerous cysts are more common in men than women and usually these cysts present as an asymptomatic swelling, found when non-eruption of a tooth is investigated or incidentally with panoramic survey radiographs. Infection is uncommon, but it may present as a dentoalveolar or facial abscess.

Radiographically, a circumscribed, unilocular, radiolucent area is seen with a thin radiopaque lamina dura associated with the crown of the involved tooth. The tooth and adjacent structures may be displaced (Fig. 20.3). Cysts within the maxilla may occupy the maxillary sinus (Fig. 20.4).

Treatment is by removal of the causative tooth and enucleation of the cyst lining and the cavity is managed as described for radicular cysts. In those with very large cysts who are infirm, marsupialization may be the treatment of choice. If the tooth is to be retained for orthodontic reasons, it may also be advantageous to marsupialize the cyst.

Eruption cyst

This soft cystic swelling, usually blue or purple in color, is seen in children. It is found on the alveolus overlying an erupting tooth. The cyst most likely arises from the enamel organ. They are uncommon

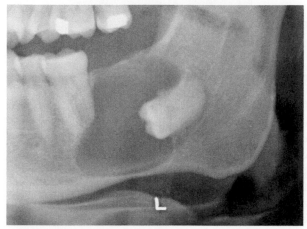

Fig. 20.3 Dentigerous cyst arising from lower left third molar. Note displacement of the tooth and the inferior dental canal by the enlarging cyst.

and many burst spontaneously. Should the cyst not resolve quickly, the overlying tissue may need to be removed to allow the tooth to erupt. Radiographs are usually unnecessary, but if taken may show a lucent lesion at the alveolar margin in association with the crown of the tooth.

Gingival cysts

Two varieties of gingival cyst are found. In newborns small nodules are frequently seen on the alveolar crest. These lesions arise from proliferation of the cell rests of Serres. In the majority of cases they resolve spontaneously but persistent lesions may require local excision or curettage. In adults, usually in the fifth decade, soft tissue cysts can occasionally be found overlying the alveolus. These may cause local resorption of bone resulting in small saucer-shaped depressions in the alveolar plate. These cysts are treated by local excision.

Odontogenic keratocyst (primordial cyst, keratocystic odontogenic tumor)

The World Health Organization reclassified the odontogenic keratocyst as a benign tumor, with the new

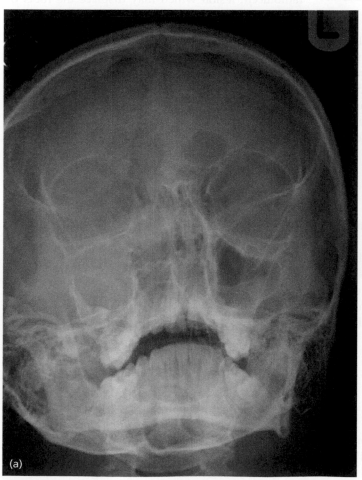

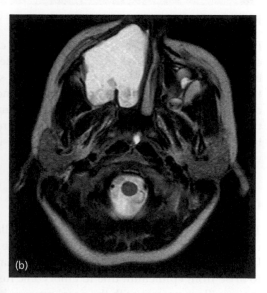

Fig. 20.4 Dentigerous cyst of maxilla involving maxillary sinus: (a) occipitomental radiograph and (b) MRI.

title of keratocystic odontogenic tumor in 2006. It is discussed under this title in Chapter 21.

Calcifying epithelial odontogenic cyst

This rare cyst, first described in 1962, may be found at any age and in either gender. It may be intraosseous or be found within the gingiva eroding the jaw. The radiographic appearance may have little calcification within it in early lesions, giving a similar appearance to other jaw cysts, but with increasing calcification may have the appearance of an odontome or calcifying odontogenic tumor. It has a benign behavior but can be aggressive and recur. Initial treatment is usually by enucleation and curettage.

Malignancy within odontogenic cysts

This is very rare but a few cases are reported of malignancy in the wall of dental cysts. Such lesions should be managed as primary malignant tumors once the diagnosis is established.

Non-odontogenic cysts

Fissural cysts

Fissural cysts were originally described to classify cystic lesions found in areas of what were believed to be embryonic fusion. With more detailed studies these lines of fusion are believed not to exist and close examination of previous cases shows that most of these cysts actually have an odontogenic or respiratory origin. However, the names are occasionally used for descriptive purposes only.

Globulomaxillary cysts

The term globulomaxillary cyst is an umbrella term used for cystic lesions appearing between the upper lateral incisor and canine tooth. It was originally felt to arise from epithelium due to embryonic fusion of the maxillary process with the nasal process, but this version of embryonic fusion has no supporting evidence. Many reported cases are in fact apical cysts related to non-vital lateral incisors or other cystic lesions. Treatment is by enucleation.

Median mandibular cyst

This is a term for cystic lesions in the midline of the jaw. Original proposals for this being of embryonic origin have now been disproved and, rather like the globulomaxillary cyst, most cases are in fact of odontogenic origin.

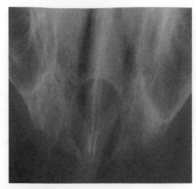

Fig. 20.5 Nasopalatine cyst.

Nasopalatine cysts

Nasopalatine or incisive canal cysts arise from the epithelial remnants of the embryonic nasopalatine ducts. This occurs during the creation of the incisive canal by the fusion of the premaxilla with the palatine processes of the maxillary bones. The etiology of cyst formation may be local inflammatory processes such as infection and trauma. Nasopalatine cysts are more common in males than females and in the fourth to sixth decades. The cyst presents as a symmetrical swelling behind the upper incisors in the midline. Rarely, a fistula can be found leading to the incisive canal. Radiographs show a midline round or oval radiolucent lesion which may displace the roots of the central incisors laterally (Fig. 20.5). Accurate vitality tests are essential to avoid misdiagnosis. It is difficult to differentiate a small nasopalatine cyst from a large incisive canal, but it has been proposed that an incisive canal of less than 6 mm on occlusal radiograph is within normal limits provided the patient has no symptoms nor abnormal clinical findings. Treatment is by enucleation, but the nasopalatine nerve may be lost in the process.

Non-epithelially lined cysts

Stafne/static bone cyst

This classic radiolucency is found in the mandible as an incidental finding on survey radiographs such as orthopantomograms and lateral obliques. A small, smooth outlined lesion is found beneath the second and third molar teeth, below the inferior dental canal. The lesion is asymptomatic and is not a true cyst. It is an invagination of the medial aspect of the mandible, usually containing salivary tissue, although lymphoid tissue has been reported. Occasional cases are reported of Stafne-type lesions occurring more anteriorly in the mandible. In difficult cases radiographic assessment can be made with either fine cut coronal computed tomography (CT) scan to determine the bony anatomy and the soft tissue signal within the cavity or by magnetic resonance imaging (MRI) scan. Biopsy and exploration are not indicated.

Aneurysmal bone cysts

This non-epithelially lined cyst-like lesion occurs occasionally in the jaws. It is more common in the mandible than maxilla. The etiology is unknown, but essentially it is a vascular malformation that arises from a prior unrelated lesion. It presents in adolescents and young adults as a swelling, which is painful in 50% of cases, or as an incidental finding on a panoramic radiograph. Radiographically it may be a uni- or multilocular lesion with irregular outline and occasional displacement of tooth roots. Histopathologically, the lesion contains many giant cells and can be indistinguishable from central giant cell granuloma. This feature has led to the idea that aneurysmal bone cysts are a vascular variation of central giant cell granuloma. Treatment is by curettage although the lesions can recur. Resection and adjuvant cryotherapy have been proposed for large or recurrent lesions.

Solitary bone cyst

Solitary bone cysts have been given many titles including simple bone cyst, traumatic bone cyst, hemorrhagic bone cyst, and latent bone cavity. All these terms refer to the same lesion, a non-epithelially lined space that may be found to contain a small amount of straw-colored fluid but may have no fluid within it. It is found most often in the long bones and rarely in the jaws. Its etiology is unknown, but trauma has been proposed, following which there is intramedullary bleeding and clot formation. However, instead of the normal process of resorption of the clot and bone formation, the clot liquefies leaving a cavity. It is then proposed that the liquid content decreases with time and the lesion becomes filled with air. The oxygen from this is absorbed into the blood leaving nitrogen that has been found on analysis. It is most commonly found in adolescents as a painless swelling or incidental finding on radiographs affecting the mandible. Females are more commonly affected than males (3:2). It has rarely been described in association with florid cemento-osseous dysplasia. Radiographs show a radiolucency that extends between the roots of involved teeth. One explanation for their rare appearance after adolescence is that these lesions spontaneously resolve. In longstanding or large lesions, treatment is by curettage of the cavity, which results in clot formation and complete bony infill.

Soft tissue cysts

Nasolabial cysts

This is a rare cyst of the soft tissues with unknown etiology. Like the globulomaxillary cyst it has been proposed to arise from embryonal fusion but this has no evidence to support it. This cyst is commonest in the fourth and fifth decades and is more common in females (male:female 1:4). It is found as a swelling at the nasal fold and can become quite large before being detected, causing distortion of the alar rim and local resorption of the maxilla. Treatment is by excision. It can be lined by squamous or respiratory epithelium.

Sublingual dermoid and dermoid cysts

Sublingual dermoid cysts are soft tissue cysts found in the midline beneath the tongue and as far down as the hyoid bone. These cysts are believed to arise from epidermal cell rests resulting from the fusion of embryonal processes. Unlike mucous retention cysts they are deeply placed and filled with keratin, giving a much firmer feel. Initially they are asymptomatic but as they increase in size they start to affect speech and swallowing if above the mylohyoid, where they bulge into the floor of the mouth. Those cysts arising below mylohyoid appear as a swelling in the neck. Treatment is by excision.

Other small dermoid cysts may be found within the skin of the head and neck and implantation dermoid cysts can arise from local trauma where skin is driven into the subepithelial layers. These lesions are treated by surgical excision.

Branchial lymphoepithelial cysts

Branchial cysts arise from incomplete obliteration of branchial clefts (most usually the second branchial cleft) or epithelial inclusions within lymph nodes. Lymphoepithelial cysts are found in the floor of the mouth and posterior tongue. Branchial cysts usually present as asymptomatic swellings in the lateral aspect of the neck at the anterior border to the sternomastoid. Rarely, they present with acute infection. Branchial cysts are commonest in children and young adults, but can occur in older patients. In those over 40 years, cysts presenting in this fashion should be investigated for tonsillar or tongue base carcinoma as cystic metastasis for such lesions is the commonest cause of lateral neck cysts in this age group. Rare cases of primary branchial cyst carcinoma are reported in the literature.

In those with simple branchial cyst the neck should be imaged with MRI scan (Fig. 20.6) and the cyst excised. Any track to the pharynx should also be excised.

Thyroglossal cysts

These cysts arise from the thyroglossal duct, which should break down following the migration of the thyroid gland from the foramen caecum in utero. These cysts present as midline swellings anywhere from the tongue base to the thyroid gland. They are usually asymptomatic. Due to the attachment of the

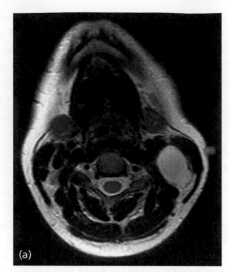

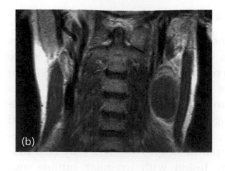

Fig. 20.6 Branchial cyst: (a) axial and coronal (b) MRI views showing cyst deep to sternomastoid.

tract to the hyoid bone and the tongue, the cysts move on swallowing and protrusion of the tongue. Investigation is by MRI scan and fine-needle aspiration. Thyroid scans will occasionally show these cysts to be active, but usually patients have other adequate functioning tissue. Solid lesions may, however, represent all of the patient's functioning thyroid tissue and a thyroid scan is required before the removal of such a lesion. Cases of carcinoma within thyroglossal cysts are reported. Treatment for uncomplicated thyroglos-

sal cyst is by the Sistrunk procedure, which involves excision of the cyst and the central portion of the hyoid bone.

Recommended reading

Goodger NM, Hendy CW. (2010) Cystic lesions of the jaws. In: *Oral and Maxillofacial Surgery* (eds, Andersson L, Kahnberg K-E, Pogrel MA). Oxford, Wiley-Blackwell.

Chapter 21

Odontogenic and Non-odontogenic Tumors of the Jaws

Introduction

Odontogenic and non-odontogenic tumors of the jaws are a relatively rare and heterogeneous group of benign and malignant neoplasms, hamartomas, and other bone-related lesions that demonstrate great variability in etiology, biologic behavior, and clinical significance. The single commonality amongst these cellular proliferations is that they may occur in the jaws. Odontogenic tumors, by definition, are derived from tooth-related tissues and, although they have been reported in tooth-bearing structures such as dermoid cysts and teratomas, they originate overwhelmingly in the maxilla or mandible. The majority of these disorders are benign, and while they may be locally aggressive, only very rarely do they have the ability to metastasize. Non-odontogenic jaw tumors, on the other hand, develop from the epithelium and/or mesenchyme of a wide variety of tissues in the body, often originate in non-tooth-bearing facial bones, and may develop in other sites outside of the head and neck. Some of these are of little clinical significance and require nothing more than observation or local excision, while many of the malignant variants mandate multimodal therapy and portend a poor prognosis for survival.

Odontogenic tumors

Odontogenic tumors (OT) are derived from tooth-forming elements and for the purposes of this chapter include lesions that are not definitively neoplastic. Even using this broad definition, OTs are rare lesions that account for <2–3% of all oral and maxillofacial specimens sent for diagnosis to oral pathology services.

Odontogenesis occurs through a complex process involving the enamel organ, the dental follicle, and the dental papilla (Fig. 21.1). The enamel organ is an epithelial structure that is derived from oral ectoderm. The dental follicle and dental papilla are derived from neural crest cells and are therefore considered ectomesenchymal in nature. Odontogenic tumors demonstrate varying inductive interactions between the odontogenic epithelium and odontogenic ectomesenchyme, and are typically subclassified by their tissue of origin.

Classification

The current WHO classification of odontogenic tumors was published in July 2005 (Table 21.1) and made a number of important changes to terminology, benign or malignant classifications, and assignment to relevant subgroups. Previous WHO classifications described only tumor histology.

Odontogenic cysts were not considered in the new 2005 classification, which means that the previous 1992 classification is still relevant for cysts of the jaws and maxillofacial region, with one notable exception: the odontogenic keratocyst (OKC) was renamed "keratocystic odontogenic tumor" (KOT or KCOT) and was added to the odontogenic tumors category. The change in terminology is a reflection of contemporary clinical, molecular, and immunohistochemical data suggesting that the KOT is a benign neoplasm rather than a cyst.

Another important change in the 2005 WHO classification is related to malignant tumors of odontogenic origin. The metastasizing ameloblastoma was incorrectly described in the previous 1992 classification. It is now clarified in the 2005 document, which provides a clear distinction between the metastasizing ameloblastoma (containing benign histological

Essentials of Oral and Maxillofacial Surgery, First Edition. Edited by M. Anthony Pogrel, Karl-Erik Kahnberg and Lars Andersson.
© 2014 John Wiley & Sons, Ltd. Published 2014 by John Wiley & Sons, Ltd.
Companion website: www.wiley.com/go/pogrel/oms

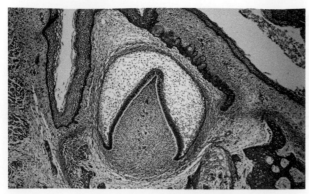

Fig. 21.1 The "bell stage" of tooth development. (Courtesy of F. James Kratochvil III, DDS.)

features) and ameloblastic carcinoma. The diagnosis of an ameloblastic carcinoma is made in the presence of malignant histological features. In addition, the clear cell odontogenic carcinoma (CCOC), formerly clear cell odontogenic tumor, has been added to the list of malignant odontogenic carcinomas due to its newly recognized aggressive behavior.

Treatment options for benign tumors of the jaws

Enucleation and curettage

Enucleation and curettage has been the traditional and time-honored method for managing odontogenic cysts and some jaw tumors. The technique offers the patient a minimally invasive procedure, with little associated morbidity and few complications. Most odontogenic cysts can be effectively removed by simple enucleation of the cystic lining and meticulous curettage of the bony cavity. However, when used alone, this technique is usually inadequate for tumors with true neoplastic potential and its use in entities such as ameloblastoma or keratocystic odontogenic tumor should be accompanied by adjuvant treatment, such as peripheral ostectomy, cryotherapy, or chemical fixation with Carnoy's solution.

Wide exposure is necessary to allow complete access to the bony cavity (Fig. 21.2). Every effort must be made to thoroughly remove the cyst lining as well as epithelial remnants that may be present between the cyst wall and overlying mucosa. One of the difficulties encountered when attempting to remove these cysts lies in the nature of the thin cystic lining which, at times, is readily removed *in toto*, but more often comes out in multiple soft tissue fragments. The inferior alveolar nerve can be routinely spared and root canal therapy is almost never indicated. Most of the time, the mucosa can be closed primarily, without the need for bone grafts or packing material. Removal of a large tumor or cyst will occasionally weaken the remaining bony integrity, placing it at risk for pathologic fracture. This can be managed with 6 weeks of

Table 21.1 WHO histological classification of odontogenic tumors. Adapted from Barnes L, Eveson JW, Reichart P, Sidransky D (2005) *World Health Organization Classification of Tumours, Pathology and Genetics of Head and Neck Tumours.* pp, 284. IARC Press, Lyon.

Malignant tumors

Odontogenic carcinomas

Metastasizing (malignant) ameloblastoma
Ameloblastic carcinoma – primary type
Ameloblastic carcinoma – secondary type (dedifferentiated), intraosseous
Ameloblastic carcinoma – secondary type (dedifferentiated), peripheral
Primary intraosseous squamous cell carcinoma-solid type
Primary intraosseous squamous cell carcinoma derived from keratocystic odontogenic tumor
Primary intraosseous squamous cell carcinoma derived from odontogenic cysts
Clear cell odontogenic carcinoma
Ghost cell odontogenic carcinoma
Odontogenic sarcomas
Ameloblastic fibrosarcoma
Ameloblastic fibrodentino- and fibro-odontosarcoma

Benign tumors

Odontogenic epithelium with mature, fibrous stroma without odontogenic ectomesenchyme

Ameloblastoma, solid/multicystic type
Ameloblastoma, extraosseous/peripheral type
Ameloblastoma, desmoplastic type
Ameloblastoma, unicystic type
Squamous odontogenic tumor
Calcifying epithelial odontogenic tumors
Adenomatoid odontogenic tumor
Keratocystic odontogenic tumor

Odontogenic epithelium with odontogenic ectomesenchyme, with or without hard tissue formation

Ameloblastic fibroma
Ameloblastic fibrodentinoma
Ameloblastic fibro-odontoma
Odontoma, complex type
Odontoma, compound type
Odontoameloblastoma
Calcifying cystic odontogenic tumor
Dentinogenic ghost cell tumor

Mesenchyme and/or odontogenic ectomesenchyme with or without odontogenic epithelium

Odontogenic fibroma
Odontogenic myxoma/myxofibroma
Cementoblastoma

Bone-related lesions

Ossifying fibroma
Fibrous dysplasia
Osseous dysplasias
Central giant cell lesion (granuloma)
Cherubism
Aneurysmal bone cyst
Simple bone cyst

intermaxillary fixation and/or placement of a reconstruction plate. Enucleation and curettage is a reasonable method for the primary treatment of small, unilocular cysts that are typically not biopsied prior to definitive treatment.

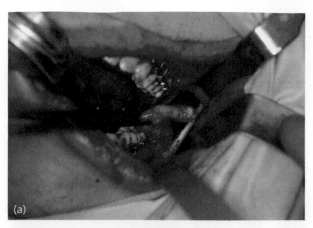

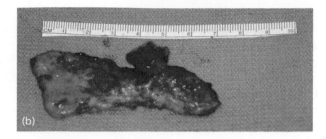

Fig. 21.2 Enucleation and curettage. (a) Exposure of the cyst to allow complete access to the bony cavity, (b) complete intact removal of the cyst.

Enucleation and peripheral ostectomy

Enucleation with peripheral ostectomy is an extension of the curettage technique described in Enucleation and curettage. It involves the use of a rotary instrument to remove bone adjacent to the cyst lining, theoretically facilitating removal of all residual epithelium and/or daughter cysts. Methylene blue staining is often used to aid in identification of appropriate bony margins. The technique can stand alone or include chemical or thermal fixation of the interior of the bony cavity. The advantage of peripheral ostectomy is that it provides an additional "margin" of bone removal during excision of the lesion and can potentially alleviate the need for adjunctive measures. The disadvantages are that it places other anatomic structures at risk of injury, i.e. teeth and the inferior alveolar nerve, and may further weaken the jaw structure. The use of peripheral ostectomy for treatment of a number of odontogenic tumors has merit in that it can facilitate a more "radical" surgery than curettage but is less morbid than resection.

Marsupialization

Marsupialization is a technique that is designed to initially decompress and shrink the cyst or tumor prior to definitive removal, generally by enucleation and curettage several months later. The primary advantage of this method is to minimize the surgical defect that is created by removal of the cystic lesion. This technique has been observed to cause inflammation and subsequent thickening of the cystic lining which facilitates its ultimate removal. Various inflammatory mediators may play a role in cyst volume reduction. Marsupialization has been shown to inhibit interleukin1-alpha expression within the lining of KCOTs, thereby halting epithelial cell proliferation and decreasing the size of the cystic tumor. The technique is performed by "de-roofing" the cyst and either repeatedly packing the cavity with gauze or by simply placing a tube, catheter or drain in order

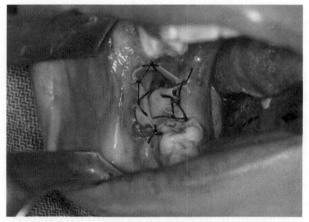

Fig. 21.3 Marsupialization of a keratocystic odontogenic tumor (KCOT).

to facilitate gradual decompression and shrinkage of the defect (Fig. 21.3). The pack or drain is left in place for 2–3.

Intralesional adjunctive therapy: chemical fixation

Remnants of the dental lamina may play a role in the etiology of some odontogenic tumors. The presence of epithelial islands within the mucosa overlying the cyst as well as the bony cavity has prompted the use of various surgical strategies to adjunctively treat the surrounding tissue in an effort to eradicate residual disease and minimize recurrence. The use of such adjuvant measures is perhaps best studied in the treatment of KCOTs. Stoelinga, Voorsmit, and colleagues advocate excision of the overlying mucosa and have popularized the use of Carnoy's solution as a chemical tissue fixative for treatment of KCOTs. Carnoy's solution is a mixture of absolute alcohol, chloroform, glacial acetic acid, and ferric chloride that penetrates bone to a predictable, time-dependent depth, without injuring the neurovascular structures, providing that it is not in contact with the inferior alveolar nerve for longer than two minutes. A 5-minute application will penetrate bone to a depth of over 1.5 mm. Because most residual cells and daughter cysts from locally recurrent lesions are adjacent to the main lesion, it is likely that fixation of vital bone need only extend for 2–3 mm beyond the enucleated lesion. Theoretically, enucleation of the cyst wall, excision of the overlying mucosa, and treatment of the surrounding tissue with Carnoy's solution should sufficiently remove the cystic lesion along with any epithelial remnants remaining in the area. Application of the Carnoy's solution can be either prior to enucleation or afterwards. Voorsmit's original description of the technique called for treatment of the cyst before enucleation which causes a "tanning effect" of the lesion thereby facilitating complete removal. The author's experience, however, is that treatment of the bony cavity after enucleation allows for easier removal of the cyst lining and better identification of soft tissue remnants.

Intralesional adjunctive therapy: cryotherapy

Cryosurgery with liquid nitrogen, a method of treating disease by the production of freezing temperatures in tissue, has been advocated as an adjunct to the surgical treatment of benign cysts and tumors of the jaws. Cryosurgery for osseous lesions produces cellular necrosis in bone while maintaining the inorganic osseous framework. Predictable cell lysis occurs at temperatures below −20°C and is caused by direct damage from intracellular and extracellular ice crystal formation, osmotic disturbances, and electrolyte imbalance. Similar to chemical fixation with Carnoy's solution, cryosurgery allows for removal of the cyst or tumor by enucleation and curettage followed by treatment of the surrounding tissue. A single 1-minute freeze produces a depth of bone necrosis of 1–3 mm depending on the technique (Figs 21.4, 21.5 and 21.6). The techniques acceptable for oral cryosurgical use include the cryoprobe with water-soluble jelly and liquid nitrogen spray. The advantage of a cryoprobe with jelly is that it is possible to freeze irregular, gravity-dependent portions of the bony cavity. The disadvantage is that there is non-uniform freezing. The advantage of liquid nitrogen spray is potent, uniform freezing. The disadvantage is the potential for damage to surrounding tissues. Immediate bone grafting has been recommended for defects greater than 4 cm that are treated with cryotherapy. Bone grafting is thought to decrease complications such as wound dehiscence and pathologic fracture, while simultaneously providing greater residual bone height and density, thus facilitating implant placement.

Resection

The aggressive clinical behavior of some odontogenic and non-odontogenic jaw tumors is well recognized.

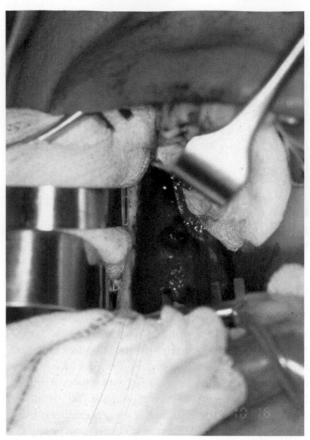

Fig. 21.4 Cryotherapy preparation. Malleable retractors are positioned so as to self-retain gauze sponges to protect and insulate the soft tissues.

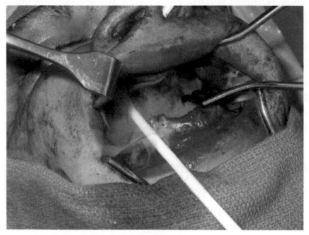

Fig. 21.5 Cryo-applicator in water-soluble jelly.

Although rare, extension into vital anatomic regions occurs and can involve the skull base, infratemporal fossa, and/or orbit. Composite, segmental or marginal resection should be considered for some large primary or recurrent benign tumors, tumors involving the orbit, posterior maxilla, pteryopalatine fossa, skull base or infratemporal fossa, and malignant tumors.

Reconstruction

Ideally, benign or malignant ablation should be followed by immediate oromandibular or palatomaxil-

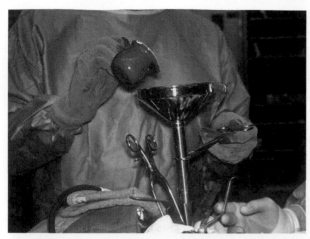

Fig. 21.6 Open funnel cryo-application system.

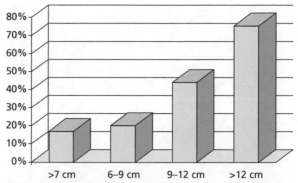

Fig. 21.7 The failure rate of non-vascularized bone grafts when related to the length of the graft. (From Pogrel MA, Podlesh S, Anthony JP, Alexander J. A comparison of vascularized and nonvascularized bone grafts for reconstruction of mandibular continuity defects. *Journal of Oral and Maxillofacial Surgery* 1997; 55: 1200–6. Copyright © 1997 Elsevier.)

lary reconstruction to re-establish function and achieve an acceptable cosmetic result. Immediate bony reconstruction of smaller defects can be performed by using non-vascularized autogenous bone grafts harvested from the ilium. Important factors that have been found to affect graft survival include the length of the mandibular defect, timing of the reconstruction (immediate versus delayed), pre- or postoperative radiation therapy, postoperative recipient site complications, malignant diagnosis, intraoral communication, estimated blood loss, the number of days on postoperative antibiotics, and the use of soft tissue flaps. In the primary setting, however, microvascular transfer of free osteocutaneous flaps from the fibula, iliac crest, radial forearm, or scapula seems to provide the most reliable means for reconstruction of composite or segmental defects with a success rate of around 95%. Length of the defect has been shown to be an important factor in bone graft survival for mandibular reconstruction. Foster *et al.* critically evaluated the use of non-vascularized grafts compared to microvascular composite free flaps in reconstruction of mandibular continuity defects and found that success was dependent in part on the length of the defect. Success rates in terms of osseous union using non-vascularized bone grafts decreased significantly in those patients with defects greater than 6 cm (Fig. 21.7). The overall success rate of non-vascularized bone grafts was approximately 69% while the overall success rate of vascularized bone flaps was 96%. Additionally, it took an average of 2.3 operations to complete the reconstruction for those patients with non-vascularized bone grafts as opposed to only 1.1 operations for those patients with vascularized bone flaps.

Surgical treatment of malignant tumors of the jaws

Malignant tumors typically require standard extra oral neck incisions in order to obtain proper access and facilitate reconstruction. A tracheostomy may be

needed depending on the location and extent of the planned surgical resection. A neck dissection is generally required and, classically, it precedes surgical resection of the primary tumor. Classically, the tumor resection should be performed *en bloc* with the neck dissection and the tumor delivered along with the lymph node-bearing tissue.

Benign tumors

Odontogenic epithelium with mature, fibrous stroma without odontogenic ectomesenchyme

Ameloblastomas

The ameloblastoma is a true neoplasm of odontogenic epithelial origin. The etiology of ameloblastoma is not known with certainty but the cells of origin are thought to be ameloblasts. Excluding odontomas, ameloblastomas are the most common odontogenic neoplasm and account for approximately 10% of all tumors that arise in the mandible and maxilla. Larsson and Almeren described an incidence of 0.3 cases per million people per year in Sweden. On the other hand, studies from Africa suggest that ameloblastomas may represent more than 60% of all odontogenic tumors in that part of the world.

Presenting symptoms may include a slow-growing submucosal mass, loose teeth, malocclusion, paresthesia, and pain. As many as 35% of patients are completely asymptomatic and the lesions are discovered as incidental findings on routine dental radiographs. The median age at presentation is 35 years (range, 4–92 years) and there is no gender predilection. Eighty percent of ameloblastomas arise in the mandible, usually in the ramus region, and are often associated with molar teeth.

Ameloblastomas have a distinctive histological appearance manifested by columnar, basally staining cells arranged in a palisaded pattern along the basement membrane (Fig. 21.8). Six histopathologic

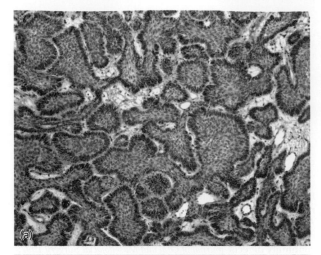

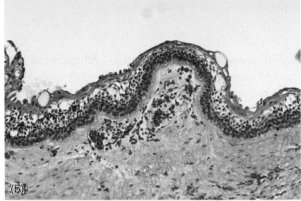

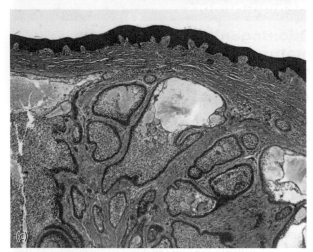

Fig. 21.8 Histologic appearance of ameloblastoma. (a) Solid/multicystic: note columnar, basally staining cells arranged in a palisaded pattern along the basement membrane. (b) Unicystic: note cystic architecture with typical ameloblastic changes confined to the cyst-lining epithelium. (c) Peripheral: note histological characteristics of intraosseous tumor. (Courtesy of Jeffery C. Stewart, DDS, MS.)

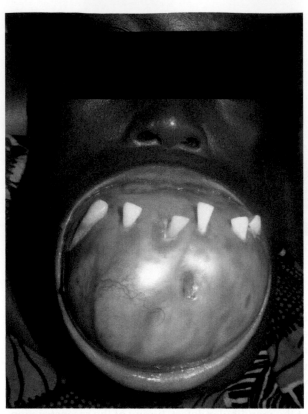

Fig. 21.9 Massive ameloblastoma of the mandible. (Courtesy of Dr J.T. Arotiba.)

subtypes are recognized, including follicular, acanthomatous, plexiform, basal cell, desmoplastic, and granular cell variants. Most tumors show a predominance of one pattern, but mixtures of different patterns are commonly observed. Granular cell ameloblastoma was at one time thought to be a more aggressive variant; however, this is no longer the case. Currently, most clinicians consider the histologi-

cal subtypes to be of academic interest only and there is no convincing evidence suggesting a significant difference in biologic behavior. All ameloblastomas are benign but locally aggressive, will occasionally metastasize, and a few have malignant potential.

Solid/multicystic ameloblastomas

These normally present as locally aggressive tumors that demonstrate inherent neoplastic cellular proliferation, are associated with high recurrence rates when inadequately treated, and represent the most clinically significant odontogenic tumor based on potential morbidity and prevalence. If left untreated, these tumors can grow to extreme sizes (Fig. 21.9). Enucleation and curettage has been associated with a recurrence rate of 60–80%. Neoplastic cells have been shown to be present several millimeters from the radiographic margin of the tumor, which has led to the recommendation that resection be performed with care to maintain 1 cm tumor-free margins. It is clear, based on the current body of evidence, that enucleation and curettage alone is inadequate for definitive treatment of solid ameloblastoma. Resection is the gold standard and currently offers the most predictable recurrence-free treatment for solid ameloblastoma (Figs 21.10 and 21.11). For many tumors, however, resection with 1 cm tumor-free margins will commit the surgeon and patient to a segmental mandibulectomy or maxillectomy, often with sacrifice of the inferior alveolar nerve or creation of an

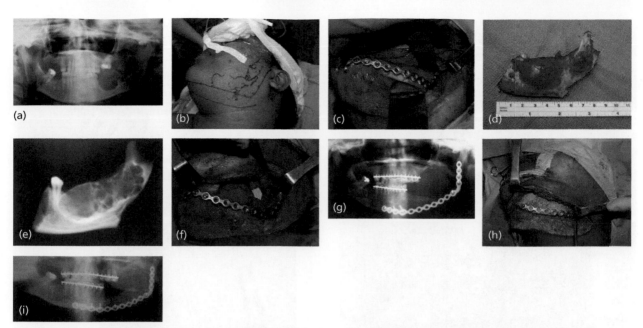

Fig. 21.10 Transcervical segmental resection for solid ameloblastoma of the mandible and delayed reconstruction with autogenous corticocancellous bone harvested from the posterior iliac crest. (a) Multilocular, expansile radiolucency of the left mandible. (b) Presurgical marking for segmental resection. (c) Transcervical approach to the mandible with application of the reconstruction plate prior to segmental resection. (d) Specimen. (e) Radiograph of the specimen demonstrating negative resection margins. (f) Reconstruction plate in situ. (g) Postoperative panoramic radiograph. (h) Secondary (delayed) reconstruction of the same patient 6 months later using autogenous corticocancellous bone harvested from the posterior ilium. (i) Postreconstruction panoramic radiograph. (Courtesy of David L. Hirsch, DDS, MD.)

oral–antral communication, and will necessitate primary or secondary reconstruction of continuity defects of the mandible or maxillectomy defects. Techniques have been described for segmental mandibular resection with inferior alveolar nerve preservation; however, this technique runs the theoretical risk of inviting perineural recurrence. Since ameloblastoma is a benign disease, many surgeons are reluctant to perform radical surgery on these patients. This understandable reserve has led to a number of other techniques including enucleation with peripheral ostectomy and/or adjuvant treatment with liquid nitrogen cryotherapy.

Although most ameloblastomas occur in the mandible, maxillary ameloblastomas are often more problematic than mandibular tumors (Fig. 21.12). Although histologically identical to their mandibular counterpart, the surrounding anatomy is more complex. Involvement of the maxillary sinus and nasal cavity commonly occurs and infiltration into the orbit, pterygomaxillary space, and skull base is distinctly possible in some patients with recurrent or uncontrolled disease. Even simple enucleation and peripheral ostectomy may result in oral–antral communication and thus require reconstruction. If it is possible to perform excision with peripheral ostectomy and treatment with liquid nitrogen therapy without creating an oral–antral/oral–nasal defect, then this is the preferred treatment for most small to medium-sized lesions. However, because of the reconstructive issues, the general approach for larger tumors is to

perform resection and immediate reconstruction using either local or regional rotational flaps, or alternatively microvascular free flaps or an obturator.

Unicystic ameloblastoma

Unicystic ameloblastoms represent a subgroup seen in approximately 6% of ameloblastomas and were first described in 1977. They tend to occur in a younger population (mean age 22.1 years) and a high percentage of these lesions are associated with an impacted tooth. They will often present as a well circumscribed, unilocular periapical radiolucency (Fig. 21.13). Histologically, the unicystic ameloblastoma shows a cystic architecture with the typical ameloblastic changes confined to the cyst-lining epithelium (Fig. 21.8b). While most pathologists accept the concept of unicystic ameloblastoma as a separate entity rather than as a precursor to solid ameloblastoma, much controversy exists over the terminology and how it should be classified.

One of the contentious issues regarding unicystic ameloblastoma is related to proliferation of the ameloblastic epithelium into the lumen of the cystic cavity or into the adjacent bone. Extension of the ameloblastic epithelium into the lumen of the cystic cavity is termed intraluminal, or mural proliferation. There seems to be general agreement that as long as the ameloblastic characteristics are confined to the lining epithelial layers or if it remains intraluminal, conservative therapy such as enucleation and curettage

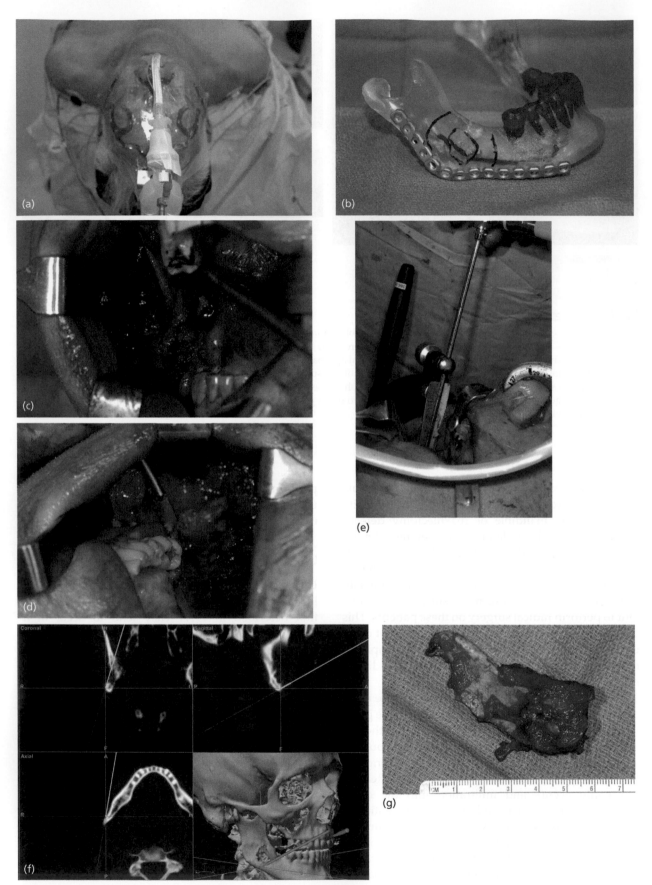

Fig. 21.11 Navigation and endoscope-assisted, transoral marginal resection for solid, recurrent ameloblastoma of the mandible and immediate reconstruction with autogenous corticocancellous bone harvested from the anterior iliac crest. (a) Preoperative set-up for intraoperative navigation. (b) Stereolithographic model for precise prebending of a load-bearing reconstruction plate, visualization of the tumor, and osteotomy design. (c) Soft tissue resection is initiated with 1 cm margins. (d) Prebent reconstruction plate is placed transorally under endoscopic visualization and navigation guidance. (e) Osteotomy is completed via a transbuccal approach under navigation guidance. (f) Intraoperative navigation confirming accurate osteotomy design with 1 cm tumor-free resection margins. (g) Resection specimen. (h) Postoperative facial appearance. (i) Postoperative occlusion. (j) Postoperative panoramic radiograph.

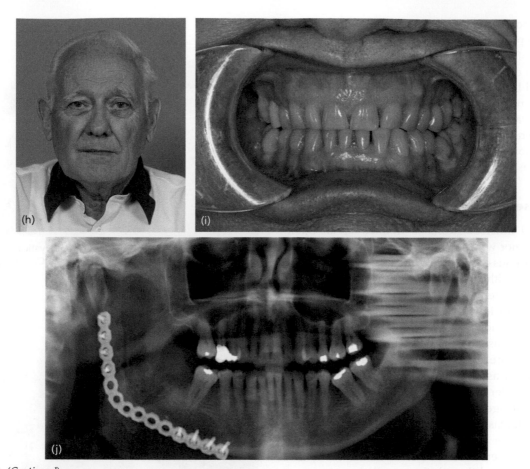

Fig. 21.11 (*Continued*)

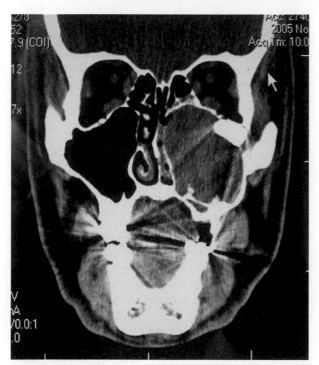

Fig. 21.12 Computed tomography (CT) scan of large maxillary ameloblastoma (solid).

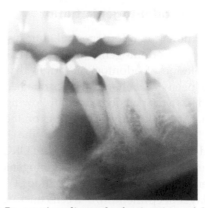

Fig. 21.13 Panoramic radiograph of unicystic ameloblastoma.

is sufficient treatment. On the other hand, transmural involvement of the epithelium and bony invasion is defined by some pathologists as solid or "invasive" ameloblastoma, a term more descriptive of its aggressive biologic behavior.

It is clear that some unicystic ameloblastomas have a better prognosis and less chance for recurrence than do multicystic or solid variants when treated with enucleation and curettage. It is also clear that the unicystic ameloblastoma is considerably more aggressive than a simple dentigerous cyst, with which it is included in a differential diagnosis.

The clinical problem rests in the fact that the diagnosis is often made retrospectively once the patient has undergone definitive treatment for a presumptive odontogenic cyst. The issue is complicated by the fact that to definitively establish a lesion as a unicystic ameloblastoma, complete microscopic evaluation of the bony margin surrounding the lesion must be performed, therefore necessitating *en bloc* resection of the osteolytic lesion. Clearly this is impractical and would represent gross overtreatment of the vast majority of lesions. Since incisional biopsy can never provide a definitive diagnosis, it is doubtful that the issue will be settled in the near future. The surgeon should consider all of the clinical, radiographic, and patient-related factors, provide an appropriately tailored therapy warranted by the benign nature of these lesions, and probably accept a small rate of recurrence.

Extraosseous/peripheral ameloblastoma

Peripheral ameloblastoma is defined as an odontogenic tumor with the histological characteristics of its intraosseous counterpart, but occurs exclusively in the gingiva without bony involvement (Fig. 21.8c). It is thought to represent between 2% and 10% of all diagnosed ameloblastomas. Similar in appearance to basal cell carcinoma, it has been suggested that some lesions previously reported as basal cell carcinoma of the gingiva are in fact peripheral ameloblastomas. They present as a painless, firm, exophytic growth without gender predilection and in all age groups, with a mean age of 52. Seventy percent of peripheral ameloblastomas occur in the mandible, more commonly anterior to the mental foramen. Simple excision with conservative margins is all that is required for treatment and these lesions rarely recur.

Keratocystic odontogenic tumor

Formerly known as odontogenic keratocyst (OKC), the keratocystic odontogenic tumor (KOT or KCOT) is a cystic lesion of odontogenic origin that demonstrates the behavioral characteristics of a benign neoplasm and has a propensity to recur following surgical treatment. A greater understanding of the clinical behavior and molecular biology of the KOT has prompted the terminology change from OKC and led to its recent classification as an odontogenic tumor. The salient histologic features include: (1) a thin, uniform layer of epithelium, 5–6 cells thick, with little or no evidence of rete ridges; (2) a well-defined basal cell layer with palisading cuboidal or columnar cells; and (3) a corrugated, keratinizing luminal surface that is primarily parakeratinized but may be orthokeratinized or a mixture of both (Fig. 21.14). The presence of "satellite" or "daughter" cysts has been recognized in a significant minority of KOTs and inflammation is an inconsistent finding. The radiographic appearance of KOTs is that of a unilocular or multilocular radiolucency, often with cortical expansion or erosion (Fig. 21.15).

Recurrence rates following initial treatment range as high as 62% and have prompted as yet unanswered questions about the pathophysiology of recurrence associated with this unique lesion. Various theories have been popularized that correlate the potential for recurrence with the presence of "daughter" or "satel-

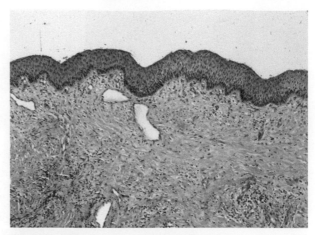

Fig. 21.14 Histological appearance of keratocystic odontogenic tumor (KCOT) (H&E). (Courtesy of Jeffery C. Stewart, DDS, MS.)

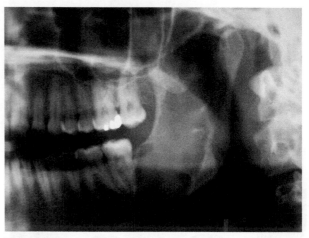

Fig. 21.15 Panoramic radiograph of keratocystic odontogenic tumor. Note multilocular appearance, cortical expansion, and erosion.

lite" cysts remaining in the epithelium following enucleation, the presence of a thin cystic lining, incomplete removal of the cyst, or remnants of dental lamina not associated with the original cyst.

There is a growing body of evidence that a distinction should be made between parakeratinized KOTs, which have a relatively high risk of recurrence, and the orthokeratinized variant, which rarely recurs. In fact, the orthokeratinized version was not redefined by WHO and is still referred to as an odontogenic keratocyst.

The aggressive nature of KOTs is well documented and is manifested by cortical erosion, soft tissue involvement, and extension into the skull base, orbit, and infratemporal fossa. Recurrence rates following initial treatment with a variety of procedures range from 2.5% to 62.5%. Myriad surgical strategies have been proposed to facilitate complete removal of the lesion and to minimize recurrent or residual disease, including more meticulous surgery with or without peripheral ostectomy, tissue fixation methods, soft tissue excision, radical treatment when necessary, and more conscientious follow-up. The optimum treatment modality has yet to be determined.

Stoelinga published the results of a prospective clinical trial conducted on 82 OKCs (KOTs) diagnosed in 80 patients over a 25-year period. Thirty-three patients underwent simple enucleation and curettage while 38 patients underwent excision of the overlying mucosa attached to the cyst where it had perforated through the bone, followed by treatment of the lesion with Carnoy's solution, enucleation of the cyst, and curettage of the bony cavity (Fig. 21.16). Five patients in the Carnoy's group presented with a recurrent tumor. With follow-up that ranged from 2 to 25 years there was an overall recurrence rate of 11%

(nine patients). Most of the recurrences (six) occurred in the patients who were treated with enucleation and curettage alone. None of the patients presenting with recurrent lesions re-recurred following treatment using the authors' protocol. Of those with recurrence, six patients presented without signs or symptoms and the cyst was noticed on routine radiograph. There did not appear to be a correlation between age, sex, or site and recurrence.

Schmidt and Pogrel published the results of 26 patients with KOTs who were treated with enucleation and cryotherapy. The majority of these cystic lesions ($n = 22$) were recurrent lesions. With follow-up of 2–10 years, recurrence was noted in three patients (11.5%). Complications were limited

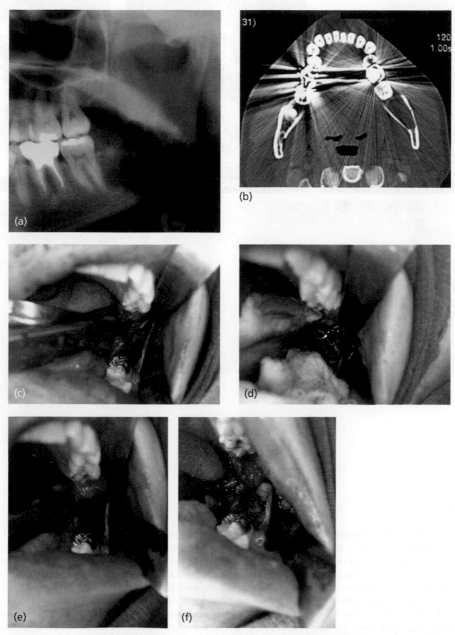

Fig. 21.16 A 34-year-old female with KCOT involving the left mandible treated with enucleation and curettage with chemical fixation using Carnoy's solution. (a) Preoperative panoramic radiograph. (b) Preoperative CT scan. (c) Intraoperative photograph following enucleation and curettage (note inferior alveolar nerve). (d) Treatment with 5 minute application of Carnoy's solution. (e) Conservative peripheral ostectomy with rotary instrument. (f) Freeze-dried, demineralized bone graft reconstruction.

to wound dehiscence and local infection. The authors concluded that enucleation and liquid nitrogen cryotherapy may offer patients improved therapy in the management of KOTs.

Keratocystic odontogenic tumors can be treated by marsupialization and decompression. They appear to respond very well to this treatment, and clinically and radiographically they shrink down considerably over 9–12 months. In many cases, they will appear to disappear completely, but it is now known that if further treatment is not added the recurrence rate can be up to 20%. For that reason, marsupialization and decompression is normally used to reduce the size of the lesion prior to a more definitive treatment.

Resection is the only predictably curative procedure for patients with KOTs that offers a recurrence rate approaching zero. The concern with this method, of course, is the functional and esthetic morbidity associated with continuity defects of the mandible and maxilla. Advances in head and neck reconstruction, microvascular surgery, and dental implants during the last two decades, however, have made this aggressive treatment modality less foreboding (Fig. 21.17).

Based on the current level of evidence, treatment of most KOTs should involve enucleation and curettage with some sort of adjunctive procedure if resection is not a consideration.

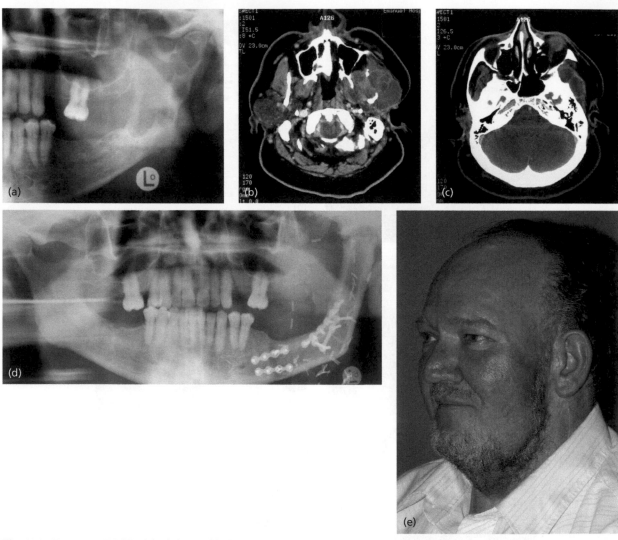

Fig. 21.17 Recurrent KCOT of the left mandibular ramus with extension to the infratemporal fossa. The patient had been treated with three previous operations during a 20-year period, two of them aggressively through a transcutaneous approach. The full extent of the recurrent lesion involves not only the mandible but also the infratemporal fossa, parotid gland, and temporalis muscle, extending to the skull base. (a) Panoramic radiograph of the patient demonstrating multilocular radiolucency; however, the extensive involvement cannot be appreciated on plain film, demonstrating the need for additional imaging. (b) Axial CT scan of the same patient demonstrating extensive involvement by KOT of the mandible, infratemporal fossa, parotid gland, and skull base. Note also the proximity of the lesion to skin. (c) CT of the same patient demonstrating cranial extension of the lesion with involvement of the temporalis muscle and skull base. (d) Panoramic radiograph demonstrates long-term result of the same patient 7 years after undergoing composite resection of the mandible and infratemporal fossa and superficial parotidectomy, with immediate reconstruction utilizing a fibular free flap. Note evidence of osseous healing, restoration of mandibular continuity, and no evidence of recurrent disease. (e) Clinical photograph of the patient 7 years after surgery. Note well healed parotidectomy scar and excellent restoration of form and function. (Courtesy of Eric J. Dierks, DMD, MD, FACS.)

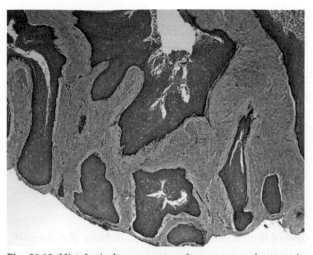

Fig. 21.18 Histological appearance of squamous odontogenic tumor. Note rounded or oval islands of well differentiated squamous epithelium within a fibrous stroma. (Courtesy of Jeffery C. Stewart, DDS, MS.)

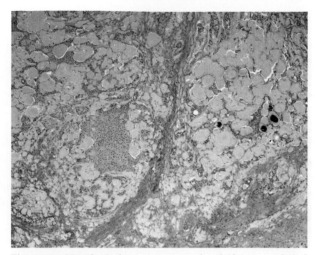

Fig. 21.19 Histological appearance of calcifying epithelial odontogenic tumor (CEOT). Note islands and sheets of polyhedral epithelial cells with abundant eosinophilic cytoplasm within a fibrous stroma. (Courtesy of Jeffery C. Stewart, DDS, MS.)

Squamous odontogenic tumor

The squamous odontogenic tumor (SOT) was first described by in 1975, with fewer than 50 cases having been reported to date. Other synonymous terms were previously used to describe this tumor, including benign epithelial odontogenic tumor, acanthomatous ameloblastoma, acanthomatous ameloblastic fibroma, hyperplasia and squamous metaplasia of residual odontogenic epithelium, and benign odontogenic tumor unclassified. SOT is defined as a locally infiltrative neoplasm consisting of islands of well differentiated squamous epithelium in a fibrous stroma (Fig. 21.18). The age range is broad (8–74 years, mean = 38.7) and there is no gender predilection. The etiology is unknown. The tumor typically presents as a localized gingival swelling or extraosseous mass in the maxilla or mandible with possible tooth mobility, pain, and gingival erythema.

Treatment is by conservative surgical excision and recurrences are rare.

Calcifying epithelial odontogenic tumor

The calcifying epithelial odontogenic tumor (CEOT) or Pindborg tumor, is defined as a locally invasive epithelial odontogenic neoplasm, characterized by the presence of amyloid material that may become calcified (Fig. 21.19). Fewer than 200 cases have been reported in the literature and it is thought to represent approximately 1% of all odontogenic tumors. The tumor has been reported to occur in patients between 13 and 80 years of age and has no gender predilection. The majority of cases occur in the mandible (3:1 ratio) and the premolar area is a common site.

The CEOT usually presents as an asymptomatic, slow-growing, expansile mass in the mandible or maxilla. More than 90% of the cases are intraosseous, but extraosseous variants have been reported. Radiographically, they have been described as a well-defined, unilocular or multilocular, mixed radiolucent/radiopaque lesion; however, these findings are variable.

CEOT is a locally invasive tumor that is associated with recurrence rates of 14–20% following enucleation and curettage. Slightly higher rates of recurrence have been associated with the clear cell variant. Although thought to be less aggressive than the solid ameloblastoma, excision with 0.5–1.0 cm margins is generally recommended.

Adenomatoid odontogenic tumor

The adenomatoid odontogenic tumor (AOT) is a unique lesion involving the jaws (centrally located), or in the soft tissue (gingival) overlying tooth-bearing areas or alveolar mucosa in edentulous regions. It is defined by the WHO as a tumor of odontogenic epithelium in a "variety of histoarchitectural patterns, embedded in a mature connective tissue stroma and characterized by slow but progressive growth". Typically the tumor is made up of a cellular multinodular proliferation of spindle, cuboidal, and columnar cells in a variety of patterns; usually scattered duct-like structures, eosinophilic material, and calcifications in several forms; and a fibrous capsule of variable thickness (Fig. 21.20). It is regarded by some authors as a benign neoplasm and by others as a developmental hamartoma.

AOTs account for approximately 2–7% of all odontogenic tumors. They occur in almost any age group (3–82 years); however, more than 90% are diagnosed prior to age 30 and half of the cases occur in adolescence. The male:female ratio is approximately 1:1.9

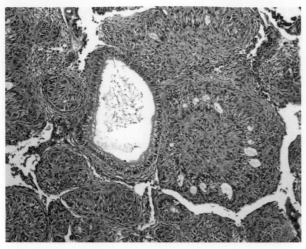

Fig. 21.20 Histological appearance of adenomatoid odontogenic tumor (AOT). Note proliferation of spindle, cuboidal, and columnar cells, scattered duct-like structures, eosinophilic material, and calcifications within a fibrous capsule (capsule not visualized). (Courtesy of Jeffery C. Stewart, DDS, MS.)

and AOT may be more prevalent in Asians. The most common site is in the anterior maxilla, with a 2:1 (maxilla:mandible) ratio.

AOTs are often detected on routine radiographic evaluation as an asymptomatic intraosseous lesion associated with an unerupted permanent tooth, commonly a maxillary canine. When intraosseous growth causes cortical expansion, it may present as a slow-growing, painless, bony mass, but peripheral variants are also described. The characteristic radiographic appearance is that of a well-defined, unicystic radiolucency associated with the crown of an impacted tooth. The radiolucency shows focal areas of radiopacity in two-thirds of the cases of intraosseous tumor.

The biological behavior of this tumor is more hamartomatous than neoplastic, although aggressive variants are occasionally encountered. Treatment is with conservative local excision and recurrences are unusual.

Odontogenic epithelium with odontogenic ectomesenchyme with or without hard tissue formation

Ameloblastic fibroma/fibrodentinoma

Along with odontoameloblastoma and dentinogenic ghost cell tumor, the ameloblastic fibroma (AF) is one of the benign "mixed" odontogenic tumors that is a true neoplasm characterized by expansile growth and potentially destructive behavior. It lies in contradistinction to the other "mixed" odontogenic tumors, ameloblastic fibro-odontoma and odontoma, which represent hamartomas that rarely result in significant morbidity. The AF consists of "odontogenic ectomesenchyme resembling the dental papilla and epithelial strands and nests resembling dental lamina and enamel organ", which distinguishes them from tumors of purely ectomesenchymal or pure epithelial

origin. Generally, no dental hard tissues are present; however, if dentin is observed, the lesion is referred to as an ameloblastic fibrodentinoma. AF tends to occur in the first two decades of life, but patients older than 22 years are not uncommon. The posterior mandible is affected in more than 70% of the cases. The tumor presents as a unilocular or multilocular radiolucency that may demonstrate cortical expansion, erosion or both (Fig. 21.21). Most authorities recommend conservative excision, particularly in young patients, and find that the lesions rarely recur.

Ameloblastic fibro-odontoma

One of the "mixed" odontogenic tumors, the ameloblastic fibro-odontoma most likely represents a hamartoma, rather than a true neoplasm. It has been suggested that the ameloblastic fibro-odontoma is simply an immature complex odontoma. Histologically, it shares the same features of ameloblastic fibroma, except that it contains dentin and enamel. The tumor typically presents as an asymptomatic, well circumscribed, mixed radiopaque/radiolucent mass involving the posterior mandible. Rarely exhibiting aggressive behavior, the tumor is treated effectively with enucleation and curettage.

Odontoma, complex and compound type

Odontomas are the most common of the odontogenic tumors, representing a benign hamartoma rather than a true neoplasm, and generally have a benign clinical course. Odontomas are described in two types: complex and compound. The difference between the two forms is that compound odontomas contain recognizable enamel, dentin, and sometimes cementum, shaped in toothlike structures; whereas complex odontomas are composed of irregular masses of dentin and enamel and have no anatomic resemblance to a tooth. Complex odontomas are typically found in the posterior maxilla or mandible and compound odontomas are predominately in the anterior maxilla. The compound odontoma is twice as common as the complex odontoma. The lesions appear as well circumscribed, radiopaque masses, often surrounded by what appears to be a periodontal ligament (Fig. 21.22). The masses are treated with simple enucleation and curettage, which is virtually always curative.

Odontoameloblastoma

According to the WHO, odontoameloblastoma (OA) "combines the clinical and histological features of ameloblastoma with those of an odontoma". This is a rare neoplasm that occurs in the maxilla and mandible with equal prevalence, usually in the first three decades of life. Clinical signs and symptoms, as well as biological behavior, may be identical to those of a solid ameloblastoma. The radiographic appearance

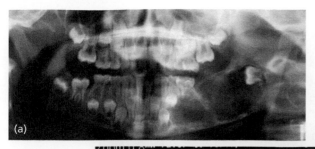

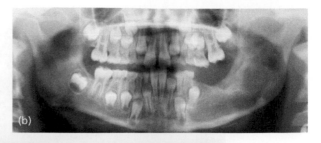

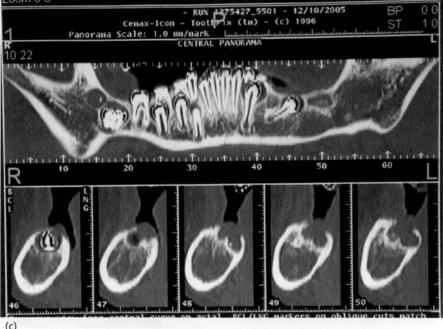

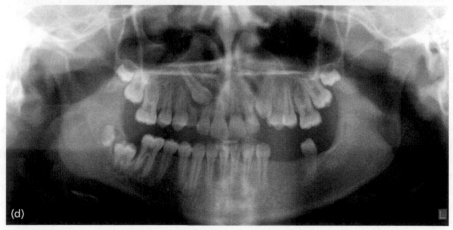

Fig. 21.21 Ameloblastic fibroma of the mandible treated by excision with peripheral ostectomy and cryotherapy. (a) Preoperative panoramic radiograph. (b) 1-year postoperative panoramic radiograph. (c) Small recurrence noted on cone-beam CT scan 2 years following treatment. (d) Postoperative panoramic radiograph 2 years following conservative, outpatient excision of recurrence. (Courtesy of Eric J. Dierks, DMD, MD, FACS.)

of this tumor differs from that of ameloblastoma by varying amounts of radiopaque material, which generally represents displaced or unerupted teeth. OA is locally aggressive and requires surgical excision with 0.5–1.0cm tumor-free margins.

Calcifying cystic odontogenic tumor

Calcifying cystic odontogenic tumor (CCOT) is a benign odontogenic neoplasm that resembles amel-

oblastoma with ghost cells that may calcify. It is also termed Gorlin cyst and calcifying odontogenic cyst. The CCOT may present as an expansile mass involving the maxilla or mandible with equal frequency, and both intraosseous and extraosseous forms occur. It can occur at any age and there is no gender predilection. It typically presents as an asymptomatic, unilocular, well-defined radiolucency; however, it can exhibit a radiopaque component as well. Histologically, the CCOT is characterized by a cyst wall

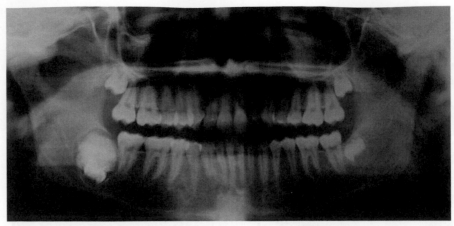

Fig. 21.22 Complex odontoma of the mandible.

that is lined by thin ameloblastomatous epithelium with the formation of ghost cells. Aggressive clinical behavior is not typical of this benign entity, and simple enucleation and curettage is generally curative.

Dentinogenic ghost cell tumor

Formerly considered a solid variant of the calcifying cystic odontogenic tumor (Gorlin cyst), the dentinogenic ghost cell tumor is a locally invasive neoplasm characterized by ameloblastoma-like islands of epithelial cells in a mature connective tissue stroma, with varying amounts of dysplastic dentin and ghost cells. The tumor typically presents as an asymptomatic hard tissue or soft tissue mass (intraosseous or extraosseous variants), showing varying amounts of bone resorption or tooth displacement. Radiographically, it may present as a radiolucent or mixed radiolucent/ radiopaque lesion with unilocular, well-circumscribed borders. It is histologically distinguished from ameloblastoma and calcifying odontogenic tumor by the presence of ghost cells with dysplastic dentin. Although malignant transformation has been described, recurrences after appropriate excision with 0.5–1.0 cm margins are rare. Similar challenges to ameloblastoma are present with regards to the most appropriate surgical treatment and the extent of resection.

Mesenchyme and/or odontogenic ectomesenchyme with or without odontogenic epithelium

Odontogenic fibroma

The odontogenic fibroma (OF) is a very rare neoplasm that is defined by the WHO as containing "varying amounts of inactive-looking odontogenic epithelium embedded in a mature fibrous stroma". The OF occurs as a radiolucent lesion involving the jaws without respect to gender, age, or site (maxilla or mandible). The radiographic appearance is that of a radiolucent lesion that may be unilocular or multi-

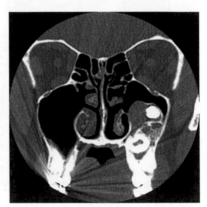

Fig. 21.23 Odontogenic myxoma. Coronal CT scan demonstrating well defined expansile mass with displacement of teeth.

locular and cause cortical expansion. They do not appear to behave in an aggressive fashion and both respond well to enucleation and curettage.

Odontogenic myxoma/myxofibroma

The odontogenic myxoma (OM) is relatively common amongst odontogenic tumors and may comprise between 3 and 20% of all such lesions. The WHO characterizes this intraosseous neoplasm as containing "stellate and spindle-shaped cells embedded in an abundant myxoid or mucoid extracellular matrix" (Fig. 21.23). The term myxofibroma is used when a relatively greater amount of collagen is evident.

Two-thirds of OMs are located in the mandible, commonly in the molar regions, and typically present in the second to fourth decade of life (age range 1–70 years) without gender predilection. It is commonly found as an incidental finding on routine panoramic radiograph. The radiographic appearance is that of a well-defined, unilocular or multilocular radiolucency, generally associated with an erupted tooth. The lesion has a rather bland histological appearance that is characterized by a loose mesenchymal fibrous tissue that lacks atypia. Randomly oriented stellate, spindle-shaped and round cells with eosinophilic cytoplasmic processes sit in a mucoid or myxoid stroma. OM has a similar histological appearance to that of hyperplastic dental follicles and the dental papilla of a developing tooth, though odontogenic epithelium is not seen. Clinical correlation is essential to avoid misdiagnosis.

The OM is a benign but locally aggressive tumor that is probably less aggressive than ameloblastoma, but can result in progressive growth with skull base involvement if left untreated. Resection with 1–1.5 cm bony margins and one uninvolved anatomic barrier margin has been advocated as the best chance for a curative treatment due to its potentially aggressive behavior.

Cementoblastoma

Cementoblastoma is characterized by the formation of a radiopaque cementum-like mass intimately associated with the root of a tooth (usually a lower second or third molar). The tooth typically remains vital and symptoms include varying degrees of cortical expansion and pain. Classically, the tumorous mass is surrounded by a radiolucent ring, that represents the periodontal ligament (Fig. 21.24). Histologically identical to an osteoblastoma, the cementoblastoma is differentiated from its bony counterpart by virtue of its intimate association with teeth. Biopsy will distinguish it from an odontoma, focal sclerosing osteomy-

elitis, and hypercementosis, all of which may have a similar clinical and radiographic appearance. Treatment is otherwise by excision with peripheral ostectomy for all but the largest tumors.

Non-odontogenic benign tumors

Ossifying fibroma

Ossifying fibroma (OF) is one of the so-called fibro-osseous lesions that include ossifying fibroma, fibrous dysplasia, and cemento-osseous dysplasia. This benign neoplasm is characterized by the replacement of normal bone by fibrous tissue and varying amounts of newly formed bone or cementum-like material. A juvenile, and possibly more aggressive variant has also been described. The WHO recognizes two distinct histological variants of juvenile ossifying fibroma, neither of which differ from each other significantly in their biological behavior or treatment: juvenile trabecular ossifying fibroma (JTOF) and juvenile psammomatoid ossifying fibroma (JPOF). The juvenile variants occur in a younger age group than the conventional type of ossifying fibroma. The mean age for JPOF is 20 years, compared with that of 35 years in cases of adult ossifying fibroma, whereas the mean age range for JTOF is 8.5–12 years.

All variants of OF generally present as painless, slow-growing, expansile osseous lesions. The radiographic appearance is typically a well-defined expansile mass with a variable degree of internal calcification (Fig. 21.25). Root displacement and root resorption may be seen.

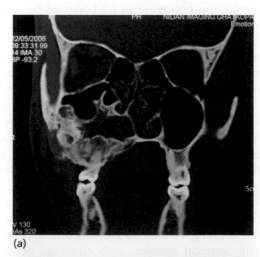

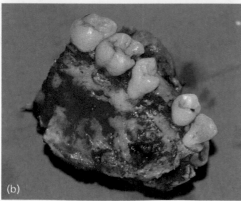

Fig. 21.24 Cementoblastoma of the maxilla. (a) Preoperative CT scan. (b) Resection specimen.

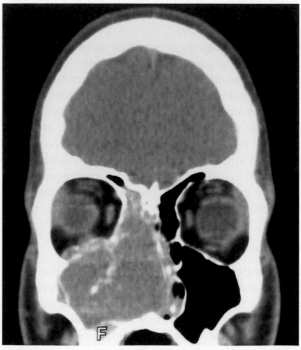

Fig. 21.25 Coronal CT scan of an ossifying fibroma of the maxilla with extension into the paranasal sinuses and anterior skull base.

Conventional therapy includes appropriate excision dependent on the extent and location of the tumor, with recurrence rates reported between 1% and 63%.

Fibrous dysplasia

Fibrous dysplasia (FD) is a genetically based sporadic, non-odontogenic disease of bone that is characterized by the replacement of bone with benign fibrous tissue that may affect single (monostotic) or multiple (polyostotic) bones throughout the human skeleton. Fibrous dysplasia involving only multiple adjacent craniofacial bones (termed craniofacial fibrous dysplasia) is regarded as monostotic.

FD presents most commonly in the long bones, followed by the jaws (maxilla more than mandible), base of skull, and ribs. Patients with craniofacial FD typically complain of painless swelling, facial asymmetry, loosening of teeth, malocclusion, and root resorption. Children that exhibit café-au-lait spots should be evaluated to rule out McCune–Albright syndrome.

The radiographic appearance has classically been described as that of a "ground glass" appearance with ill-defined borders and cortical expansion (Fig. 21.26). In fact, there is a spectrum of appearances that includes an early-phase radiolucent appearance, a midphase appearance characterized by sclerosis, and a later phase that demonstrates a mixed radiolucent/radiopaque character. Computed tomography (CT) is the imaging modality of choice, and three-dimensional reconstructions and stereolithographic models are useful in determining the extent of involvement and in planning surgery.

The histological appearance of FD is that of cellular fibrous tissue with spindle-shaped cells and immature, trabeculated woven bone (Fig. 21.27). Bundles of collagen fibers can be identified that are characteristically oriented perpendicular to the bony surface. Osteoblastic rimming can be noted, which may represent long-standing, mature lesions.

FD can often exhibit aggressive, destructive behavior prior to skeletal maturity; however, it often becomes indolent in adulthood. Surgical recontouring or complete excision/resection can also be contemplated in cases of persistent deforming growth or in those patients that request it due to esthetic or functional concerns.

Osseous dysplasias

Osseous dysplasias (ODs) are defined by the WHO as "idiopathic processes located in the periapical region of the tooth-bearing jaw areas, characterized by a replacement of normal bone by fibrous tissue and metaplastic bone". The terminology for this lesion is confusing due to the numerous synonyms that are used based on the site of occurrence within the jaws: in the anterior mandible the lesion has been referred to as periapical osseous dysplasia; and in the posterior mandible it is known as focal osseous dysplasia (formerly focal cemento-osseous dysplasia); periapical cemental dysplasia is a term used to describe this lesion in association with the roots of teeth; and florid osseous dysplasia describes widespread involvement of the mandible in multiple quadrants. The latter form may present with symptoms of pain or secondary infection, but the vast majority of these lesions are asymptomatic and are of no clinical significance. The histological appearances of the various expressions of this lesion are identical: cellular fibrous tissue surrounding sheets and strands of woven and lamellar bone interspersed between masses of cementum-like material. The common age range is 25–60 and it appears more frequently in people of African American heritage. OD does not require treatment unless complications occur. Biopsy should be performed in cases that demonstrate progression, cortical expansion or bony erosion. Aggressive surgical treatment is rarely needed except in the extremely unusual case of gigantiform cementoma.

Osteoblastoma and osteoid osteoma

These are probably variants of the same tumor and only differ in size. Lesions less than 2 cm in diameter are normally termed osteoid osteoma whilst larger ones are termed osteoblastoma. They are both felt to be true tumors occurring in all bones of the body including the jaws. The cementoblastoma is identical but associated with teeth and felt to derive from the cementoblasts. The interesting feature of these tumors is that they are painful, and often this is the presenting feature. The pain is worse at night and is relieved very effectively with aspirin. Clinically they grow rapidly and generally appear as a mixed radiolucency/radiopacity on radiographs with a clearly-defined margin with a thin radiolucent zone surrounding the variably calcified contents. Histologically, they show trabeculae of osteoid and immature bone in a vascular stromal network. Calcification is variable and there is some resemblance to fibro-osseous lesions from which they must be differentiated. Treatment is normally surgical excision with curettage or local excisions. Recurrences are rare, and examples of malignant transformation even rarer. Spontaneous regression has also been reported after biopsy, which puts doubts on the histogenesis of the lesion.

Central giant cell lesion

The central giant cell lesion (CGCL) is a benign but potentially aggressive proliferation of fibroblasts and multinucleated giant cells that cause osteolysis and reactive bone formation. The proliferating cell in this lesion appears to be the fibroblast. Controversy exists with regards to whether the CGCL is unique to the jaws or whether it represents a continuum of the

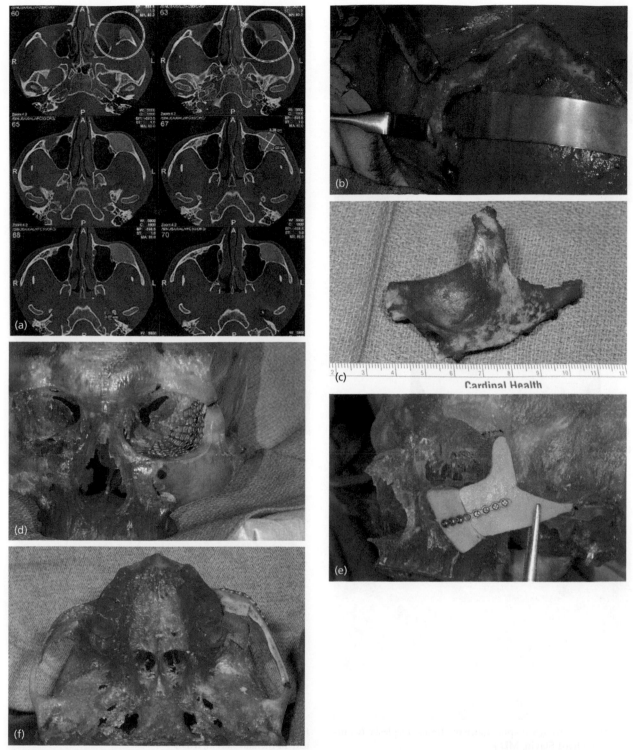

Fig. 21.26 Craniofacial fibrous dysplasia exhibiting active growth and progressive deformity in a 25-year-old male. (a) CT scan demonstrating homogeneous, expansile bony lesion with "ground glass" appearance. (b) Coronal approach combined with transoral and periorbital incisions to facilitate complete resection of the involved bone. (c) Resection specimen. (d) Stereolithographic model ground down to normal anatomic contours and resected according to the planned surgery. (e) Full-thickness calvarial bone harvested, milled to reproduce the ground down model, and inset into the stereolithographic model to achieve proper fit and symmetry. (f) Stereolithographic model demonstrating proper arch projection and symmetry. (g) Inset of the neo-zygoma construct. (h) Postoperative axial CT scan of the patient demonstrating excellent symmetry. (i) Postoperative appearance of the patient.

same disease process that affects the long bones (termed giant cell tumor).

CGCL of the jaws is most often diagnosed in children and young adults under the age of 30 years. One-third of the patients are diagnosed under 20

years of age. The mandible is more often involved than the maxilla and the posterior mandible is affected more often than the anterior aspect of the jaws or the ascending ramus. The lesion typically consists of spindle-shaped fibroblastic cells loosely arranged in

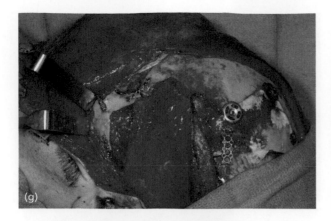

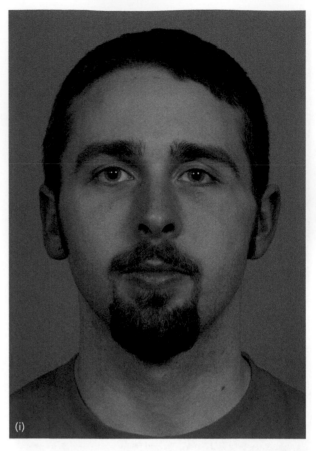

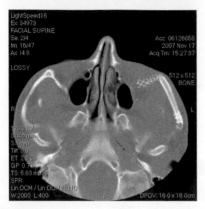

Fig. 21.26 (*Continued*)

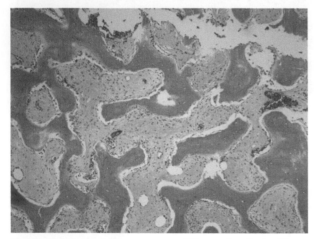

Fig. 21.27 Histological appearance of fibrous dysplasia. (Courtesy of Richard Slavin, MD.)

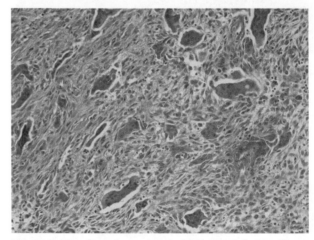

Fig. 21.28 Histological appearance of giant cell lesion. (Courtesy of Richard Slavin, MD.)

a fibrous connective tissue stroma with areas of hemorrhage, hemosiderin deposits, macrophages, lymphocytes, granulocytes, and plasma cells (Fig. 21.28). Small clusters of osteoclast-like giant cell are found dispersed within the lesion. Mitoses are frequently observed. Brown tumor of hyperparathyroidism is histologically indistinguishable from CGCL, therefore a serum calcium, phosphate and parathyroid hormone level is often recommended to rule out primary or secondary forms of parathyroid dysfunction.

Clinical manifestations of the disease may include painless cortical expansion, facial asymmetry, cortical perforation, and/or root resorption (Fig. 21.29).

Complete excision of the tumor is required to prevent the sequela of persistent bony growth. Enucleation and curettage has been the primary mode of treatment, but is associated with an overall recurrence rate of between 15 and 50%. The first nonsurgical modality to be successfully applied was intralesional corticosteroid injections. Weekly injections of triamcinolone for 6 weeks have resulted in

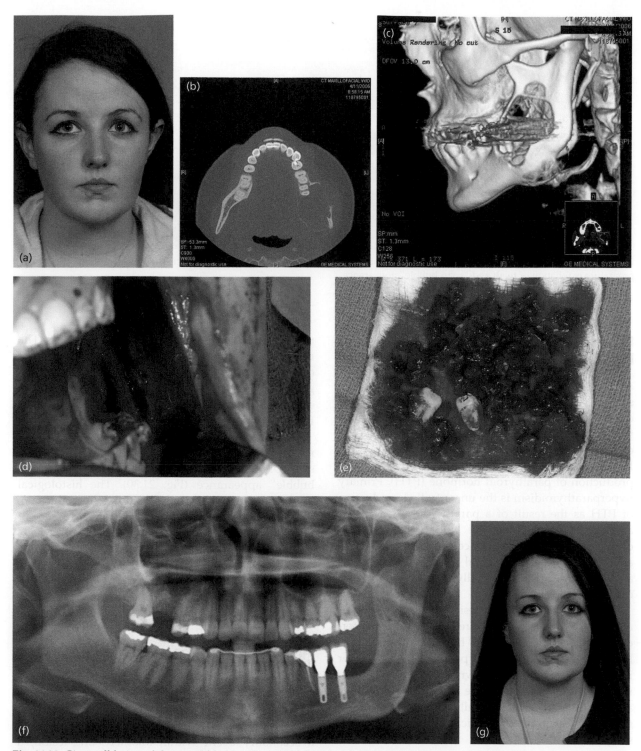

Fig. 21.29 Giant cell lesion of the mandible in a 17-year-old female. (a) Preoperative appearance with mild facial asymmetry. (b) Preoperative cone-beam CT scan demonstrating multilocular, expansile lesion with cortical erosion. (c) Axial CT scan demonstrating cortical expansion and mandibular deformity. (d) Transoral excision with peripheral ostectomy and immediate anterior iliac crest bone graft reconstruction. (e) Specimen. (f) Postoperative panoramic image of the patient 2 years following surgery with maintenance of mandibular continuity and no evidence of tumor recurrence. (g) Postoperative appearance 2 years after surgery.

partial or complete resolution in some patients. Experience with this technique is varied, however, and response to therapy is unpredictable. Calcitonin has also been proposed as a definitive, non-surgical treatment for giant cell lesions, presumably based on its inhibition of osteoclastogenesis. Daily subcutaneous injections of human or salmon calcitonin injections are carried out for approximately 18 months, and have caused resolution of these lesions. Alpha-interferon, given by subcutaneous injection as an adjunct to surgical excision, has also been used. The data thus far suggest that alpha-interferon treatment may result in less radical surgery and a reduced rate of recurrence, however this is not yet conclusive. Furthermore, treatment with alpha-interferon is associated with significant side-effects and potential morbidity.

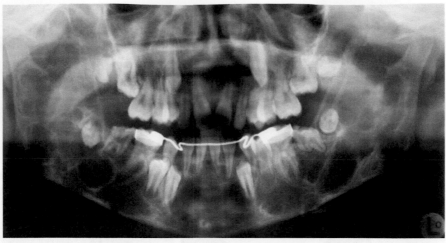

Fig. 21.30 Cherubism. Panoramic radiograph demonstrating bilateral multilocular radiolucencies exhibiting cortical expansion, premature exfoliation of teeth and "soap bubble" appearance.

Brown tumor of hyperparathyroidism

Altered calcium regulation resulting from primary or secondary hyperparathyroidism or renal dysfunction can result in the formation of giant cell lesions of bone termed "brown tumors" due to the hemosiderin deposition within the lesion that causes a brown color. Hyperparathyroidism is characterized by the overproduction of parathyroid hormone (PTH). Primary hyperparathyroidism is the uncontrolled production of PTH as the result of a parathyroid adenoma or adenocarcinoma. Secondary hyperparathyroidism occurs in response to hypocalcemia and is most often associated with chronic renal failure. These lesions are clinically and histologically identical to those of central giant cell lesions.

Patients with giant cell lesions should be evaluated for the presence of altered PTH levels, hypercalcemia (seen in primary hyperparathyroidism), hypocalcemia (secondary hyperparathyroidism), or impaired renal function. Brown tumors will typically resolve with treatment of the underlying metabolic abnormality. Persistent, locally destructive lesions that are recalcitrant to medical therapy should be surgically excised.

Cherubism

Cherubism is a rare hereditary condition that is characterized by giant cell lesions which cause symmetrical expansion of the jaws. First described in 1933, it follows an autosomal dominant pattern of inheritance with 100% penetrance in males, 50–75% penetrance in females, and variable expressivity. The genetic defect has been mapped to chromosome 4p16.3, which encodes the binding protein SH3BP2.

Cherubism is generally diagnosed in early childhood. Mandibular involvement is most prominent, although both jaws may be affected and the process may extend into the anterior and inferior orbits. The mandibular condyles are spared. With involvement of the maxillary contribution to the orbital floor, the globes may be displaced upward, resulting in scleral show and the "looking toward Heaven" appearance that inspired the lesion's name.

The radiographic appearance is that of bilateral mulilocular radiolucencies exhibiting cortical expansion, premature exfoliation of teeth, and a "soap bubble" appearance (Fig. 21.30). The histological appearance is similar to the central giant cell lesion, but may usually be distinguished by the presence of hemosiderin deposits, stromal fibrosis, and perivascular cuff-like collagen deposits.

The clinical course is generally indolent. The lesions regress as the patient approaches skeletal maturity. Treatment is not recommended unless severe dysfunction is present.

Aneurysmal bone cyst

The aneurysmal bone cyst (ABC) is defined by the WHO as an osteolytic lesion "with blood filled spaces separated by fibrous septa containing osteoclast-type giant cells and reactive bone". ABCs often present as a secondary event within another bone lesion, a finding that has led some authors to question the existence of this lesion as a separate entity. Furthermore, as it often occurs within a central giant cell lesion and itself contains giant cells, other authors have suggested that the ABC is simply part of the spectrum of development in giant cell lesions. While many of these lesions are thought to be reactive, there are some cytogenetic data that suggest ABCs are indeed a distinct entity.

ABC is rare, with an incidence estimated to be 0.014 per 100 000. It occurs in young patients, generally below age 30 and with a peak incidence in the second decade. ABC may occur in virtually any bone in the body, and involvement of the jaws occurs in

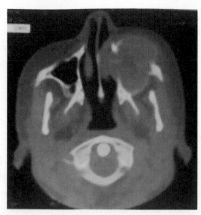

Fig. 21.31 Aneurysmal bone cyst. Axial CT scan of ABC demonstrating expansion and cortical erosion through the anterior and medial wall of the maxillary sinus.

less than 3% of the cases. When present in the maxilla or mandible, it may present as an asymptomatic radiolucency discovered incidentally on routine dental radiography, or may present with marked facial swelling, similar to fibrous dysplasia (Fig. 21.31). Teeth remain vital and the same functional problems regarding encroachment on vital structures or foramina that exist in fibrous dysplasia are also of concern with ABC.

The histological appearance of ABC is that of hemorrhagic, multilocular, well-circumscribed blood-filled cavities that are lined by macrophages, not endothelial cells. Fibroblasts, osteoclast-like giant cells, and reactive bone are dispersed within osteoid, occasionally containing hemosiderin deposits and nuclear mitoses.

Genetic evidence supporting the classification of ABC as a distinct pathological entity is derived primarily from research in extracranial lesions: a 17p-rearrangement with balanced translocation with 16q has been reported by a number of investigators. These translocations have been regarded by some authors as resulting from acquired aberrations that provide evidence that some ABCs are clonal proliferations.

ABCs are typically treated with enucleation and curettage. The lesions can be highly vascular, therefore removal in an office setting is generally ill-advised for all but very small lesions.

Malignant tumors

Odontogenic carcinomas

Malignant odontogenic tumors are classified by the WHO as odontogenic carcinomas and odontogenic sarcomas. All of these tumors are exceedingly rare and many are still reportable cases. They are classified as odontogenic if the tumor demonstrates epithelium that histologically resembles that seen in a developing tooth or recognizable odontogenic tumor, such as ameloblastoma or ameloblastic fibroma.

Ameloblastic carcinoma

Malignant ameloblastoma is subclassified into four distinct entities, three of them only of academic importance: (1) metastasizing ameloblastoma; (2) ameloblastic carcinoma – primary type; (3) ameloblastic carcinoma – secondary type (dedifferentiated), intraosseous; and (4) ameloblastic carcinoma – secondary type (dedifferentiated), peripheral. Metastasizing ameloblastoma is differentiated from ameloblastic carcinoma by its benign histologic appearance, despite its ability to metastasize. Ameloblastoma with metastatic deposits that exhibit cellular atypia is defined as ameloblastic carcinoma. Secondary ameloblastic carcinoma, either intraosseous or peripheral, arises in a pre-existing benign ameloblastoma.

The incidence of ameloblastic carcinoma is unknown, as fewer than 70 cases have been reported. The median age is 44 years; however, the tumor occurs in a wide age range of patients, with a sex ratio of 1.75 male to 1 female. The mandible is involved more frequently than the maxilla (ratio 2.14 : 1). Ameloblastic carcinoma seems to behave similarly to squamous cell carcinoma in terms of local invasion, regional lymph node metastasis, and distant metastasis. The 5-year disease-specific survival rate is around 68%.

Optimal treatment of ameloblastic carcinoma is unknown, but there is general agreement that it should be managed in similar fashion to squamous cell carcinoma of the oral cavity, consisting of composite resection with 1 cm tumor-free margins, neck dissection, and immediate reconstruction with microvascular free flaps. Adjuvant radiation therapy should be considered for all patients, especially those cases exhibiting unfavorable histologic characteristics, such as positive resection margins, perineural invasion, and lymph node metastasis.

Primary intraosseous squamous cell carcinoma

Primary intraosseous squamous cell carcinoma (PIOSCC) is a central jaw carcinoma derived from epithelium arising within benign odontogenic cysts or tumors, usually a dentigerous cyst or keratocystic odontogenic tumor. The incidence of malignant transformation of odontogenic cysts has been estimated to be approximately 0.12%. The most common sites are generally the same as for non-malignant cysts, most commonly the mandibular third molar, maxillary canine and third molar, and mandibular second premolar regions.

Treatment is similar to that of invasive squamous cell carcinoma with bony involvement: radical resection with ipsilateral neck dissection and immediate reconstruction using microvascular composite free flaps. Although data are lacking, adjuvant radiation therapy or chemoradiation therapy should be considered depending on the tumor's histopathological characteristics, margin status, and the status of the regional lymph nodes.

Clear cell odontogenic carcinoma

Clear cell odontogenic carcinoma (CCOC) is defined by the WHO as a malignant odontogenic tumor that is characterized by sheets and islands of vacuolated and clear cells. Previously known as clear cell ameloblastoma or clear cell odontogenic tumor, fewer than 40 cases have been reported. There is a strong female predilection and it tends to occur in the mandible of older patients, with a mean age at diagnosis of 60 years.

Regional and distant metastasis have been described and should be treated in similar fashion to squamous cell carcinoma. Adjuvant radiation therapy should be considered following composite resection, neck dissection, and microvascular free flap reconstruction.

Ghost cell odontogenic carcinoma

Ghost cell odontogenic carcinoma is a malignant odontogenic epithelial tumor that is defined by the WHO as having "features of calcifying cystic odontogenic tumor and/or dentinogenic ghost cell tumor". This tumor is extremely rare, having been reported less than two dozen times in the English literature. It may be more common in Asia, appears to affect more men than women, and occurs in a wide age range. Twice as many tumors occur in the maxilla as in the mandible, similar to that of the calcifying odontogenic cyst.

Histological diagnosis is based on the identification of malignant epithelial cells within the histological architecture of a calcifying cystic odontogenic tumor. Ghost cells are found in varying numbers.

The clinical presentation is typical of the malignant osseous lesions. Imaging may demonstrate an osteolytic radiolucency with or without calcifications, which is poorly defined, may displace or destroy tooth roots, and extend into adjacent tissues. Treatment data are lacking; however, presumably the lesion should be managed with radical resection, neck dissection, and immediate reconstruction using composite free tissue transfer. Adjuvant radiation therapy or chemoradiation therapy should be considered, depending on the histopathologic features, margin status, and status of the cervical lymph nodes.

Odontogenic sarcomas

Odontogenic sarcomas are very rare tumors. The WHO defines two distinct types: ameloblastic fibrosarcoma and ameloblastic fibrodentinosarcoma and fibro-odontosarcoma.

Ameloblastic fibrosarcoma

The ameloblastic fibrosarcoma (AFS) is the malignant counterpart of the ameloblastic fibroma. An odontogenic tumor with a benign epithelial and a malignant ectomesenchymal component, the etiology is unknown. Many of these tumors appear to represent malignant transformation of pre-existing ameloblastic fibroma.

Ameloblastic fibrodentinosarcoma and fibro-odontosarcoma

These rare tumors show the histological features of ameloblastic fibrosarcoma, together with dysplastic dentin (fibrodentinosarcoma) and/or enamel/enameloid and dentin/dentinoid (fibro-odontosarcoma). Treatment is radical resection and the prognosis appears to be good.

Non-odontogenic malignant jaw tumors

Osteosarcoma

Osteosarcoma (OS) is a malignant tumor of bone characterized by the formation of osteoid by neoplastic cells. OS is the most common primary sarcoma of bone and only plasma cell neoplasms outnumber this tumor in the category of all primary bone tumors. It has been classified as central type, which is more common and arises from the medullary portion of the bone, and peripheral or juxtacortical type, which is less common and originates on the surface of bone. OS may develop from pre-existing bone disorders such as Paget's disease, giant cell tumors, or fibrous dysplasia, or from prior radiation therapy, but most arise *de novo*.

Central osteosarcomas most often involve the distal femur and proximal tibia of patients in their second decade of life. OS involving the jaws accounts for 5–7% of all OS, but the presentation appears to be older, more often presenting in the third or fourth decade of life. There is a slight male predilection and the mandible is more commonly affected than the maxilla.

The clinical presentation of OS is commonly that of jaw pain and swelling. Paresthesia is common in mandibular lesions, as is loosening of teeth. Nasal obstruction, epistaxis, proptosis, or diplopia may all be presenting signs or symptoms in advanced maxillary lesions. The radiographic appearance of central OS is classically that of an osteolytic lesion that is associated with symmetrical widening of the periodontal ligament and extracortical bone producing a "sunburst" appearance.

Treatment consists of radical resection (Fig. 21.32). The most important prognostic indicator of successful outcome is negative resection margins. Consequently, bone margins of up to 3 cm have been recommended. Well-designed, prospective outcome data for OS of the jaws are lacking. Radiation therapy, either as definitive treatment or in the adjuvant

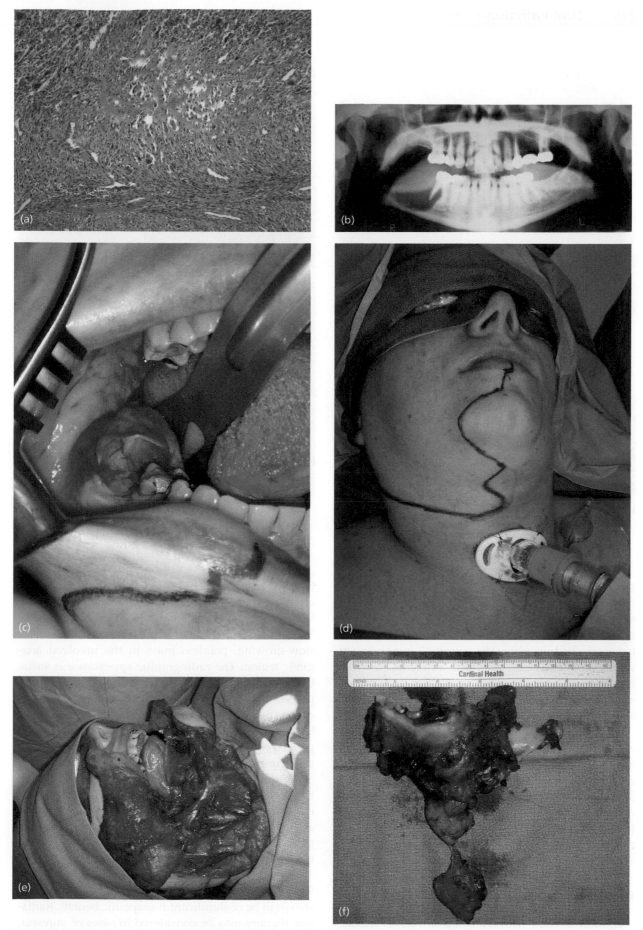

Fig. 21.32 Osteogenic sarcoma in 48-year-old female. (a) Histological appearance (courtesy of Richard Slavin, MD). (b) Preoperative panoramic radiograph demonstrating aggressive features of cortical destruction and root resorption. (c) Clinical appearance of the tumor. (d) Outline of lip-splitting incision used to facilitate composite resection. (e) Composite resection of the floor of mouth and mandible with selective neck dissection, primarily for vascular access. (f) Resection specimen. (g) Stereolithographic model to prebend reconstruction plate prior to ablative surgery. (h) Inset of a fibular osteocutaneous free flap for reconstruction of the ablative defect. (i) Fibular flap harvested. (j) Inset of the flap.

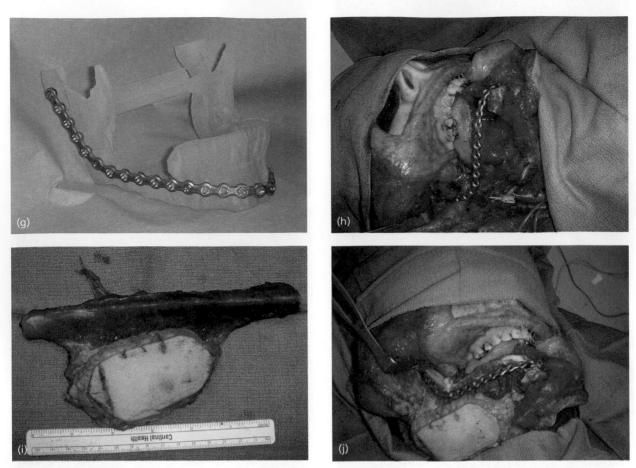

Fig. 21.32 (*Continued*)

setting, has not been shown to be beneficial. Current treatment strategies that employ a multimodal approach incorporating preoperative and postoperative chemotherapy for cases involving the long bones have resulted in dramatic survival improvement when compared with previous outcomes. Current recommendations for craniofacial OS include preoperative and postoperative chemotherapy in addition to radical resection and free flap reconstruction.

In contrast to the central medullary OS, the peripheral OS may be less aggressive and is associated with a more favorable prognosis in long bones. Most reports cite an overall 5-year survival rate for head and neck OS of 40–70%. Metastasis occurs in approximately 18–50% of cases, generally occurring in the lungs. The hematogenous route does not invite regional lymph node involvement and therefore cervical lymphadenectomy is not advocated.

Chondrosarcoma

A chondrosarcoma (CS) is a malignant tumor characterized by the formation of cartilage by malignant tumor cells. Only 1% or 2% of all chondrosarcomas are located in the head and neck. Unlike osteosarcoma, chondrosarcoma is more frequent in the maxilla than the mandible. The maxillary lesions occur most often in the anterior region and the mandibular tumors occur most often in the posterior mandible. The most common clinical presentation is that of a slow-growing, painless mass in the involved anatomic region. The radiographic appearance is variable, although most lesions demonstrate an osteolytic process with ill-defined margins, cortical erosion, and destructive behavior. Radiopacities are often present. Similar to osteosarcoma, there may be a "sunburst" pattern with symmetrical widening of the periodontal ligament space around involved teeth.

The histological appearance of CS is characterized by variable amounts of cartilage formation, but not osteoid or bone, emanating from a sarcomatous stroma. If the malignant cellular elements are noted to produce osteoid or bone in any portion of the tumor, it is considered an osteosarcoma.

The treatment of choice for CS is radical resection. Unlike osteosarcoma, chemotherapy has not been shown to be of significant therapeutic benefit. Radiation therapy may be considered in cases of unresectable, residual, or recurrent tumors. The prognosis for CS of the jaws is worse than that for tumors of the axial skeleton. The overall 5-year survival for CS of the jaws ranges from 32 to 81%. Like osteosarcoma, the lung is the most common site of metastasis and cervical lymph nodes are generally not involved. Neck dissection is therefore not recommended.

Ewing sarcoma

Ewing sarcoma (ES) is one of the "small, round, blue cell" tumors and is in the family of tumors that includes the primitive neuroectodermal tumors. The pelvis and lower extremities are most commonly affected. Jaw tumors account for less than 3% of ES. ES primarily presents in children and young adults, usually under 20 years of age. A male predilection exists.

The clinical signs and symptoms usually include rapidly progressing pain and swelling. Tumor expansion may also cause paresthesia or tooth mobility. The radiographic appearance is that of other malignant jaw tumors, including an osteolytic process with ill-defined borders and displacement or resorption of teeth or tooth roots. Growth may be rapid and progressive.

The histological appearance is that of closely packed cells that may be compartmentalized by fibrous bands, with round to oval nuclei, and finely dispersed chromatin. The cytoplasm of the tumor cell frequently stains with periodic acid-Schiff stain.

Treatment of patients with Ewing family of tumors (EFT) requires systemic chemotherapy in conjunction with either surgery or radiation therapy or both modalities for local tumor control.

About 60% of patients with localized disease can be cured. For patients with metastatic disease at diagnosis, the prognosis is much worse, with only 30–40% surviving long-term.

Malignant peripheral nerve sheath tumor

Malignant peripheral nerve sheath tumors (MPNSTs) comprise a rare group of tumors that arise from peripheral nerves or that display differentiation along the lines of the various elements of the nerve sheath, including Schwann cells, perineural fibroblasts, or fibroblasts. This group of tumors was previously referred to as malignant schwannoma, neurofibrosarcoma, or neurogenic sarcoma. Although approximately half of the patients with this disorder will have a history of neurofibromatosis type 1, many cases will arise *de novo*, or as a postradiation sarcoma. The most common site in the head and neck for intraosseous tumors is the mandible, although skull base tumors originating various cranial nerves are relatively frequent. Patients generally present with a rapidly growing mass, pain, and/or neurosensory disturbance within the anatomic distribution of the involved region or nerve.

Radiographically, tumors of the mandible may produce widening of the inferior alveolar canal or the mental foramen. More commonly, they invade the mandible from adjacent structures or cranial nerves. The microscopic appearance is that of fascicles of spindle cells that closely resemble the cells of fibrosarcoma.

Based on the current body of evidence, treatment recommendations are as follows: (1) complete surgical removal with as wide a margin of normal tissue as is feasible to achieve negative margins; (2) adjuvant radiation therapy and chemotherapy based on residual disease after initial surgery, tumor size, and grade; (3) immediate reconstruction with free tissue transfer as appropriate.

Metastatic carcinoma

Metastatic carcinoma is the most common form of malignancy affecting bone. While the jaws are relatively uncommon sites for distant metastasis, bones with active marrow spaces such as vertebrae, ribs, pelvis, and skull are generally considered preferential sites for dissemination. Metastatic carcinoma has previously been thought to represent approximately 1% of all malignant jaw lesions. More recent data based on autopsied carcinoma cases, however, demonstrate that 16% of the mandibles have microscopic deposits of metastatic tumor cells, despite the lack of radiographic evidence of osteolysis. Metastatic spread of carcinoma to the jaws occurs by a hematogenous route, most commonly from the breast or lung (Fig. 21.33), but also from the kidney, prostate, thyroid, colon, and rectum. Emboli of primary carcinomas may enter the venous circulation and bypass the lungs via the valveless prevertebral venous plexus of Batson to deposit in the jaws.

Treatment is usually palliative and aimed at controlling symptoms and local extension into vital structures. This is commonly in the form of focused radiotherapy or systemic therapy based on the histopathologic diagnosis. Occasionally, surgery may be indicated to provide local control for radioresistant tumors or in patients that have developed pathological fracture.

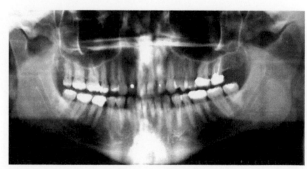

Fig. 21.33 Panoramic radiograph demonstrating bronchogenic carcinoma metastatic to the left mandibular condyle.

Recommended reading

Bell RB. (2010) Odontogenic and non-odontogenic tumors of the jaws. In: *Oral and Maxillofacial Surgery* (eds, Andersson L, Kahnberg K-E, Pogrel MA). Oxford, Wiley-Blackwell.

Foster RD, Anthony JP, Sharma A, Pogrel MA. (1999) Vascularized bone flaps versus nonvascularized bone grafts for mandibular reconstruction: an outcome analysis of primary bony union and endosseous implant success. *Head and Neck*, 21, 66.

Ladeinde AL, Ajayi OF, Ogunlewe MO, *et al.* (2005) Odontogenic tumors: a review of 319 cases in a Nigerian teaching hospital. *Oral Surgery, Oral Medicine, Oral Pathology, Oral Radiology, and Endodontology*, 2, 54–9.

Larsson A, Almeren H. (1978) Ameloblastoma of the jaws. An analysis of a consecutive series of all cases reported to the Swedish Cancer Registry during 1958–1971. *Acta Pathologica et Microbiologica Scandinavica*, 86, 337–49.

Pogrel MA. (1993) The use of liquid nitrogen cryotherapy in the management of locally aggressive bone lesions. *Journal of Oral and Maxillofacial Surgery*, 51, 269.

Schmidt BL, Pogrel MA. (2001) The use of enucleation and liquid nitrogen cryotherapy in the management of odontogenic keratocysts. *Journal of Oral and Maxillofacial Surgery*, 59, 720–5.

Stoelinga P. (2001) Long-term follow-up on keratocysts treated according to a defined protocol. *International Journal of Oral and Maxillofacial Surgery*, 30, 14–25.

Voorsmit RACA, Stoelinga PJW, Van Haelst JGM. (1981) The management of keratocysts. *Journal of Maxillofacial Surgery*, 9, 228–36.

Chapter 22

Potentially Malignant Disorders of the Oral Mucosa

Many terms have been used to describe oral premalignancies that may have a potential to transform into cancers of the oral mucosa. These include "precancer", "premalignant", "precursor lesions", "intraepithelial neoplasia", and "potentially malignant". The World Health Organization (WHO) Collaborating Center proposed that oral mucosal presentations recognized as precancerous can be classified into two major groups: as precancerous lesions and precancerous conditions. A precancerous lesion was defined as "a morphologically altered tissue in which oral cancer is more likely to occur than in its apparently normal counterpart". On the other hand, a precancerous condition is defined as "a generalized state associated with a significantly increased risk of cancer". This classification was based on the concept that the origin of malignancy in the oral mucosa of a patient with a precancerous lesion would correspond with the specific local site of precancer; whereas a malignancy may arise in any part of the oral mucosa in a precancerous condition.

Precancerous lesions include leukoplakia, erythroplakia, and palatal keratosis associated with reverse smoking, and precancerous conditions include sideropenic dysphagia, lichen planus, oral submucous fibrosis, syphilis, discoid lupus erythematosus, xeroderma pigmentosum, and epidermolysis bullosa.

There may need to be some modification of this concept since it is now known that even clinically normal-looking oral mucosa in patients with a precancerous lesion on one side of the oral cavity may have dysplasia or molecular abnormality on the contralateral side, suggesting the possibility of malignant transformation, and that cancer could subsequently develop in the normal-appearing mucosa.

Histology (grading of dysplasia)

Histological changes that may be observed in potentially malignant disorders of the oral mucosa can be expressed as oral epithelial dysplasia. Although the clinical appearance of oral epithelial dysplasia is variable, oral squamous malignancies of the lining mucosa are known generally to develop from dysplastic surface epithelium of the oral mucosa. The grade of epithelial dysplasia can be expressed in several categories, such as no dysplasia, mild dysplasia, moderate dysplasia, and severe dysplasia. The relationship of epithelial dysplasia in various grades to the subsequent development of cancer has not been fully clarified. However, it is generally believed that any degree of epithelial dysplasia, even a mild form, indicates an increased risk, and severe dysplasia suggests a very high risk of the subsequent development of cancer.

Histologically, grade 1 (mild dysplasia) demonstrates general architectural disturbance limited to the lower third of the epithelium accompanied by cytological atypia (Fig. 22.1). Grade 2 (moderate dysplasia) demonstrates architectural disturbance extending into the middle third of the epithelium (Fig. 22.2). Grade 3 (severe dysplasia) starts with greater than two-thirds of the epithelium showing architectural disturbance with associated cytological atypia. However, architectural disturbance extending into the middle third of the epithelium with sufficient cytological atypia is upgraded from moderate to severe dysplasia (Fig. 22.3).

The term carcinoma in situ (CIS) denotes that malignant transformation has occurred but invasion is not present.

Essentials of Oral and Maxillofacial Surgery, First Edition. Edited by M. Anthony Pogrel, Karl-Erik Kahnberg and Lars Andersson.
© 2014 John Wiley & Sons, Ltd. Published 2014 by John Wiley & Sons, Ltd.
Companion website: www.wiley.com/go/pogrel/oms

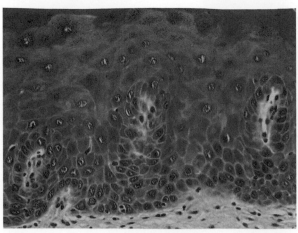

Fig. 22.1 Mild dysplasia. There is hyperplasia of basal and parabasal cells with weak loss of polarity showing slightly increased nuclear size and increased nuclear:cytoplasmic ratio. The architectural changes are limited to the lower third of the epithelium.

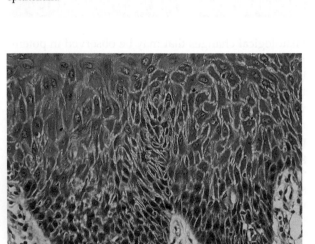

Fig. 22.2 Moderate dysplasia. The epithelial cells demonstrate variation in nuclear size and shape with increased number and size of nucleoli with some disturbance in epithelial stratification and polarity of basal and parabasal cells. The architectural changes extend into the middle third of the epithelium.

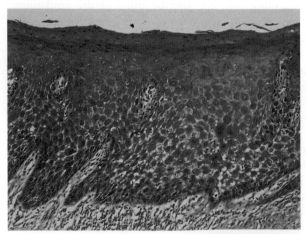

Fig. 22.3 Severe dysplasia. The architectural disturbance with cytological atypia including loss of intercellular adhesion extends to more than two thirds of the epithelium.

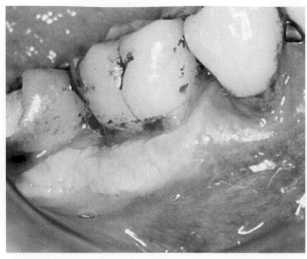

Fig. 22.4 Homogeneous leukoplakia in the lower gingival mucosa.

Potential molecular biological markers or molecular genetics of potentially malignant disorders of the oral mucosa, which may have special association with progression of oral epithelial dysplasia to carcinoma, have been studied. Loss of heterozygosity (LOH) at 3p and 9p increase the risk of progression of dysplasia to squamous cell carcinoma (SCC). Mutation of p53 tumor suppressor gene is one of the most common genetic events in carcinogenesis. Although LOH at the p53 loci appears to be associated with progression, mutation of the p53 gene is rare in dysplasia and appears to be a late event. The p53 protein and other markers of apoptosis appear in basal and parabasal layers of dysplastic lesions that progressed to SCC.

Potentially malignant disorders of the oral mucosa

Leukoplakia

The WHO working group defines leukoplakia as: *"The term leukoplakia should be used to recognize white plaques of questionable risk having excluded (other) known diseases or disorders that carry no increased risk for cancer."*

Leukoplakia itself has no specific histology, it may show atrophy or hyperplasia (acanthosis), and may or may not demonstrate epithelial dysplasia.

Oral leukoplakia occurs most frequently on the lip vermillion, buccal mucosa, lateral border of tongue, floor of mouth, and gingival mucosa. The clinical finding of leukoplakia has been reported using various terms, but classification into two types is generally accepted: homogeneous and non-homogeneous leukoplakia, based on surface color and morphologic characteristics. Homogeneous leukoplakias look uniformly flat and thin (Fig. 22.4). Non-homogeneous leukoplakias include several subtypes:

- Speckled type – mixed appearance of white and red, but still retaining predominantly white character.
- Nodular type – small polypoid outgrowths with rounded red or white excrescences.
- verrucous type – wrinkled or corrugated surface appearance.
- Erythroleukoplakia is one type of non-homogeneous leukoplakias. It is very similar to speckled type leukoplakia and appears white and red, with red areas of minimal keratin production interspersed among the background of white areas with thickened keratin. The red areas of erythroleukoplakia are larger than in speckled type leukoplakia, and erythroleukoplakia shows a rather thin epithelial layer with some dysplasia (Fig. 22.5). An alternative term for this is erosive leukoplakia.
- Proliferative verrucous leukoplakia (PVL) is another type of oral leukoplakia. PVL develops nodular, papillary or verrucous surface projections (Figs 22.6 and 22.7), which gradually spread laterally to encompass large areas of oral mucosa. Sometimes it presents at multifocal sites in the same oral cavity. PVL occurs predominantly (74%) in females, unlike other leukoplakia, and 63% of

patients do not use tobacco products. In histology almost half of all PVL patients demonstrate epithelial dysplasia and more than 70% of them will develop SCC later. PVL is an aggressive form of oral leukoplakia with considerable morbidity and a strong prediction for malignant transformation. Conservative management of these lesions has been unsuccessful and wide surgical excision offers the best hope for control.

Malignant transformation rates from oral leukoplakia reported in the literature vary greatly. In the large-scale community-based surveys in India, estimates of the malignant transformation rate range from 0.13–0.9%. In contrast, reports from hospital-based sample studies derived from patients referred to selected special units by primary health care workers show much higher rates, ranging widely between 1.8 and 17.5%. In general terms, non-homogeneous leukoplakias present a greater risk of malignant change than the homogeneous types.

Erythroplakia

Oral erythroplakia is defined as "*a fiery red patch that cannot be characterized clinically or pathologically as any other definable lesion*". Erythroplakia is a clinical term, just like in leukoplakia, and it does not have any specific histopathological connotation. Oral erythroplakia has the highest risk of malignant transformation compared to all other oral potentially malignant disorders – these red lesions often show invasive carcinoma and CIS or severe dysplasia. Transformation rates vary from 14% to 50% (Figs 22.8 and 22.9).

Oral submucous fibrosis

Oral submucous fibrosis (OSF) is a chronic disorder of the upper digestive tract including the oral cavity, oropharynx, and often the upper third of the esophagus, characterized by fibrosis of the mucosa and sub

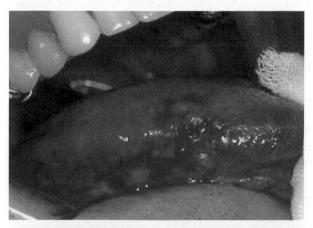

Fig. 22.5 Erythroleukoplakia on the lateral surface of the tongue. The red area is larger than in speckled type leukoplakia.

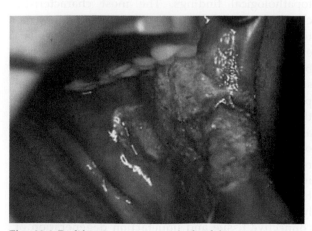

Fig. 22.6 Proliferative verrucous leukoplakia (PVL) on the buccal mucosa with papillary and verrucous surface projection in female who does not use tobacco. This patient later developed squamous cell carcinoma.

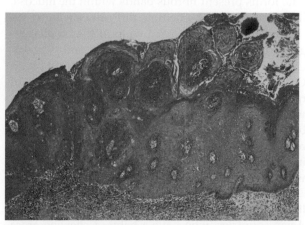

Fig. 22.7 Histopathologic findings of proliferative verrucous leukoplakia (PVL) showing papillary exophytic proliferation of squamous epithelium with little dysplasia but no stromal invasion.

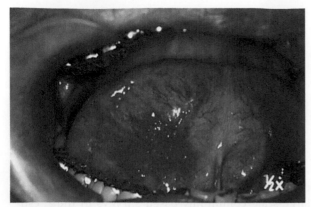

Fig. 22.8 Erythroplakia on the ventral surface of the tongue showing red, smooth, flat patch.

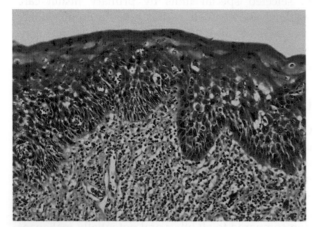

Fig. 22.9 Histopathologic findings of erythroplakia with severe dysplasia. The architectural disturbances include decreased epithelial layer, irregular epithelial stratification, irregular polarity of basal and parabasal cells with loss of intercellular adhesion and some cellular atypia.

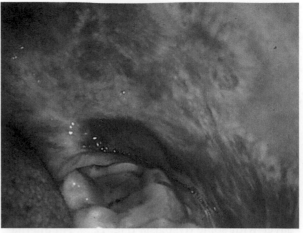

Fig. 22.10 Typical clinical feature of oral lichen planus (OLP) showing white striations with linear, reticular, and anular shapes in light erythematous or erosive background. This patient has bilateral symmetrical lesions.

mucosa. Clinical presentations in early forms include a burning sensation with exacerbation by spicy food, vesiculation or ulceration of the oral mucosa, blanching of the mucosa, and "leathery" mucosa, which shows thickened, firm tissue with a wrinkled surface. Late forms present fibrous bands within the mucosa, limitation of mouth opening, difficulties with mastication and phonation, narrowing of the oropharyngeal orifice with distortion of the uvula, and "woody" changes to the mucosa and tongue. In histopathology, OSF shows epithelial atrophy, with metaplasia of non-keratinized areas to para- or ortho-keratinization, with various degrees of dysplasia. Thickening of the basement membrane is common, and there is marked reduction in vascularity of the connective tissues in inverse proportion to increased density of collagen, which appears hyalinized.

OSF has been reported mainly among subjects living on the Indian subcontinent, and neighboring Asian countries, who have a habit of chewing areca nut. A clear dose-dependent relationship is observed for both frequency and duration of chewing areca nut in the development of OSF. The commercially avail-

able freeze-dried products such as pan masala, guthka, and mawa (areca and lime) have high concentrates of areca nut per chew and appear to cause OSF more rapidly than self-prepared conventional betel quid. Areca alkaloids, such as arecoline and its active metabolite arecaidine, cause fibroblast proliferation and increase collagen synthesis. In addition, tannin present in areca nut reduces degradation of collagen by inhibiting collagenases; and the copper content in areca nut is high and copper is known to stimulate fibroblast proliferation. Epithelial dysplasia in OSF tissues appears to vary from 7% to 26%, depending on the population. Malignant transformation rate of OSF to oral cancer may be around 7.6% over a 15-year period.

Oral lichen planus

Oral lichen planus (OLP) is one of the most prevalent diseases of the oral mucosa. Diagnosis of OLP should be based on both clinical features and histopathological findings. The most characteristic clinical feature of OLP is the presence of white striations and/or papules, which often appear in bilateral areas of the oral mucosa (Fig. 22.10). These bilateral, often symmetrical reticular lesions are strong determining components of the clinical profile of OLP. In addition to the white lesions, erythematous lesions with plaque-type, atrophic, ulcerative or sometimes bullous appearance may also be observed during the course of the disease, but these red lesions are not OLP specific and can also be seen in other similar disorders. Essential histological criteria for diagnosing OLP are a band-like dense lymphoid cell infiltrate confined to subepithelial connective tissue and liquefaction degeneration of the epithelial basal layer. The epithelium may develop hyperkeratosis, atrophy, hyperplasia, acanthosis, and saw-toothed rete ridges (Fig. 22.11).

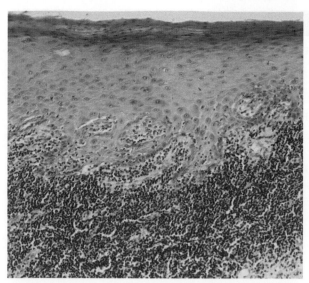

Fig. 22.11 Histopathologic findings of oral lichen planus (OLP). The dense band-like zonal cellular infiltration of lymphocytes with some macrophages is evident just under the epithelial tissue. The epithelium shows acanthosis with a little hyperparakeratosis, liquefaction degeneration in the basal cell layer, and some saw-tooth rete ridges, but no dysplasia.

The malignant transformation rate for oral lichen planus varies from 0.4% to 6.4% overall, and 0.07–0.74% per year, though this remains controversial. The erosive or ulcerative form may have a higher malignant transformation rate than the reticular form.

Others

Actinic keratosis of the lip is considered to be a potentially malignant condition. The squamous epithelium of the vermillion of the lip may be atrophic or hyperplastic with disordered maturation showing varying degrees of keratinization, atypia, and increased mitosis.

Early detection, diagnosis, and management of potentially malignant disorders of the oral mucosa

The potentially malignant disorders (PMD) of the oral mucosa can arise not only from preceding lesions but also from any part of normal-looking mucosa, and most PMD must be confirmed by histopathological diagnosis.

Conventional oral examination

A conventional oral examination under normal light by inspection and palpation is the standard method for screening PMD or oral cancers, but a variety of adjunctive aids are available including the use of toluidine blue, tissue reflectance, fluorescent imaging and the brush biopsy. These are discussed in more detail in Chapter 19, including their advantages and disadvantages.

Scalpel biopsy

Histological diagnosis made by taking a sample tissue material from the lesion by means of a scalpel biopsy is still considered the gold standard for definitive diagnosis.

A scalpel biopsy should be performed in cases of dysplasia to avoid false-negative results in cases of carcinoma. An incisional biopsy is performed by taking a small piece of tissue for the purpose of making the definitive diagnosis. In the biopsy of PMD, the most malignancy-suspected part of the lesion, such as indurated, erosive, ulcerative, verrucous, or red areas, rather than a white area, is the preferred site to perform the biopsy. Vital staining by toluidine blue or iodine may help to define the most malignancy-suspected site of the PMD. If the lesion has a homogeneous appearance a marginal area of the lesion, including a normal-looking area, is a preferred site to make the incision. On the other hand, an excisional biopsy is performed to remove the whole area of the lesion for both treatment and definitive diagnosis. Therefore, it is indicated for smaller lesions, and the excision line must be placed outside the lesion, including peripheral normal mucosa.

Management

The main concept of the management of PMD is to avoid malignant transformation. As the most common PMD encountered in clinical practice is oral leukoplakia, the major focus of management of PMD can be considered to be that of leukoplakia. The management of other PMD can be modified according to the biological nature of each PMD and the histopathological characteristics of each PMD, including the degree of epithelial dysplasia.

Surgical removal is generally considered to be the recommended first choice and the most reliable way of management of PMD, especially for lesions with high malignant potential such as erythroplakia, proliferative verrucous leukoplakia, erythroleukoplakia, speckled type leukoplakia, palatal lesions in reverse smokers, and oral submucous fibrosis. The hypothesis that removing PMD by active surgical intervention can prevent the onset of oral cancer, however, remains unproved, and it is also considered reasonable that more conservative treatments or "wait and see" policy are options if the lesion is considered to have low malignant potential.

The CO_2 laser, NdYAG laser, and KTP laser have been employed for excision or vaporization for the treatment of PMD, especially oral leukoplakia. The main advantages of laser surgery are the hemostatic effects, limited tissue contraction and scarring after therapy, reduced postoperative pain, swelling, and infection. These advantages may permit the treatment of large or multiple lesions. Vaporization does not provide a tissue specimen for histological diagnosis, which is a major disadvantage. Surgical excision of PMD offers significant advantages over laser vaporization. The most important advantage is that excision generates a surgical specimen that provides the patient and surgeon with histological evidence of the entire lesion upon which to base future treatment planning.

Cryosurgery has been utilized, but does not seem to be of any particular benefit in the management of leukoplakia, since the margin of the treated area is only apparent some days later, when necrosis becomes clear, and, again, there is no histological specimen.

Recommended reading

El Naggar AK, Reichart PA. (2005) Proliferative verrucous leukoplakia and precancerous conditions. In: *World Health Organization Classification of Tumours: Pathology & Genetics of Head and Neck Tumours* (eds, Barnes L, Everson JW, Reichart P, Sidransky D), pp. 180–1. Lyon, IARC Press.

Fujibayashi T. (2010) Mucosal lesions (potentially malignant disorders of the oral mucosa). In: *Oral and Maxillofacial Surgery* (eds, Andersson L, Kahnberg K-E, Pogrel MA). Oxford, Wiley-Blackwell.

Kramer IRH, Lucas RB, Pindborg JJ, Sobin LH and World Health Organization Collaborating Center for Oral Precancerous Lesions. (1978) Definition of leukoplakia and related lesions: an aid to studies on oral precancer. *Oral Surgery, Oral Medicine, Oral Pathology*, **46**, 518–39.

Chapter 23

Principles of Oral Cancer Management

Epidemiology and risk factors

The incidence of oral squamous cell carcinoma, particularly in younger patients, is increasing in North America and the UK. In certain regions of the world, such as India, oral cancer is one of the most common malignancies. In these regions of the world the use of betel nut and betel quid clearly contribute to the high incidence of oral cancer. However, the etiology in the western portions of the world is less clear. Survival rates for oral cancer patients have not changed significantly. The roles of tobacco and alcohol are firmly established as risk factors for oral cancer. However, approximately 33% of oral squamous cell carcinoma patients were never smokers. Our understanding of the role of smokeless tobacco in oral carcinogenesis has gone through considerable evolution over the last three decades. The conclusion of a recent review of 32 relevant studies published between 1920 and 2005 concluded that smokeless tobacco, at most, plays only a minor role in the development of oral cancer. There has been considerable confusion regarding the role of human papillomavirus (HPV) in the development of oral cancer. Based on the available studies there is a lack of reproducible molecular data supporting the role of HPV in the development of oral cancer. This is in contrast to oropharyngeal carcinogenesis where HPV has a much stronger etiologic role.

Histologic grading, tumor staging, and clinical behavior

Ninety-five percent of oral cancers are squamous cell carcinoma (SCC). Different histologic variants of SCC include verrucous SCC, basaloid SCC, and papillary SCC (Fig. 23.1). Clinicians and investigators have attempted to use the combination of clinical information and histologic findings to predict the behavior of oral SCC. The histologic features that have been evaluated include tumor differentiation, tumor thickness, tumor size, and tumor invasive pattern.

Proliferative verrucous leukoplakia

Most oral SCCs are preceded by clinically evident precancerous oral lesions, most often oral epithelial dysplasia, which appears as white (leukoplakia) or red patches (erythroplakia) that are characterized microscopically by varying degrees of dysplasia (from mild to severe). Other oral SCCs are preceded by proliferative verrucous leukoplakia (PVL), a condition which is persistent, recurrent, and multifocal (Fig. 23.2). Dysplasia has an unpredictable transformation rate to oral SCC that is thought to be approximately 16%, whereas the transformation rate for PVL is much higher (50–70%). In contrast to oral dysplasia, PVL is not associated with tobacco or alcohol consumption. In addition, whereas dysplasia is more common in men, the female to male ratio for PVL is about 4 to 1. At initial presentation, PVL lesions are white, irregular areas on the attached gingiva, buccal mucosa, and tongue. Histologically, PVL exhibits no dysplasia or mild dysplasia. In spite of the bland clinical and histologic appearance of early lesions, PVL is characterized by relentless growth and irreversible progression through a continuum of lesions, namely, hyperkeratosis, verruciform hyperkeratosis, verrucous hyperplasia, verrucous carcinoma, and ultimately SCC (Fig. 23.3). Repeated surgical excisions of all clinically and histologically appearing abnormal tissue can slow the transformation to carcinoma. However, such treatment results in significant disfigurement and morbidity.

Essentials of Oral and Maxillofacial Surgery, First Edition. Edited by M. Anthony Pogrel, Karl-Erik Kahnberg and Lars Andersson.
© 2014 John Wiley & Sons, Ltd. Published 2014 by John Wiley & Sons, Ltd.
Companion website: www.wiley.com/go/pogrel/oms

Preoperative assessment, staging, and work-up

Most oral cancers are painful, and it is the most common presenting symptom. For oral cancer patients, pain severely limits oral function including eating, drinking, and talking. Pain is rated as the oral cancer patient's worst symptom and is the primary determinant of a poor quality of life. Opioids, such as morphine, are the only drugs that have any efficacy for oral cancer pain. Morphine provides minimal relief, does not restore oral function and progressively larger doses are required; therefore, tolerance

rapidly develops. Pain management should be tailored to provide relief when patients are required to function. Total resection of the oral cancer produces near complete relief. Overall, approximately 50% of oral cancer patients will not be cured with surgery, chemotherapy, or radiation therapy.

The tobacco history should be reviewed and the patient should be classified as a never smoker, nonsmoker, or smoker. If the patient is a smoker or nonsmoker the pack-years of use should be calculated. If the patient is a non-smoker the time since the patient's last cigarette should be determined. While there is conflicting data in the literature as to whether marijuana use contributes to oral carcinogenesis, patients should be asked whether and how much marijuana they use.

Systematic palpation of the neck should be performed on every patient at every visit. Palpation of the neck should be performed on one side of the neck at a time and should always be performed from behind the patient. The sensitivity of clinical examination to detect metastasis, however, is little better than 50%. A panoramic radiograph should be performed in almost all cases of oral cavity SCCs. Even if the carcinoma does not involve the maxilla or the mandible, the dentition should be evaluated prior to surgery to determine whether extractions will be

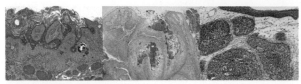

Fig. 23.1 Histologic variants of oral squamous cell carcinoma. Papillary SCC (left) shows mild degrees of atypia with invasive islands seen in the lamina propria. Verrucous carcinoma (center) is characterized by proliferation with broad, deeply pushing epithelial rete with parakeratin plugging and no atypia. Basaloid SCC (right) demonstrates islands of invasive, basaloid appearing malignant epithelial cells with palisading peripheral cells and comedo (central) necrosis.

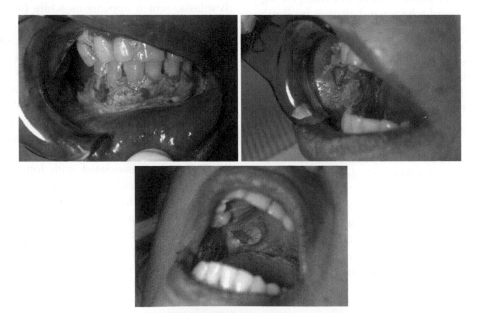

Fig. 23.2 Photograph of a patient with PVL. All three photographs are from the same patient. The patient has extensive involvement of the maxillary and mandibular gingival, buccal mucosa and palate. As depicted here PVL is characterized by extensive verrucous-appearing lesions with areas of ulceration.

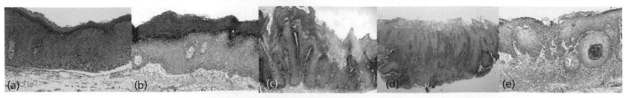

Fig. 23.3 Histologic progression of PVL. The stages of histologic progression of PVL include (a) hyperkeratosis, (b) verruciform hyperkeratosis, (c) verrucous hyperplasia, (d) verrucous carcinoma, and (e) squamous cell carcinoma.

required at the time of surgical resection if postoperative radiation therapy is anticipated. Nasopharyngoscopy can be easily and painlessly performed with proper preparation of the nasopharyngeal membranes with local anesthetic and a topical vasoconstrictor. Nasopharyngoscopy can be used to evaluate the nasopharynx, base of tongue, and supraglottic structures.

The significant limitations of imaging for detecting carcinoma need to be considered when evaluating the oral cancer patient, particularly when attempting to identify metastasis in the oral cancer patient who is N0 on clinical exam. Imaging, in the forms of computed tomography (CT), magnetic resonance imaging (MRI), ultrasound (US), or now PET (positron emission tomography)/CT, has been used to assess primary tumors. Unfortunately, despite improved resolution and software analysis, all imaging techniques are still insufficiently sensitive for detecting occult neck metastases, with 20–45% of patients staged as N0 using these techniques having occult nodal involvement on pathologic evaluation of the neck.

Preoperative imaging of the primary cancer and the head and neck should include CT or MRI. MRI is often more helpful than CT in evaluating the primary cancer because of the high soft tissue resolution which MRI provides (Fig. 23.4). Moreover, MRI is less obscured by the dental artifact that occurs with high density materials such as dental amalgam. CT can aid in the evaluation of bone involvement; however, its usefulness is often limited by dental artifact in the area of interest (Fig. 23.5).

PET imaging with fluorine-18 fluorodeoxyglucose (FDG) has been shown to have a higher sensitivity and specificity than traditional CT or MRI in the evaluation of the patient with head and neck SCC. However, the results of PET scan rarely change the treatment decision in the management of oral SCC. In the case of an N0 neck in a patient with oral SCC, the ^{18}F-FDG PET scan does not have a clear role. The poor resolution of PET/CT makes it difficult to use for surgical planning.

PET has been proposed to evaluate for distant metastasis but distant metastasis is rare in oral SCC. PET scans are also associated with a false-positive rate which often obligates the clinician to pursue "hot spots", often leading to a delay in treatment. PET scans theoretically could impact on the decision to perform a neck dissection; however, micrometastasis is unlikely to produce a positive PET result. The rate of occult metastasis for almost all oral cavity SCCs dictates that a neck dissection should be performed regardless of the results of a CT, MRI, or PET scan. The PET scan can be helpful in evaluating oral cancer patients with symptoms suggestive of recurrence when no clinically apparent lesion is found; it also clearly has a role in the patient with an occult primary head and neck cancer.

The neck can also be evaluated with ultrasound. However, it appears that diagnosing occult metastasis with ultrasound is highly technique-sensitive and user specific.

A chest radiograph is part of the standard workup recommended by the National Comprehensive Cancer Center Network for head and neck cancer patients. The role of the chest radiograph is for the evaluation of distant metastasis. Approximately 1% of patients with a head and neck SCC will have a synchronous primary in the lung. For patients with oral cavity SCC, a chest CT would only be indicated in the setting of advanced cervical involvement or if a suspicious lesion were identified on the chest radiograph. The use of panendoscopy is dependent on the provider and concern regarding a second primary. The cost effectiveness of panendoscopy is questionable given the relatively low incidence of second primaries.

Following the history and physical examination, each patient should be staged according to the AJCC staging system. Clinical tumor staging should be based on all clinical, imaging, and pathologic data. Every oral cancer patient deserves to be presented at a multidisciplinary tumor board. Management of oral cavity SCC almost always involves surgical resection with consideration of adjunctive chemotherapy and radiation therapy. Because of the

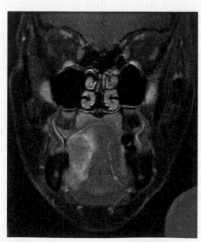

Fig. 23.4 Coronal view of MRI of lateral tongue squamous cell carcinoma. MRI can provide high resolution and anatomic detail which aids in clinical staging and surgical planning.

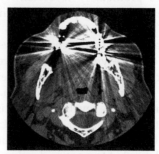

Fig. 23.5 Dental artifact from amalgam obscuring CT. One of the significant drawbacks of CT in the evaluation of an oral cavity primary is the artifact generated by dental materials.

significant, progressive side-effects, radiation therapy should be avoided if possible, as discussed under the heading Surgery and postoperative radiation.

In planning for surgery, patient preference should be evaluated. The patient's goals for treatment should be discussed and considered. The wishes of the patient and family must be weighed heavily when considering treatment options. The question is often raised of what to do with an elderly patient with a limited life expectancy. It is often a mistake to not treat the cancer since many of these patients will live much longer than expected and if the cancer is not treated patients will progress to endure profound pain. Surgical resection offers significant pain relief. Nutritional support has many benefits for the surgical patient, including improved healing following surgery, decreased complications, lean body mass preservation, and improved quality of life.

Management of the neck

Surgery is the treatment of choice for almost every oral cavity SCC. The data overwhelmingly support elective neck dissection for even small T1 lesions given the high rate of occult metastasis with oral cavity SCCs. The goals of treating the N0 neck are twofold: (1) to therapeutically remove the lymph nodes that might harbor carcinoma; and (2) to histopathologically review the surgically resected neck specimen leading to accurate staging which would potentially warrant adjuvant treatment leading to improved cancer control. The "wait and see" practice is the opposing approach to the elective neck dissection and refers to the practice of closely following patients who are N0 at the time of surgery rather than performing a neck dissection. With this approach once a patient fails in the neck a salvage of the patient is attempted. "Wait and see" approaches for the N0 neck have been associated with high failure rates. Salvage rates for the failed neck in patients with oral SCC are extremely poor.

Extent of neck dissection for the N0 neck

When oral cancer metastasizes to the cervical region, it metastasizes predictably to certain lymph node groups. Since Crile's description of the neck dissection in 1906, treatment of the neck has evolved to become less radical and more conservative, including the sparing of non-lymphatic structures such as the spinal accessory nerve, the sternocleidomastoid muscle, and the internal jugular vein. Also, the number of lymph node levels that are dissected has decreased with no change in outcome. Limiting the dissection to the node levels and structures that are at greatest risk has led to a marked reduction in postoperative morbidity, particularly with avoiding sacrifice of the spinal accessory nerve and avoiding

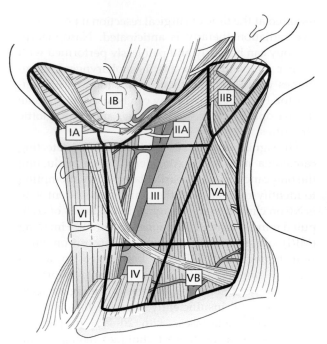

Fig. 23.6 Illustration of the levels and sub-levels of the neck. Notice that level II is divided into IIA and IIB by the spinal accessory nerve and level V is divided by a horizontal plane from the inferior border of the cricoid arch into VA and VB.

trauma to this nerve by foregoing dissection of the posterior triangle. For the N0 oral SCC patient levels I–III should be removed. Figure 23.6 illustrates the levels of neck dissection.

Sentinel node biopsy

Perhaps the best example of the shift towards ultraselectivity in management of the N0 neck is the application of the sentinel node biopsy technique. The sentinel lymph node biopsy technique involves injection of radiolabeled tracer around the periphery of the tumor, allowing the tracer to drain via the lymphatic system to the first echelon of nodes. The sentinel node or nodes are then delineated using a gamma probe, followed by the surgical removal of the node(s) in a manner that is oncologically safe. These nodes are then examined by frozen section. If micrometastases are identified on frozen section, the patient receives a selective neck dissection (SND). Postoperatively, the nodes from the permanent specimen are then examined thoroughly by serial sectioning, as opposed to bisectioning, which is the technique typically used to sample lymph nodes for histopathologic review. If micrometastases are located in the permanent serial sections, the patient is brought back to the operating room for a conventional SND if it has not already been performed.

This technique, which has been used effectively in the treatment of melanoma and breast cancer, has been advocated for treatment of the N0 neck in oral SCC. There have been some concerns regarding the use of sentinel node biopsy in the management of the N0 neck. The radiolabeled tracer which is injected into the oral SCC tumor, especially tumors involving the floor of mouth and oral tongue, would obscure gamma probe readings in the first echelon nodes due to their proximity to the primary tumor, negating any benefit from the exercise. Another criticism of the sentinel lymph node technique is that if micrometastasis is detected later after serial sectioning of the permanent specimen, the patient would be required to undergo a second surgery. Knowing the high rates of occult metastasis, this would likely result in 20–45% of patients requiring second surgeries. Although the sentinel node biopsy warrants further investigation, it is still too early to recommend it as a treatment for the N0 neck.

Managing the N+ neck

For the patient with clinically palpable nodes a fine needle aspiration can be performed to determine if there is malignant involvement of the neck. If neck involvement is either suspected or confirmed then a modified radical neck dissection (MRND) with preservation of the spinal accessory nerve should be performed. Appropriate muscle flap coverage of the carotid artery with a scalene muscle should be considered, especially if the patient is to receive postoperative radiation therapy. Preservation of the internal jugular might be required for free flap reconstruction. Sacrificing the spinal accessory nerve should be reserved for cases where there is direct involvement of the nerve with carcinoma. Shoulder dysfunction is a common complaint following neck dissection. Complications following neck dissection, while rare, include hematoma, lymphocele, ear numbness, and shoulder dysfunction. Given that ear numbness is one of the primary complaints following neck dissection, the greater auricular nerve should be preserved if possible.

Surgery and postoperative radiation

The role of radiation therapy in the management of oral cancer is adjuvant. Oral cavity SCCs are poorly responsive to radiotherapy as primary treatment. Surgical salvage, frequently required following radiation therapy, is extremely difficult and postoperative complications are more frequent and more difficult to manage. Preoperative radiation therapy is not generally given for oral cavity carcinoma. In certain cases preoperative radiation therapy, in the dose range of 50 Gy, is used for sinonasal or paranasal carcinomas to improve resectability. Preoperative radiation therapy is associated with wound healing complications. The surgical margins would not change following radiation therapy for oral cavity carcinoma.

Possible indications for postoperative radiation therapy include positive or close margins, perineural invasion, extensive bone invasion, and neck involvement (strong indication of more than one lymph node involved or extracapsular spread). While these recommendations are commonly used, each case must be evaluated independently and there is not universal agreement on these indications. Timing of radiation therapy is critical and should be started as soon as possible following healing. Multiple studies have demonstrated that recurrence rates increase when there is a delay in starting radiation therapy. A delay of greater than 6 weeks after surgery leads to increased recurrence rates.

Chemotherapy and radiation therapy

The addition of chemotherapy (principally Cisplatin) to postoperative radiation therapy has improved both locoregional tumor control and survival rates.

Follow-up

Most recurrences and locoregional failures will occur within the first 2 years. Follow-up appointments are recommended every month for the first year, every 2 months for the second year, every 3 months for the third year and every 6 months thereafter. There is little available data to guide the surgeon in making evidence-based decisions regarding interval imaging. This decision should be made by the surgeon based on the clinical behavior of the cancer and the pathologic findings. Patients with oral cancer are at risk for second primaries. The risk for a synchronous or metachronous second head and neck primary in patients with oral SCC ranges is 21%, a rate that is higher than patients with pharyngeal or laryngeal SCC. Studies show a substantial impact of smoking on the development of second primary tumors and survival. Therefore, an aggressive smoking cessation program should be implemented with oral cancer patients who continue to smoke.

Recommended reading

Gillison ML. (2004) Human papillomavirus-associated head and neck cancer is a distinct epidemiologic, clinical, and molecular entity. *Seminars in Oncology*, **31**, 744–54.

O'Dowd A. (2007) Skin cancer is on the increase but incidence of lung cancer is falling. *British Medical Journal*, **335**, 322.

Schmidt BL. (2010) Principles of oral cancer management. In: *Oral and Maxillofacial Surgery* (eds, Andersson L, Kahnberg K-E, Pogrel MA). Oxford, Wiley-Blackwell.

Schmidt BL, Dierks EJ, Homer L, Potter B. (2004) Tobacco smoking history and presentation of oral squamous cell carcinoma. *Journal of Oral and Maxillofacial Surgery*, **62**, 1055–8.

Shiboski CH, Schmidt BL, Jordan RC. (2005) Tongue and tonsil carcinoma: increasing trends in the US population ages 20–44 years. *Cancer*, **103**, 1843–9.

Weitkunat R, Sanders E, Lee PN. (2007) Meta-analysis of the relation between European and American smokeless tobacco and oral cancer. *BMC Public Health*, **7**, 334.

Chapter 24

Management of Patients Undergoing Radiation and Chemotherapy

Radiotherapy

The aim and purpose of radiation therapy in the treatment of head and neck cancer may be two-fold:

- the target (cancer) is either a primary tumor with or without regional spread to the regional lymph nodes;
- the target is clinically and radiologically tumor-free lymph nodes of the neck, but with a high risk of micrometastasis.

Occasionally radiotherapy may also be used to treat benign tumors, such as ameloblastomas or pleomorphic adenomas, when other treatments may be detrimental.

The intention of radiotherapy may either be curative or palliative. When the intention is to cure the patient from the disease, the radiation may be given either as a single modality if the cancer is small, i.e. stage I and II, or as a complement to surgery. When combined with surgery, it may be given prior to, or after surgery. Radiotherapy can also be given in combination with chemotherapy, with a curative intention. When the radiotherapy has a curative intention, the radiation is given at small doses (1–2 Gy) once or twice a day for a period of 3–7 weeks.

When the cancer is not curable, the intention of radiotherapy may be palliative, i.e. it can be used to reduce the symptoms of the disease, e.g. reducing pain emanating from skeletal metastasis, relieving pressure on vital organ systems. When the radiotherapy has a palliative intention, higher doses are given each time, to reach an effect faster. Palliative radiotherapy can improve the quality of life during the last months of life of a patient with an incurable cancer.

Radiation involves the transport of energy, either as electromagnetic waves (photons) or as a beam of particles (electrons or protons). The position of the tumor determines which type of radiation to be used. Particle beams normally have a shorter range, implying that such radiation is used when the cancer is located relatively superficially in the tissues. In contrast, photon radiation is used when the tumor is located more deeply in the tissues.

When radiotherapy is given as a single modality therapy, a lower dose is given to local lymph nodes in order to prevent and sterilize micrometastasis and a higher dose is administered to the known primary tumor, i.e. the cancer. If, on the other hand, radiation is combined with surgery, a smaller dose is given with the aim of sterilizing potential micrometastasis in local lymph nodes.

Conventional radiotherapy implies that the primary tumor as well as the larger lymph nodes of the neck are irradiated with up to 70 Gy. The radiation is given in single fractions of 1.8–2.0 Gy on a daily basis for 6–7 weeks.

Altered fractions have recently been shown to achieve better control both locally and regionally. Hyperfractionation is where 1.2 Gy is given twice a day for about 6–7 weeks, and accelerated fractionation means that 1.6 Gy is given twice a day for about 6 weeks. A third alternative may be accelerated fractionation with a concomitant boost given as 1.8 Gy a day for 6 weeks and during the last 12 days an additional 1.5 Gy is given daily as the boost.

Recently a new form of radiotherapy has been introduced, IMRT (intense modulated radiotherapy). This technique is built on a computer-generated three-dimensional image which allows delivery of high doses of radiotherapy to clinical target volumes, still preserving some critical normal structures, for instance salivary glands.

Essentials of Oral and Maxillofacial Surgery, First Edition. Edited by M. Anthony Pogrel, Karl-Erik Kahnberg and Lars Andersson.
© 2014 John Wiley & Sons, Ltd. Published 2014 by John Wiley & Sons, Ltd.
Companion website: www.wiley.com/go/pogrel/oms

Brachytherapy

Interstitial radiotherapy, or brachytherapy, is administration of irradiation by implantation of a radioactive material very close to, or inside, the primary tumor. A frequently used substance is iridium (^{192}Ir). The time-span of the treatment may vary between a few seconds to a few days, depending on the type of cancer.

Small tumors, without a risk of spreading to the regional nodes, may be treated with brachytherapy only. In cases where the tumor is of larger size or invades surrounding tissues or structures, as well as when there is a risk of spread to regional lymph nodes, brachytherapy is used to deliver a final boost to the primary tumor after an initial more moderate external dose. Brachytherapy is sometimes used as the final part in the treatment of cancer in the base of the tongue and in the tonsils. Brachytherapy can also be used when there is a palliative intention, for instance in the treatment of laryngeal cancer.

Chemotherapy

The use of drugs in the treatment of head and neck cancer is still a matter of debate. Despite considerable research, there is no drug or combination of drugs available today that can cure solid cancers in the head and neck region. In general oncology, chemotherapy is given either to cure cancer, or to reduce the speed of progression, or to ameliorate the symptoms. Sometimes chemotherapy is also administered to reduce the risk of recurrences, so-called adjuvant treatment.

Chemotherapy is generally used prior to (induction), or parallel (concomitant) to radiotherapy. The purpose of chemotherapy is to kill the cancer cells, or at least impede their growth.

Side-effects

Radiotherapy

The side-effects of radiation therapy can be divided into acute, but mostly reversible, effects, and late, more commonly irreversible, conditions. The acute side-effects almost always decline within 4–6 weeks after completion of radiation, whereas the late effects can develop after different periods of time and they will also almost always last for the rest of the patient's life.

Among the acute effects, an inflammatory reaction in the mucosa (Fig. 24.1) of the oral and pharyngeal mucosa – mucositis – is the most common. The appearance of the mucosa can vary from an increased redness, to an intense reddish appearance, to white necrotic lesions. The damage to the oral mucosa can also make it more susceptible to both bacterial and

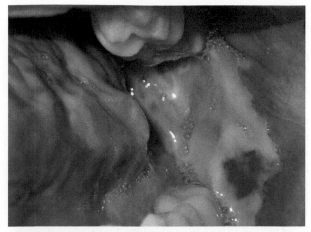

Fig. 24.1 Intraoral mucositis, degree 3–4, observed at the later stages of external, and after interstitial, radiotherapy.

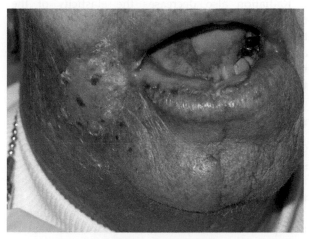

Fig. 24.2 Clinical appearance of a burn-like wound of the skin after termination of external radiation therapy.

fungal infections. These conditions are almost always associated with varying degrees of pain, and may need relatively strong analgesics.

The skin reactions can vary between a tan-like appearance to almost burn-like (Fig. 24.2) wounds. Softening and lubricating lotions are recommended for the affected skin. Males should be recommended to use an electrical shaver in order to spare the skin as well as not to use aftershave, since the alcohol may add to dryness of the skin.

An increased production of sticky mucus can also be observed after radiation of cancers in the pharyngeal region. Both still and sparkling water seem to be effective in dissolving the mucus. The use of milk products should be minimized. Pilocarpine (a parasympathomimetic agent taken orally) may also help.

Nutritional problems are frequently seen, and are almost always as a result of local reactions in the mucosa as well as a result of the pain. A loss of appetite may also be caused by a loss of, or change in, taste.

A majority of the patients undergoing radiotherapy to the head and neck region need professional assistance with nutrition. Some people may need some type of gastric tube to be able to feed themselves.

Tiredness and nausea are other side-effects which are frequently observed during radiotherapy.

Among the irreversible side-effects observed after radiotherapy for head and neck cancer, xerostomia is the most common. The degree differs between different patients. A majority of all saliva is secreted by the large salivary glands, and frequently these glands are within the field of irradiation. A secondary effect of increased oral dryness may be an altered taste and increased sensitivity to different tastes. Some patients need to avoid some type of spices, for instance pepper. The mucosa can also be more sensitive to different types of food, i.e. its consistency. Xerostomia carries an increased risk for development of dental caries and other dental problems.

Radiation also decreases the elasticity of the tissues, which can result in both dysphagia and trismus. The negative effect of radiation on vessels is also well recognized; decreased vascularity can lead to necrosis of both the soft tissues and the bone within the irradiated area.

Chemotherapy

Chemotherapy is also associated with a number of side-effects. Loss of hair is the most well-known and is usually observed between 1 and 2 weeks after the treatment.

All mucous membranes are susceptible to chemotherapy due to the quick turnover of cells. Wounds and dryness of the mouth, nausea, and diarrhea may be the result of chemotherapy. Nausea is observed more often in women and younger people. The condition can, however, be reduced effectively with medications.

Loss of appetite is another side-effect, resulting in weight loss. Professional nutritional counseling is frequently needed. It is, however, not unusual for a patient to gain weight during chemotherapy due to the fact that they may feel better with food in the stomach.

Another vital organ affected by chemotherapy is the bone marrow. The effect may be low blood counts for all types of blood cells, resulting in anemia, increased susceptibility to infections, and increased risk of spontaneous bleeding, e.g. nose bleeds and gingival bleeding. Transfusions may be necessary during chemotherapy.

Tiredness is also a frequently seen side-effect. Lack of energy and problems with concentration may be related to the tiredness. It is of great importance to rest when necessary, to eat as good and well-balanced food as possible, and to exercise.

The most positive fact related to chemotherapy is, however, that all side-effects almost always subside after termination of the treatment.

Management of oral health during radiation

Prior to the start of radiation therapy for treatment of head and neck cancers, it is of great importance to survey the oral health of the patient. A thorough oral examination, including radiographs, with special attention to marginal and apical periodontitis, calculus, and dental caries, is necessary. All infections should be treated, i.e. teeth may be either extracted or treated endodontically. Calculus should be removed, i.e. the teeth should be scaled and cleaned professionally. All caries should be excavated and the teeth should, at least, be supplied with temporary fillings. Daily rinsing with sodium fluoride solutions is recommended and prescribed to each patient as a complement to the use of fluoridated toothpaste.

By taking impressions of both the upper and the lower jaw, the dental technician can make casts on which different devices can be produced. These devices, the mouth-opening device (Fig. 24.3) and the mandibular protection device (Fig. 24.4), are used in

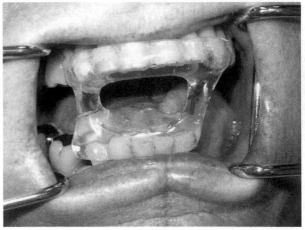

Fig. 24.3 A clinical picture of a patient with a mouth-opening device used to protect parts of the head in no need of radiation.

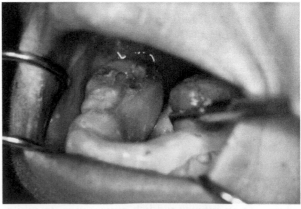

Fig. 24.4 A clinical picture of a patient wearing a mandibular protection device used during interstitial radiation (brachytherapy).

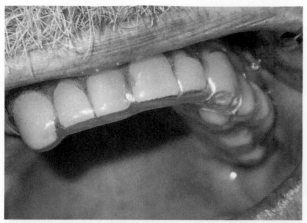

Fig. 24.5 A clinical picture of a patient wearing fluoride gel trays.

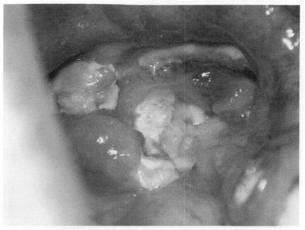

Fig. 24.6 A clinical view of a severe case of osteoradionecrosis in the anterior part of the mandible.

order to reduce the effect of irradiation on, or to protect, the surrounding tissues not in need of treatment. The casts can also be used to produce trays (Fig. 24.5) to administer high-concentration (0.2%) sodium fluoride gel on a daily basis.

The mouth-opening device can be designed with and without a tongue depressor. A device without a tongue depressor is used during the radiotherapy when the cancer is located in the floor of the mouth, in the submandibular gland, or in the chin. In contrast, a device supplied with a depressor is used when the cancer is located in the tongue, in the base of the tongue, in the maxillary sinus, in the nose, in the upper lip, in the palate, and sometimes also in the floor of the mouth.

The mandibular protection device is used during interstitial radiotherapy to displace the tongue, the cheek or the lip away from the implanted radiation source. It also protects the mandibular bone. This device is used during interstitial radiation of carcinomas in the tongue, the base of the tongue, the tonsils, the floor of the mouth, and the lips. The mandibular protection device is made of approximately 6 mm thick plastic with 2 mm of lead included. The device can also be used to protect the bone of the maxilla, although it is most frequently used to protect the mandible.

During the period of radiation, at least weekly professional cleaning of the teeth and mouth is recommended. As treatment continues, i.e. radiation accumulates within the tissues, the patient will have more discomfort, making it hard to maintain proper oral hygiene.

Management of oral health during chemotherapy

As with patients scheduled for radiotherapy, it is important to thoroughly examine the oral health of patients who will receive chemotherapy. The impor-

tance of maintaining good oral hygiene during the period of chemotherapy cannot be overstressed.

Mucositis normally develops after 5–10 days of chemotherapy. At later stages, ulcers can develop. The ulcers can be infected secondarily with bacteria, viruses or fungi. They can also be very painful, resulting in nutritional problems.

Management of postradiation conditions

To reduce the xerostomia the patient should be recommended frequent intake of small amounts of water. There are a number of saliva replacement products, artificial saliva, and salivastimulatory products available on the market, which have many positive effects on oral well-being. The use of such products can also be of benefit for taste. Life-long use of additional sodium fluoride products, i.e. daily rinsing, should be recommended in order to prevent rapid development of dental caries. Frequent and scheduled visits to a general dentist and/or a dental hygienist are desirable.

Reduced mouth-opening capacity is another late side-effect of irradiation. Different training programs are available to prevent early development of this condition. Sometimes it can be of benefit to begin the training prior to radiation, and continue it as soon as possible after termination of treatment. A very strict and frequent use of these training programs is desirable since the effect is quickly reduced and even eliminated if they are not followed. Today, a number of mouth-training devices are also available.

Soft tissue and bone necrosis (osteoradionecrosis) are the side-effects that usually develop last (Figs 24.6 and 24.7). It is not possible to predict which patient is at risk for development of these conditions, though they rarely occur in tissues subjected to less than 55 Gy of radiation. To prevent the development of these conditions it is of benefit to treat dental problems

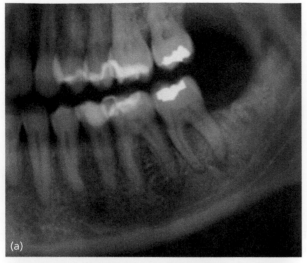

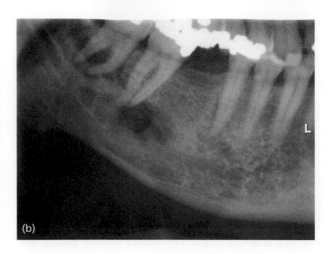

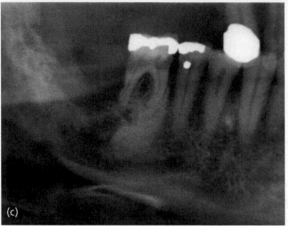

Fig. 24.7 Radiographical appearances of osteoradionecrosis. (a) At an early stage. (b) At an intermediate stage. (c) At a late and severe stage. In the late stage the mandible has fractured.

immediately and conservatively, i.e. regular visits to a general dentist to prevent development of both periodontal disease and dental caries. Dental extractions should be avoided as long as possible. Instead, endodontic treatment should be the treatment of choice when apical periodontitis has developed. If extraction is the only alternative, it should be performed surgically with the aim of covering the area with soft tissue. Systemic use of antibiotics for 7–10 days is recommended.

When, and if, osteoradionecrosis has developed, it is important to maintain good dental hygiene, to prevent development of infections in the affected area.

Some alternatives are available to reduce the speed of development, although controversy remains. Hyperbaric oxygen treatment has been used to reduce the development of, and also to treat, osteoradionecrosis.

In later stages of osteoradionecrosis it may be necessary to carry out surgical resection, with or without adjunctive hyperbaric oxygen. Microvascular reconstruction, using free flap technology after surgical resection of the affected area, is today a relatively common treatment in order to restore both function and esthetics in this group of patients.

Recommended reading

Kjeller G. (2010) Management of patients undergoing radiation and chemotherapy. In: *Oral and Maxillofacial Surgery* (eds, Andersson L, Kahnberg K-E, Pogrel MA). Oxford, Wiley-Blackwell.

Marx RE, Johnson PP. (1987) Studies in the radiobiology of osteoradionecrosis and their clinical significance. *Oral Surgery, Oral Medicine, Oral Pathology*, **64**, 379–90.

Chapter 25

Salivary Gland Disorders

Salivary gland disorders usually present to clinicians as enlargements (local or generalized), underactivity (xerostomia) or overactivity (ptyalism). Table 25.1 lists pathological entities by clinical classification.

Investigations

The salivary glands are easily accessible and open to a wide range of investigative techniques. The first-line investigation is often high-resolution B-mode ultrasonography. It can reliably distinguish between intra-and extraglandular masses, accurately recognize calculi/strictures and can demonstrate changes within the parenchyma. Doppler flow studies can identify vascular pathology. Conventional plain radiographs are virtually obsolete except for the ability to show small (<2mm diameter) calculi within the ductal orifice. Traditional sialograms are still useful when investigating stones and evaluating strictures. Further evaluation can be carried out by MRI (with modest superiority over computed tomography (CT)) and recent developments such as diffusion-weighted and dynamic contrast-enhanced MRI may, in the future, permit routine visualization of the facial nerve, although at present this is still a research tool. Salivary gland scintiscans assess glandular function.

The second most useful investigation is fine-needle aspiration cytology (FNAC). The prospect of a reliable tap can be improved by ultrasound or CT-guided aspiration. A cytology service should be able to distinguish between benign and malignant disease in over 85% of cases. A correct histological diagnosis is more problematic and results cannot be relied on but the technique has particular value when a neoplasm is not suspected and if this is confirmed surgery can be avoided.

Etiology

Infection (bacterial and viral)

Acute viral sialadenitis

Over a third of all pediatric salivary gland disorders are of an inflammatory nature, with either an obstructive or non-obstructive etiology.

There is a wide range of viral infections that can involve the salivary glands (Coxsackie A and B3, parainfluenza B, ECHO type 9, and Epstein–Barr). The most common is mumps. It is caused by a highly infectious paramyxovirus with an incubation period of 2–3 weeks. The subject is infectious from 5 days prior and 10 days after the onset. In adults, the condition may be more severe and complicated by orchitis or oophoritis and varying degrees of meningoencephalitis are relatively common (25%). In rare instances, occurrence may be unilateral.

Juvenile recurrent parotitis

Juvenile recurrent parotitis (JRP) is a unique, non-obstructive, non-suppurative, usually unilateral variant of sialadenitis and occurs in young children. Traditionally it is considered a self-limiting condition but continual problems can occur into adult life in approximately 30–40% of cases.

It is probable there is more than one etiology: incompetent parotid ducts, juvenile Sjögren's syndrome, lymphoma, HIV-SGD, amongst others. Congenital ductal malformations, genetic factors, bacterial or viral infection, allergy or autoimmune congenital immunoglobulin deficiency have also been postulated. The symptom-free interval may be increased following duct lavage.

Essentials of Oral and Maxillofacial Surgery, First Edition. Edited by M. Anthony Pogrel, Karl-Erik Kahnberg and Lars Andersson.
© 2014 John Wiley & Sons, Ltd. Published 2014 by John Wiley & Sons, Ltd.
Companion website: www.wiley.com/go/pogrel/oms

Table 25.1 Pathological entities by clinical classification.

Discrete single or multiple masses within a salivary gland
Granulomas and chronic infections
Tuberculosis (TB)
Non-TB mycobacterial infections
Actinomycosis
Cat scratch disease
Syphilis
Hydatid disease
Inflammatory conditions
Kim-Kimura's disease
Castleman's disease
Kuttner tumor
Inflammatory pseudotumor
Cystic lesions
Simple cysts
HIV-SGD
Dermoid cysts
Congenital duct cysts
Polycystic disease of the parotid gland

The diffusely enlarged gland
The intermittently swollen gland (unilateral)
The obstructed gland
Sialolithiasis
Strictures
Polyps/mucus plugs
Impacted foreign bodies
Pneumoparotid
Persistent swollen gland (unilateral)
Infection
Acute
Subacute
Chronic
Autoimmune salivary disease
Benign lymphoepithelial lesions
Sjögren's syndrome
Wegener's granulomatosis
Graft-versus-host disease
Non-autoimmune salivary gland disease
Amyloid
Sarcoidosis Churg–Strauss syndrome
Metabolic salivary gland disease
Endocrine
Liver, gastrointestinal disease and malnutrition
Bulimia nervosa
Cystic fibrosis
Miscellaneous

Bacterial sialadenitis

This condition is uncommon today and when it does occur it is invariably related to salivary calculi and/or a predisposing medical condition (immune suppression). It may also arise as an acute exacerbation of chronic sialadenitis. First-line treatment consists of antibiotics targeted at staphylococci and streptococci. Surgical intervention (drainage) is seldom required apart from stone removal.

Chronic/subacute sialadenitis

Chronic sialadenitis is usually unilateral, recurrent, and secondary to an underlying obstruction (stone or foreign body). Approximately 2% of patients with Sjögren's syndrome are affected each year.

Autoimmune salivary disease

Sjögren's syndrome

Primary Sjögren's syndrome has the histological features accompanied by dry eyes and mouth; if accompanied by a connective tissue disorder (systemic lupus erythematosus (SLE), polyarteritis nodosa, CREST (calcinosis, Raynaud phenomenon, esophageal dysmotility, sclerodactyly, and telangiectasia), dermatomyositis, systemic sclerosis) or primary biliary cirrhosis, it is secondary Sjögren's. Other supposed symptom complexes have been identified (sialadenitis, nodal osteoarthritis and xerostomia, SOX). Sjögren's syndrome subjects have a 44 times increased risk of developing lymphoma with an incidence of 5–10% of cases. It is estimated that 1% of the adult population (mean age 50 years: female predominance of 10:1) have Sjögren's syndrome.

Salivary mucosa-associated lymphoid tissue (MALT) lymphomas

These tumors are uncommon (about 1 case per million population per annum). Mikulicz (1888) described painless enlargement of the major salivary glands and lacrimal glands, which in hindsight was probably a MALT lymphoma. They are the most common lymphoma to affect salivary tissue and the third most common of the non-Hodgkin lymphomas. In the head and neck most occur in the parotid (Fig. 25.1).

Obstructive salivary gland disease

In the last decade a revolution has occurred in the management of obstructive salivary gland disease with the introduction of minimally invasive techniques. Stone clearance is achieved in 80% of cases and gland removal considerably reduced. Historically the rationale for gland removal was that a calculus induces irreversible parenchyma damage, which, in turn, leads to chronic sialadenitis. There is, however, increasing evidence that salivary glands recover function following stone removal and remain asymptomatic.

Investigation

A history of repeated preprandial swelling (mealtime syndrome) is almost pathognomonic of salivary gland obstruction. Stagnant saliva leads to mucus plugs which become impacted in the stricture so symptoms typically follow a period of reduced gland activity such as sleep. The obstruction is frequently released after massage, which, in turn, is followed by a gush of salty saliva.

Ultrasonography

The main salivary glands (parotid, submandibular, and sublingual) are assessable to sonographic evaluation (frequencies of 7.5–13.5 MHz). A stone >2 mm diameter is reliably detected as an echo opaque reflection with distinct distal shadowing (Fig. 25.2). A dilated duct proximal to the echo confirms the diagnosis and dilation without an echo suggests the stricture. Consequently, ultrasound imaging can be used to monitor recovery following treatment, and portable ultrasound machines are an invaluable adjunct to current clinical practice.

Sialography

A sialogram is also a valuable investigation (Fig. 25.3) for it can identify the size, position, and mobility of a stone (the latter has an impact on the choice of treatment) but its main advantage over ultrasound is its

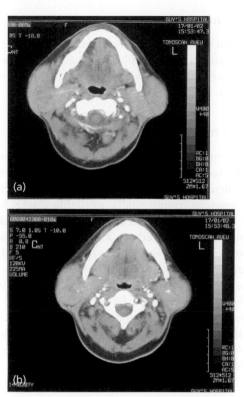

Fig. 25.1 Long-standing parotid swelling (10 years plus) initially thought to be due to sarcoid. Tail of parotid biopsy confirmed MALT lymphoma.

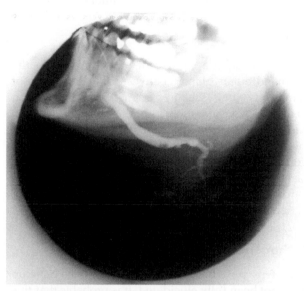

Fig. 25.3 Submandibular sialogram showing calculi. The fact that the duct is dilated along its length suggests the stones are mobile and suitable for basket retrieval.

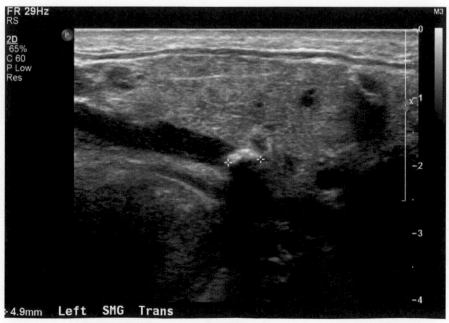

Fig. 25.2 Ultrasound scan demonstrating a 4.9 mm calculus at the hilum of the submandibular gland.

ability to provide information on the number and shape of strictures.

Plain film radiography

The average submandibular duct stone can be easily demonstrated by a mandibular true lower occlusal view, while large hilar stones can be seen on the panoramic or an oblique lateral radiograph.

CT and MRI scans

CT and, particularly, MRI imaging can be used, in the absence of simpler modalities, to demonstrate stones and chronic inflammation, but they should be reserved for evaluating salivary tumors.

Sialolithiasis

There is usually a significant delay (greater in the submandibular gland) between the initiation of symptoms and seeking a medical consultation (parotid 4.8 years, submandibular gland 5.4 years) and this correlates with submandibular stones being larger than parotid calculi. The anatomical distribution of calculi shows that 63–94% occur in the submandibular gland and the remainder occur in the parotid gland. Multiple stones occur in about 10% of patients.

Pathogenesis of salivary stones

The steps by which salivary gland stones develop have not been fully elucidated. It is probable that this process is multifaceted with one important item being the anatomical configuration of the salivary ducts. Both duct systems have kinks and stones seem to congregate at these kinks (Fig. 25.4).

It is hypothesized that a calculus forms from a nidus of debris. Calcium-binding proteins are present in both the salivary and the renal systems and a deficit of crystallization inhibitors has been proposed as a cause of kidney stone formation. No such association has been demonstrated in the salivary glands nor is water hardness relevant.

The submandibular stone has a significant inorganic component (80%) and tends to be radiopaque (94%) whereas the parotid sialolith is formed of 50% organic material and 43% are radiopaque.

Pathogenesis of salivary strictures

The origin of salivary strictures is unclear. Strictures can be pinpoint, multiple (giving a sausage-like appearance) or diffuse along the length of the duct (Fig. 25.5).

Modern management of salivary calculi

The advent of minimally invasive salivary therapy was ushered in by innovations in the management of renal calculi. A salivary extracorporeal lithotripter (ECL) became commercially available (Storz Minilith®: Storz Medical, Kreuzlingen, Switzerland) in the mid-1990s followed in 2000 by first-generation microendoscopes (Fig. 25.6) which then raised the possibility of intracorporeal lithotripsy (ICL).

The armamentarium available for minimally invasive therapy includes an ECL (Storz Minilith), salivary endoscopes, microballoons, and an array of wire baskets and microforceps (Fig. 25.7). These instruments should be used in combination and treatment is governed by stone size (Fig. 25.8).

Lithotripsy

The shockwave generated by the ECL (Fig. 25.9) produces a compressive wave which passes through the

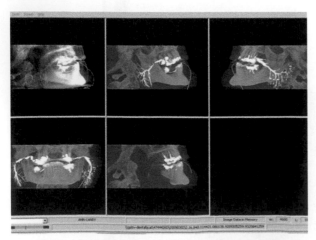

Fig. 25.4 Long cone-beam CT sialogram demonstrating the parotid duct system.

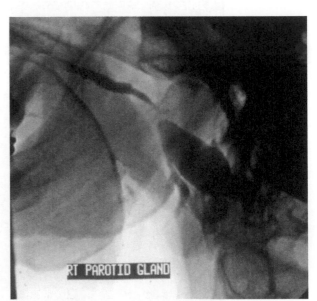

Fig. 25.5 Sialogram showing a point stricture in a parotid duct with gross proximal dilatation.

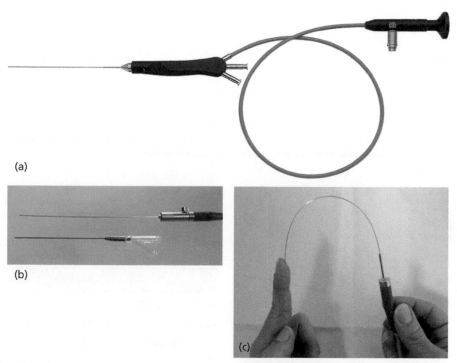

(a)

(b)

(c)

Fig. 25.6 Examples of third generation endoscopes produced by Storz (a) and Polydiagnost (b, c). One is based on a reusable multichannel unit (Storz), the other on a disposable design that minimizes concerns with sterilization. Both are delicate instruments but possess greater flexibility than their predecessors.

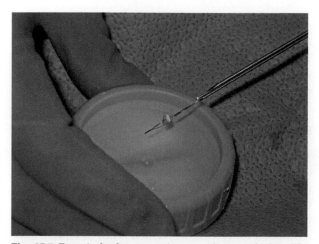

Fig. 25.7 Dormia basket to retrieve a salivary calculus. The basket is advanced unexpanded along the duct, past the calculus. It is then activated and expanded and withdrawn back along the duct, bringing the calculus with it. Usually the punctum has to be incised to release the calculus.

calculus producing stress fractures. At the same time, the pressure wave induces vapor bubbles at the stone's surface. As the bubble collapses a jet of water strikes the stone, drilling tiny holes in its surface.

It has become apparent that the chance of stone clearance is better in the parotid gland and with stones <8 mm in diameter. The stone clearance rate averages about 45%.

Gland-preserving surgery (endoscope-assisted stone retrieval)

Gland-preserving surgery is the treatment of choice for large or fixed submandibular stones and is usually reserved for those 10% of patients with parotid stones that remain symptomatic after extracorporeal shock wave lithotripsy (ESWL). The success rate for both techniques is in the region of 95% stone retrieval.

Endoscope-assisted retrieval of submandibular calculi

This technique is reserved for stones in the middle or proximal portion of the submandibular gland. It can be performed in the outpatient or preferably a day-case setting. Palpable stones in the floor of mouth are ideally suited to this technique.

Endoscopic-assisted removal of parotid calculi

The sialoendoscope helps to identify the duct for the light at the end of the endoscope acts as a beacon to direct the surgeon on to the stone (Fig. 25.10). The direct transcutaneous technique is applicable to large calculi situated on the anterior edge of the masseter muscle where the parotid duct is superficial. The light at the end of the endoscope is used to mark the position of the stone and a preauricular skin flap is raised

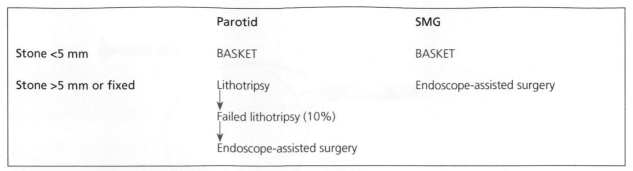

	Parotid	SMG
Stone <5 mm	BASKET	BASKET
Stone >5 mm or fixed	Lithotripsy	Endoscope-assisted surgery
	↓	
	Failed lithotripsy (10%)	
	↓	
	Endoscope-assisted surgery	

Fig. 25.8 Flow diagram demonstrating the management protocol for salivary stones.

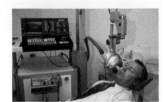

Fig. 25.9 Storz sialo-lithotripter.

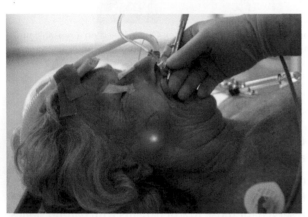

Fig. 25.10 The light at the end of the sialoendoscope is used as a guide to identify the duct and the position of the stone prior to surgical release.

to expose the duct and stone. The buccal branch of the facial nerve runs parallel to the parotid duct and is easily visualized in the dissection. Prophylactic antibiotics are prescribed and a stent is optional.

Salivary gland tumors

New developments

- Warthin's tumor is a polyclonal lesion and not a neoplasm.
- Benign parotid tumors can be safely treated by procedures less than the traditional superficial parotidectomy.
- Management of malignant salivary tumors should be governed mainly by stage rather than grade (+ histological type).

Table 25.2 shows the distribution of 517 salivary gland tumors seen over a 9-year period in two hos-

Table 25.2 The proportions of benign and malignant salivary gland tumors in a defined UK population by anatomic site (1988–1997). The traditional 10:1:1 rule holds true for distribution of tumors between parotid, submandibular, and minor salivary glands. Figures in parentheses are percentages.

	Benign	Malignant	Total
Major salivary glands			
Parotid gland	397	26 (6)	423
Submandibular gland	35	12 (34)	47
Minor salivary glands	32	10 (24)	42
Sublingual gland	0	5 (100)	5
Total	464	53	517

pitals in the UK. The incidence of benign tumors was 7.2, and of malignant tumors 0.8 per 100 000 people. The causes of salivary gland tumors are unknown, with the exception of previous exposure to ionizing radiation.

Benign parotid tumor

The majority of benign tumors (93%) are represented by two histological types – pleomorphic adenoma (71%) and Warthin's tumor (22%). In the last decade there has been a fundamental reappraisal of these two tumors. Pleomorphic adenomas had a fearful reputation for recurrence, which is not deserved, and the rationale for wide excision was based on this reputation. Similarly it is now appreciated that Warthin's tumor is a polyclonal lesion and not a neoplasm, which may manifest with synchronous or metachronous lesions. In both instances a more conservative approach to treatment is possible.

Investigation

Complex salivary gland masses that run deep to the mandible or are suspected of being malignant should be visualized by CT or, preferably, MRI scans. MRI offers superior soft tissue contrast and artifacts caused by dental fillings usually play a minor role on scanning. The greatest drawbacks with MRI are the long scan times and the claustrophobic environment that it demands. These imaging modalities should be complemented by the use of fine-needle aspiration cytology.

Traditional parotidectomy

An essential step in traditional superficial parotidectomy is the identification of the facial nerve and a prerequisite for safe surgery is wide exposure. This is achieved through a variety of preauricular incisions (lazy S: facelift). It is a useful exercise to release the parotid gland from the confines of the deep cervical fascia by freeing the fascia from the sternomastoid muscle, mastoid process, and tragus (the greater auricular nerve is ideally preserved). The increased mobility allows tumors wedged between the mandible and the mastoid to become more accessible. Using the avascular pretragal plane of dissection, the parotid is displaced anteriorly to identify the facial nerve. The main trunk is located halfway between the bony external auditory meatus and the tip of the mastoid at the medial aspect of the tympanomastoid fissure. The extent of the nerve dissection is governed by the location of the tumor. If the tumor is small only a quadrant of the parotid gland need be removed (partial superficial parotidectomy). The parotid duct is normally preserved. Parotid surgeons should be equally adept at both retrograde and antegrade nerve dissection. Intraoperative neurophysiological monitoring has been advocated in this type of surgery. The equipment is relatively inexpensive, easy to use, minimally invasive, and may on occasion reduce the extent (rather than incidence) of nerve injury through constant feedback during surgery.

A total parotidectomy (TP) accompanies tumors deep to the facial nerve where the exposed branches of the nerve are lifted to access the tumor. With this additional stripping of the nerve comes an increased risk of permanent and temporary nerve injury. Occasionally a parotid tumor extends into the parapharyngeal space and is usually removed following a total parotidectomy. This may necessitate a vertical subsigmoid mandibular osteotomy and division of the stylomandibular ligament or posterior belly of the digastric, either alone or in combination in order to improve access. Once these binding structures are released the tumor can usually be displaced inferiorly, where by necessity it is freed by a form of extracapsular dissection.

Extracapsular dissection

The practice of surgery in general is moving down a minimally invasive pathway and in the parotid this has found expression in extracapsular dissection (ECD) of benign parotid tumors. ECD should be reserved for discrete benign parotid lumps (>2 cm diameter) in the superficial portion of the parotid gland. The nature of the lump should be confirmed by FNAC since the main risk in ECD is not tumor recurrence but the inadvertent treatment of a low-grade malignant salivary gland tumor masquerading as a benign lump. The initial surgical approach and exposure of the parotid is similar to that for superficial parotidectomy. In the majority of cases (60%) the greater auricular nerve can be preserved.

Recurrences of pleomorphic adenoma

Recurrences of pleomorphic adenoma are rare, following the abandonment of local enucleation. Rupture of the tumor capsule may occur during surgery, especially if there is a significant myxoid component, or pseudopodia or satellite nodules in the "bare area". However, macroscopic spillage carries only an 8% risk of recurrence, compared to 2.5% if no recognizable spillage was noted. Therefore the concept of spillage may not be as important as previously believed.

On average, recurrences occur 8 years after the initial treatment, presenting as either uninodular or multinodular lesions. MRI in combination with mandatory FNAC will confirm the recurrence of benign disease. Single nodules may be safely removed by nerve-preserving additional surgery, with a 15% risk of further recurrence at 10 years. Surgery alone is insufficient for the more common multinodular recurrences, which may be dispersed over the surgical field. Forty-five percent of multinodular recurrences will recur within 10 years of surgical removal; adjuvant postoperative radiotherapy will significantly reduce this to 4%. Malignant progression is very rare.

Benign tumors of the submandibular and minor salivary glands

A submandibular gland adenoma should be removed in continuity with the gland. The situation to be avoided is an adenectomy for apparent sialoadenitis when the lesion is a malignant tumor.

The commonest intraoral site for benign salivary gland tumors is the junction of the hard and soft palate. Most present as rubbery lumps and the diagnosis can be established by FNAC or ideally a dermatological punch biopsy. The latter retrieves a small core (2–4 mm diameter) of tissue without violating the tumor margins. Those tumors situated on the junction of the soft and hard palate do not require a through-and-through dissection into the nasal cavity but can be safely dissected in a subperiosteal plane. It is advisable to cover the raw area with a dental healing plate.

Malignant tumors

Parotid tumors

The object of treatment is to excise the tumor with an adequate rim of normal tissue but this may not be feasible because of the complex anatomy of the parotid area since adequate surgical clearance of tumor is not possible with large masses. It is for this reason that adjuvant radiotherapy plays an important part in the management of salivary gland cancer. The traditional approach to a malignant parotid tumor is a total parotidectomy.

Submandibular gland

Submandibular gland cancers carry a 20% worse prognosis than malignant tumors in the parotid or mouth, and, again, comprehensive extracapsular excisional surgery is the primary treatment.

Minor salivary gland tumors

Minor salivary gland cancers within the oral cavity are managed in the same way as squamous cell carcinomas in the mouth.

Radiotherapy

Postoperative radiation therapy shows improvement in local control when compared with surgery alone. It is generally acknowledged that adjuvant radiotherapy reduces local recurrence but does not have a significant impact on overall survival due to distant metastasis.

Recommended reading

Iro H, Zenk J, Escudier MP, *et al.* (2009) Outcome of minimally invasive management of salivary calculi in 4,691 patients. *Laryngoscope*, **119**, 263–8.

McGurk M, Sherman J. (2010) Salivary gland disorders. In: *Oral and Maxillofacial Surgery* (eds, Andersson L, Kahnberg K-E, Pogrel MA). Oxford, Wiley-Blackwell.

McGurk M, Escudier MP, Brown JE. (2005) Modern management of salivary calculi. *British Journal of Surgery*, **92**, 107–12.

McGurk M, Renehan AG, Gleave EN, Hancock BD. (1996) Clinical significance of the tumour capsule in the treatment of parotid pleomorphic adenomas. *British Journal of Surgery*, **83**, 1747–9.

Pease CT, Charles PJ, Shattles W, Markwick J, Maini RN. (1993) Serological and immunogenetic markers of extraglandular primary Sjögren's syndrome. *British Journal of Rheumatology*, **32**, 574–7.

Yoshimura Y, Morishita T, Sugihara T. (1989) Salivary gland function after sialolithiasis: scintigraphic examination of submandibular glands with 99mTc-pertechnetate. *Journal of Oral and Maxillofacial Surgery*, **47**, 704–11.

Part 5: Trauma

(Section Editor: Lars Andersson)

Introduction: Oral and Maxillofacial Traumatology

At least five million people die from trauma every year; half of all deaths are in the age group 10–24 years, and trauma is the number one killer of individuals up to 40 years of age. Moreover, several hundred million people are injured by trauma every year. Trauma has a multitude of consequences for the traumatized individual, family members, and society. The impact is not only physical but also psychosocial and economical. The maxillofacial region is important, with vital functions such as breathing, eating, talking, smelling, and vision. Moreover, it is also an esthetically important region. Injuries to the maxillofacial region may, therefore, have serious consequences for the individual's quality of life.

In developing countries road traffic accident is the main cause of maxillofacial injuries: in more developed countries, despite more cars, there has been a decrease in the proportion of road traffic accidents as etiologic factors, especially in the past three decades, due to a more developed and safer traffic environment and the use of seat belts. Many studies have reported that a lifestyle with high alcohol consumption is a major contributing factor resulting in assault injuries due to interpersonal violence.

Oral injuries are most frequent during the first 10 years of life, decreasing gradually with age, and are very rare after the age of 30, in contrast to bodily injuries which are seen most frequently in adolescents and young adults and are common throughout life.

Although the oral region comprises as small an area as 1% of the total body area, it accounts for 5% of all bodily injuries. In preschool children oral injuries make up as much as 17% of all bodily injuries, with injuries to the head being the most common in contrast to later in life where injuries to hands and feet are the most common, as shown in many studies.

Simultaneous injuries to different oral tissues are commonly seen in patients presenting with oral trauma. Dental injuries are the most common injuries to the oral region, and are seen in as many as 92% of patients presenting with oral injuries, whereas soft tissue injuries to the same patients are seen in 28%. Fractures involving the jaws are seen in 6% of all patients presenting with oral injuries.

In Chapter 26, *traumatic dental injuries* are presented in detail, because these are the injuries that most clinicians should be able to treat themselves. In Chapter 27, *maxillofacial fractures* are covered, which are injuries treated by specialists in oral and maxillofacial surgery. However, all clinicians must be aware of how to diagnose such injuries and have some knowledge of principles of treatment. In Chapter 28, *soft tissue injuries* are covered, which are injuries where clinicians, although not treating all such injuries themselves, must know how to diagnose and understand the principles of treatment.

Essentials of Oral and Maxillofacial Surgery, First Edition. Edited by M. Anthony Pogrel, Karl-Erik Kahnberg and Lars Andersson.
© 2014 John Wiley & Sons, Ltd. Published 2014 by John Wiley & Sons, Ltd.
Companion website: www.wiley.com/go/pogrel/oms

Chapter 26

Traumatic Dental Injuries

Traumatic dental injuries (TDI) are the most common of the oral and maxillofacial injuries. More or less all clinicians, general practitioners and specialists, meet such patients, either in the emergency phase or later as a consequence of the trauma. The prognosis for some TDI depends very much on correct early emergency management at the place of accident and at the clinic immediately after the accident. This chapter presents how to diagnose, classify, and treat TDI with emphasis on the emergency phase.

Epidemiology of traumatic dental injuries and relation to oral and somatic injuries

Oral injuries (dental, soft tissue, and bone) caused by trauma occur very frequently. They are most common during the first 12 years of life and are rare after the age of 30. In contrast, other bodily injuries are most frequently seen at ages 15–25 years and occur throughout life (Fig. 26.1).

Of all patients presenting with oral injuries, TDI is the most common oral injury (92%), followed by orofacial soft tissue injuries (28%); whereas fractures of the maxillofacial bones are relatively rare and seen in only 6% of such patients. The annual incidence of TDI is 1–2% of the population. The prevalence is high and every fourth boy and every fifth girl will have already sustained dental injuries by the age of 14. One in five children has sustained a TDI to the permanent teeth before leaving school and one in four adults has evidence of TDI. Due to the high number of injured individuals and often complex treatment, TDI are associated with high costs for society and the individual.

The prognosis of treatment for some dental injuries, and especially for avulsed teeth, depends very much on early and correct management at the place of the accident and during emergency treatment at the clinic.

Examination and diagnosis of dental injuries

History taking is important with regard to when, where, and how the injury occurred, as well as to the patient's general health and possible medication. Be alert to other injuries and symptoms indicating more serious injuries. It is also of value to ask what has been done before the patient reached the clinic, such as any treatment carried out elsewhere and how avulsed teeth have been stored.

A brief summary is given here of the important issues for emergency examination and for TDI. For an overview of evaluation of patients with more severe maxillofacial injuries, see Chapter 27. As for oral and maxillofacial injuries, it is important to examine and treat TDI in a systematic way. "Examine from the outside towards the inside and treat from the inside towards the outside" is a helpful principle for a systematic approach for examining oral injuries. Suturing of lips should ideally be carried out after intraoral emergency examination and emergency treatment has been performed, otherwise it may be difficult to enter the oral cavity once edema has started to develop.

The possibility of inhaling or swallowing teeth at the time of injury should always be considered when teeth, parts of the teeth, or prosthetic appliances are missing. This is especially important in the unconscious patient; if there is reason to suspect inhalation or swallowing of a tooth or dental appliance, it is important that radiographs of the chest and the abdomen are considered. Inhalation of foreign bodies

Essentials of Oral and Maxillofacial Surgery, First Edition. Edited by M. Anthony Pogrel, Karl-Erik Kahnberg and Lars Andersson.
© 2014 John Wiley & Sons, Ltd. Published 2014 by John Wiley & Sons, Ltd.
Companion website: www.wiley.com/go/pogrel/oms

is normally associated with symptoms such as coughing but may also occur in a conscious patient without producing symptoms.

Examination of crowns of teeth should be carried out in order to look for presence and extent of fractures and pulp exposures. Crown–root fractures in the molar and premolar regions should be expected when there has been an indirect trauma such as a blow to the chin. Crown–root fractures in one quadrant are very often accompanied by similar fractures on the same side of the opposing jaw. For this reason it is therefore necessary to examine occlusal fissures of all molars and premolars to detect possible fractures (Fig. 26.2).

The fracture surface should be carefully examined for the extent of fracture in dentin and pulp exposures (Fig. 26.3). When pulp is exposed, the size and location should be recorded. In some cases, the dentin layer may be so thin that the outline of the pulp can be seen through the dentin wall. One should take care not to perforate the thin dentinal layer during the examination.

Displacement and avulsion of teeth are usually evident by visual examination; however, minor abnormalities can often be difficult to detect. In such cases, it is helpful to examine the occlusion as well as radiographs taken at various angulations. In cases of tooth luxation, the direction of the dislocation as well as extent should be recorded. It is important to remember that, apart from displacement and interference with occlusion, laterally luxated and intruded teeth present very few clinical symptoms (Fig. 26.4). Moreover, these teeth are normally firmly locked in their displaced position and do not usually demonstrate tenderness to percussion. While radiographs can be of assistance, diagnosis is confirmed by the percussion tone, when tapping on the tooth with the handle of an instrument. A high, bony percussion

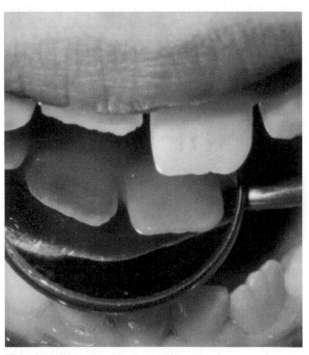

Fig. 26.3 Right central incisor with crown fracture of dentin showing pulpal exposure.

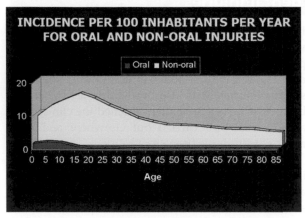

Fig. 26.1 Incidence per 100 inhabitants per year for oral and non-oral injuries. Source: Eilert-Petersson, E., Andersson, L. and Sörensen, S. (1997) Traumatic oral vs non-oral injuries. An epidemiological study during one year in a Swedish county. *Swedish Dental Journal*, 21, 55–68.

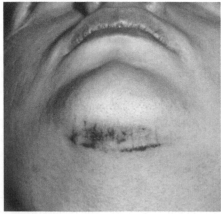
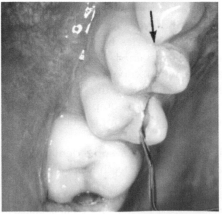

Fig. 26.2 Induced dental trauma. (a) Impact was transferred via the chin to the dental arches. (b) Crown–root fractures were inflicted in both right premolars by the forceful occlusion. From Andreasen *et al.* 2007.

tone is registered compared to the normal sound of uninjured teeth. In contrast, when a Le Fort I level midface fracture is present a change in percussion sound to a crack-like sound can be noticed.

In the primary dentition, it is of utmost importance to diagnose the direction of dislocation of the apex of a displaced primary tooth, since this tooth is located in close relationship to the permanent successors and can impinge on the development of the permanent successor (Fig. 26.5). This diagnosis is often best made by palpating the alveolar process from a vestibular approach.

The patient may also react with pain to percussion of a tooth which is indicative of damage to the periodontal ligament. As with all examination techniques used at the time of injury, the percussion test should be started on a non-injured tooth to ensure a reliable patient response. In smaller children, the use of a fingertip can be a gentler diagnostic tool.

Patients can usually detect and guide the examiner to the place where there has been a change in the occlusion. Abnormalities in occlusion can indicate fractures of the jaw, alveolar process or a lateral luxa-

tion (Figs 26.6, 26.7, 26.8). All teeth should be tested for abnormal mobility, both horizontally and axially. It should be remembered that erupting teeth and primary teeth undergoing physiologic root resorption always exhibit some mobility. The typical sign of alveolar fracture is movement of adjacent teeth when the mobility of a single tooth is tested (Fig. 26.6). Palpation of the alveolar process is important for detection of fractures with dislocations.

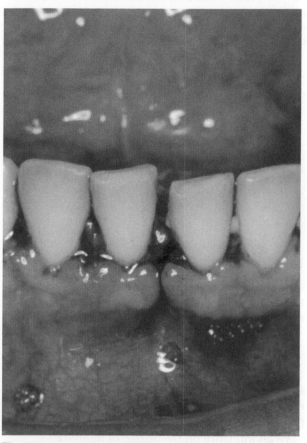

Fig. 26.6 A step in the mandibular incisor level indicating mandibular body fracture.

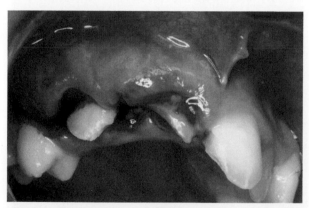

Fig. 26.4 Intruded incisors. The teeth are impacted and locked in the bone and show no signs of tenderness to percussion. A high, bony percussion sound is registered. From Andreasen *et al.* 2007.

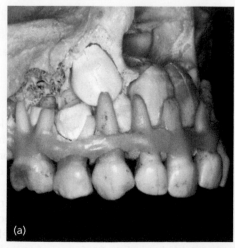
(a)

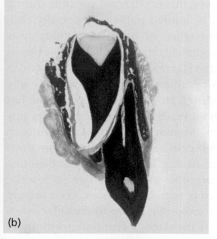
(b)

Fig. 26.5 (a) Anatomic relationship between primary incisor and its permanent successor in a human skull. (b) Histologic relationship between primary incisor and its permanent successor. From Andreasen *et al.* 2007.

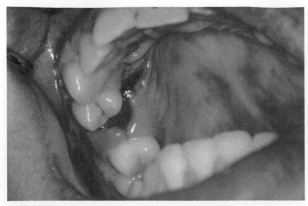

Fig. 26.7 A rift in the palatal mucosa and a step in the premolar occlusal level indicating a fracture of the maxillary alveolar process.

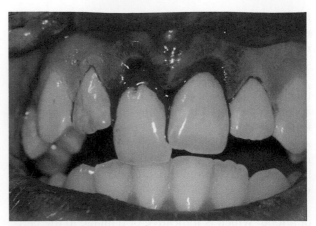

Fig. 26.9 Central incisors with root fractures.

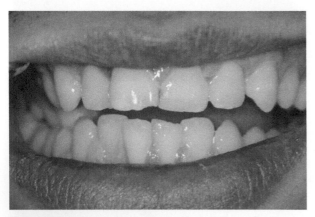

Fig. 26.8 Primary contact in premolar region indicating an alveolar process fracture in the maxilla.

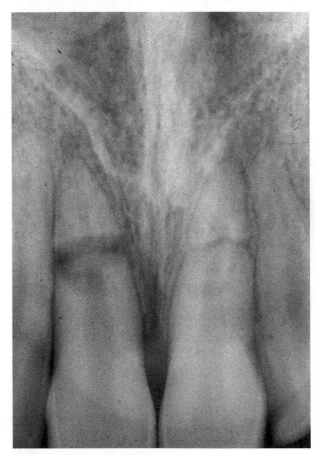

Fig. 26.10 Radiograph showing fractures of the roots 11 and 21.

When mobility of a tooth is detected it is not possible to discriminate between luxation injuries and root fractures without radiographic examination (Figs 26.9, 26.10). The site of the root fracture will have an influence on the degree of mobility.

Pulp testing following traumatic injuries is a controversial issue. These procedures require cooperation and a relaxed patient, in order to avoid false reactions. However, this is often not possible during initial treatment of injured patients, especially children. The interpretation of pulpal sensibility tests performed immediately after traumatic injuries is complicated by the fact that sensitivity responses can be temporarily or permanently decreased, especially after luxation injuries. However, repeated testing has shown that normal reactions can return after a few weeks or months. Moreover, teeth which have been loosened can elicit pain responses merely from pressure of the pulp testing instrument. It is therefore important to reposition and immobilize such teeth, e.g. root-fractured or extruded incisors, prior to pulp testing. Another important factor to consider when testing the pulp is the stage of eruption; teeth under root development sometimes show an unreliable response. Teeth undergoing orthodontic movement

display higher excitation thresholds. If local anesthetics are to be administered for various treatment procedures, pulp testing should be performed prior to doing this. Pulpal sensibility testing is difficult in the emergency situation but it is helpful, as such tests have a strong predictive value for later pulp healing complications. For this reason it is important to carry out a sensibility test within the first week after trauma to establish a point of reference for evaluating pulpal status at later follow-up examinations.

Radiographic examination of TDI

This is an overview of suitable examinations for patients who have been subjected to dentoalveolar trauma.

Dental films

All injured teeth should be examined radiographically to diagnose injuries and to reveal the stage of root formation which is important for the choice of treatment method. The ideal method is the use of different angulations for each traumatized tooth, using a standardized projection technique. Thus, a traumatized anterior region of the maxilla is covered by one occlusal film, projected steeply superiorly, and three periapical exposures perpendicular to the long axes of the teeth, where the central beam is directed between the central incisors and for each lateral incisor. This procedure ensures diagnosis of even minor dislocations or root fractures. It is important to bear in mind that a steep occlusal exposure is of special value in the diagnosis of root fractures and lateral luxations with oral displacement of the crown.

Most root fractures are disclosed by radiographic examination provided that they are steeply superiorly projected. A widening of the periodontal space is seen in lateral and extrusive luxations, whereas intruded teeth often demonstrate a lack of periodontal space.

Extraoral radiographs may be of value for determining the direction of dislocation of intruded primary incisors. Dislocated tooth fragments within a lip laceration can be demonstrated radiographically by the use of an ordinary film placed between the dental arches and the lips (Fig. 26.11). A short exposure time is advocated for this situation.

Panoramic technique

This method gives an excellent overview of the dentoalveolar region. It is especially useful in cases where a jaw fracture is suspected.

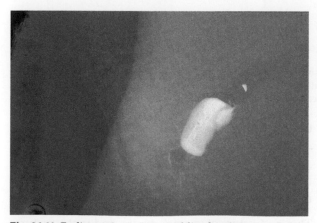

Fig. 26.11 Radiograph of a lacerated lip showing coronal fragment of a fractured incisor.

Computed tomography scanning

This is a very useful method in the diagnosis of maxillofacial fractures; however, the resolution is not high enough and radiation exposure is too high to make it useful for dental trauma diagnosis. Cone-beam CT has high enough resolution to be a valuable tool for diagnosis of different dental injuries (Fig. 26.12).

Classification and clinical findings

TDI can be classified in many ways but the following system based on World Health Organization classification, modified by Andreasen, is well suited to the clinical situation; following this system facilitates treatment.

Injuries to the hard dental tissues and the pulp

A schematic overview of hard tissue injuries is presented in Figure 26.13.

Crown infraction

This is incomplete fracture of the enamel without loss of tooth substance (Fig. 26.13a mesial side). Various patterns of craze lines can be detected depending on the location and direction of trauma, e.g. vertical, horizontal, or oblique lines.

Uncomplicated crown fracture

This is a fracture with loss of tooth substance (Fig. 26.13a distal and Fig. 26.13b). It involves enamel or enamel and dentin without pulp exposure. The exposed

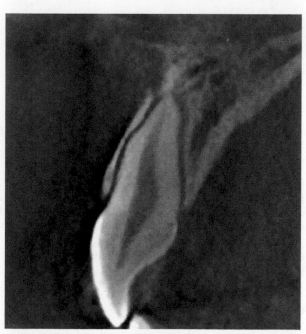

Fig. 26.12 Cone-beam CT of a central incisor showing a lateral luxation with fracture of the labial bone plate. From Andreasen *et al.* 2007.

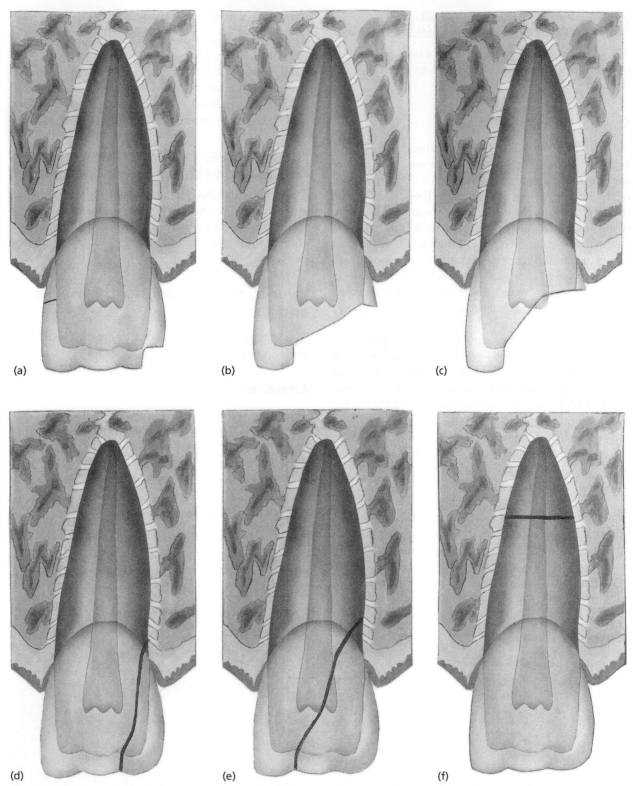

(a)   (b)   (c)

(d)   (e)   (f)

Fig. 26.13 Injuries to the hard dental tissues and pulp. (a) Crown infraction and uncomplicated fracture without involvement of dentin. (b) Uncomplicated crown fracture with involvement of dentin. (c) Complicated crown fracture. (d) Uncomplicated crown–root fracture. (e) Complicated crown–root fracture. (f) Root fracture. From Andreasen *et al.* 2007.

dentin usually gives rise to symptoms such as sensitivity to hot and cold stimuli and mastication.

Complicated crown fracture

This is a fracture with loss of enamel and dentin with pulp exposure (Fig. 26.13c). The exposed pulp often gives rise to pain and sensitivity.

Uncomplicated crown–root fracture

This is a fracture of enamel, dentin, and root structure without pulp exposure (Fig. 26.13d).

Complicated crown–root fracture

This is a fracture of enamel, dentin, and root structure with pulp exposure (Fig. 26.13e). Vitality testing is usually positive. Even with pulp exposure, symptoms are usually few and limited to pain upon heat and cold exposure when touching the fragment or biting on the fragment.

Root fracture

This is a horizontal root fracture comprising dentin, cementum, and pulp (Fig. 26.13f). The fracture is located within the alveolus. The coronal fragment may be mobile and displaced. The tooth might be slightly extruded and tender to percussion.

Injuries to the periodontal tissues

A schematic overview of injuries to the periodontal tissues is presented in Figure 26.14.

Concussion

This is an injury to the tooth-supporting structure without abnormal loosening or displacement of the tooth (Fig. 26.14a). The tooth has not been displaced and does not have increased mobility. It is tender to touch or tapping.

Subluxation

Subluxation is injury to the tooth-supporting structure with abnormal loosening, but without displacement of the tooth (Fig. 26.14b). The tooth is tender to touch or tapping and has increased mobility. There might be bleeding from the gingival sulcus.

Extrusive luxation (extrusion)

This is partial displacement of the tooth out of its socket (Fig. 26.14c). The tooth appears elongated and is excessively mobile. There is bleeding from the gingival sulcus.

Lateral luxation

Displacement of the tooth occurs in a direction other than axially (Fig. 26.14d). The tooth is displaced in its socket, most commonly with the crown in a retroclined position. The tooth is most often immobile due to its locked position in the socket and there is a high ankylotic percussion tone.

Intrusive luxation (intrusion)

The tooth has been displaced axially into the alveolar bone through the alveolar socket (Fig. 26.14e). The crown appears shortened. There is usually bleeding from the gingiva. Percussion tone is high and metallic similar to that of an ankylosed tooth. The percussion tone can be used to distinguish an intruded tooth from a partially erupted or unerupted tooth.

Avulsion (exarticulation, total luxation)

This is complete displacement of the tooth out of its socket (Fig. 26.14f, Fig. 26.15; see also Fig. 26.20). There is bleeding from the socket, which is empty.

Treatment

An overview on the treatment that should be carried out for permanent teeth is given under the individual headings for the emergency situation. The treatment recommended is according to the International Association of Dental Traumatology (IADT) guidelines, which are regularly updated on the internet (www.iadt-dentaltrauma.org). Another very informative web page is the Dental Trauma Guide (www.dentaltraumaguide.org), which presents an interactive guide for diagnosis and treatment of TDI. For more detailed information regarding treatment after the emergency situation see current textbooks and manuals.

Infraction

No treatment is necessary. In case of marked infractions, they might later be sealed with resin to prevent future discoloration.

Crown fracture

Uncomplicated crown fracture

If the fracture is confined to enamel; a slight grinding or smoothening of sharp edges may be sufficient. With more extensive loss of enamel, a composite restoration is necessary as contouring is not sufficient. If the enamel fragment is available it can be bonded to the tooth. Fracture comprising dentin and enamel and the fragment is found: the fragment can immediately or later be bonded to the tooth (Fig. 26.16). If the decision is made perform the bonding later, it is important to cover the exposed dentin with a thin layer of, for example, glass ionomer cement or other restorative material. Save the fragment by keeping it moist in saline. Fracture comprising dentin and enamel but the fragment is not found: the exposed dentin should be covered with glass ionomer as an emergency treatment. It is possible to make a permanent composite restoration using a bonding agent in the emergency situation, or this treatment can be performed at a later stage.

Complicated crown fracture

Exposed vital pulp
Open root apex
In young patients with immature, still developing roots it is very important to preserve pulp vitality by pulpotomy; this technique-sensitive procedure can be

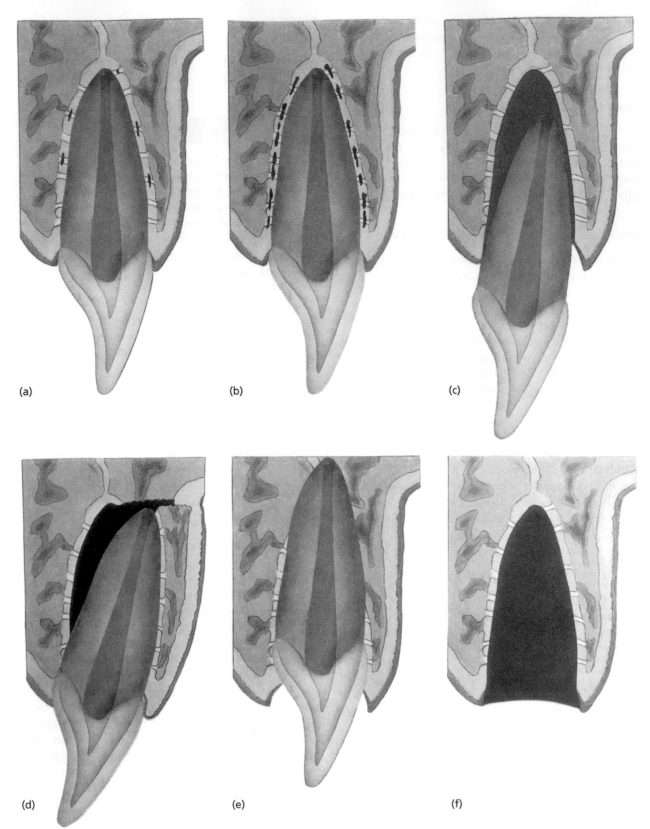

Fig. 26.14 Injuries to the periodontal tissues. (a) Concussion. (b) Subluxation. (c) Extrusive luxation. (d) Lateral luxation. (e) Intrusive luxation. (f) Avulsion. From Andreasen *et al.* 2007.

performed later, when optimal facilities are available. In the emergency phase pulp capping with calcium hydroxide can be performed.

Pulpotomy is performed by removal of 1–2 mm of the exposed pulp tissue below the exposure site. The pulp is removed using a sterile round diamond bur in a high-speed handpiece then irrigated with sterile saline. After hemostasis, $Ca(OH)_2$ or white mineral trioxide aggregate (MTA) can be applied. A thin layer of glass ionomer is placed to achieve a tight seal.

Composite restoration can be performed either in the emergency phase or later. If the crown fragment is available, bonding of the crown fragment to the tooth can be performed.

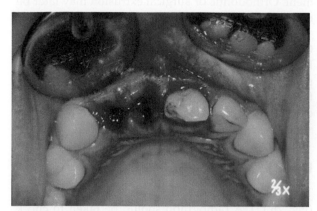

Fig. 26.15 Avulsed right central and lateral incisor.

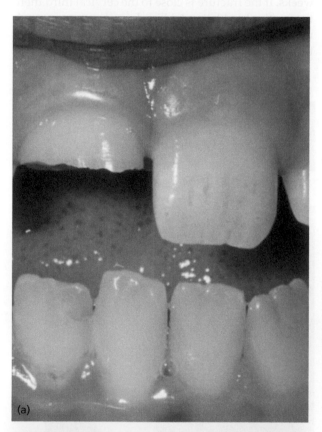

(a)

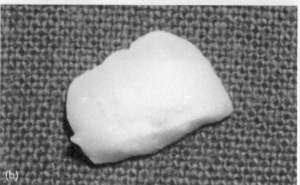

(b)

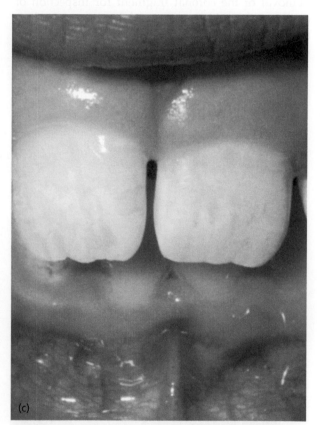

(c)

Fig. 26.16 (a) Crown fractured right central incisor. (b) Tooth fragment found. (c) Fragment bonded back to its original position using a dentin-bonding technique.

Closed root apex

In young patients when crown substance loss is not too extensive, pulp capping or pulpotomy can be performed. If there is severe loss of crown substance or if too much time has elapsed between the injury and treatment, pulp extirpation is carried out and $Ca(OH)_2$ placed to save the tooth in the emergency phase. Root canal treatment is carried out later.

Necrotic pulp
Open root apex

An apexification procedure is performed using $Ca(OH)_2$ paste or a root-end closure procedure is performed using MTA. Follow-up is important.

Closed root apex

Canal debridement is carried out and $Ca(OH)_2$ is applied; root canal treatment is completed within 2 weeks.

Crown–root fracture

Uncomplicated crown–root fracture

Removal of the coronal fragment for careful inspection of the fracture level is necessary in order to take a final decision on whether restoration is possible for the remaining fragment. This can be done in the emergency phase. An alternative in the emergency phase is to temporary stabilize the coronal fragment to the tooth by bonding. The definitive treatment depends on the extent of the fracture. To later restore the tooth, gingivectomy, ostectomy, or orthodontic extrusion may later be required. Surgical extrusion is not recommended because of risk of devitalizing the pulp. If post space is required, elective root canal treatment should be carried out.

Complicated crown–root fracture

Removal of the coronal fragment for inspection of the fracture level is necessary. If there is a deep fracture or longitudinal fracture making the tooth non-restorable, extraction of the tooth must be performed.

Pulp treatment
Closed root apex

Pulp extirpation and Ca(OH)₂ application is the first alternative in teeth with completed root development. Orthodontic or surgical extrusion may later be required to enable restoration of the tooth.

Open root apex

Regardless of the size of the exposure a superficial pulp, pulp capping or partial pulpotomy is performed. To restore the tooth later, gingivectomy, ostectomy, orthodontic extrusion, or surgical extrusion can be performed.

Root fracture

The displaced coronal fragment may be repositioned (Fig. 26.17). A radiograph should be taken to check for correct repositioning. The tooth is splinted for 4 weeks. If the fracture is close to the cervical third then the tooth should be stabilized for longer (up to 4 months). Root canal treatment is not performed in the emergency phase of the treatment, because pulp

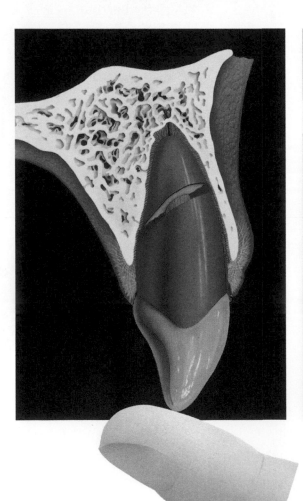
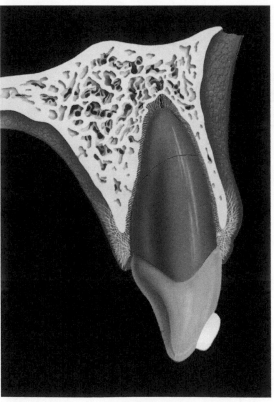

Fig. 26.17 Treatment of root fracture by repositioning the coronal fragment and splinting. From Andreasen *et al.* 2007.

healing is possible, even in cases with discoloration of the coronal fragment. Signs of pulp necrosis are watched for at follow-up visits. If pulp necrosis later develops then root canal treatment of the coronal segment is performed, as the apical fragment normally contains vital pulp tissue.

Concussion

No treatment is needed. However, the injury should be documented in the records for follow-up purposes or later insurance claims.

Subluxation

Splinting is generally not necessary but a flexible splint to stabilize the tooth for patient comfort can be used for up to 2 weeks.

Lateral luxation

The tooth is repositioned manually with a finger in the vestibule, or with forceps to disengage it from its bony lock and gently reposition it into its original location (Fig. 26.18). The tooth is stabilized for 4 weeks using a flexible splint. The pulpal condition is monitored in the weeks after trauma. If the pulp becomes necrotic, root canal treatment is indicated to prevent root resorption. In immature, developing teeth, revascularization can be confirmed radio-graphically by evidence of continued root formation and possibly by positive sensibility testing.

Extrusive luxation (extrusion)

Extruded teeth should be manually repositioned in the tooth socket and stabilized for 2 weeks using a flexible splint.

Intrusive luxation (intrusion)

Teeth with incomplete root formation
Spontaneous re-eruption is allowed to take place. If no movement is noted within 3 weeks, rapid orthodontic repositioning is recommended. If the teeth is intruded more than 7 mm, reposition surgically or orthodontically (Fig. 26.19).

Teeth with completed root formation
- If tooth is intruded less than 3 mm allow spontaneous eruption.
- If no movement after 2–4 weeks, reposition surgically or orthodontically to avoid ankylosis.
- If tooth is intruded 3–7 mm, the tooth should ideally be repositioned orthodontically or surgically as soon as possible (Fig. 26.19).
- If the tooth is intruded more than 7 mm, surgical repositioning is the treatment of first choice.
- If the tooth has been repositioned, stabilize with a flexible splint for 4–8 weeks.

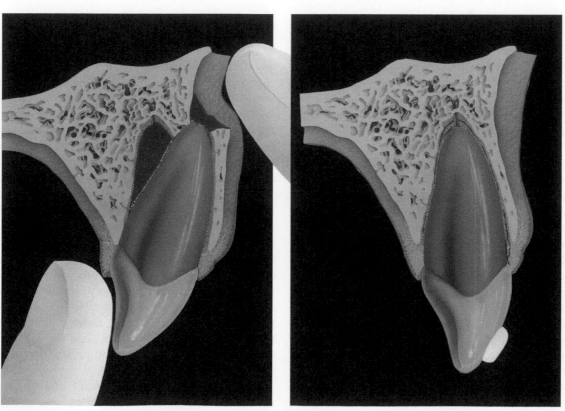

Fig. 26.18 Treatment principle for lateral luxation: repositioning and splinting. From Andreasen *et al.* 2007.

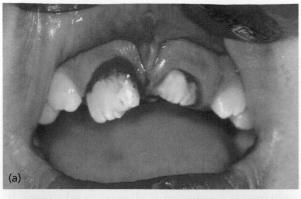
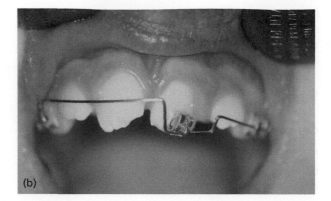
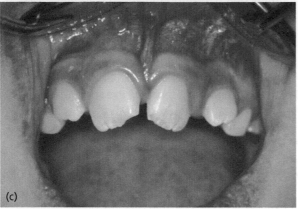

Fig. 26.19 (a) Intruded left central incisor. (b) Orthodontic repositioning. (c) Final result after 2 months.

Avulsion

See Figure 26.20.

Advice immediately after the accident

An avulsed permanent tooth is a very critical injury since the prognosis depends very much on what is done immediately after the injury. Clinicians should always be prepared to give appropriate advice to the public. Instructions may have to be given by telephone to the patient or other people at the place of accident, e.g. parents, guardians, teachers, etc. The following instructions should be given:

1. Make sure it is a permanent tooth. (Primary teeth should not be replanted because of the risk of injury to the underlying permanent tooth.)
2. Keep the patient calm.
3. Find the tooth and pick it up by the crown (the white part) and avoid touching the root.
4. If the tooth is dirty, wash it briefly (max 10 seconds) under cool running water and reposition it. Try to encourage the patient/guardian to replant the tooth. Hold it in position or bite on a handkerchief.
5. If this is not possible, place the tooth in a suitable storage medium, e.g. a glass of milk or in saline. The tooth can also be transported in the mouth, keeping it between the molars and the inside of the cheek if the patient is conscious, or spit in a container and store the tooth in saliva. Avoid storage in water.

6. If there is access to special storage media (tissue culture/transport medium, Hank's balanced salt solution (HBSS) or saline) such media can preferably be used.
7. Seek emergency dental treatment immediately.

At the clinic

A patient may come to the clinic with the tooth already replanted or with the tooth outside the mouth stored in a medium. Treatment must be related to the status of the root development (closed or open apex) and the status of the periodontal ligament cells. Assessing these factors is of utmost importance in the emergency situation for the choice of correct treatment. If the tooth has been immediately replanted or replanted within the first hour, or stored in a suitable storage medium, such as milk, saliva, or a special storage medium, there is a chance for healing. However, if the tooth has been stored dry for more than 1 hour the periodontal ligament cells will be necrotic, healing with normal periodontal ligament cannot be expected, and the tooth will be subjected to later root resorption. Such teeth should still, in the majority of cases, be replanted in the emergency phase and final decisions on more definitive treatment should be taken at a later stage when all factors can be taken into consideration and preferably in a multidisciplinary approach.

For the clinician it is important first to roughly assess the condition of the cells by classifying the avulsed tooth into one of the following categories:

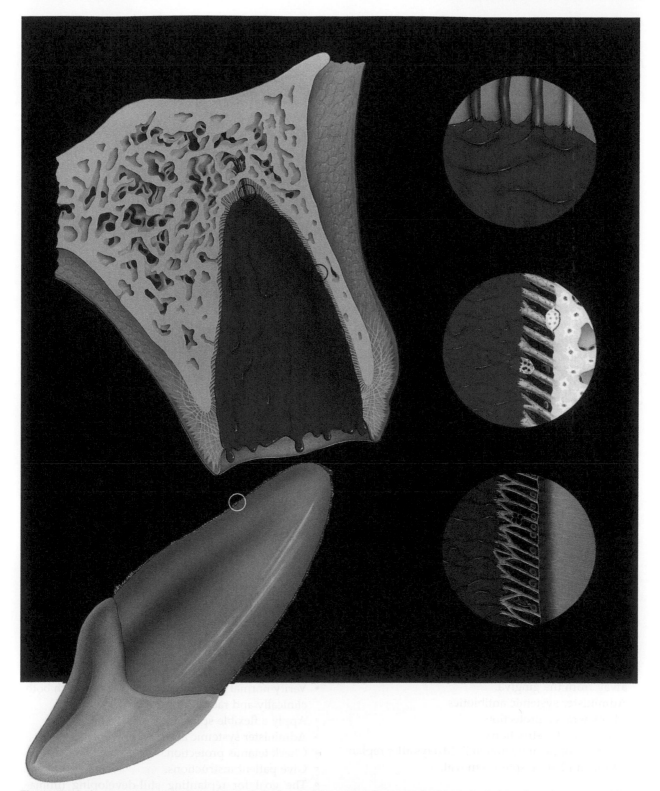

Fig. 26.20 Mechanism of avulsion. Frontal impacts lead to avulsion with subsequent damage to both the pulp and periodontal ligament (PDL). The vascular supply of the pulp is interrupted, the PDL attaching to the alveolar socket and the root surface is damaged. The extraoral time and environment determine the fate of the PDL and pulp after replantation. From Andreasen *et al.* 2007.

1. The PDL cells are most likely viable (i.e. the tooth has been replanted immediately or after a very short time at the place of accident).
2. The PDL cells may be viable but compromised. The tooth has been kept in storage medium (e.g. tissue culture medium, HBSS, saline, milk or

saliva) and the total drying time is less than 60 minutes.
3. The PDL cells are non-viable. Total extra oral dry storage time is more than 60 minutes, regardless of additional storage medium, or if the storage medium was non-physiologic.

Avulsed permanent tooth with *closed apex*

The tooth has been replanted before the patients arrival at the clinic

- Leave the tooth in place;
- Clean the area with water spray, saline, or chlorhexidine;
- Suture gingival lacerations, if present;
- Verify normal position of the replanted tooth both clinically and radiographically;
- Apply a flexible splint for up to 2 weeks;
- Administer systemic antibiotics;
- Check tetanus protection;
- Give patient instructions;
- Initiate root canal treatment 7–10 days after replantation and before splint removal.

The tooth has been kept in a physiologic storage medium or osmolality balanced medium and if also stored dry, the extraoral dry time is less than 60 minutes

Physiologic storage media include, for example, tissue culture medium and cell transport media. Examples of *osmolality balanced media* are HBSS, saline and milk. Saliva can also be used.

- Clean the root surface and apical foramen with a stream of saline and soak the tooth in saline thereby removing contamination and dead cells from the root surface.
- Administer local anesthesia.
- Irrigate the socket with saline.
- Examine the alveolar socket. If there is a fracture of the socket wall, reposition it with a suitable instrument.
- Replant the tooth slowly with slight digital pressure. Do not use force.
- Suture gingival lacerations, if present.
- Verify normal position of the replanted tooth both clinically and radiographically.
- Apply a flexible splint for up to 2 weeks, keep away from the gingiva.
- Administer systemic antibiotics.
- Check tetanus protection.
- Give patient instructions.
- Initiate root canal treatment 7–10 days after replantation and before splint removal.

Dry time longer than 60 minutes or other reasons suggesting non-viable cells

Delayed replantation has a poor long-term prognosis. The periodontal ligament will be necrotic and not expected to heal. The goal in delayed replantation is, in addition to restoring the tooth for aesthetic, functional and psychological reasons, to maintain alveolar bone contour. However, the expected eventual outcome is ankylosis and resorption of the root and the tooth will be lost eventually.

The technique for delayed replantation is:

- Remove attached non-viable soft tissue carefully e.g. with gauze. The best way to this has not yet been decided.
- Root canal treatment to the tooth can be carried out prior to replantation or later.
- In cases of delayed replantation, root canal treatment should be done either on the tooth prior to replantation, or it can be done 7–10 days later like in other replantation situations
- Administer local anesthesia.
- Irrigate the socket with saline.
- Examine the alveolar socket. If there is a fracture of the socket wall, reposition it with a suitable instrument.
- Replant the tooth.
- Suture gingival lacerations, if present.
- Verify normal position of the replanted tooth clinically and radiographically.
- Stabilize the tooth for 4 weeks using a flexible splint.
- Administration of systemic antibiotics.
- Check tetanus protection.
- Give patient instructions.

In order to slow down osseous replacement of the tooth, treatment of the root surface with fluoride prior to replantation has earlier been suggested (2% sodium fluoride solution for 20 min) but it should not be seen as an absolute recommendation.

Avulsed permanent tooth with an *open apex*

The tooth has been replanted prior to the patients arrival at the clinic

- Leave the tooth in place.
- Clean the area with water spray, saline or chlorhexidine.
- Suture gingival lacerations, if present.
- Verify normal position of the replanted tooth both clinically and radiographically.
- Apply a flexible splint for up to 2 weeks.
- Administer systemic antibiotics.
- Check tetanus protection.
- Give patient instructions.
- The goal for replanting still-developing (immature) teeth in children is to allow for possible revascularization of the pulp space. If that does not occur, root canal treatment may be recommended.

The tooth has been kept in physiologic storage medium or osmolality balanced medium and if also stored dry the extraoral dry time is less than 60 minutes

Physiologic storage media include e.g. tissue culture medium and cell transport media. Examples of *osmo-*

lality balanced media are HBSS, saline, milk. Saliva can also be used.

- If contaminated, clean the root surface and apical foramen with a stream of saline.
- Topical application of antibiotics has been shown to enhance chances for revascularization of the pulp and can be considered if available.
- Administer local anesthesia.
- Examine the alveolar socket.
- If there is a fracture of the socket wall, reposition it with a suitable instrument.
- Remove the coagulum in the socket and replant the tooth slowly with slight digital pressure.
- Suture gingival lacerations, especially in the cervical area.
- Verify normal position of the replanted tooth clinically and radiographically. Apply a flexible splint for up to 2 weeks.
- Administer systemic antibiotics.
- Check tetanus protection.
- Give patient instructions.
- The goal for replanting still-developing (immature) teeth in children is to allow for possible revascularization of the pulp space. The risk of infection-related root resorption should be weighed up against the chances of revascularization. Such resorption is very rapid in teeth of children. If revascularization does not occur, root canal treatment may be recommended.

Dry time longer than 60 minutes or other reasons suggesting non-viable cells

Delayed replantation has a poor long-term prognosis. The periodontal ligament will be necrotic and not expected to heal. The goal in delayed replantation is to restore the tooth to the dentition for aesthetic, functional and psychological reasons and to maintain alveolar bone crest contour. The eventual outcome, however, will be ankylosis and resorption of the root.

The technique for delayed replantation is:

- Remove attached non-viable soft tissue carefully e.g. with gauze.
- Root canal treatment to the tooth can be carried out prior to replantation or later
- Administer local anesthesia.
- Remove the coagulum from the socket with a stream of saline. Examine the alveolar socket. If there is a fracture of the socket wall, reposition it with a suitable instrument.
- Replant the tooth slowly with slight digital pressure. Suture gingival laceration. Verify normal position of the replanted tooth clinically and radiographically.
- Stabilize the tooth for 4 weeks using a flexible splint.
- Administer systemic antibiotics.
- Check tetanus protection.
- Give patient instructions.

It is beyond the scope of this book to cover complications and follow-up. For more detailed information regarding follow-up and complications we refer to textbooks and manuals of dental traumatology or recent IADT guidelines (www.iadt-dentaltrauma .org) or visit the web page Dental Trauma Guide (www.dentaltraumaguide.org – see Recommended reading).

Splinting of TDI

After emergency treatment of TDI where teeth and/ or root fragments have been repositioned, there is a need for splinting to stabilize the injured tooth in the initial healing period. However, splinting may also have adverse effects on healing, such as increased risk for ankylosis and osseous replacement resorption or compromised revascularization of the pulp if splinting is not done well. Bars used for maxillomandibular fixation in jaw fracture treatment are not suitable for splinting of luxated or replanted teeth because there is a risk for extrusion of teeth because the preformed bar does not have any occlusal curve built in. Hence, the preformed bar will extrude any repositioned luxated anterior teeth.

Since the discovery of adhesive techniques, dental splints have been made by an acid-etched bonding technique which fulfills most requirements of a modern splint. An optimal splint should enable the injured tooth to move slightly during the healing phase. This can be achieved either by the splint being flexible, by combining the bonding material with a wire to allow for flexibility, or by not stretching out the splint too far.

The bonding material can be combined with a steel wire, twist flex wire, nylon fishing line, fiberglass or titanium splint. Some examples of splints can be seen in Figures 26.21, 26.22 and 26.23. The splinting period should ideally be related to the type of TDI. The periods shown in Table 26.1 have been recommended by an expert group of IADT.

TDI in the primary dentition

Similar diagnosis and classification principles are applied to primary teeth. However, the treatment of primary teeth is often modified and consideration must always be given to the underlying permanent tooth germs. For this reason primary teeth must never be replanted. Moreover, a primary tooth that has been dislocated in the direction of the permanent underlying tooth germ should be extracted, while dislocation away from the underlying tooth germ may allow the primary tooth to be repositioned and kept. A primary tooth should not be kept if it poses a risk for the permanent tooth because of infection. Other modifying factors when treating traumatized

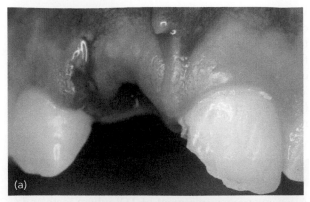

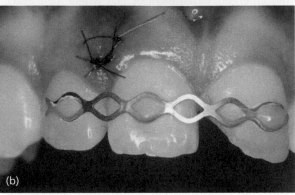

Fig. 26.21 Titanium trauma splint. (Courtesy of Dr von Arx, Bern, Switzerland.)

primary teeth are maturity of the child, caries, tooth development, occlusion, and time for exfoliation. For more detailed information regarding treatment of primary teeth after trauma, see textbooks and manuals of dental traumatology or recent IADT guidelines for primary teeth (free download at www.iadt-dentaltrauma.org or visit the interactive web page Dental Trauma Guide: www.dentaltrauma guide.org).

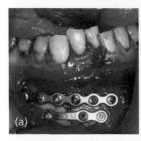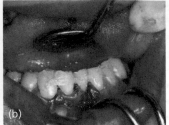

Fig. 26.22 Patient with mandibular body fracture and luxated incisors. (a) The mandibular fracture has been splinted by plate and screw osteosynthesis. (b) A separate fiberglass splint has been applied to the luxated and repositioned teeth. The use of separate splints will enable optimized splinting time and type.

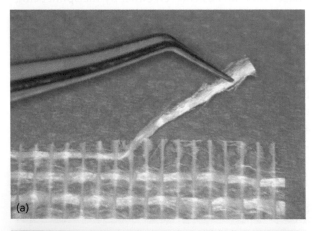

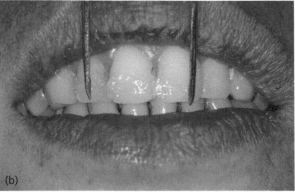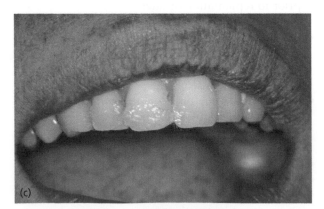

Fig. 26.23 Splinting using fiberglass and resin. (a) A string of fiberglass. (b) The fiberglass is bonded to the acid-etched enamel of the luxated tooth and the adjacent teeth. (c) Finished splint.

Table 26.1 Splinting periods for various TDI requiring fixation.

TDI	Splinting period
Subluxation	(2 weeks)
Extrusive luxation	2 weeks
Avulsion	2 weeks
Lateral luxation	4 weeks
Intrusion (if surgically repositioned)	4–8 weeks
Root fracture (middle third)	4 weeks
Root fracture (cervical third)	4 months

Summary

TDI occur frequently and are often seen simultaneously with other oral and maxillofacial injuries. The prognosis for some TDI is highly dependent on prompt and correct emergency management. Hence the clinicians in oral and maxillofacial surgery should have knowledge to manage dental injuries in the emergency phase. This chapter has presented the basic knowledge needed for such management.

Recommended reading

Andersson L. (2013) Epidemiology of traumatic dental injuries. *Journal of Endodotics*, **201**, 39(3 Suppl), S2–5.

Andersson L, Andreasen JO. (2010) In: Traumatic dental injuries. In: *Oral and Maxillofacial Surgery*. (eds, Andersson L, Kahnberg K-E, Pogrel MA). Oxford, Wiley-Blackwell.

Andreasen JO, Andreasen FM, Andersson L, eds. (2007) *Textbook and Color Atlas of Traumatic Injuries to the Teeth*, 4th edn. Oxford, Blackwell Publishing.

Andreasen JO, Andreasen FM, Bakland LK, Flores MT, Andersson L. (2011) *Traumatic Dental Injuries: a Manual*, 3rd edn. Oxford, Wiley.

Dental Trauma Guide. Online. Available from: <www.dentaltraumaguide.org> [18 November 2013].

DiAngelis AJ, Andreasen JO, Ebeleseder K, *et al.* (2012) International Association of Dental Traumatology guidelines for the management of traumatic dental injuries: 1. Fractures and luxations of permanent teeth. *Dental Traumatology*, **28**, 2–12.

Glendor U, Andersson L. (2007) Public health aspects of oral diseases and disorders: dental trauma. In: *Community Oral Health* (eds, Pine C, Harris R). Pp 203–11. London, Quintessence Publishing.

International Association of Dental Traumatology. Online. Available from: <www.iadt-dentaltrauma.org> [18 November 2013].

Malmgren B, Andreasen JO, Flores MT, *et al.* (2012) International Association of Dental Traumatology guidelines for the management of traumatic dental injuries: 3. Injuries in the primary dentition. *Dental Traumatology*, **28**, 174–82.

Petersson EE, Andersson L, Sörensen S. (1997) Traumatic oral vs non-oral injuries. An epidemiological study during one year in a Swedish county. *Swedish Dental Journal*, **21**, 55–68.

Chapter 27

Maxillofacial Bone Fractures

Evaluation of patient with maxillofacial injuries

Maxillofacial fractures are often seen in combination with more severe, sometimes life-threatening, injuries, and often require hospital resources. When a trauma patient with maxillofacial injuries arrives in a hospital emergency room, life-threatening injuries must be addressed first. In most hospitals today there are trauma teams with many specialists participating. Specialists dealing with trauma patients undergo special training and work according to guidelines for advanced trauma life support (ATLS), where the principle is treating the greatest threat of life first and indicated life-threatening emergency treatment should not wait for definite diagnosis. Airways must first be secured, either by inserting a nasopharyngeal or oropharyngeal airway. Sometimes an endotracheal intubation, or even surgical access to the trachea, has to be performed. Excessive bleeding must be stopped and evaluation of neurological injuries and the cervical spine are important at an early stage. The patient must be stabilized and the vital signs, such as pulse and blood pressure, checked before all regions of the body are carefully evaluated.

After the lifesaving phase, a brief history can be taken from the patient, if conscious. However, if the patient is unconscious an accompanying person or a witness to the accident may give some information. It is important to register when, where and how the injury occurred as well as symptoms and changes. The patient may guide you to the correct examination if you listen to their history carefully. It is also important to obtain a medical history with information about, for example, medication and allergies.

A full maxillofacial examination is performed which includes the facial skeleton, scalp, eyes, ears, nose and oral cavity. Examining and treating the oral and maxillofacial region must be done in a sequential way. The principle is to examine from outside towards inside, whereas treatment of the oral and maxillofacial region is best performed from inside towards outside, if possible.

The evaluation comprises inspection and palpation. Vision, pupils and ocular movements may indicate injuries in the orbital region. Motoric function of facial muscles and masticatory muscles and sensoric evaluation of the facial region is performed. Inspection for hematoma and ecchymoses is included in the examination (Fig. 27.1) and palpation of all bone margins and rims, looking for tenderness or steps in bone contours or crepitation sounds. The naso-orbital-ethmoidal (NOE) region is carefully assessed for hematoma, telecanthus (widening of intercanthal distance medially) or changes in the lateral canthus indicating fracture (Fig. 27.2). The mandibular opening capacity is assessed and the TMJ region is palpated. Finally, the intraoral examination is carried out with inspection for hematomas, teeth and occlusion and palpation of the alveolar process. For evaluation and treatment of traumatic dental injuries and soft tissue injuries, see Chapters 26 and 28, respectively.

Mandibular bone fractures

Fractures of the mandible comprise 10–25% of all facial fractures. Figure 27.3 depicts the percentage of mandibular fractures based on anatomic location. The condyle, angle and body are the most common anatomic locations. Frequent combinations of multiple mandibular fractures are angle and contralateral body, bilateral angle or body, and condylar and contralateral body.

Essentials of Oral and Maxillofacial Surgery, First Edition. Edited by M. Anthony Pogrel, Karl-Erik Kahnberg and Lars Andersson.
© 2014 John Wiley & Sons, Ltd. Published 2014 by John Wiley & Sons, Ltd.
Companion website: www.wiley.com/go/pogrel/oms

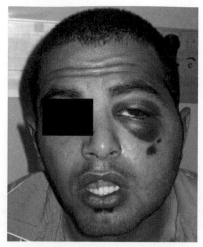

Fig. 27.1 Edema, periorbital hematoma, and temporal subconjunctival suffusion develop shortly after zygomatico-maxillary complex fracture (ZMC) fracture.

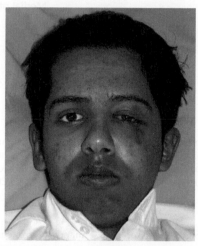

Fig. 27.2 Downward slant of the palpebral fissure in the horizontal plane as a consequence of displacement of lateral palpebral canthus.

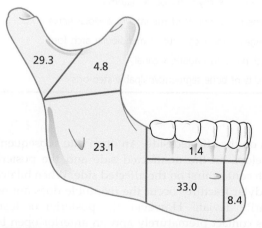

Fig. 27.3 Percentage of mandibular fractures based on anatomic location. (From Chacon G, Larsen P. (2004) Principles of management of mandibular fractures. In: *Peterson's Principles of Oral and Maxillofacial Surgery* (ed, Miloro M), 2nd edn, Vol. 1, p. 413. Decker Inc., Hamilton, Ontario. Reproduced with permission.)

Classification and terms of mandibular fractures

Mandibular fractures are classified and named after anatomic region or fracture pattern and there are also terms associated specifically with temporomandibular joint (TMJ) fractures (Table 27.1). Angle and body fractures can be classified as favorable or non-favorable.

Table 27.1 Classification of mandibular fractures.

Anatomic region

Symphysis – fracture involving the area between the lateral incisors extending vertically through the inferior border of the mandible

Parasymphysis – fracture between the mental foramen and the mesial aspect of the canine extending through the inferior border of the mandible

Body – fracture between the mental foramen and the distal aspect of the second molar extending through the inferior border of the mandible

Angle – fracture between the distal aspect of the second molar and the posterior attachment of the masseter muscle extending through the inferior border of the mandible

Ramus – fracture extending horizontally through the anterior and posterior borders of the ramus or extending vertically from the sigmoid notch to the inferior border of the mandible distal to the second molar

Condylar process – fracture extending from the sigmoid notch to the posterior border of the ramus

Coronoid process – fracture involving the coronoid process

Alveolar – fracture confined to the tooth-bearing segment of bone

Fracture pattern

Greenstick – fracture through one cortex and no discontinuity of bone. No mobility of fractured segments. Common in children

Simple – fracture does not communicate with the external environment. A closed fracture

Compound – fracture communicates with the external environment either through the skin or the periodontal ligament of a tooth. An open fracture

Comminuted – multiple segments of bone as a result of greater force from the trauma

Complex – fracture involving damage to adjacent structures

Telescoped or impacted – one fractured segment is driven into the other segment

Pathologic – fracture resulting from normal function in an area of diseased bone

Terms associated with temporomandibular joint (TMJ) fractures

Displaced – movement of the condylar (proximal) segment relative to the remainder of the mandible. Although the condyle is malpositioned, it is still within the confines of the glenoid fossa and has not ruptured the capsule of the TMJ

Dislocated – the condylar (proximal) segment is no longer within the confines of the glenoid fossa

Extracapsular – fracture not involving the capsule of the TMJ

Intracapsular – fracture occurring within the TMJ capsule

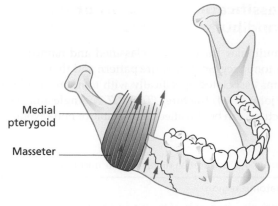

Fig. 27.4 Horizontally favorable fracture. (From Barber HD, Bahram R, *et al*. (2005) Mandible fractures. In: *Oral and Maxillofacial Trauma* (eds, Fonseca R, Walker RV, *et al*.), 3rd edn. Vol. 1, p. 488. Elsevier Saunders, St Louis. Copyright © 2005 Elsevier.)

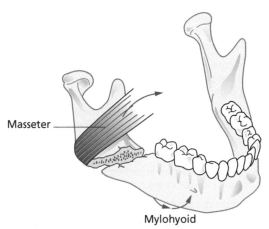

Fig. 27.5 Horizontally unfavorable fracture. (From Barber HD, Bahram R, *et al*. (2005) Mandible fractures. In: *Oral and Maxillofacial Trauma* (eds, Fonseca R, Walker RV, *et al*.), 3rd edn. Vol. 1, p. 488. Elsevier Saunders, St Louis. Copyright © 2005 Elsevier.)

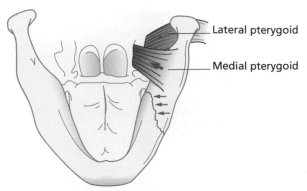

Fig. 27.6 Vertically favorable fracture. (From Barber HD, Bahram R, *et al*. (2005) Mandible fractures. In: *Oral and Maxillofacial Trauma* (eds, Fonseca R, Walker RV, *et al*.), 3rd edn. Vol. 1, p. 488. Elsevier Saunders, St Louis. Copyright © 2005 Elsevier.)

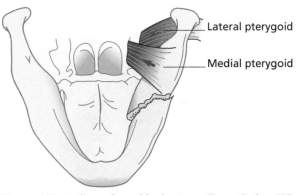

Fig. 27.7 Vertically unfavorable fracture. (From Barber HD, Bahram R, *et al*. (2005) Mandible fractures. In: *Oral and Maxillofacial Trauma* (eds, Fonseca R, Walker RV, *et al*.), 3rd edn. Vol. 1, p. 488. Elsevier Saunders, St Louis. Copyright © 2005 Elsevier.)

Table 27.2 Signs and symptoms of mandibular fractures.

Occlusal changes
Deviation on opening
Altered range of motion
Localized pain
Lacerations, ecchymosis, or hematoma
Neurosensory deficits of the inferior alveolar nerve
Changes in facial contour or mandibular arch form
Blood in external auditory canal
Mobility of bone segments/palpable step-offs

If the fracture resists the pull of the segment by the muscles it is considered a favorable fracture. If the muscles tend to pull the segments apart it is an unfavorable fracture (Figs 27.4, 27.5, 27.6, 27.7).

Patient evaluation

A number of signs and symptoms are highly suggestive of a mandibular fracture (Table 27.2). Occlusal changes are one of the most common physical findings in patients with fractures of the mandible. Occlusal changes may be the result of dental fractures, fractures of the alveolus, trauma to associated structures of the TMJ, fractures of the maxilla, or contusions of the masticatory muscles. It is important to consider that the patient may have had a pre-existing malocclusion prior to the injury.

Deviation of the mandible on opening is indicative of a condylar fracture. In a unilateral condylar fracture, the mandible deviates to the side of the fracture due to the unopposed action of the lateral pterygoid muscle on the unaffected side and the lack of transla-

tion on the affected side. An open bite subsequently develops on the unaffected side and the posterior teeth contact first on the affected side. When bilateral condylar fractures occur the mandible does not necessarily deviate. However, the posterior occlusion does contact prematurely and an anterior open bite subsequently develops.

An altered range of motion can occur with mandibular fractures. The most common cause of limited opening is from pain and reflex guarding associated with the trauma. Decreased opening also occurs when a depressed zygomatic arch fracture mechanically impinges upon the coronoid process of the mandible. Muscle contusions and edema overlying any fracture site can also contribute to limited mouth opening.

Hematoma from contusion injuries or lacerations may be associated with either dental or alveolar fractures or they may indicate an underlying mandibular fracture. A laceration to the chin should raise the surgeon's suspicion for not only a symphysis fracture, but also subcondylar fractures. Sublingual ecchymosis is also consistent for a mandibular fracture.

Imaging

When an isolated mandibular fracture is suspected, the routine radiographic assessment may consist of a panoramic radiograph. A panoramic radiograph is the single most comprehensive image and usually allows for satisfactory visualization of all regions of the mandible (condyle, ramus, body, and symphysis). It is also useful for examining the existing dentition, and showing the presence of impacted teeth with respect to the fracture, the alveolar process, and the position of the mandibular canal.

Currently, computed tomography (CT) scans offer the most detailed and comprehensive view of the facial skeleton. Current protocols allow for axial, coronal, sagittal, and even reconstructed three-dimensional (3D) images to be formatted, as shown in Figures 27.8, 27.9, 27.10 and 27.11. A CT scan is

typically reserved for cases involving complex (comminuted, avulsive, etc.) mandibular injuries or concomitant midfacial or orbital injuries. In some cases where a dislocated condylar fracture is suspected, the CT scan will allow for detailed 3D imaging.

Treatment

Mandibular fractures can be treated by closed or open reduction.

Closed reduction of mandibular fractures

Closed reduction means that the fracture is repositioned and stabilized without surgical opening. Indications for closed reduction are listed in Table 27.3. Most non-displaced stable mandibular fractures lend themselves to closed treatment. There are fewer complications when closed reduction is performed, but the balance between advantages and disadvantages of a closed versus open technique must be individualized, as it should be with the use of all evidence-based decisions.

The majority of mandibular fractures in children are best treated with closed techniques. Developing tooth buds occupy a significant portion of the mandible

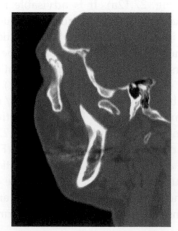

Fig. 27.10 Sagittal CT scan depicting an anteriorly displaced condylar fracture.

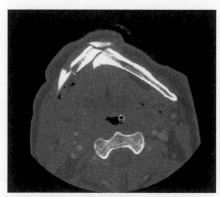

Fig. 27.8 Axial CT scan depicting comminuted symphysis fractures.

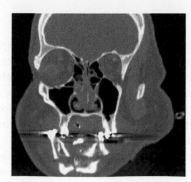

Fig. 27.9 Coronal CT scans of patient in Fig. 27.8.

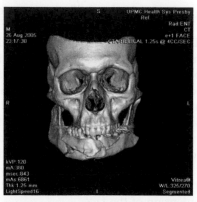

Fig. 27.11 3D reconstructed image of the patient in Figs 27.9 and 27.10. Note additional left angle and right subcondylar fractures.

Table 27.3 Indications for closed reduction techniques of mandibular fractures.

Non-displaced mandibular fracture

Grossly comminuted mandibular fracture

Atrophic edentulous mandibular fracture

Loss of soft tissue coverage over a fracture

Mandibular fractures in children

Condylar fracture

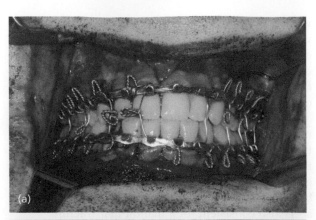

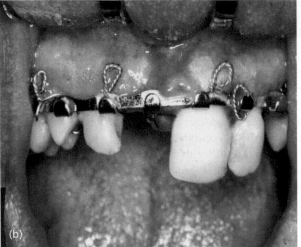

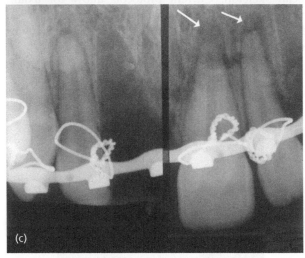

Fig. 27.12 (a) Erich arch bars and interdental stainless steel 25-gauge wires. (b,c) Displacement of an originally subluxated left central and lateral incisors by an Erich's arch bar (see arrows).

and are at risk of injury with the placement of hardware commonly used in open techniques Most studies also support the treatment of condylar fractures in both children and adults with closed techniques. Regardless of the degree of radiographic displacement of the condylar segment, closed reduction and early postoperative physical therapy achieved excellent clinical results. These same studies also concluded that no correlation exists between radiographic alignment of the fracture and postoperative function.

Closed reduction of fractures is most commonly achieved by applying arch bars to maxillary and mandibular dentition circumdental soft stainless steel wires (Fig. 27.12a). It is advisable not to use Erich bars for splinting some simultaneously occurring dental injuries. For example, repositioned and replanted and root-fractured incisors can be extruded by Erich bars, since these bars are straight and have no occlusal curve built in (Fig. 27.12b,c). In these cases it may better to give the repositioned/replanted tooth a separate splint (see Fig. 26.22). Other closed reduction methods include loops (Fig. 27.13) and intermaxillary fixation (IMF) bone screws (Fig. 27.14). Edentulous and partially edentulous patients with severe fractures may benefit from the use of splints wired around the mandible to maintain an interocclusal dimension and re-establish arch form.

Open reduction of mandibular fractures

Several clinical scenarios support the use of open reduction in the repair of mandibular fractures (Table 27.4).

A displaced and unfavorable fracture of the mandible cannot be adequately treated with maxillomandibular fixation alone. If a patient sustains multiple fractures of the facial bones and/or the mandible, open reduction of the mandibular fractures allows for a more stable foundation for further reconstruction, especially if other facial bones are involved. When bilateral condylar fractures occur in conjunction with midfacial fractures, at least one of the condylar fractures must be opened and fixated to re-establish the vertical dimension of the face.

Most condylar fractures are best treated with closed reduction for approximately 2 weeks. Then the mandible is actively mobilized to avoid an altered range of motion. When a condylar fracture occurs concurrently with another mandibular fracture, it is favorable to open the non-condylar fracture to allow for the necessary postoperative mobilization of the mandible after the 2-week period of maxillomandibular fixation.

With the advent of miniplates and bone screws, it has become widely accepted that most fractures involving the craniomaxillofacial skeleton are now

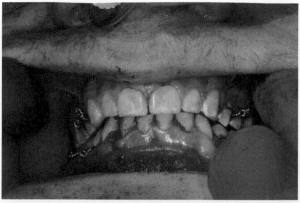

Fig. 27.13 Ivy loops made with 25-gauge stainless steel wires.

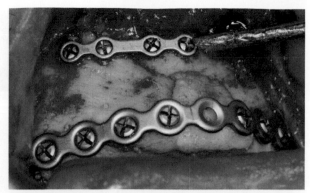

Fig. 27.15 Rigid fixation of symphysis fracture via a transoral approach.

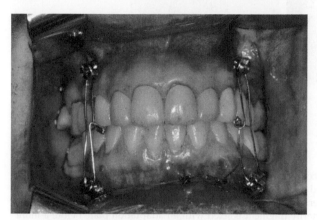

Fig. 27.14 Intermaxillary fixation (IMF) bone screws and maxillomandibular fixation wires.

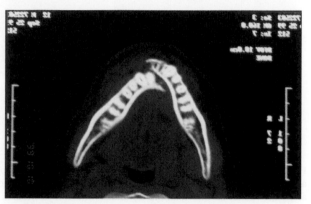

Fig. 27.16 Axial CT scan of a symphysis fracture that will be reduced and fixated with the lag screw technique.

Table 27.4 Indications for open reduction techniques of mandibular fractures.

Systemic disorders

Displaced unfavorable fractures

Multiple facial and/or mandibular fractures

Bilateral condylar fractures and midface fractures

Delayed treatment with soft tissue in between the fracture

Malunion/non-union

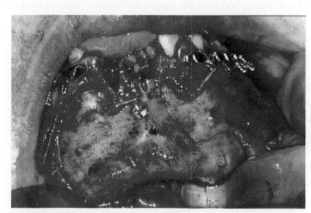

Fig. 27.17 Placement of a lag screw through the symphysis fracture in Fig. 27.16.

treated with open reduction and rigid internal fixation techniques. An open approach gives the surgeon optimal visualization of the fracture segments, therefore allowing the best possible anatomic reduction. Fractures involving the mandibular symphysis, parasymphysis, body, and occasionally the angle, may be successfully approached through a transoral approach (Fig. 27.15). There are also several techniques used to approach the mandible using an extraoral incision.

The primary advantage of rigid internal fixation is that it usually obviates the need for postoperative maxillomandibular fixation and allows for a faster return to function. Other advantages of rigid internal fixation include better anatomic reduction, greater stability across the fractured segments, improved

healing, and decreased mobility, which further reduce the incidence of infection.

An alternative technique for fixation of mandibular fractures is the lag screw technique. This technique compresses the fracture segments by placing screws through two intact and stable cortices (Figs 27.16, 27.17).

Due to recent development of endoscopic instruments, especially chip camera technology, endoscope-assisted techniques have become more widely accepted in oral and maxillofacial surgery, such as in TM)

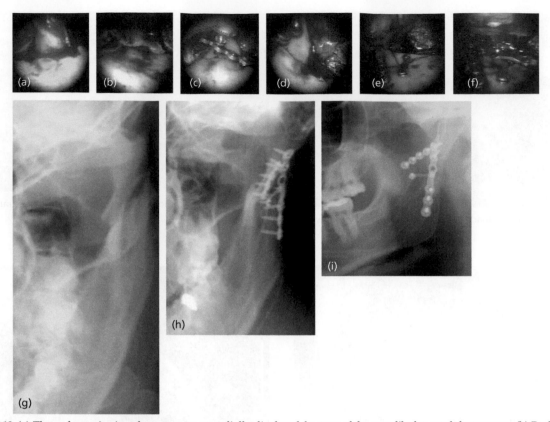

Fig. 27.18 (a) The endoscopic view demonstrates a medially displaced fracture of the mandibular condylar process. (b) By forward and downward rotation of the mandible, the TMJ area is distracted and the fragment is reduced in a lateral displacement before anatomic reduction and fixation. (c) Transoral osteosynthesis is performed using an angulated drill and screwdriver. (d) Note a butterfly fragment is missing at the posterior border. (e, f) The butterfly fragment is fixed with an adaptation plate before a more rigid plate is placed at the posterior aspect of the ascending mandibular ramus. Fracture reduction including the realignment of butterfly fragment is recommended to allow for a load-sharing situation, to reduce the stress of functional loading on the osteosynthesis. Townes' radiographs preoperatively (g), postoperatively (h), and a panoramic radiograph (i) demonstrate the displaced fracture before and after the minimally invasive reduction and fixation.

arthroscopy and sialoendoscopy. Superior visibility can be achieved through limited incisions with the transoral approach for endoscope-assisted surgical reduction of mandibular condyle fractures (Fig. 27.18). The endoscope-assisted transoral approach has developed in recent years and is today a reliable surgical approach for some displaced and dislocated condylar fractures. In non-dislocated fractures and fractures of the condylar head, non-surgical treatment still remains the treatment of choice.

Midfacial bone fractures

Midfacial skeleton as a three-dimensional structure

The midface skeleton (Fig. 27.19) is a complex structure of bone linked by sutures. The midface can be viewed as a labyrinth of air-containing cavities (Fig. 27.20). Rims constitute a system of pillars and struts resembling the framework of a building, and the position and stability of each is interrelated (Fig. 27.21). The midface buttress system comprises verti-

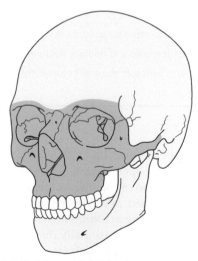

Fig. 27.19 Midfacial area highlighted.

cal, horizontal, and sagittal components. The main objective of fracture repair of the midface is the reconstruction of these buttresses using osteosynthetic devices. Most of these buttresses are robust enough bony structures to allow secure insertion of screws.

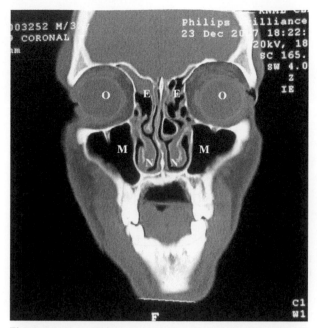

Fig. 27.20 The midface as a system of cavities: O, orbits; E, ethmoidal sinuses; M, maxillary sinuses; N, nasal cavities.

Classification

From a clinical point of view it is practical to use the classification system in Table 27.5. This is a classification based on anatomic location.

Le Fort classification system distinguishes three fracture patterns (Fig. 27.22):

- Le Fort I separates the whole complex of alveolar and palatal processes of the maxilla, horizontal plates of the palatal bones and lower parts of the pterygoid plates just above the pterygo-maxillary junction;
- Le Fort II (also known as "pyramidal" fracture) separates the whole maxilla with part of the nasal bones and the lower part of the pterygoid plates;
- Le Fort III separates both zygomatico-maxillary complexes plus the nasal bones, palatal bones and most of the pterygoid plates, from the rest of the cranium.

However, in clinical practice Le Fort types of fractures are very rarely encountered in pure forms, as described in the classification system. In most

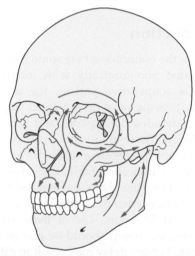

Fig. 27.21 Projection of masticatory forces through the vertical pillars of the midface.

Table 27.5 Classification of midface fractures with regards to anatomic location and clinical relevance.

Frontal bone
Zygomatic arch
Zygomatico-maxillary complex
Orbit
Nasal
Naso-orbito-ethmoidal fractures
Le Fort I, Le Fort II, Le Fort III
Maxillary sinus walls
Maxillary alveolar process
Palate

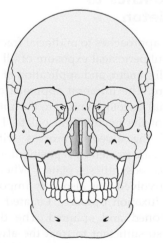
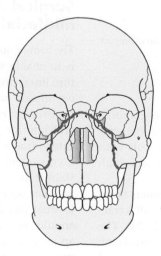
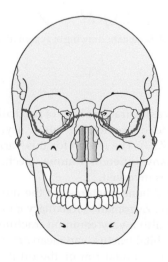

Fig. 27.22 Le Fort fracture patterns.

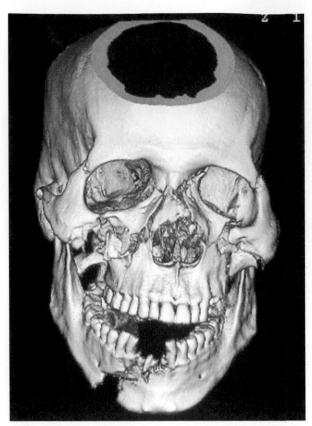

Fig. 27.23 3D CT of panfacial fracture with patterns of all three Le Fort fractures recognizable.

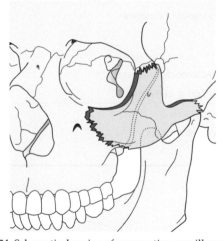

Fig. 27.24 Schematic drawing of zygomatico-maxillary complex fracture.

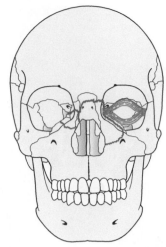

Fig. 27.25 Schematic drawing of naso-orbito-ethmoidal fracture.

instances the fracture lines of particular types combine in quite unpredictable, often asymmetric patterns (Fig. 27.23). The reason for this variability rests with the many different trauma mechanisms and high energies involved.

Nasal bone fractures are the most common facial fracture. Zygomatico-maxillary complex (ZMC) fracture is also a very common fracture (Fig. 27.24). The term orbital fracture can mean any fracture involving either the orbital rim or the orbital wall. In clinical practice it is usually understood to be a fracture of the orbital walls. Another common fracture is the naso-orbito-ethmoid (NOE) fracture (Fig. 27.25).

Open reduction

In contrast to the mandible where some fractures can still be treated non-surgically with intermaxillary fixation in a cooperative patient, the majority of midface fractures are most often treated surgically.

In recent decades bone plates and screws have been developed. These are mostly made of titanium but biodegradable plates are also used. The principle is to expose, reduce, and stabilize the fractures by rigid fixation using the plates and screws. Treatment should ideally be carried out in the emergency phase within the first 24 hours, and if these conditions cannot be met, treatment should be planned within the first week. Longer delay may result in difficulties in repositioning the fragments. To be able to do this, a surgical approach must be made.

Surgical approaches to midfacial skeleton

The aim of surgical approaches to midfacial fractures is to enable wide subperiosteal exposure of all fracture lines, precise alignment, and application of osteosynthesis hardware. The intraoral approach offers exposure of midfacial skeleton limited to the anterior and inferior parts of the maxilla and palate. Dislocated fractures of the alveolar process without involvement of teeth are treated by repositioning and stabilization with osteosynthesis plates. When the alveolar socket is involved it is also very important to treat the dental luxation properly. Luxated teeth should be repositioned and splinted. The dental splint is usually also sufficient to treat the alveolar process fracture. For details on treatment of dental

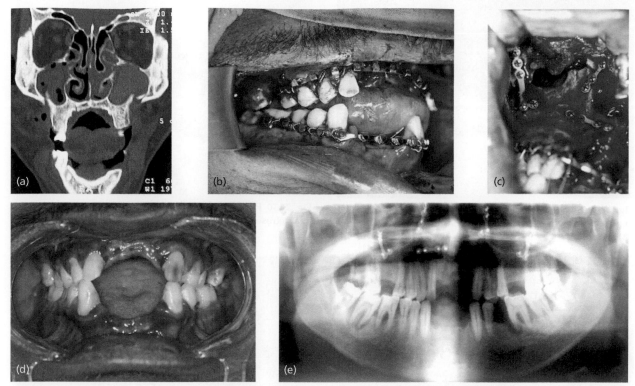

Fig. 27.26 Le Fort I fracture. (a) Coronal CT scan; note superior displacement of the fragment with comminution of fracture lines and linear fracture of hard palate. (b) Anterior open bite in the same patient. (c) Osteosynthesis of zygomatico-alveolar, paranasal, and sagittal fracture lines with titanium miniplates. (d) Normal occlusion after treatment. (e) Postoperative panoramic radiograph.

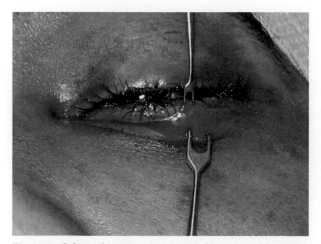

Fig. 27.27 Subtarsal incision: incision in skin crease of lower lid.

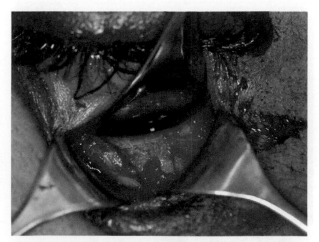

Fig. 27.28 Subtarsal incision: exposure of fracture of inferior orbital rim.

trauma see Chapter 26. Most Le Fort 1 fractures can be treated by an intraoral approach (Fig. 27.26).

In order to reach the levels of the infraorbital rims and more superior, periorbital incisions are made through the skin (Figs 27.27, 27.28, 27.29), or trans-conjunctival incisions are sometimes combined with lateral canthotomy (Figs 27.30, 27.31, 27.32).

Orbital fractures are challenging because of the complex geometry of the orbit. The anatomy of the orbit must be carefully reconstructed and any volume deficiency of the orbit post trauma will result in enophthalmos. For this reason virtual 3D reconstruction is now used.

A fully developed coronal flap by an incision over the scalp from ear to ear region will provide access to the frontal bone, zygomatic arches, bodies of the zygomatic bones, medial, superior and lateral orbital margins, and much of the corresponding orbital walls, as well as the nasal bones (Figs 27.33, 27.34). By preauricular extension it is possible to also address the temporomandibular joint and the upper neck of the condylar process of the mandible.

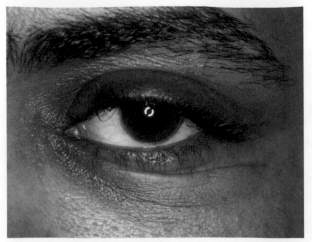

Fig. 27.29 Subtarsal incision: appearance of scar camouflaged in skin crease 6 months after operation.

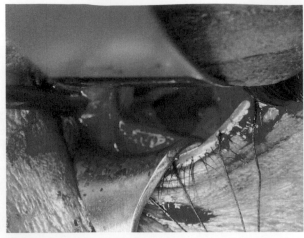

Fig. 27.30 Exposure of the orbital floor through transconjunctival retroseptal approach.

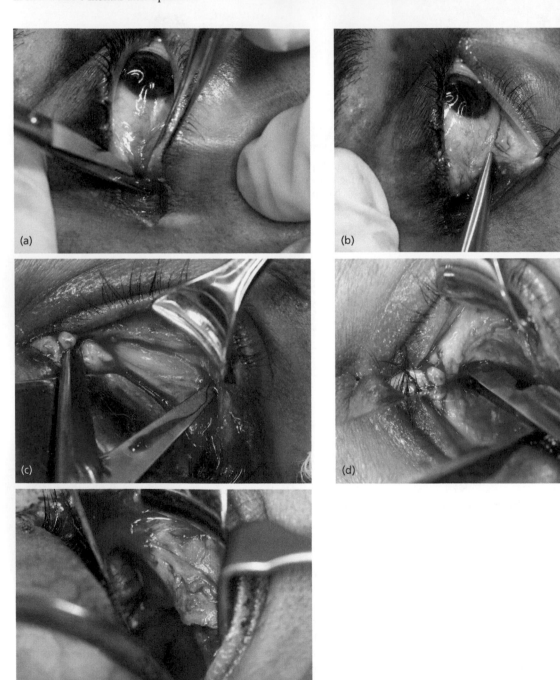

Fig. 27.31 Lateral canthotomy. (a) Division of inferior limb of lateral canthal ligament. (b) Incision of conjunctiva. (c) Dissection through capsulo-palpebral fascia and lower lid retractor. (d) Incision of periosteum of inferior orbital margin. (e) Fracture of inferior orbital rim and orbital floor exposed. (Courtesy of Dr Sabriyah Al-Saleh, Ophthalmology Department, Al-Adan Hospital, Kuwait.)

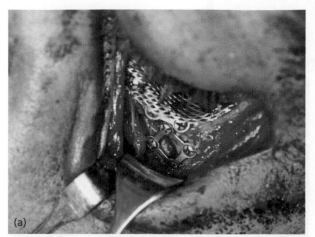

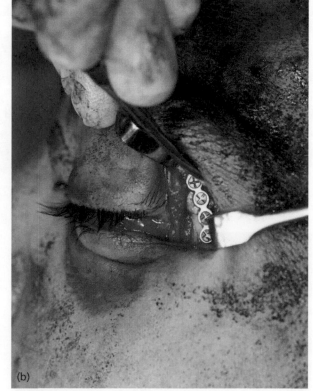

Fig. 27.32 Lateral canthotomy used for simultaneous approach to inferior and lateral orbital rim. (a) Inferior orbital rim plated and orbital floor reconstructed with titanium mesh. (b) Lateral orbital rim plated from the same approach. (Courtesy of Dr Sabriyah Al-Saleh, Ophthalmology Department, Al-Adan Hospital, Kuwait.)

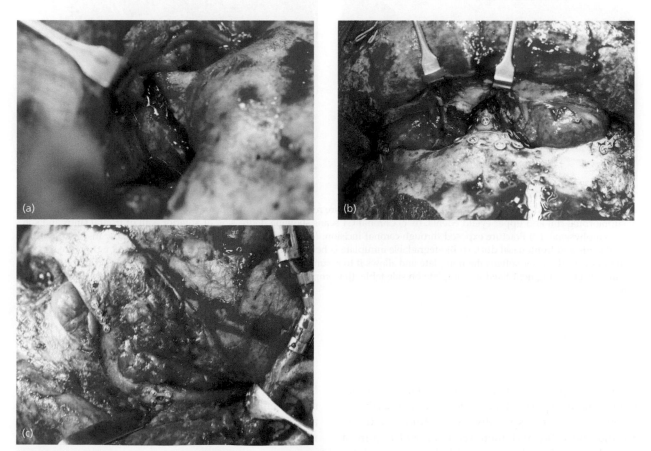

Fig. 27.33 Le Fort III fracture. (a) Frontonasal fracture exposed through a coronal incision. (b, c) Miniplate fracture repair in areas of frontonasal and zygomatico-frontal sutures, as well as zygomatic arch.

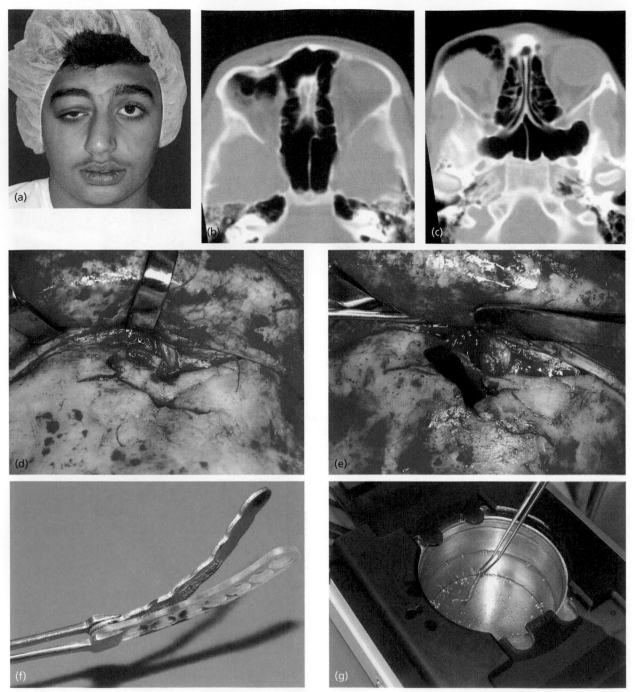

Fig. 27.34 Use of biodegradable miniplates in frontal bone fracture repair. (a) Clinical appearance of patient with marked deformity of supraorbital rim and upper eyelid edema. (b, c) Coronal CT scans showing depression of anterior wall of frontal sinus and soft tissue emphysema. (d) Fracture exposed through coronal incision. (e) Fragments temporarily removed to allow inspection of the frontal sinus and frontonasal duct. (f) Biodegradable miniplate is held together with template that was molded in fracture site. (g) Bath of hot sterile water softens the miniplate and allows it to assume the shape of the template. (h) Template and miniplate after cooling. (i) Bone fragment fixed to miniplate on side-table. (j) Completed reconstruction. (k) Appearance of patient 1 month after surgery.

Titanium plates are usually left in place but sometimes patients report palpable and/or visible hardware through the skin, especially in the thin soft tissue around the orbit and their removal will require a second entry. For this reason biodegradable plates have been introduced. These plates will resorb and a second entry is not necessary (Fig. 27.34). Biodegradable plates are also used in growing children, where metal plates would interfere with growth.

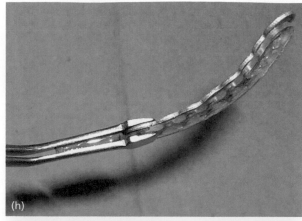

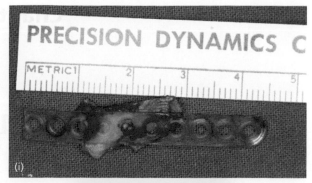

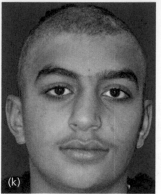

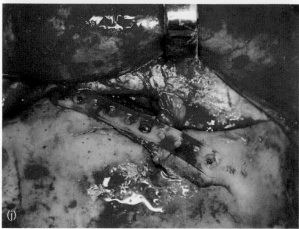

Fig. 27.34 (*Continued*)

Recommended reading

Andersson L, Andreasen JO. (2010) Traumatic dental injuries. In: *Oral and Maxillofacial Surgery* (eds, Andersson L, Kahnberg K-E, Pogrel MA). Oxford, Wiley-Blackwell.

Bast B. (2010) Assessment of the injured patient. In: *Oral and Maxillofacial Surgery* (eds, Andersson L, Kahnberg K-E, Pogrel MA). Oxford, Wiley-Blackwell.

Chung W, Costello BJ. (2010) Assessment of the injured patient. In: *Oral and Maxillofacial Surgery* (eds, Andersson L, Kahnberg K-E, Pogrel MA). Oxford, Wiley-Blackwell.

Fonseca R, Walker RV, *et al.* (2005) *Oral and Maxillofacial Trauma*, 3rd edn. St Louis, Elsevier Saunders.

Hupp JR, Ellis EE, Tucker MR. (2013) *Contemporary Oral and Maxillofacial Surgery*. St Louis, Elsevier Mosby.

Metzger MC, Weyer N, Schön R, Schmelzeisen R. (2010) Orbital reconstruction and panfacial fractures. In: *Oral and Maxillofa-*

cial Surgery. (eds, Andersson L, Kahnberg K-E, Pogrel MA). Oxford, Wiley-Blackwell.

Miloro M, Ghali GE, Larsen P, Waite P (2012) In: *Peterson's Principles of Oral and Maxillofacial Surgery*, 3rd edn. Hamilton, ON, BC Decker Inc.

Petersson EE, Andersson L, Sörensen S. (1997) Traumatic oral vs non-oral injuries. An epidemiological study during one year in a Swedish county. *Swedish Dental Journal*, **21**, 55–68.

Schutz P, Andersson L. (2010) Midfacial fractures. In: *Oral and Maxillofacial Surgery*. (eds, Andersson L, Kahnberg K-E, Pogrel MA). Oxford, Wiley-Blackwell.

Schön R, Schmelzeizen R. (2010) Transoral endoscope assisted endoscopic treatment of displaced condylar mandibular fractures. In: *Oral and Maxillofacial Surgery*. (eds, Andersson L, Kahnberg K-E, Pogrel MA). Oxford, Wiley-Blackwell.

Chapter 28

Soft Tissue Injuries

Soft tissue injuries are one of the most common problems treated in the emergency rooms and the facial region is an esthetically sensitive area with a complex variety of tissues. Around one-third of patients presenting with oral injuries have sustained soft tissue injuries.

Soft tissue in the oral and maxillofacial region absorbs a lot of energy when the region is subjected to impact from trauma. This may result in various injuries such as contusions, abrasions, lacerations and tissue avulsion. Foreign bodies are often found in the tissue. Teeth often penetrate the soft tissue and parts of the teeth may be found as foreign bodies in lacerations. Correct emergency treatment is a prerequisite for uneventful healing and the oral and maxillofacial region is an esthetically sensitive area. Failure to remove foreign bodies may result in permanent tattoos and unesthetic scarring and delayed healing and infection.

Types of soft tissue trauma

Soft tissue injuries can be divided into the following types of injuries:

- Contusion
- Abrasion
- Laceration
- Tissue avulsion.

Contusion

A contusion is a bruise without a break in the skin or mucosa. Subcutaneous or submucosal hemorrhage in the tissue results in hematoma and swelling of tissue is seen (Figs 28.1, 28.2). A contusion may be isolated to the soft tissue but often indicates a deeper injury, such as an underlying bone fracture.

Abrasion

An abrasion is a superficial wound in the skin or mucosa produced by rubbing and scraping of the skin or mucosa leaving a raw, bleeding, and often very painful surface (Fig. 28.3).

Laceration

Laceration is a wound in the skin or mucosa penetrating into the soft tissue (Fig. 28.4). A laceration may disrupt blood vessels, nerves, muscles, and involve salivary glands. The most frequently occurring lacerations in the maxillofacial region are seen in lips, oral mucosa, and gingiva. More seldom the tongue is involved.

Avulsion

Avulsion (loss of tissue) injuries are rare but seen with bite injuries or as a result of a very deep and extended abrasion (Fig. 28.5).

Emergency management of soft tissue injuries

Besides medical history and history of medications it is important to determine the mechanisms of injury and time of occurrence to provide information of any potential foreign bodies that may affect healing. Moreover, it is important to know the tetanus immunization status of the patient.

Abrasion

Abrasions require thorough lavage and irrigation along with careful inspection and removal of any solid remnants and necrotic epithelium. Remaining

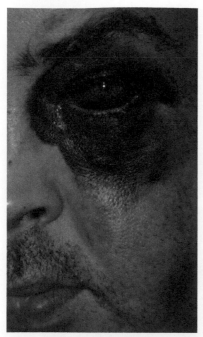

Fig. 28.1 Contusion injury with periorbital hematoma. In this patient there was an underlying bone fracture. (From Andersson and Andreasen 2007.)

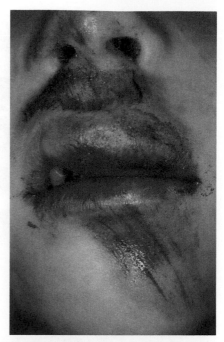

Fig. 28.3 Abrasion of the upper and lower lip. (From Andersson and Andreasen 2007.)

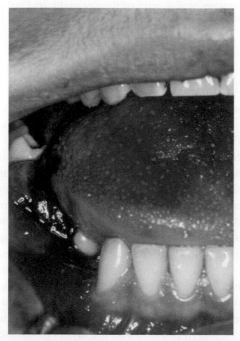

Fig. 28.2 Hematoma of soft tissue. Perimandibular hematoma may indicate underlying bone fracture as in this patient. (From Andersson and Andreasen 2007.)

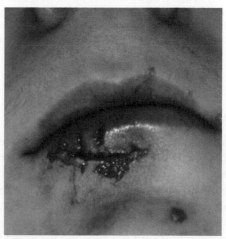

Fig. 28.4 Laceration of upper lip. (From Andersson and Andreasen 2007.)

irritants may be the source of prolonged inflammation, infection, and discoloration following healing, if they are not removed. Abrasions are generally more painful than lacerations or puncture wounds and more aggressive forms of pain management should be considered. Remove all dirt, gravel, asphalt and other foreign bodies. The only chance for a complete removal is in the emergency situation and these inju-

ries should be treated as soon as possible after the injury. Failure to do so may result in future permanent tattoo and scarring in the skin. Apply local anesthesia as topical and/or terminal injection. Rinse the abrasion with saline. Use a scrub brush, gauze swabs or a soft tooth brush. With severe contamination a mild soapy solution may be used. Remove all foreign bodies with a small *excavator* or a surgical blade (Fig. 28.6 a–g). Irrigation with saline should be performed. Then the wound should be dressed with antibiotic ointment and covered with sterile gauze if necessary to maintain wound moisture until reepithelialization is complete. Intra oral abrasions do not have to be treated other than removal of any foreign bodies.

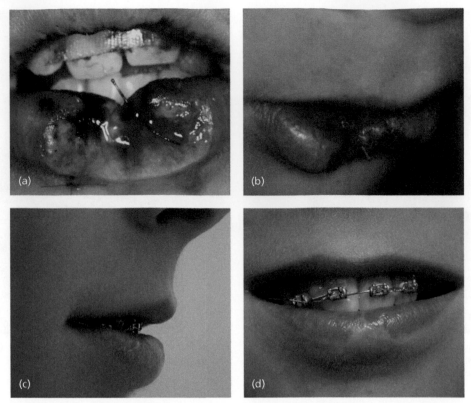

Fig. 28.5 (a) Avulsion injury of lower lip showing 2 cm wide avulsion injury. (b) Avulsion injury of lower lip showing considerable anterior loss of tissue of the vermillion. Nevertheless this was left for spontaneous healing without flaps or grafts. (c) Final result 1 year after trauma. A normal contour of the lip is seen. (d) Scar tissue is seen centrally in a circular area (9 mm diameter) at the vermillion border. (From Andersson and Andreasen 2007.)

Contusion

No treatment is necessary for contusions when the injury is limited to soft tissue injury. Blunt trauma and contusion to the soft tissues of the head and neck result in hematoma formation, or a self-limiting bleeding within the subcutaneous tissue which resorbs spontaneously. Make sure that there is no ongoing deep bleeding if a swelling is located in the floor of the mouth or tongue with risk for blocking of airway. Such patients should be observed. Contusions often indicate underlying bone fractures (see Figs 28.1, 28.2) therefore it is important to always carry out radiographic examination to detect bone fractures, which may require separate treatment.

Laceration

Administer local anesthesia. Inspect the laceration wound for foreign bodies or tooth fragments, which is the most common reason for lip lacerations. With deep wounds, supplement with radiographic examination. Place a dental film between the lip and the alveolar process with lowest exposure time (Fig. 28.7).

Remove all foreign bodies in the emergency phase to prevent infection and disfiguring scarring or tattooing in the skin. Use a syringe with saline under high pressure, a scrub brush, gauze swabs soaked in saline, a surgical scalpel blade or a small spoon excavator (Fig. 28.7).

Although many different ways of closing wounds have been presented, such as suturing, gluing, taping and using staples, in the oral and maxillofacial region suturing is still the most frequently used method of wound closing. Suturing is carried out with simple interrupted sutures in the oral mucosa and gingiva. Use absorbable synthetic material suture material in sizes 4-0 to 5-0 for intra oral sutures. For skin sutures a thinner suture, 5-0, 6-0, is preferable in esthetically sensitive areas. Absorbable or non-absorbable sutures may be used in the skin. With deep lacerations suture in layers. It is important that the layers of the laceration be reapproximated to their appropriate counterpart. Intracutaneous (intradermal, subcuticular) suturing technique may be preferred for cutaneous closure in esthetically sensitive areas (Fig. 28.8). Scars contract with time, so a slight wound-edge eversion is an important principle. A technique that slightly raises the wound edges above the skin plane will ultimately result in a cosmetically acceptable closure. Adhesive tape/strips may be used to relieve tension. Penetrating lacerations engaging both the skin and the oral cavity are complex lacerations necessitating layered closure. After thorough debridement, cleaning and irrigation, repair begins with alignment of

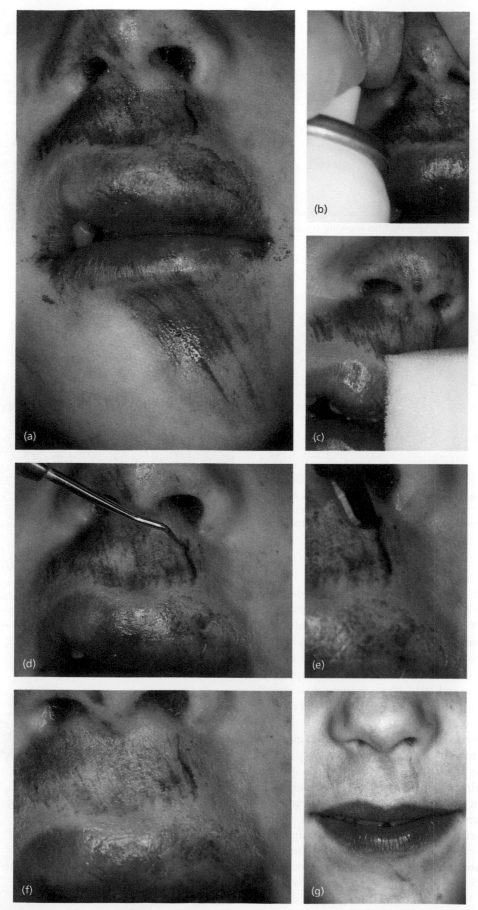

Fig. 28.6 (a, b) In order to adequately cleanse the abrasions, a topical anesthetic is necessary. (c) Washing the wounds. The lips are washed with surgical sponges or gauze swabs. *Removing of asphalt particles* (d, f). The impacted foreign bodies cannot be adequately removed by scrubbing and washing, but should be removed with a small excavator (a surgical blade held perpendicular to the direction of the abrasions). *Cleaned wound and follow-up.* (g) Two weeks after injury, the soft tissue wound has healed without scarring. (From Andersson and Andreasen 2007.)

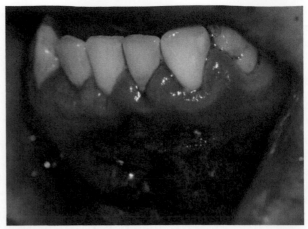

Fig. 28.7 Radiograph of a lacerated lip showing coronal fragment of a fractured incisor.

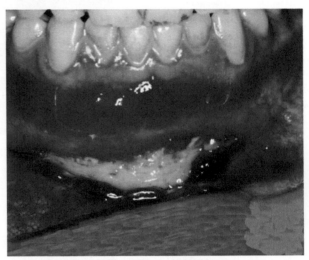

Fig. 28.9 Severely contaminated vestibular laceration. All soil and foreign bodies have to be removed. (From Andersson and Andreasen 2007.)

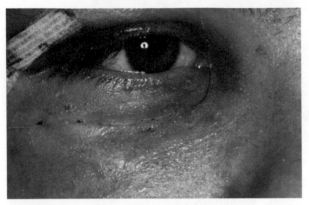

Fig. 28.8 Intracutaneous suture of an infraorbital soft tissue wound. Note the excellent adaptation of tissue without stitch marks 5 days after suturing. (From Andersson and Andreasen 2007.)

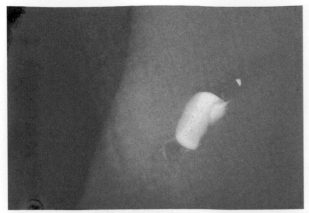

Fig. 28.10 Despite meticulous cleaning, bone exposure is seen after 2 weeks. This exposure was treated by daily rinsing by patient and weekly follow-up at the clinic. A superficial sequestration was seen after 3 weeks. (From Andersson and Andreasen 2007.)

the vermillion (the red part of the lip) border and white roll (the prominent ridge just above where the lip meets the facial skin), if involved. Special attention must be paid to carefully approximate the transition of skin to mucosa (vermillion border) as any inaccuracy in wound closure will be very apparent and compromise esthetics. Next, the muscle is closed with absorbable sutures followed by mucosal closure and, finally, skin closure.

Ideally, lacerations in the maxillofacial region are repaired in order for healing to occur by primary intention. This type of healing takes place quickly and with minimal scar formation. The consensus is that uncomplicated clean lacerations of the face can be closed primarily up to 24 hours after injury. Delayed primary closure is a method of management of dirty or infected traumatic wounds or wounds that have gone unrepaired for a considerable amount of time (Figs 28.9, 28.10, 28.11). Severely dirty wounds are converted to fresh wounds through debridement and removal of tissue edges and can later be closed if no infection is evident. When a wound is left open, a more prolonged healing process, healing by secondary intention, occurs. This will result in scar contrac-

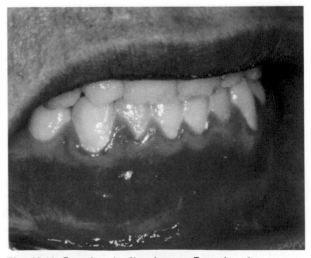

Fig. 28.11 Complete healing is seen 7 weeks after trauma. (From Andersson and Andreasen 2007.)

tion and can be sometimes be accepted in the oral mucosa but should be avoided in the skin because of compromised esthetical result.

Avulsions

Administer local anesthesia. Clean the wound. Small defects can be left for spontaneous healing especially in young individuals who have a higher regeneration capacity than older individuals (see Fig. 28.5). With large tissue loss, excision and primary closure with flaps or skin grafts may be necessary for coverage. With animal bites, usually dogs, antibiotics should always be administered regardless of duration. Rabies vaccine should be considered, depending on the status of the dog.

Antibiotics to prevent wound infection

Bacterial infection is the most common complication and is highly related to time between trauma and wound closure. There is no convincing evidence that antibiotics are useful for preventing infections in simple lacerations. However, there are situations when antibiotics should be given:

- heavily contaminated wound;
- compromised wound cleansing;
- delayed treatment >24 hours;
- injuries penetrating through the whole lip or cheek;
- human or animal bite wounds;
- simultaneous extensive surgery such as open reduction of fracture;
- when general defense system of the patient is compromised e.g. diabetes and immunocompromised patients.

Tetanus

In case of contaminated wounds, especially wounds occurring outdoors, tetanus prophylaxis should be considered. Tetanus has declined considerably since the use of widespread vaccination. However, tetanus has a high morbidity so it is important to always check if the patient is immunized. If there is more than 10 years since last immunization, a booster dose should be given.

Recommended reading

Andersson L, Andreasen JO. (2007) Soft tissue Injuries. In: *Textbook and Color Atlas of Traumatic Injuries to the Teeth*. (eds, Andreasen JO, Andreasen FM, Andersson L) , 4th edn. Oxford, Blackwell Publishing.

Andreasen JO, Andreasen FM, Bakland LK, Flores MT, Andersson L. (2011) *Traumatic Dental Injuries. A Manual*, 3rd edn. Oxford, Wiley.

Serafin B, Koshgerian P, Haug RH. (2010) Soft tissue trauma. In: *Oral and Maxillofacial Surgery*. (eds, Andersson L, Kahnberg K-E, Pogrel MA). Oxford, Wiley-Blackwell.

Part 6: Dentofacial Deformities

(Section Editor: Karl-Erik Kahnberg)

Chapter 29

Cleft Lip and Palate: An Overview

Global burden of birth defects: cleft lip and palate

More than four million children are born with birth defects worldwide every year. Craniofacial anomalies comprise a large fraction of all human birth defects, less frequent only than congenital heart disorders and clubfoot. Cleft lip with or without palate (CL/P) is the most common craniofacial birth defect with an estimated quarter of a million affected babies born each year in the world. This malformation shows considerable variation across geographic regions and ethnic groups and has significant medical, psychological, social, and economic ramifications. It is a costly public health problem with an average lifetime treatment cost per child in the US estimated to be roughly $101 000.

The World Health Organization (WHO) and most cleft organizations across the globe recommend interdisciplinary care by a team of specialists. In reality, however, surgical and non-surgical treatment is often fragmented and dictated by socio-economic factors and access to medical facilities. In developing countries, particularly in rural areas, care is often neglected due to social beliefs and lack of awareness, or initiated late due to restricted resources and inadequate access. The delay in treatment and intermittent care by local or overseas cleft mission surgeons, combined with incomplete follow-up, results in poor outcomes with unnecessary complications. More recently, some humanitarian non-profit organizations supporting cleft care have changed their aid philosophy. They are identifying centers with a potential to deliver quality care in low- and middle-income countries and providing support for the physicians, staff, and hospital infrastructure, helping to establish parameters of care, as well as monitoring treatment outcomes at these centers.

Birth defects are emerging as a cause of neonatal mortality in countries that have made progress in controlling infectious diseases and malnutrition. The strategies proposed to reduce the global impact of birth defects include: (1) effective family planning, genetic counseling, and prenatal diagnosis; (2) education for couples to decrease maternal exposure to avoidable environmental risk factors such as tobacco, alcohol, and teratogenic medications; (3) improving periconception maternal intake of micronutrients such as folic acid (400 µg); and (4) improving the availability of medical and surgical care locally for the affected infants. National leadership and commitment are essential for proper surveillance of birth defects, infant mortality, and to monitor the clinical and cost effectiveness of various interventions.

The WHO initiative for collaborative craniofacial anomalies research has identified areas of uncertainty in clinical care and efforts are being made to conduct trials with sufficiently large samples of patients to provide evidence for treatment strategies. Initial research efforts have focused on addressing surgical, anesthetic, and nursing care for patients with craniofacial anomalies in developing countries. Surgical techniques for repair of various cleft sub-types and correction of velopharyngeal insufficiency are being evaluated. Adjunctive services such as use of prophylactic ventilation tubes, presurgical orthopedics, psychological counseling, speech therapy, and feeding interventions before and after surgery are also being monitored and assessed. An international database of craniofacial anomalies has been established to improve answers to questions relevant to individuals with cleft and craniofacial anomalies, their families, and health care providers.

Essentials of Oral and Maxillofacial Surgery, First Edition. Edited by M. Anthony Pogrel, Karl-Erik Kahnberg and Lars Andersson.
© 2014 John Wiley & Sons, Ltd. Published 2014 by John Wiley & Sons, Ltd.
Companion website: www.wiley.com/go/pogrel/oms

Table 29.1 Epidemiology of oral clefts.

Distribution of oral clefts
Cleft lip and palate 46%
Cleft palate only 33%
Cleft lip only 21%
Cleft lip with or without palate
Average birth prevalence 1 : 700
More common in males
Unilateral > bilateral
Left side > right side
Association with other anomalies 10%
Cleft palate only
Average birth prevalence 1 : 2000
More common in females
Association with other anomalies 50–60%

Epidemiology

Cleft lip with or without palate (CL/P) has an average birth prevalence of 1:700 ranging from 1:500 to 1:2000, depending on the race (Table 29.1). There are wide ethnic variations with highest occurrence in Native Americans (3.6:1000), followed by Asians (2.1:1000 Japanese births and 1.7:1000 Chinese births), Caucasians (1:1000), and lowest in those of African descent (0.3:1000). Cleft of palate only (CP), which differs genetically from CL/P, has a birth prevalence rate of 1:2000 and is more similar across all populations. About half of the oral clefts involve lip and palate (46%), a third of the clefts involve only the palate (33%), and clefts of lip alone account for 21%. CL/P is more often unilateral than bilateral and more common in males than females. The unilateral defects occur more often on the left side than the right side. Clefts of lip occur in the ratio of 6:3:1 for unilateral left, unilateral right, and bilateral. CP is more common in females and more often associated with other developmental anomalies.

Clefts are referred to as non-syndromic and syndromic, based on their association with other anomalies. About 50% of CP and 10% of CL/P are associated with a syndrome. Some common syndromes associated with cleft lip and palate include Van der Woude, Treacher Collins syndrome, Down syndrome, oro-facial digital syndrome, Opitz syndrome, craniofacial microsomia, and fetal alcohol syndrome. Nearly half of the syndromic cleft palate presentations are associated with the triad of micrognathia, glossoptosis, and airway obstruction (Pierre Robin sequence). The most common syndromic presentations of this triad are Stickler's syndrome, accounting for 25%, and velo-cardiofacial (VCF) syndrome, accounting for 15% of all syndromic cleft palate individuals.

Etiology and genetics

Non-syndromic CL/P is a complex trait with multifactorial etiology, resulting from gene–gene and gene–environmental interactions. Identification of key genes contributing to the genesis of orofacial clefts will help in early diagnosis, disease prevention, or possibly developing adjunctive therapies. The most recent estimates suggest that anywhere from 3 to 14 genes contribute to cleft lip and palate. Candidate genes and loci responsible for non-syndromic CL/P have been identified on chromosomes 1, 2, 4, 6, 11, 14, 17, and 19. Two genes *IRF6* and *MSX-1* now seem to explain about 15% of non-syndromic CL/P. Mutations in *IRF6* lead to Van der Woude and popliteal pterygium syndromes. Mutations in other genes, *TBX22*, *FGFR1*, and *P63*, also contribute to syndromic clefts. Aberrant transforming growth factor beta-3 (TGF-β3) signaling plays a role in the pathogenesis of cleft palate.

Environmental factors that contribute to the etiology of facial clefting disorders include cigarette smoking, folic acid deficiency during the periconceptional period, and maternal exposure to alcohol and teratogenic medications such as retinoids, corticosteroids, and anticonvulsants (phenytoin and valproic acid). Co-sanguinous marriages, maternal diabetes, and obesity have also been linked to an increased risk of orofacial clefts. Less consistent associations have been found between clefts and maternal viral infections such as rubella and varicella.

Studies conducted to determine the risk of having a child with CL/P show that every parent has about a 0.14% (1:700) chance of having a child with a cleft. The risk of recurrence of a cleft condition is determined by a number of factors, including the number of family members with clefts, their relationship to family members with clefts, race and sex of the affected individuals, and the type of cleft. Studies show that the recurrence risk for first-degree relatives is about 3.3% for CL/P and for isolated CP it is 2%. Once parents have a child with a cleft the risk of having a second child with a cleft is about 2–5%, and after two affected children that risk rises to 9–12%. In twins with CL/P and those with isolated CP, the concordance is far greater for monozygotic twins than for dizygotic twins. Parents and young adults should be counseled appropriately by a geneticist so that they are in a better position to make decisions about future pregnancies.

Embryology

The embryologic development of the face begins at 4 weeks after conception from the neural crest ectomesenchyme that forms five prominences; the frontonasal process, and paired maxillary and mandibular processes surrounding a central depression. During the fifth and sixth weeks of embryonic development,

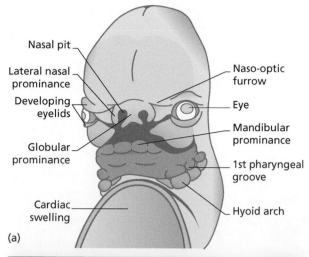

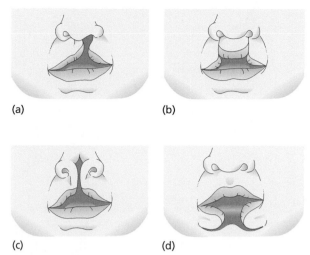

(a)   (b)

(c)   (d)

Fig. 29.2 Orofacial clefts resulting from errors during embryonic development of face. (a) Unilateral cleft of upper lip. (b) Bilateral cleft of the upper lip. (c) Midline cleft of the upper lip and nose. (d) Median mandibular cleft. (Adapted and redrawn from Sperber GH. *Craniofacial Development*. Hamilton: BC Decker Inc, 2001. Reproduced with permission.)

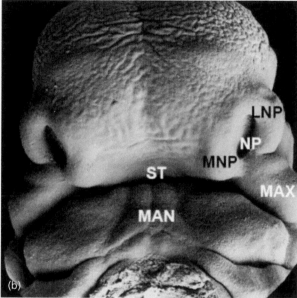

Fig. 29.1 (a) Schematic diagram showing embryonic development of face at 6 weeks. (b) Electron microscopy showing the development of face of a 37-day-old human embryo. The nasal pit (NP) is surrounded by the medial nasal process (MNP) and lateral nasal process (LNP) and maxillary process (MAX). (Adapted and redrawn from Sperber GH. (2001) *Craniofacial Development*. BC Decker Inc, Hamilton. Reproduced with permission.)

bilateral maxillary processes derived from first brachial arch fuse with the medial nasal process to form the upper lip, alveolus, and the primary palate (Fig. 29.1). The lateral nasal process forms the alar structures of the nose. The lower lip and jaw are formed by the mandibular processes.

This process of formation of the face is the consequence of a cascade of processes that involve cell proliferation, cell differentiation, cell adhesion, and apoptosis. Failure or error in any of these cellular processes that lead to fusion of the medial nasal process with the lateral nasal and maxillary process can cause orofacial clefts (Fig. 29.2). The molecular events that underlie these cellular processes are under the control of a strict array of genes that include fibroblast growth factors (FGFs), sonic hedgehog

(*SHH*), bone morphogenic proteins (BMPs), and members of the transforming growth factor beta (TGF-β) superfamily and other transcription factors. The formation of the secondary palate begins during the sixth week after conception from the two palatal shelves, which extend from the internal aspect of the maxillary processes. During the eighth week, these bilateral maxillary palatal shelves after ascending to an appropriate position above the tongue, fuse with each other and the primary palate. A disruption in the fusion of these embryonic components can occur due to delay in elevation of the palatal shelves from vertical to horizontal, defective shelf fusion, or postfusion rupture resulting in a cleft of the secondary palate (Fig. 29.3).

Classification

In order to standardize documentation and communicate effectively, various types of classification systems have been described. The early Veau classification included groups 1–4 with increasing severity of clefting:

- group 1 – cleft of the soft palate;
- group 2 – cleft of the hard and soft palate up to incisive foramen;
- group 3 – complete unilateral cleft lip and palate;
- group 4 – complete bilateral cleft lip and palate.

However, this classification is not always adequate to document the variations. The more sophisticated schematic diagrams, such as the one described by Kernahan and Stark have been used recently (Fig. 29.4). Berkowitz used a simple classification for labio-palatine clefts:

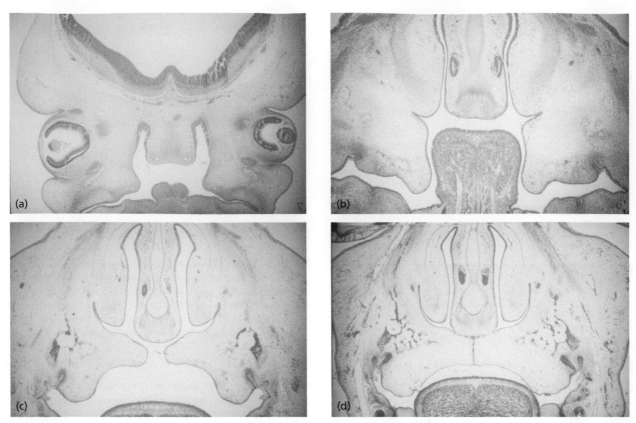

Fig. 29.3 Coronal scanning electron microscopy photos of human embryo showing the stages of formation of the palate at 8–9 weeks. (a) Development of palate showing palatal shelves and tongue position. (b) The vertical orientation of the palatal shelves on either side of tongue. (c) Palatal shelves elevate and (d) fuse with each other and the nasal septum in the midline.

1. Clefts of lip and alveolus.
2. Clefts of primary (including lip) and secondary palate.
3. Clefts of secondary palate only.
4. Submucous cleft.

Interdisciplinary management of the cleft individual

The idea of interdisciplinary care is to coordinate treatment by multiple specialists in a timely fashion with an aim of achieving normality in all aspects, including feeding, breathing, speech, hearing, alignment of teeth, appearance, and overall psychological and physical development. The timing of surgical and non-surgical interventions should coincide with the physical, cognitive, and social development of the child (Table 29.2). Cleft teams generally include a craniomaxillofacial surgeon, pediatrician, nurse practitioner, speech pathologist, orthodontist, social worker, and geneticist. Experience in Scandinavian countries and a multicenter Euro-cleft study have demonstrated that standardization, centralization, and participation of surgeons who perform a large number of cleft procedures produce better surgical results in terms of speech, appearance, and facial

growth. However, this cannot be applied to all countries, particularly those with a high volume of cleft individuals and a limited number of care facilities.

Prenatal diagnosis

Interdisciplinary team care begins with prenatal diagnosis and parental counseling. With the advent of sophisticated high resolution three-dimensional (3D) ultrasonography and genetic tests for screening of birth defects, intrauterine diagnosis of cleft lip is possible. Early diagnosis of a cleft of the lip should alert the obstetrician to the possibility of other malformations that may require further investigations. While early diagnosis may help parents to be better prepared, the advent of such a capability raises both ethical and psychological issues, such as dilemma of termination of birth. Physicians and surgeons have to inform parents that CLP in the absence of other major systemic anomalies is a treatable non-life-threatening condition. The cleft team also can discuss feeding issues and timing of lip and palate surgery, and can help establish contact with support groups for the family.

Transvaginal ultrasonography may reveal a cleft of lip as early as 11 weeks whereas 16–20 weeks is ideal for transabdominal ultrasonography. Several

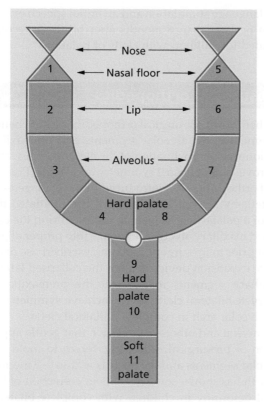

Fig. 29.4 Kernahan and Stark classification of clefts. Kernahan's striped-Y classification: areas 1 and 5 represent the right and left sides of nasal floor, 2 and 6 represent the right and left sides of the lip, respectively. The alveolus is represented by areas 3 and 7, the hard palate anterior to the incisive foramen by areas 4 and 8, the hard palate posterior to the incisive foramen by areas 9 and 10, and the soft palate by area 11. (From Millard, Jr, DR. (1977) The unilateral deformity. In: *Cleft Craft: The Evolution of its Surgery*, Vol 1, p52. Little, Brown, Boston. Reproduced with permission. Copyright © D. Ralph Millard, Jr.)

Table 29.2 Timing of treatment in the cleft patient.

Prenatal

Diagnosis and parental counseling

0–6 months

General assessment for associated anomalies

ENT evaluation – breathing, feeding, swallowing, and hearing

Presurgical orthopedics (0–3 months)

Primary lip repair (3–4 months)

6 months–2 years

Speech and oral sensory motor assessment

Grommets/ear tubes (as needed)
Primary palate repair (9–12 months)

Preschool: 3–5 years

Dental care

Speech assessment and therapy (continue as needed)

Assess need for lip revision

Childhood: 6–12 years

Correction of velo-pharyngeal dysfunction (as needed)

Orthodontic treatment – phase I

Alveolar cleft repair (8–11 years)

Adolescence: 13–18 years

Orthodontic treatment – phase II

Orthognathic surgery (if needed) – 14–16 years (female),
16–18 years (male)
Revision chielorhinoplasty

Replacement of missing teeth (as needed)

factors may influence the accuracy of ultrasound studies: sophistication of the scanning equipment; experience and skill of the sonographer; number of weeks into pregnancy; position of the baby while scanning; amount of amniotic fluid; maternal body structure; and severity of cleft.

Premaxillary protrusion is an important clue to the presence of cleft lip and cleft palate and may be more conspicuous than the cleft itself. The presence of a paranasal echogenic mass favors the presence of bilateral cleft lip and cleft palate. Clefts of palate alone are rarely visualized on ultrasound. The majority of the cases of orofacial clefts are detected antenatally. A recent study by Johnson *et al.* showed that the frequencies of prenatal diagnosis for cleft lip and palate, cleft lip only, and CP only were 33.3%, 20.3%, and 0.3%, respectively. Although the benefits of fetal healing have been well documented, at this time there is no indication for intrauterine repair of the cleft lip deformity as the risk of fetal surgery is far too high both for the fetus and mother for correction of this non-life-threatening condition.

General assessment

Every child born with a CL/P should be thoroughly assessed by complete physical examination and necessary diagnostic tests to check for associated systemic abnormalities, including congenital heart, renal, or airway anomalies. If the child is delivered in a non-medical facility or a small hospital they should be referred to a tertiary hospital with specialists or a craniofacial team for further evaluation. A proper airway assessment, and counseling for nutrition and feeding should be initiated immediately.

Feeding and nutrition

Feeding is one of the first concerns in a child born with a CL/P. Parents should be taught how to feed the baby and informed about various feeding nipples that can deliver more milk under less pressure. The goal is to provide adequate nutrition to satisfy the caloric requirements and avoid failure to thrive. The team nurse generally provides the parents with information on feeding before birth or immediately after birth. Children with cleft lip only without a cleft palate may have some difficulty in creating a seal around the nipple but generally can be breast fed before and after lip surgery. However, the presence of a cleft palate makes it difficult to create a negative pressure that is necessary to feed. Four randomized clinical trials conducted with a total of 232 babies showed that squeezable bottles may be easier to use than rigid bottles for children with CL/P. There was no statistical difference found in growth outcomes of children with CL/P who were fitted with a passive palatal appliance to help with feeding and those without an appliance. A feeding tube is rarely necessary except in infants with other associated anomalies, particularly airway anomalies.

Ear, nose, and throat evaluation

A proper airway assessment should be priority for a newborn with congenital craniofacial anomalies. Infants are obligate nasal breathers. It is important to check if there is obstruction at any level in the upper or lower airway, including the nares and choanae. Children born with a cleft of the palate may have associated micrognathia, glossoptosis, and airway obstruction (Fig. 29.5). In these children, one should look for signs of increased effort while breathing, stridor, weight loss, and failure to thrive. Parents should be informed to watch for an abnormal breathing pattern or respiratory distress, particularly during upper respiratory tract infection. If there are signs of airway obstruction, a pediatric otolaryngologist should be consulted to perform an endoscopic evaluation of upper and lower airway to look for possible cause of obstruction.

An audiology assessment is recommended soon after birth to check for hearing abnormalities. Children with cleft palate exhibit a higher frequency of otitis media prior to palate repair than those without clefts. Middle ear ventilation disorders due to Eustachian tube dysfunction can cause conductive hearing loss. This can also contribute to speech and language delay in these children. Although not as common as conductive hearing loss, sensorineural hearing deficits exist within the cleft population, and it has an effect on speech perception and clarity, as well as auditory comprehension skills. Early speech

and language stimulation and an initial speech evaluation no later than 6 months after birth are recommended for children with clefts of palate.

Presurgical orthopedics

The benefits of presurgical orthopedics include better alignment of the alveolar segments and premaxilla, tension-free approximation of the cleft lip edges, and improvement of nostril symmetry and shape. Presurgical orthopedics was introduced in the management of clefts by McNeill and Burston. They initiated the use of a palatal acrylic plate in order to bring the collapsed maxillary alveolar segments into proper alignment prior to lip surgery. Latham described use of an active expansion device to align the collapsed lateral maxillary segments and retract the premaxilla in complete bilateral clefts, and to achieve symmetry of the alveolar arch in complete unilateral clefts.

Grayson and others have shown that gentle application of presurgical orthopedic forces to mold the alveolar segments and the nostrils within 0–3 months of birth has shown some benefits in correction of the nasal deformity in children with complete bilateral CLP and wide unilateral clefts. Nasoalveolar molding increases the surface area of the nasal mucosal lining, and also helps with elongation of the columella and making the columella upright. This preoperative expansion of the nasal lining allows suturing of interdomal cartilages without tension and decreases widening of the nose (Fig. 29.6).

There is a wide variation in the availability of expertise and cost of treatment when it comes to infant presurgical orthopedics or nasoalveolar molding. In recent years, several centers have reported the adoption of this technique to improve the outcomes of lip and nose repair, especially in complete bilateral CLP. It is important to evaluate these recent studies critically for their overall clinical and cost effectiveness. Non-surgical lip adhesion with tape is a cost-effective and simple technique that can bring the alveolar segments closer to facilitate cheiloplasty in infants with wide clefts of the lip and palate (Fig. 29.7).

Cleft lip repair

The goal of primary lip repair is to reconstruct a functional lip with minimal scarring and normal appearance. The timing for primary lip repair is usually between 3 and 6 months after birth. Most craniofacial centers follow the "rule of 10s" to ensure that the infant is fit for the surgical procedure. This rule implies that the infant should be at least 10 weeks of age, weigh at least 10 lb, and have a hemoglobin level of at least 10 g/100 mL. Some centers have reported lip repair in children with lower hemoglobin levels (8 g/100 mL) with no deleterious effects. In low- and

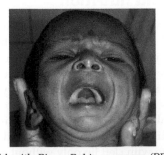

Fig. 29.5 Child with Pierre Robin sequence (PRS) showing a wide cleft of palate, small lower jaw, and a retropositioned tongue in the cleft obstructing the airway.

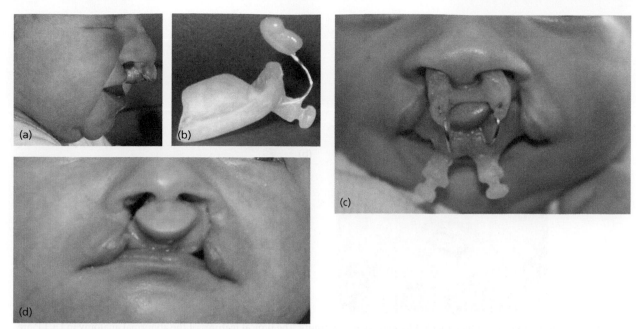

Fig. 29.6 (a) Baby with a bilateral cleft lip and palate showing protrusion of premaxilla before nasoalveolar molding. (b) Nasoalveolar molding appliance. (c) Nasoalveolar molding appliance in position to expand nasal soft tissues and align the alveolar cleft segments. (d) Note the position of premaxilla in frontal and view after nasoalveolar molding. (Courtesy of Dr Oberoi, UCSF Center for Craniofacial Anomalies.)

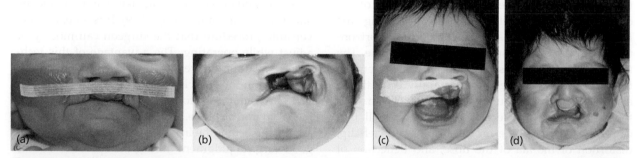

Fig. 29.7 (a–d) These photos illustrate that simple presurgical orthopedic techniques, such as lip taping, can be used to align the cleft alveolar segments prior to lip repair.

middle-income countries, infants are often malnourished and proper feeding and nutrition counseling is essential to prepare them for lip surgery by 3 months. Lip repair is performed under general anesthesia with an Oral RAE® endotracheal tube taped to the midline of lower lip without distorting the commissure. Postoperative care includes keeping the wound clean by preventing crusting and using antibiotic cream; in some centers arm restraints are also used for 7–10 days.

A surgical lip adhesion may be preferred as an initial surgical procedure within 6–8 weeks after birth in some centers. Lip adhesion helps to align the maxillary alveolar segments and achieve a tension-free definitive lip repair at a later date. Good approximation of the alveolar segments also allows the surgeon to perform a gingivoperiosteoplasty at the time of definitive cheiloplasty. The disadvantages of convert-

ing the complete cleft lip to an incomplete one by lip adhesion are: the need for an extra operation and the possibility of excising more tissue at the time of definitive lip repair. Non-surgical orthopedic techniques during the first 6–8 weeks after birth, as described earlier in this chapter, can produce good alignment of the alveolar segments.

Unilateral cleft lip

Surgical anatomy

Unilateral cleft lip is an asymmetric deformity that presents with a multitude of inherent anatomic variations (Fig. 29.8). The most visible anatomic abnormalities of the complete unilateral cleft lip and nose deformity are due to the abnormal position of the orbicularis oris muscle. After fetal dissections, Fara

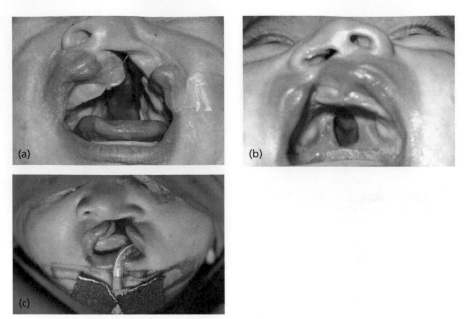

Fig. 29.8 (a–c) Variations of the unilateral cleft lip and palate deformity. The typical features of the abnormal anatomy in UCLP are seen in these photos. There is vertical shortening of the lip at the cleft margins, orbicularis oris muscle fibers terminate medially beneath the base of the columella and laterally beneath the alar base. Fibers of orbicularis oris in the lateral segment are more hypoplastic and do not extend up to the cleft margin. Note the discrepancy of vermillion width with excess vermillion at the cleft margin on the lateral side compared with the medial side. The maxillary alveolus exhibits asymmetry with an upward and outward rotation of the greater segment.

noted that in a complete cleft lip, the fibers of the orbicularis oris muscle turn upward along the margins of the cleft instead of proceeding horizontally from the commissure towards the midline. The fibers of the orbicularis terminate medially beneath the base of the columella and laterally beneath the alar base and periosteum of the piriform rim. It is these abnormal muscle attachments and pull that cause the typical bulge on the unrepaired cleft lip, distortion of the ala of the nose, and deflection of anterior nasal spine and septum of the nose. The nasal deformity is proportionate to the severity of clefting. In the complete unilateral cleft lip and palate deformity, there is slumping of the alar cartilage on the cleft side resulting in an asymmetric nasal tip. The alar base is displaced laterally, inferiorly, and posteriorly leading to a widened nasal aperture. There is shortening of the medial crus of the alar cartilage and lack of overlap of upper and lower lateral cartilages. The columella and the caudal edge of the septum and anterior nasal spine are deviated to the non-cleft side.

Evolution of unilateral cleft lip repair

Several surgeons, including Rose (1891), Thompson (1912), Blair (1930), Le Mesurier (1949), Tennison and Randall (1952), and Skoog (1974), have contributed to the evolution of cleft lip repair, but the most popular technique was introduced by Millard (1955) who described the rotation–advancement concept. Today various modifications of the rotation–advancement technique by Millard are used to repair the unilateral cleft lip deformity. In Millard's technique the medial

flap is rotated downward to achieve length, while the lateral flap is advanced (Fig. 29.9). It is an extremely versatile procedure that the surgeon can modify or adjust while operating. The advantage of this technique is that the suture line lies on the recreated philtral column and incision allows easy access for primary rhinoplasty to reposition the nasal septum, lower lateral cartilage, and alar base. The main disadvantage is that the inexperienced surgeon requires good surgical judgment during the operation as it is not based on exact measurements. The triangular flap technique, described by Tennison and Randall, is based on exact measurements, can be reproduced well, and used more easily in wide clefts of the lip.

Principles of repair of unilateral cleft lip and nose

An adequate repair of the unilateral lip deformity should correct the alignment of the orbicularis oris muscle, and create a cupid's bow and philtral column on the affected side. In the unilateral defect the normal side can be used as a guide to identify the key points and to plan the incisions on the cleft side. Despite inherent variations there are some similarities that form the basis of the guiding principles in surgical repair of this deformity (Fig. 29.10).

1. *Rotation or lengthening of shortened vertical height of lip.* The difference in the vertical length of the lip from the height of the cupid's bow to the base of the columella between the non-cleft side and the cleft side indicates the amount of rotation and

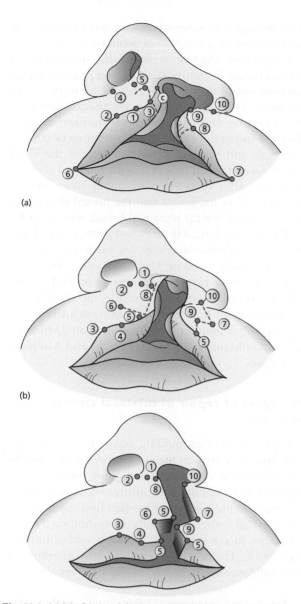

(a)

(b)

Fig. 29.9 (a) Markings of the key points and incisions for repair of the unilateral cleft lip using the Millard rotation–advancement principle: lengthening the shortened vertical height of the lip on the medial side to match the lateral, and advancing the flap of tissue from lateral to medial. (b) Markings of the key points and incisions for repair of the unilateral cleft lip using the triangular flap technique.

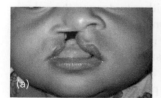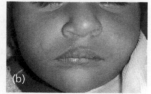

Fig. 29.10 Unilateral cleft lip repair. (a) Preoperative and (b) postoperative views of lip repair performed by a modified Millard technique.

back cut necessary. The medial lip element (non-cleft side) is rotated inferiorly to achieve adequate length and symmetry of the cupid's bow.

2. *Advancement of flap of tissue from lateral to medial.* The flap of tissue from lateral should be advanced in

to the lip on the medial segment. It is important to release the abnormally inserted paranasal and facial muscles at the alar base by subperiosteal dissection in order to approximate the edges without tension.

3. *Retaining cupid's bow and creating a philtral column.* Approximation of the cleft edges should be achieved without loss of natural landmarks: the cupid's bow, philtral dimple, and philtral column. The scar of union of cleft edges should be placed along a natural line – the philtral column. Creating a good philtral column requires proper approximation of the muscle and tension-free closure of the overlying skin.

4. *Muscle reconstruction.* The muscle bellies should be dissected within the skin and mucosal envelope. The muscles should be approximated with interrupted mattress sutures. The muscles at the base of the columella and ala should be dissected and approximated to help reposition the distorted nasal structures.

5. *Restoration of the alveolar continuity.* If the alveolar segments are closely approximated a gingivoperiosteoplasty can be performed at the time of primary lip repair to achieve a continuous alveolar arch.

6. *Primary repair of the distorted nasal anatomy.* This requires wide undermining of the skin drape over the lateral crura of the alar cartilages and repositioning of the nasal septum with a suture (Fig. 29.11). Long-term results of primary rhinoplasty by McComb and others show that the outcomes are better and there is no decrease in overall size or nasal growth inhibition after primary correction.

Bilateral cleft lip

Surgical anatomy

Bilateral cleft lip repair is much more challenging and the results are often less satisfactory than those of unilateral cleft lip. Complete bilateral clefts of lip are rare, accounting for only 10% of cleft lips and therefore the experience in treating these deformities is limited. The typical anatomical abnormalities that make the bilateral cleft lip deformity so difficult to repair are the absence of muscle in the prolabial segment, resulting in lack of philtral dimple, philtral columns, white roll margin, and the median tubercle. The prolabium lacks the angular peaks and the typical cupid's bow. The premaxilla is protuberant and sometimes deviated to one side, making tension-free approximation of muscle and cleft margins difficult. The orbicularis oris muscle which is in the lateral lip elements inserts at the alar base on each side. The accompanying nasal deformity consists of a columella that is abnormally short, a wide nasal tip, and a flared alar base due to the malpositioned, splayed alar cartilages. The variations of bilateral CLP deformity are shown in Figure 29.12.

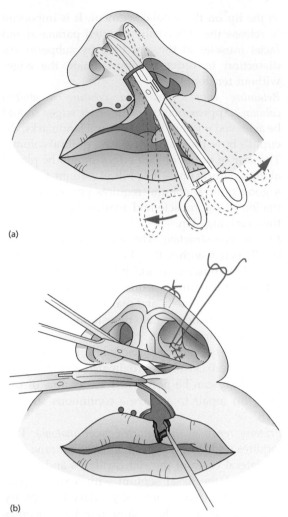

(a)

(b)

Fig. 29.11 Primary nasal deformity correction in the unilateral cleft lip. (a) Wide undermining of the skin drape over the medial and lateral crura of the alar cartilages. (b) Suturing of the alar dome.

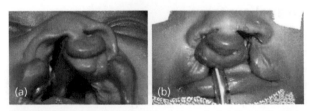

Fig. 29.12 (a, b) Variations of the bilateral cleft lip and palate deformity. These photos show the typical anatomical abnormalities seen in individuals with complete bilateral clefts of lip and palate: lack of muscle in the prolabium, lack of the angular peaks and typical dip of cupid's bow, lack of a definite philtral ridge or dimple in the prolabium, abnormally short and wide columella, lack of adequate labial sulcus depth in the premaxillary area, and flat nasal tip and flared alar base.

Evolution of bilateral cleft lip repair

The evolution of repair of the bilateral cleft lip over the years has shown that it is best to repair both sides of the cleft lip at the same time. In many centers today, primary nasal correction is performed along with the repair of the lip. The observation that the alar cartilages are splayed and rotated caudally was important in the evolution of primary rhinoplasty in cleft lip repair. The fear of growth interference when nasal cartilage is manipulated during primary repair has been one of the reasons for delaying nasal repair. For many years forked flaps were used to lengthen the columella, but McComb and Mulliken emphasized the importance of early repositioning of the alar cartilages and unraveled the problem of the short columella and broad nasal tip in the bilateral cleft lip. McComb, after reviewing his initial work over a period of 15 years, found that the nostril shape was still abnormal, the tip remained broad, and the columella was very long. He proposed primary nasal correction by repositioning the alar cartilages through a vertical skin incision. Over the years, the techniques that have been used for repair of the bilateral cleft lip and nose deformity include: the straight line closure or veau III operation; Tennison's triangular flap technique (similar to unilateral repair); Millard's technique; Manchester, Skoog, Black, and Mulliken techniques.

Principles of repair of bilateral cleft lip and nose

The basic principles guiding repair of the bilateral cleft lip deformity are: maintaining symmetry; establishing muscle continuity; designing the prolabial flap to achieve appropriate philtral width and shape; forming a cupid's bow and median tubercle from the lateral labial tissue; and, finally, repositioning the alar cartilages to construct the nasal tip and columella (Fig. 29.13). The principles outlined here are those of the Mulliken simultaneous lip and nose repair.

1. *Establishing symmetry.* Performing both sides simultaneously allows achievement of symmetry.
2. *Designing a prolabial flap of appropriate width.* The design and width of the prolabial flap should be narrow and biconcave to avoid a wide abnormal philtrum as the child grows. This width should be roughly 4 mm at the columella base and 6 mm at the peak of the cupid's bow. The mucosa of the prolabium can be used either to deepen the sulcus in the premaxillary region or to reconstruct the lip. The author's preference is to use it to deepen the labial sulcus, which is usually shallow.
3. *Forming the cupid's bow and median tubercle from lateral lip elements.* The prolabium usually has a very narrow strip of vermillion and hence, in the majority of cases, reconstruction of the vermillion in the mid-portion of the lip presents a difficult problem. The incision on the prolabium is made at the mucocutaneous junction and lateral lip vermillion flaps are used to reconstruct the central portion of the vermillion or the tubercle.
4. *Establishing muscle continuity.* In a complete bilateral cleft the prolabium is devoid of muscle fibers. Establishing continuity of muscle beneath the skin

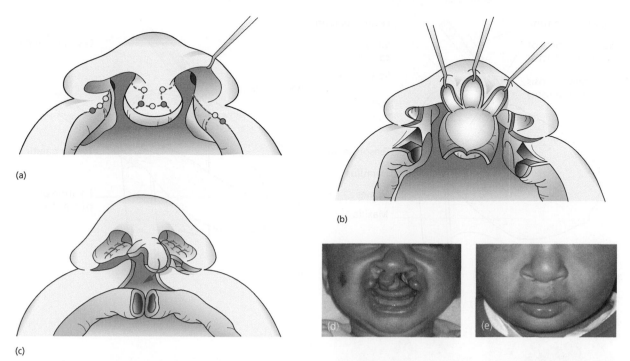

Fig. 29.13 Repair of bilateral cleft lip and palate. (a) Key points to be marked for bilateral cleft lip repair. (b) Designing prolabial flap. (c) Forming cupid's bow and median tubercle from lateral lip elements. (d) Preoperative and (e) postoperative views of a child with bilateral cleft lip repaired by modified Mulliken technique.

of the prolabium is the only way to reconstruct a normal functioning lip. The muscle fibres that are inserted at the alar base on each side are released and reoriented to be approximated in the midline with vertical mattress sutures. This may be difficult, particularly at the upper edge of the lip in wide clefts or a cleft with protruding premaxillae. While a sulcular incision bilaterally beneath the lateral lip elements is essential to mobilize the lip and achieve tension-free closure, the debate has centered on whether the incision should be subperiosteal or supraperiosteal. The author's preference is to perform a subperiosteal dissection following Delaire's principles.

5. *Reconstruction of the nasal tip and columella.* The lower lateral cartilages should be mobilized adequately from the overlying skin by wide dissection and undermining. The splayed cartilage domes can be approached by combining rim incisions with the prolabial flap. The lower lateral cartilages are repositioned anatomically and fixed with interdomal mattress sutures to create the tip and columella.

6. *Repositioning the alar base.* The nasal musculature must be mobilized by performing a subperiosteal dissection along the piriform rim and the wide alar base must be cinched with a suture to the base of the anterior nasal spine.

7. *Management of the premaxilla.* A protruding premaxilla in a complete bilateral CLP can impede the approximation of the lip wound edges with a tension-free closure. This can result in a wide scar and a poor cosmetic result. It is therefore important to reposition the premaxilla in the appropriate

position with presurgical orthopedics whenever possible.

Repair of cleft palate

The goals of palate repair are to normalize speech by surgical approximation and realignment of the aberrant attachments of the palatal muscles, and to seal the communication between the oral and nasal cavities without fistulae.

Timing of palate repair

The timing of palate repair to achieve optimal speech with minimal facial growth disturbance has been one of the more debated issues in cleft literature. Historically, cleft repair of the hard palate was delayed to minimize impairment of maxillofacial growth. It is now well accepted, and evidence in the literature shows, that speech outcomes are better when soft and hard palate repair is completed before speech development. Palate surgery is therefore timed according to the infant's speech developmental stage rather than chronologic age. For most children developing normally, this is around 9–12 months. The majority of the surgeons repair the palate (i.e. hard and soft palate) in one stage before 12 months of age. Some recommend a two-stage repair with soft palate repair as early as 3–6 months, at the time of primary lip repair, and hard palate by 12–15 months of age. Children with cleft palate often have other anomalies and it may be necessary to modify the timing of repair in

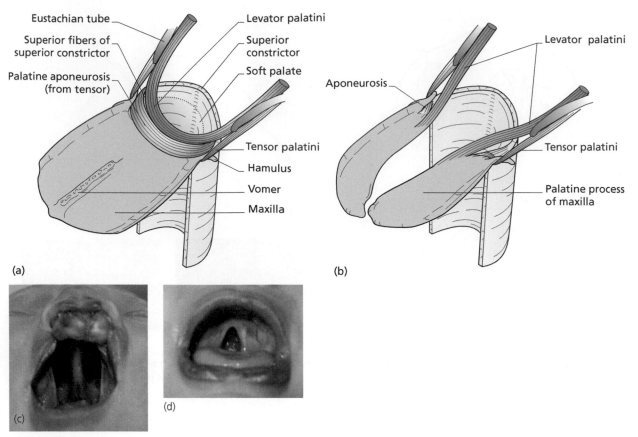

Fig. 29.14 (a) The muscle attachments in a normal palate. (b) Note abnormal attachments of muscle in a cleft palate. (c) A cleft of the secondary palate. (d) A bilateral cleft palate where neither palatal shelves fuse with the nasal septum, leaving a wide cleft in the midline.

the presence of comorbidities, particularly airway anomalies. Repair of the palate may be delayed up to 14–16 months of age if there are concerns of airway obstruction. Premature babies and infants with micrognathia are particularly at increased risk for postoperative episodes of apnea after palate repair.

Surgical anatomy

Cleft of the palate can range from a minor submucous cleft affecting only the soft palate to a complete bilateral cleft affecting the primary and secondary palate. It is important to look for overt signs of a submucous cleft if there is any suspicion. These signs include a bifid uvula, notching of the posterior nasal spine, or translucency in the mid-palatine region of the soft palate due to lack of muscle.

The muscles of soft palate that help with the function of speech and swallowing include the levator palatini, tensor palatini, palatopharyngeus, palatoglossus, and musculus uvulae. The soft palate in a non-cleft individual acts as a muscular valve that can lift superiorly and posteriorly to appose the pharyngeal wall and achieve velopharyngeal closure during speech. In a child with an unrepaired cleft, the soft palate cannot function as a muscular valve. This is due to the abnormal orientation and attachment of the muscles, primarily the levator palatini. The bundles of the levator on each side are longitudinally

directed to insert into the posterior edge of the palatine bone instead of joining in the midline in a transverse orientation and inserting into the palatine aponeurosis (Fig. 29.14). In addition, the sphincter action of the palatoglossus, palatopharyngeus, and superior constrictor muscles at oropharyngeal aperture is compromised leading to velopharyngeal insufficiency. The tensor palatini muscle fibers, which control the opening of the Eustachian tube and aerate the middle ear, do not function optimally, often leading to chronic otitis media.

Principles and techniques of palate repair

The main principle of cleft palate repair is to detach and retropose the abnormal insertion of the levator palatini and join the muscles of both halves of the soft palate in the midline at the junction of the middle and posterior third of the soft palate, in order to achieve proper elevation of the soft palate. In the hard palate, the most important principle is to reflect mucoperiosteal flaps based on the grater palatine arteries, which emerge from the greater palatine foramen bilaterally at the postero-lateral area of the hard palate.

Cleft palate surgical treatment dates back to the 1760s when a French dentist, Le Monnier, first attempted repair. Several other surgeons, including Philbert Roux, Carl Ferdinand Von Graefe, and

Johann Dieffenbach, subsequently described techniques to repair the palate. It was Von Langenbeck, who first described the use of mucoperiosteal flaps for cleft palate surgery. Kriens, in 1969, first introduced the concept of an anatomical approach to veloplasty by restoring the levator sling. The choice of surgical technique depends on the type of cleft. At the time of the primary palatoplasty the ears should be inspected. If there is evidence of serous otitis, a myringotomy is performed and fluid aspirated with placement of grommets or ventilating tubes in the myringotomy incisions.

The two-flap palatoplasty is a commonly used surgical technique for repair of the complete unilateral and bilateral cleft of the palate. The edges of the cleft are incised from the alveolus to the base of the uvula and bilateral full-thickness mucoperiosteal flaps are reflected (Fig. 29.15). The levator palatini muscles are

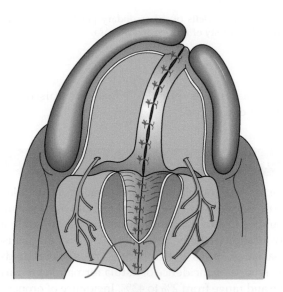

(a)

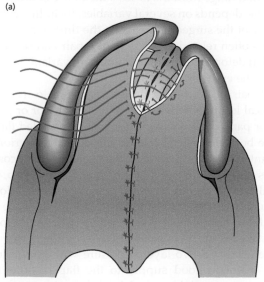

(b)

Fig. 29.15 (a) Classic two-flap palatoplasty showing two pedicled palatal mucoperiosteal flaps and closure of muscle and nasal mucosa. (b) The two flaps are brought together by good approximation of the oral layer over the nasal layer.

released and dissected to be repositioned horizontally and sutured. Bilateral releasing incisions are made to decrease the tension in the midline.

For the cleft of the secondary palate a Von Langenbeck repair can be used. In this technique bilateral releasing incisions are made and the mucoperiosteum is elevated to complete the stripping and closure of nasal layer, muscle, and oral layers as shown in Figure 29.16a. The Veau–Wardwill–Kilner (V–Y pushback) technique, named after Thomas Kilner, Victor Veau, and William Wardwill, is used less often for repair of cleft of secondary palate. In this technique the oral mucosa is divided anteriorly, which may lengthen the palate but leaves areas of exposed bone in the anterior hard palate that can potentially cause maxillary growth disturbances. The double reversing Furlow Z-plasty was introduced by Dr Leonard Furlow Jr ins 1978. This technique uses two reversed Z-plasties of the oral and nasal mucosa to repair the cleft. It has two advantages: restoring the normal anatomic position of the levator palatini in the middle and posterior third of soft palate and increasing soft palate length (Fig. 29.16b). Complications of palatoplasty include postoperative bleeding, airway obstruction, wound dehiscence, and fistula formation. Care should be taken to achieve adequate intraoperative hemostasis and careful postoperative monitoring is essential to avoid airway obstruction.

Speech and velopharyngeal dysfunction

Children with palatal clefts are at risk for a wide range of speech problems related to resonance, articulation, phonation, learning, and language delay. These speech abnormalities can be caused by velopharyngeal insufficiency, oronasal fistula, weak lip pressure, abnormal tongue pressure, malpositioned teeth, abnormal jaw relationship, neuromuscular dysfunction, and conductive or sensorineural hearing loss. It is important to identify and associate the cause with effect. Assessment of speech should begin as early as 6 months of age and be monitored throughout adolescence.

Speech in cleft individuals often has a nasal quality. This perceived hypernasality during speech is typically due to incomplete closure of the velopharyngeal port which separates the nasal cavity from the oral cavity during speech production. Typically, velopharyngeal insufficiency (VPI) refers to the inability of the soft palate and the posterior and lateral pharyngeal walls to come together to create a seal during speech production. Nasal air escape during speech may be due to an unrepaired submucous cleft of the palate. This can also occur after repair of the palate, due to improper position of palatal musculature impeding movement and/or insufficient soft palate length.

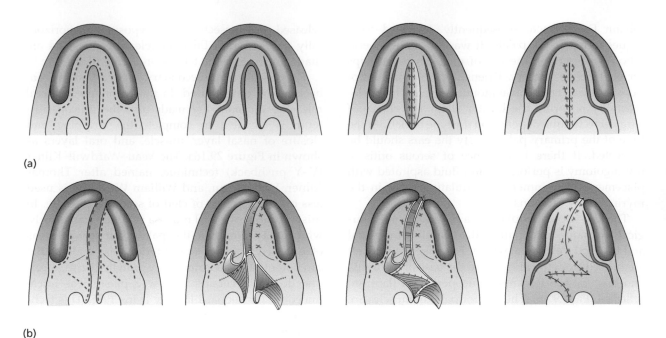

(a)

(b)

Fig. 29.16 (a) The Von Langenbeck technique of palatoplasty is generally used for clefts of the secondary palate. (b) Schematic diagram of Furlow Z-plasty technique, showing the reverse opposing double Z-plasty of muscle and mucosa.

Assessment of speech for VPI has to be both clinical and instrumental. Clinical assessment of resonance characteristics is best performed as a child's articulatory repertoire develops. Non-instrumental testing utilizing visualization of airflow with a reflecting mirror and nasal pinching often assists with the prediction of velopharyngeal function during speech. If deficits are identified, then further assessment using nasendoscopy to assess posterior and lateral pharyngeal wall motion or videofluoroscopy is indicated. Nasopharyngoscopy is a diagnostic tool for evaluation of velopharyngeal function that helps the surgeon to make a decision regarding the need for therapeutic intervention. Small-diameter pediatric flexible endoscopes with a good light source and topical anesthetic for nasal mucosa will help children become more compliant with this procedure.

Studies show that the need for surgical correction of VPI ranges from 4% to 30%. The most effective method for correction of VPI is controversial but the choice of the procedure depends on cause and where abnormality is found: lateral or posterior pharyngeal wall. A posterior flap pharyngoplasty is indicated when there is limited or lack of posterior wall motion. The flap may be superiorly or inferiorly based. A superiorly based flap, with the base at the level of the tubercle of the atlas and insertion into the soft palate, is more popular than the inferiorly based flap. A lateral pharyngoplasty is advocated for managing decreased lateral wall motion by creating a dynamic sphincter to control the size of the pharyngeal orifice. This was first by described Orticochea and modified by Jackson. The sphincter is created by posterior tonsillar pillars, including the

palatopharyngeus muscle, which are raised and sutured end to end.

Correction of oronasal fistulae

One of the complications of primary cleft palate repair is failure of healing or breakdown of wound resulting in oronasal fistulae. Fistulae can occur at any location in the hard or soft palate and may cause nasal air escape as well as regurgitation of oral fluids. The reports on incidence of fistula formation are variable and range from 2% to 43%. Incidence of oronasal fistulae depends on several variables, including experience of the surgeon and age at the time of repair; it is less often related to the type of repair and severity of cleft deformity. The most significant variable seems to be the experience of the surgeon.

Repair of the fistula varies according to its anatomical location, whether it is in the anterior or posterior part of the palate. Various local pedicled flaps have been described to close the defect. Posteriorly or anteriorly based tongue flaps, musculo-mucosal flaps based on the facial artery, a temporalis flap, or local palatal mucoperiosteal flaps can be used to close fistulae. More recently, interpositional grafts made of acellular dermis have been used to achieve tension-free closure of oronasal fistulae. It is important to have at least a two-layered closure without tension and maintain good supply to the flap in order to achieve a watertight seal of the defect without recurrence. Almost all of the fistulae can be repaired by local pedicled flaps. However, occasionally a vascularized flap may be helpful in closure of a scarred palate with a large defect.

Table 29.3 Orthodontic management in cleft individuals.

Age	Treatment
2–10 weeks	Presurgical orthopedics
6–10 years	Phase I orthodontics: Maxillary expansion for alveolar bone grafting Maxillary protraction with face mask when indicated
10–14 years	Maintain maxillary expansion and alignment of teeth Monitor facial growth and eruption of permanent teeth Orthodontic treatment with distraction of maxilla if deficiency is severe
14–18 years	Phase II orthodontics: Orthodontic treatment with full fixed appliances to align teeth Prepare for orthognathic surgery when indicated Extract teeth if mandibular arch is crowded Decide whether to replace/substitute the absent maxillary lateral incisor

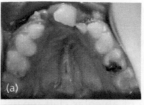
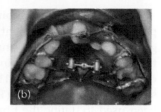
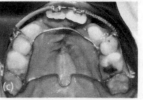

Fig. 29.17 Orthodontic expansion in a bilateral cleft of lip and palate. (a) Collapsed alveolar cleft segments with decreased anterior maxillary arch width. (b) This maxillary expansion device allows greater increase in arch width in the anterior region more than the posterior region. (c) Maxillary width being maintained after expansion.

Orthodontic management of the cleft individual

The orthodontist plays an important role in the care of the cleft individual during infancy, mixed dentition and permanent dentition (Table 29.3). Presurgical orthopedic treatment is facilitated by the orthodontist between 2 and 10 weeks after birth in infants with wide clefts and poorly aligned alveolar segments or a protruding premaxilla. In the early mixed dentition phase, children with complete clefts of lip and palate often have a posterior and anterior crossbite. The crossbite is asymmetric in unilateral clefts, affecting mainly the lesser segment or cleft side. In bilateral clefts, there is collapse of both lateral segments with a bilateral posterior crossbite and protrusion of the premaxilla. The goal of orthodontic treatment in this phase is to prepare for repair of the alveolar cleft by expanding the maxillary alveolar segments, and correcting the position of rotated maxillary incisors. The use of a quad helix or a screw expansion device allows greater expansion in the anterior maxillary arch (Fig. 29.17).

Monitoring facial growth during childhood and early adolescence helps to identify early signs of maxillary hypoplasia and allows intervention if indicated. Maxillary growth may be restricted in the vertical, transverse, and antero-posterior dimensions in children with complete CLP. These children may benefit from maxillary protraction using a reverse-pull headgear or early maxillary osteotomy and distraction osteogenesis to minimize the severity of deformity. The typical orthodontic treatment for a cleft patient following the eruption of the permanent teeth consists of maintaining maxillary arch width after repair of alveolar cleft, and alignment of teeth with full fixed appliances. This should be timed appropriately based on need for orthognathic surgery, the individual's growth potential, and ability to cooperate and maintain oral hygiene. Extraction of teeth may be necessary, particularly in the mandibular arch, if there is arch length deficiency. When surgery is indicated orthodontic treatment is coordinated with timing of growth completion, which is around age 15–16 years for females and 17–19 years for males. It is important to integrate the plan for the replacement or substitution of the absent maxillary lateral incisor and any other missing teeth into the orthodontic treatment plan.

Alveolar cleft repair

The primary goal of alveolar cleft repair is to establish bony continuity of the maxillary alveolar ridge, provide bone support for the teeth adjacent to the cleft, and seal the communication between the nose and oral cavity when there is a patent oronasal fistula. A successful alveolar bone graft should facilitate eruption and orthodontic movement of teeth in the line of the cleft (most often the maxillary canine), maintain the health of the periodontium of teeth adjacent to the cleft, provide alar base support, and improve nasal symmetry. Gingivoperiosteoplasty performed at the time of primary lip repair may seal the oronasal communication but does not always preclude the need for a bone graft. Some studies show that at least 40–50% of these patients require bone grafting in the future. More recently, Meazzini *et al.* have shown that patients who had a gingivoperiosteoplasty at the time of primary repair did not require bone grafting at a later date; however, they report a greater need for surgical correction of maxillary hypoplasia.

The timing, source of bone, the surgical technique, perioperative management, and outcome of bone grafting have all been studied and debated. The terms primary bone grafting (2–5 years of age) secondary bone grafting (7–11 years of age), and late secondary bone grafting (14–18 years of age) have been used to define the time of alveolar cleft repair. The majority of the centers use secondary alveolar bone grafting in the mixed dentition phase between the ages of 7 and 11 years, after maxillary expansion. Typically, this coincides with one-half to two-thirds of root development of the maxillary canine or lateral incisor (if present) in the line of the cleft. Completion of the maxillary expansion prior to grafting provides adequate access to the cleft defect and aligns the cleft segments better.

The gold standard for the grafting material has been particulate corticocancellous bone marrow harvested from the iliac crest, which was first described by Boyne and Sands. Other sites that have been described include rib, symphysis, calvarium, and tibia. More recently, the use of bone growth factors, such as recombinant human bone morphogenic protein-2 (rhBMP-2), has been shown to be effective in grafting the defect. BMP-2 promotes differentiation of pluripotential cells into cells that can form new bone in the defect. This eliminates donor site morbidity and minimizes hospital stay and postoperative pain and discomfort.

New imaging techniques, such as cone-beam computed tomography, allow more accurate assessment of the volume of the bony defect before surgery and radiographic outcome of the grafted alveolus after surgery, when compared with the conventional two-dimensional periapical and panoramic radiographs.

The principles of surgical repair are the same for unilateral and bilateral clefts and include: proper closure of nasal floor mucosa to seal the communication between the nose and oral cavity; removal of supernumerary teeth in the cleft defect; filling the defect with cancellous bone; and approximation of the oral mucosa on the labial and palatal aspects to achieve a watertight closure over the grafted bone, as illustrated in Figure 29.18. In the bilateral cleft, the position of the premaxilla makes the repair more technically challenging. The premaxilla is often inferiorly positioned, and retruded with the incisors located below the level of the occlusal plane. In some instances, the position of the premaxilla can be corrected by presurgical orthodontics; however, in others it may have to be corrected by performing a vomerine osteotomy at the time of surgical alveolar cleft repair. The osteotomized premaxilla has to be maintained in position with a splint for 4–6 weeks postoperatively.

The amount of maxillary arch expansion prior to surgery should be planned and monitored. Too much presurgical expansion of the lateral segments leaves a large palatal defect making it difficult to advance the scarred palatal mucoperiosteal flaps to cover the bone graft, and too little expansion limits surgical

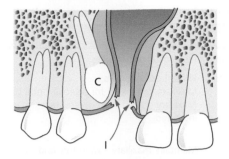

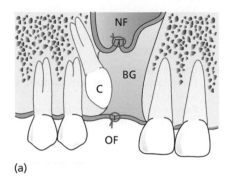

(a)

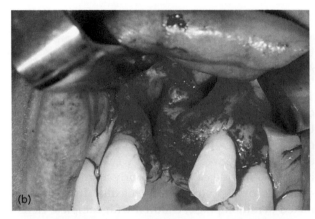

(b)

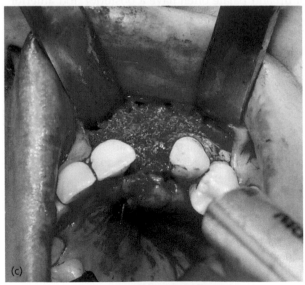

(c)

Fig. 29.18 Alveolar cleft repair. (a) Schematic diagram of the alveolar cleft showing closure of the nasal and oral mucosa. (Reproduced from Assael L. (1995) Cleft lip and palate. *Atlas of the Oral and Maxillofacial Clinics of North America* 3(1), p. 31. Copyright © 1995 Elsevier.) (b) The alveolar cleft deformity is visible and nasal mucosa is closed to seal the communication between the oral and nasal cavities. (c) Cancellous bone is packed into the defect after closure of the palatal oral mucosa.

access to the alveolar cleft. After alveolar cleft repair, orthodontic tooth movement, if necessary, can be initiated in 3–4 months. The maxillary width achieved by presurgical expansion should be maintained after surgery with a palatal retainer until phase II orthodontic treatment begins at a later date.

Replacement of absent teeth in the line of the cleft

Congenital absence of the maxillary lateral incisor in the line of the cleft can be managed appropriately by closing the space and substituting the adjacent canine in its position or by opening space and replacing it with a fixed or removable prosthesis. The experience at the center for cleft and craniofacial anomalies at the University of California has shown success of implants in grafted unilateral clefts is better than in bilateral clefts. In the bilateral cases the periodontal health of the central incisors is very often compromised, and the lateral incisors are also absent. The substitution of the lateral incisor with the adjacent canine is cost-effective; however, it can result in loss of arch length and decrease in transverse dimension of the maxillary arch. It can also be unesthetic due to the asymmetry in tooth size and shape in unilateral cases. Replacement with an endosseous implant is an option when there is adequate space and bone quantity. There may be inadequate bone at the time of placement of the implant even if the alveolar cleft was repaired previously. Alveolar ridge augmentation with a cortical onlay graft performed about 4 months prior to placement of the implant will provide adequate bone height and width for placement of the implant (Fig. 29.19). A removable prosthesis should also be considered when there is loss of premaxilla, severe deficiency of bone height and width with scarring of the overlying soft tissue, and lack of lip support. Use of teeth-supported fixed prosthetic restorations, such as a bridge, across the unrepaired alveolar cleft segments should be avoided, as movement of the cleft segments results in failure of the prosthesis and loss of abutment teeth.

Surgical correction of maxillary hypoplasia

Cleft lip and palate patients exhibit varying degrees of maxillary hypoplasia due to restriction of midfacial growth that is apparent in the sagittal, vertical, and transverse dimensions. This midface deficiency can be attributed partly to the intrinsic reduction in growth potential due to the congenital malformation and, partly, to scar contracture following primary palate surgery. The maxillary deficiency caused by the cleft deformity is superimposed upon the genetically inherited skeletal growth pattern. Hence, an underlying inherited pattern of excessive mandibular growth can present as severe midfacial deficiency and a class III malocclusion in a cleft patient. Regardless of the etiology of maxillary hypoplasia, approximately 25% (reported range 14–50%) of cleft individuals undergo surgical correction of maxillary hypoplasia. This wide range highlights the differing indications for skeletal correction by cleft team specialists. Their decisions are influenced by differing treatment philosophies (orthodontic management with dental compensation versus surgical maxillary advancement to address facial esthetics and occlusion more comprehensively), the availability of appropriately trained surgeons, and hospital/government funding. Good *et al.* reported that the frequency of a Le Fort I osteotomy for correction of maxillary hypoplasia correlated with the severity of clefting.

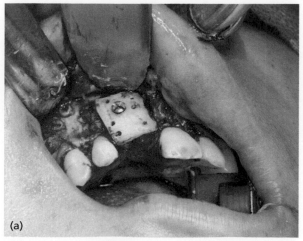

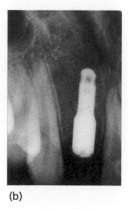

(b)

(a)

Fig. 29.19 Replacement of missing lateral incisor. (a) Alveolar ridge augmentation with a cortical bone onlay is often necessary to increase width and height, before placement of an implant in the grafted cleft site. (b) Unilateral cleft with a missing lateral incisor replaced with an endosseous implant.

Summary

An esthetic smile and normal speech are two important characteristics which give an individual his or her identity, confidence and self-esteem. The ability to restore lip and palate function without jeopardizing growth with various surgical interventions is the key to management of cleft deformities. This requires a thorough understanding of the embryological, physical and psychological development of the child.

Recommended reading

Chigurupati R, Heggie A, Bonanthaya K. (2010) Cleft lip and palate: an overview. In: *Oral and Maxillofacial Surgery*. (eds, Andersson L, Kahnberg K-E, Pogrel MA). Oxford, Wiley-Blackwell.

Cohen MM. (2000) Etiology and pathogenesis of orofacial clefting. *Oral and Maxillofacial Surgery Clinics of North America*, **12**, 379–97.

Eppley BL. (2005) The spectrum of orofacial clefting. *Plastic and Reconstructive Surgery*, **115**, 101–14e.

Hagberg C, Larson O, Milerad J. (1998) Incidence of cleft lip and palate and risks of additional malformations. *Cleft Palate-Craniofacial Journal*, **35**, 40–5.

Mulliken JB. (2004) The changing faces of children with cleft lip and palate. *New England Journal of Medicine*, **351**, 745–7.

Chapter 30

Correction of Dentofacial Deformities

The art and science of correcting dentofacial deformities by means of orthodontic tooth movement and surgical repositioning of the jaw structures is called orthognathic surgery. Orthodontic treatment is primarily the treatment of a malocclusion by the movement of the teeth within their bony base. Most patients with a malocclusion and normal jaw relation can be managed by means of orthodontic treatment alone. However, successful correction of a malocclusion combined with a skeletal discrepancy between the upper and lower jaw is often not possible by orthodontic means alone.

Over the last three decades orthognathic surgery has developed into a science and an art form through the combination of the skills of the specialities of orthodontics and oral and maxillofacial surgery. To optimise the treatment outcomes the support of the general dentist, prosthodontist, endodontist, periodontist and our medical colleagues are, however, often required. Patients with dentofacial deformities are treated with three prime goals in mind:

1. *Function.* Apart from establishing normal masticatory function, the clinicians should also consider other problems caused by an abnormal jaw relationship such as: speech defects; sleep apnoea; attrition of the teeth; periodontal problems; and temporomandibular joint (TMJ) problems.
2. *Stability of results.* Definitive orthognathic treatment is a change for life and it is important to achieve dental and skeletal stability following treatment. Experience has shown that certain orthodontic tooth movements may not be stable in the long term while neuromuscular influence on a repositioned jaw may cause relapse.
3. *Aesthetics.* Facial appearance is often the patient's main concern. Leo Tolstoy said in *Childhood*, "I am convinced that nothing has so marked influence on the direction of a man's mind as his appearance, and not his appearance itself so much as his conviction that it is unattractive". Aesthetic imbalance is often the result of dento-skeletal imbalance.

The human face is a three-dimensional soft tissue structure supported by bone and teeth and all three dimensions should be considered when evaluating the relationship of the facial soft tissues, the upper and lower jaws to each other and the occlusion. The three basic dimensions are:

1. *Vertical* – The height of the upper and lower jaws and their relationship to facial proportions.
2. *Horizontal* – The antero-posterior relationship between the jaws and its effect on the profile.
3. *Transverse* – The widths of the dental arches, symmetries of the jaws and associated soft tissues.

A surgical orthodontic treatment is the only approach indicated for the successful correction of severe dentofacial deformities. However, the treatment of some malocclusions combined with mild skeletal disharmony is possible by orthodontic compensation of the dentition. Inappropriate dental compensation may, however, lead to poor long-term dental stability and compromised facial aesthetics. Borderline cases, therefore, require meticulous assessment before finally deciding on orthodontic treatment alone or a combination of orthodontics and surgery as treatment approach. Which treatment plan to adopt should be discussed with the patient (and perhaps the parents or spouse) and all the advantages and disadvantages of each approach explained. The decision may also be influenced by factors such as: the orthodontists experience; financial insurance cover; available surgical expertise; and the patient's attitude and preferences.

Essentials of Oral and Maxillofacial Surgery, First Edition. Edited by M. Anthony Pogrel, Karl-Erik Kahnberg and Lars Andersson.
© 2014 John Wiley & Sons, Ltd. Published 2014 by John Wiley & Sons, Ltd.
Companion website: www.wiley.com/go/pogrel/oms

The family dentist is often the first clinician to recognize and diagnose the patient's dentofacial deformity. It is most helpful if the dentist has a basic knowledge of the diagnosis, treatment planning, sequence of treatment, treatment possibilities and outcomes, and an overview of orthognathic surgery procedures to begin the process of educating the patient. This instils confidence in the patient *vis-á-vis* future treatment and subsequent referral to a specialist.

A meticulous and comprehensive assessment of the patient is required before formulating a treatment plan. An orthognathic assessment will consist of the following:

History. The patient's medical history can be obtained by means of a questionnaire that the patient fills out at the first visit. Previous restorative, orthodontic, and periodontal treatment and facial pain including TMJ pain should be reviewed.

Clinical evaluation. The clinical assessment of the face is probably the most valuable of all diagnostic procedures. While an astute clinical diagnosis can be made at the chair side, photographs are essential for accurate assessment and record purposes. The face is systematically assessed from a frontal view, profile view, three-quarter view. Figures 30.1, 30.2, 30.3 and 30.4 illustrate some angular and linear parameters used during the clinical assessment of the face.

Special investigations. Cephalometric and panoramic radiographs and dental casts are essential; however, TMJ investigations, Technetium bone scans, hand wrist radiographs, CT scans, etc. may be required. The lateral cephalometric radiograph allows the clinician to analyze and evaluate the soft tissue,

skeletal and dental relations of a dentofacial deformity (Fig. 30.5).

Diagnosis and problem list. A diagnosis is made following the clinical evaluation of the patient, a radiographic evaluation and cephalometric analysis, model analysis and other indicated evaluations. The data base is used to compile a problem list.

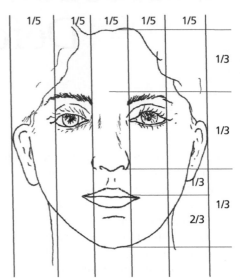

Fig. 30.2 Transverse facial proportions. The "rule of fifths" is a convenient method for evaluating transverse facial proportions. The widths of the nasal base and mouth are related to the eyes. Vertical relations. The face can be divided into three equal parts. Upper third (Trichion to Glabella), middle third (Glabella to Subnasale) and lower third (Subnasale to Menton). The lower third of the face is further divided into an upper third (Subnasale to upper lip Stomion) and a lower two-thirds (lower lip Stomion to Menton).

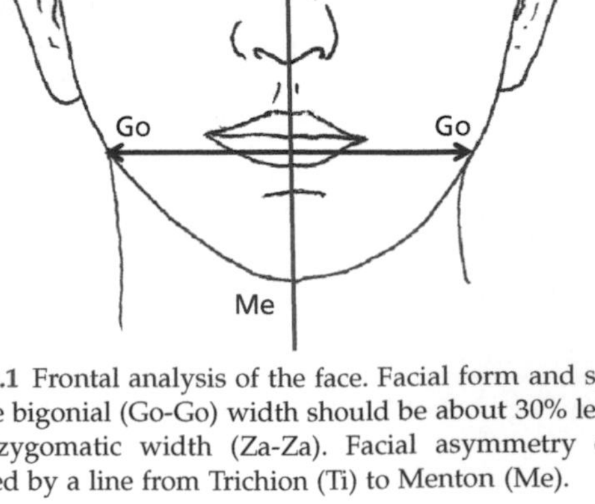

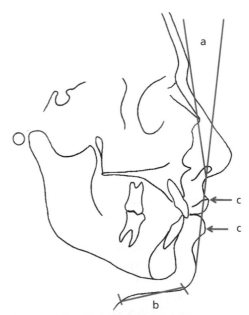

Fig. 30.3 Profile analysis of the face. (a) Facial contour angle: the angle is formed by the upper and lower facial planes. It is an indication of facial convexity or concavity and should be ±13 for females and ±11 for males. (b) Chin-throat length relates to the size of the mandible (±57 mm). (c) Lip position. The upper lip should be ±3.5 mm and the lower lip ±2.2 mm ahead of the lower facial plane.

Fig. 30.1 Frontal analysis of the face. Facial form and symmetry: the bigonial (Go-Go) width should be about 30% less than the bizygomatic width (Za-Za). Facial asymmetry can be assessed by a line from Trichion (Ti) to Menton (Me).

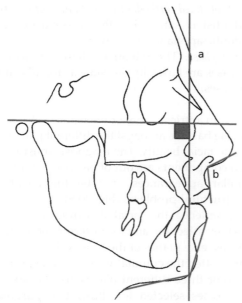

Fig. 30.4 (a) The zero-meridian (a line perpendicular to the Frankfort plane through soft tissue Nasion) indicates the ideal position of the chin. (b) The naso-labial angle (100 ± 11) is an indicator of upper lip support. (c) Lower lip-chin-throat angle (110 ± 8). The angle is usually acute in Class III (mandibular excessive) cases and obtuse in Class II (mandibular deficient) cases.

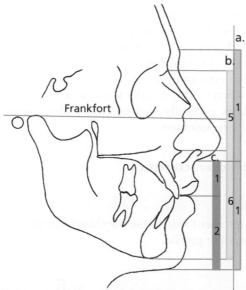

Fig. 30.5 Vertical facial proportions. (a) The soft tissue middle third (Glabella to Subnasale) should be equal to the lower third (Subnasale to Menton). (b) The skeletal middle third (Nasion to anterior nasal spine) to the lower third (anterior nasal spine to Menton) should have a ratio of 5 to 6. (c) The soft tissue of the lower third is divided into an upper third (Subnasale to Stomion) and a lower two-thirds (Stomion to Menton). Orthognathic surgery basically alters the lower third of the face.

Treatment objectives. Clear orthodontic and surgical treatment objectives regarding soft tissue, skeletal and dental structures should be identified and noted.

Development of a visual orthodontic and surgical cephalometric treatment objective. The lateral cephalometric radiograph tracing is used to develop an orthodontic visual treatment objective to predict orthodontic tooth movements. This is followed by the development of a surgical visual treatment objective predicting the required jaw repositioning and expected soft tissue changes (see individual Cases).

Treatment plan. All the factors identified in the diagnosis and problem list as well as patient concerns and reasons for considering orthognathic surgery are taken into account to formulate a final treatment plan. The sequence of treatment and the treatment to be performed by all health care professionals concerned are outlined. It is essential that when defining the treatment plan, a thorough knowledge of the many types of dentofacial deformities and the treatment modalities available to correct them is essential.

Treatment. Although the orthodontist and the oral and maxillofacial surgeon are the main role players, comprehensive correction of dentofacial deformities may involve several members of the health care team. It is mandatory that the therapeutic management is carried out as planned and any problem or change in treatment plan should be communicated to the treatment team.

Explanation of a typical treatment profile

Once a definitive treatment plan has been formulated, it is discussed with the patient and, once accepted, treatment can commence. A typical orthognathic treatment profile consists of six phases:

1. *Placement of orthodontic bands and attachments on the teeth.* Any extractions of teeth (including third molars) are performed 2–3 weeks before the orthodontic appliances are placed.
2. *Preoperative orthodontic phase.* The teeth are now aligned in their optimal positions according to the treatment plan. This phase usually takes 9–18 months. Once the orthodontist is satisfied that the preparation is complete, the patient is referred back to the surgeon.
3. *Surgical phase.* Before surgery a new set of orthognathic records are obtained. A final surgical cephalometric visual treatment objective is developed and the exact required surgical movements measured on the tracing (Fig. 30.6). Modern technology allows the surgeon to obtain three-dimensional images through CT scanning of the face. Surgical planning can be performed using these images. For the treatment of more intricate dentofacial deformities three-dimensional models can be fabricated from the CT scans to further enhance planning. New dental moulds are taken and the casts accurately articulated on an adjustable articulator. The intended surgical movements are performed

on the plaster models and the surgical movements of the jaws and teeth again measured (Fig. 30.7). Acrylic surgical splints are now fabricated on the models. The surgical splints will guide the surgeon during surgery. The jaws are now surgically repositioned according to the treatment plan. Immediately following surgery light intermaxillary elastics (3.5 oz, 2.5 mm) are placed to guide the teeth into the new occlusion and the patient is advised to maintain a soft diet for 3–6 weeks. Modern orthognathic surgery practice very seldom requires intermaxillary wire fixation. The patient is referred back to the orthodontist 2–3 weeks after surgery.

4. *Postoperative orthodontic phase.* The occlusion is now refined until the orthodontist is satisfied that maximum intercuspation has been achieved.

5. *Removal of fixed orthodontic appliance.* Once the orthodontist is satisfied with the occlusion, the orthodontic appliance is removed.

6. *Retention phase.* The retention phase for orthognathic cases are basically the same as for all orthodontic cases.

The face is an intricate three-dimensional structure and restoring balance amongst the different parts will re-constitute facial beauty. The diagnosis must identify which components are out of balance, for apparently similar appearances may be the result of differing structural problems (Fig. 30.8).

For convenience the facial deformities are discussed as they affect the antero-posterior, the vertical and the transverse planes of the face. Although facial deformity is often the cumulative effect of disproportion in two or three different planes, for the sake of clarity the cases selected for illustrative purposes have disproportion limited primarily to a single plane.

Antero-posterior problems

Mandibular excess

Mandibular prognathism describes an excessive protrusion of the lower jaw relative to the midface and cranium. True prognathism should be carefully differentiated from *pseudo prognathism* which results from occlusal interferences and a subsequent forward postural slide of the lower jaw into a habitual protrusion. An *overclosure* of the mandible, such as may occur when many posterior teeth are lost or when the maxilla is vertically deficient, may also produce a Class III appearance.

Clinical characteristics

Facial:

- A prominent chin is the dominant feature.
- A concave profile.

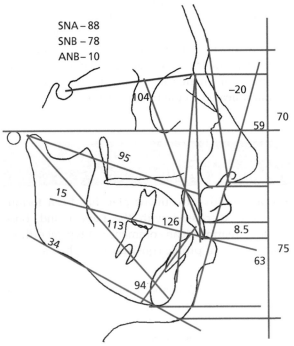

SNA – 88
SNB – 78
ANB – 10

Fig. 30.6 A tracing of a lateral cephalometric radiograph is used to analyze the hard and soft tissue structures. It is also used to develop an orthodontic and surgical visual treatment objective.

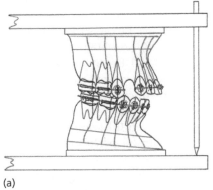

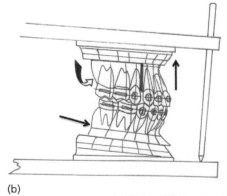

(a)   (b)

Fig. 30.7 Model surgery. The intended surgery is accurately simulated in the articulated dental casts. (a) The presurgical positions of the teeth and jaws are first measured and marked. (b) The osteotomies are performed and the teeth and dentoalveolar segments are positioned into the planned occlusion. An acrylic surgical splint is fabricated and the surgical movements recorded and used during surgery. Source: Reproduced from Reyneke (2010) with permission. © Quintessence Publishing Co Inc, Chicago.

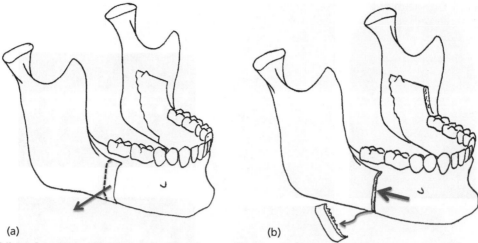

(a)   (b)

Fig. 30.8 The bilateral sagittal split ramus osteotomy for mandibular setback. A small segment of bone is removed proximally (arrow) to allow for the setback of the distal segment. The segments are fixated by either bicortical screws or bone plates.

- The midface appears relatively deficient.
- A more horizontal mandibular plane (lower border) will be associated with a more protrusive chin and a steeper mandibular plane with a less prominent but more vertically excessive chin.
- The lower third of the face appears broad and heavy.
- The lips may be incompetent and poorly supported especially in cases having severe anterior crossbites.
- The alar base of the nose may appear narrow.

Dental features:

- An angle Class III occlusion.
- Anterior and posterior crossbites are common.
- The mandibular incisor teeth are often lingually inclined. This reduces the negative overjet and is therefore a dental compensation for the unfavorable relationship of the jaw.

Treatment

Presurgical orthodontic preparation
The placement of fixed appliances is mandatory in order to level, align and decompensate all the teeth. The upper and lower arches are coordinated so that they will interdigitate properly at the time of surgical correction. The planned orthodontic tooth movement (which may include tipping lower incisors forward – decompensation) in many instances exaggerates the Class III occlusion making the problem appear worse.

Surgery
The bilateral sagittal split osteotomy is the commonest of several popular techniques for reducing the excessive mandible (see Fig. 30.9). Bicortical screws or bone plates are used to provide rigid fixation. Should the chin be excessive, the prominence may be corrected by a reduction genioplasty.

Postoperative orthodontics
Following the fixation period orthodontics is continued in order to perfect the occlusion. The teeth are retained in their new positions using conventional orthodontic techniques.

Case 1

This case comprised an 18-year-old female patient complaining of an uncomfortable bite and strong lower jaw. The diagnosis of a Class III occlusion and skeletal mandibular antero-posterior excess was made. Following a 12-month period of preoperative orthodontic treatment her mandible was set back by means of a bilateral sagittal split osteomy. After a total treatment time of 16 months the orthodontic appliance was removed (Fig. 30.9).

Mandibular deficiency

Mandibular deficiency is a common mandibular deformity and is associated with Class II malocclusion.

Clinical characteristics
Facial:

- A convex profile.
- Retruded "weak" chin.
- An everted lower lip which wedges behind the protruding upper incisor teeth, resulting in a deep labiomental fold when the jaws are closed.
- The upper lip often appears short, curled and protrusive at rest.
- The lips are generally strained when the patient attempts closure. There is noticeable puckering and flattening of the skin over the mentalis muscle area.

Dental features:

- Angle Class II occlusion.
- Increased overjet.

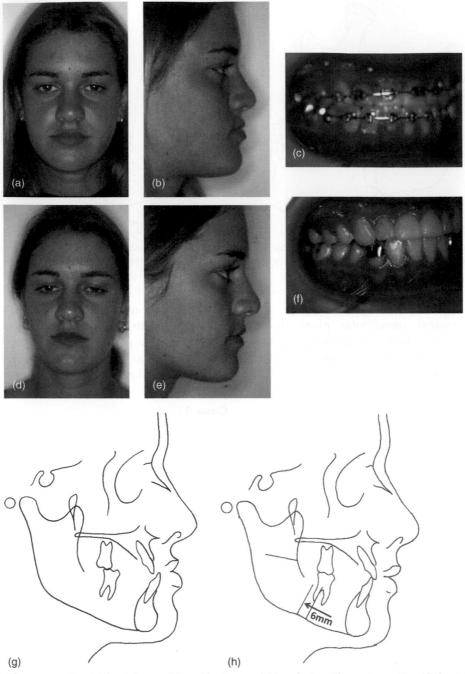

Fig. 30.9 Case 1. The preoperative (a) frontal view, (b) profile view, and (c) occlusion. The postoperative (d) frontal view, (e) profile view, and (f) occlusion. The (g) presurgical cephalometric tracing and the (h) surgical visual treatment objective indicating a 6 mm mandibular setback.

- Accentuated curve of Spee.
- Lower anterior teeth may be tipped forward and crowded.

Treatment

Presurgical orthodontic preparation
The basic orthodontic principles are to level and align the arches, and this may require extractions to provide the necessary space. All the teeth should be up-righted over basal bone and the dental arches coordinated.

Surgery
A bilateral sagittal split osteotomy of the mandibular ramus is the procedure of choice (Fig. 30.10). Should the diagnosis include a particularly retrusive chin, an advancement genioplasty will enhance the appearance.

Case 2

A 32-year-old female patient was refered from the orthodontist for surgical correction of her skeletal Class II malocclusion. The surgery involved man-

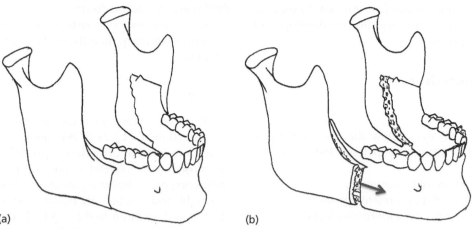

Fig. 30.10 The bilateral sagittal split ramus osteotomy for mandibular advancement. The distal segment is advanced while the condyle-fossa relationship is maintained.

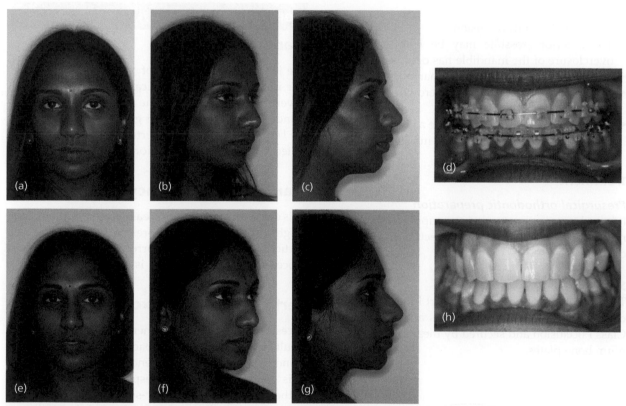

Fig. 30.11 Case 2. The pre-surgical (a) frontal view, (b) three-quarter view, (c) profile view, and (d) occlusion. The post-treatment (e) frontal view, (f) three-quarter view, (g) profile view, and (h) occlusion.

dibular advancement by means of a bilateral sagittal split osteotomy (Fig. 30.11).

Maxillary excess

Skeletal maxillary antero-posterior excess is not a common skeletal deformity; however, if it does occur it is usually dentoalveolar in origin. This can often corrected by orthodontic treatment alone.

Maxillary deficiency

In the past, maxillary deficiency was frequently misdiagnosed as mandibular antero-posterior excess, because of the similarity in facial appearance. Maxillary antero-posterior deficiencies are often also accompanied by deficiency in width and height. In these cases, closure of the lower jaw into centric occlusion brings the chin upward and forward, exaggerating the prominence of the lower jaw. It is not uncommon that antero-posterior disproportionate development may affect both jaws.

Clinical characteristics

Facial:

- The sclera of the eyes below the iris is often distinctly visible when the patient looks straight ahead.
- The paranasal areas are flattened.
- The upper lip is flat and relatively short.
- The upper incisors are seldom displayed.
- The chin may be in a good position or may *appear* prominent, especially if there is some degree of mandibular overclosure.
- The profile is concave.

Dental features:

- An Angle Class III occlusion.
- The anterior crossbite may be increased when overclosure of the mandible has occurred.
- The maxillary arch tends to be narrow.
- The maxillary teeth are more crowded than the lower.
- The lower incisor teeth may have a normal inclination, but are in crossbite with the maxillary incisors.

Treatment

Presurgical orthodontic preparation

It may be necessary to align the upper arch in segments to enable the surgical correction of posterior crossbites.

Surgery

The operation of choice is a Le Fort I maxillary osteotomy (Fig. 30.12). The maxilla is advanced into a Class I occlusion and secured by means of small titanium bone plates.

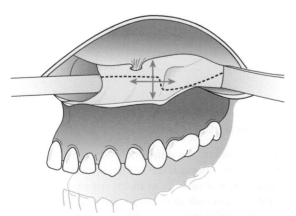

Fig. 30.12 The Le Fort I maxillary osteotomy. Once the maxilla has been down-fractured and mobilized it is repositioned according to the treatment plan.

Postoperative orthodontics

In order to enhance the postoperative stability and to maximize intercuspation the occlusion is refined and retained.

Case 3

A 20-year-old male patient was referred for the surgical correction of a Class III asymmetric malocclusion, after 16 months of orthodontic preparation. He was diagnosed with skeletal maxillary antero-posterior deficiency, mandibular asymmetry of his mandible to the right and a Class III malocclusion with lower dental midline 4 mm to the right. He required surgical advancement of his maxilla combined with a unilateral sagittal split mandibular osteotomy on the left for the correction of the asymmetry of his lower jaw (Fig. 30.13).

Vertical plane

Mandibular excess

The increase in the height of the lower third of the face in these patients is typically due to an increase in vertical development of the alveolar process of the mandible, but the exuberant growth may also affect the *body* of the mandible. Vertical chin excess is corrected by means of a reduction genioplasty.

Mandibular deficiency

This deformity causes a decrease of the anterior facial height, producing a squat, foreshortened appearance. Vertical chin deficiency is corrected by a genioplasty procedure whereby the chin is down grafted.

Vertical maxillary excess

Excessive vertical development of the maxilla will result in a downward and backward rotation of the mandible, resulting in tendency to a convex profile. This "long face" deformity responds particularly well to the combined orthodontic-surgical approach. Two varieties of this deformity have been defined:

1. *Without open bite:* usually demonstrating dental compensations with over-eruption of incisors and a long mandibular ramus.
2. *With open bite type:* due to either excessive posterior maxillary vertical growth or short mandibular ramus.

Vertical maxillary excess without open bite

Facial:

- Increased height of the lower third of the face.
- Recessive paranasal areas.

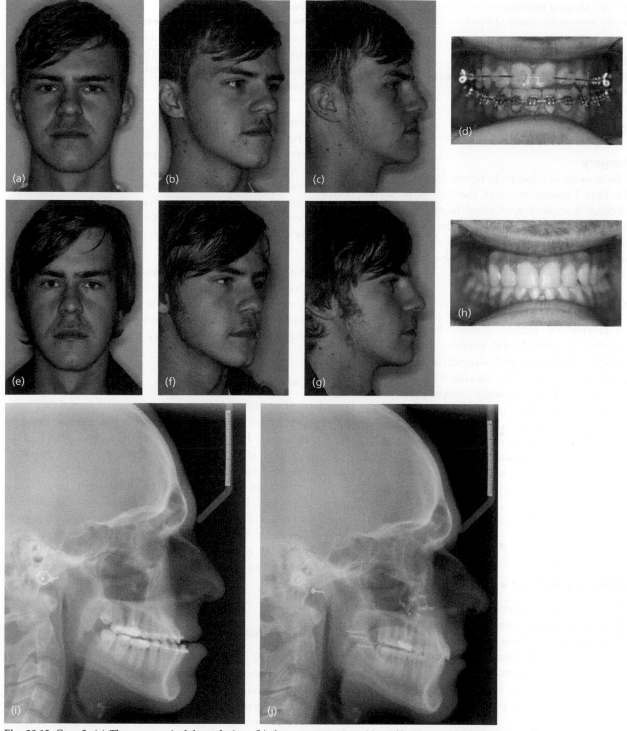

Fig. 30.13 Case 3. (a) The pre-surgical frontal view, (b) three-quarter view, (c) profile view, and (d) occlusion. The post-treatment (e) frontal view, (f) three-quarter view, (g) profile view, and (h) occlusion. (i) The pre-surgical and (j) post-treatment lateral cephalometric radiographs.

- Narrow alar base.
- Large interlabial gap (more than 4 mm) with the lips in repose.
- Severe strain when lips are closed.
- Excessive exposure of the upper incisor teeth (more than 4 mm).
- Excessive amount of gum showing when smiling ("gummy smile").

- There is a general tendency for a Class II skeletal relationship as a result of the relative downward and backward position of the mandible.
- The chin may be retruded.

Dental:

- An angle Class II occlusion in most cases.
- A high arched palate.

- "V" shaped maxilla.
- Accentuated curve of Spee.

Treatment
Presurgical orthodontic preparation

Routine orthodontic treatment aligns the arches separately, without attempting to correct the inter-arch positions.

Surgery

The maxilla is superiorly repositioned by means of a Le Fort I osteotomy and the key is to accomplish skeletal harmony and ideal tooth/lip relationship. The mandible will automatically rotate closed. Any antero-posterior discrepancies can be corrected by mandibular advancement or setback.

Case 4

A 16-year-old female patient had undergone 16 months of orthodontic preparation following her initial orthodontic and surgical consultations. Her profile was convex, the maxilla was vertically excessive, the mandible rotated clockwise, her chin deficient and she had a Class II occlusion. Her treatment plan consisted of initial orthodontic alignment of her teeth. The surgical correction involved superior repositioning of her maxilla by means of a le Fort I osteotomy. The mandible would rotate counter clockwise (forward and upward) improving the occlusion to a Class I relationship. Final aesthetic correction required advancement of her chin by means of a genioplasty (Fig. 30.14).

Maxillary vertical excess with open bite

The aetiology of anterior open bite is multifactorial. Skeletal open bite usually develops as a result of vertical maxillary excess or vertical mandibular deficiency. However, there are many factors such as genetic factors, neuromuscular effects, sucking habits, macroglossia etc. that may play a role in the development of an anterior open bite.

Clinical characteristics
Facial:

- The lower third of the face is usually elongated, with a retruded chin.
- Narrow alar base.
- Incompetent lips.

Dental features:

Although open bite deformity is most frequently associated with a Class II malocclusion, these patients can present with a Class I or even a Class III occlusal relationship.

Treatment
Presurgical orthodontic preparation

Teeth are aligned on the basal bone without any attempt to close the bite. The alignment is usually performed in sections, an anterior, and left and right posterior segments.

Surgery

The vertical dentoalveolar discrepancy is corrected by differential vertical movement of the maxilla, in segments or in one piece. Any residual antero-posterior discrepancy is corrected by mandibular surgery once the maxilla is in an ideal antero-posterior position. Anterior open bites may also be corrected by means of mandibular surgery only.

Postoperative orthodontics

Once the maxillary segments have been aligned during surgery, a complete arch wire is place to finally align the teeth. Light vertical elastics are used to hold the upper and lower teeth in occlusion.

Case 5

A 17-year-old female patient's main complaint was that when she "bit a sandwich the tomato stayed behind". Her profile was convex and she had a Class II anterior open bite. The posterior maxilla was vertically excessive and narrow with bilateral crossbites. The orthodontic treatment plan consisted of levelling and alignment of both dental arches without expanding the upper arch beyond the bony base. The upper arch was prepared for surgical expansion by means of an interdental osteotomy between the central incisor teeth (Fig. 30.15).

Maxillary deficiency

A patient with vertical maxillary deficiency has a square, short face appearance. This deformity could be misdiagnosed as mandibular antero-posterior excess, as over closure of the mandible results in relative protrusion of the chin.

Clinical characteristics

Facial:

- A short, square shaped face.
- A decreased lower third of the face.
- The mandible appears square and prominent due to overclosure.
- The incisor teeth remain concealed under the upper lip when the patient smiles or speaks, giving an edentulous appearance.
- The nasolabial angle is acute.

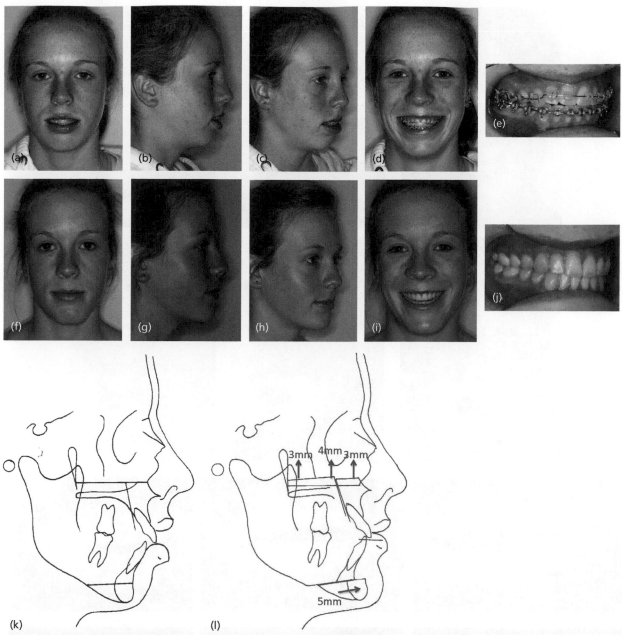

Fig. 30.14 Case 4. The pre-surgical (a) frontal view, (b) profile view, (c) three-quarter view, (d) "gummy smile", (e) occlusion. The post-treatment (f) frontal view, (g) profile view, (h) three-quarter view, (i) smile with ideal amount of tooth exposure, and (j) occlusion. (k) Pre-surgical cephalometric tracing and (l) surgical prediction tracing.

Dental features:

- An angle Class III occlusion.
- The heavy musculature and over closed mal occlusion frequently predispose to severe attrition.

Treatment

Presurgical orthodontic preparation
- Alignment of the dental arches and positioning the teeth over their bony base.
- Coordination of the upper and lower dental arches.

Surgery
A Le Fort I osteotomy is performed and the vertical dimension of the maxilla increased by a down graft-ing or a down sliding procedure. Bone harvested from the iliac crest is used when grafting is required.

Postoperative orthodontics
The occlusion is refined to establish optimum inter-digitation of the teeth.

Case 6

A 21-year-old patient had undergone orthodontic treatment and a functional and stable result had been achieved. She was, however, concerned about her "toothless" look and that her mandible appeared too prominent. She did not show any upper incisor teeth under her lip at rest. Although she had a Class I

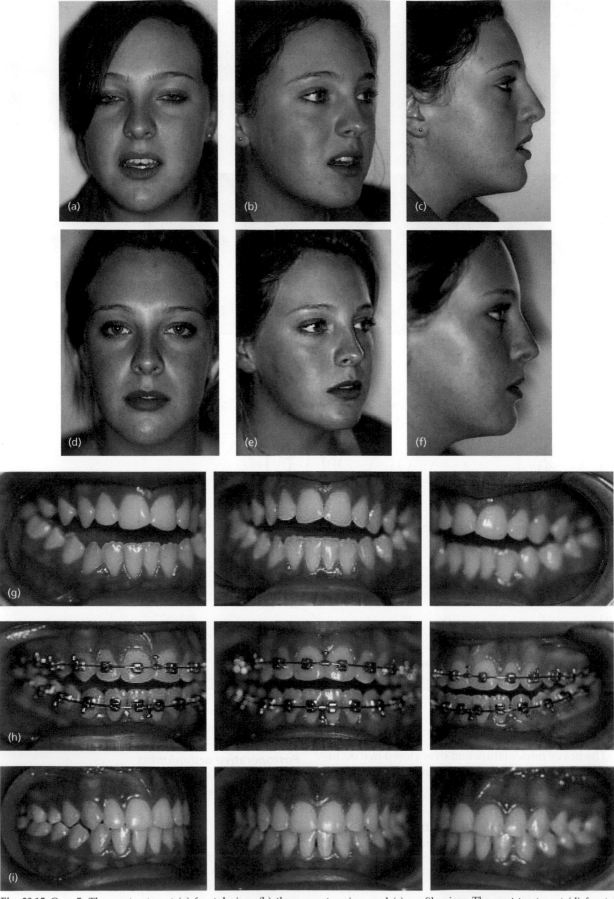

Fig. 30.15 Case 5. The pre-treatment (a) frontal view, (b) three-quarter view, and (c) profile view. The post-treatment (d) frontal view, (e) three-quarter view, and (f) profile view. The (g) pre-treatment, (h) pre-surgical, and (i) post-treatment occlusion. The (j) pre-treatment cephalometric tracing, and (k) the surgical prediction tracing indicating superior repositioning and expansion of the maxilla. Source: Reyneke and Ferretti (2007). Reproduced with permission of Elsevier Inc.

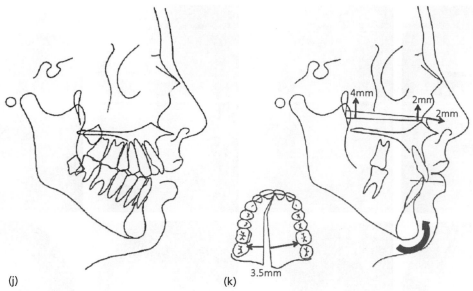

(j)   (k)

Fig. 30.15 (*Continued*)

occlusion, she appeared over closed. The diagnosis of vertical maxillary deficiency was made. Her maxilla was down grafted by means of a Le Fort I osteotomy and bone from the right Iliac crest was harvested and used as interpositional grafting material. Her existing occlusion was maintained (Fig. 30.16).

Transverse discrepancy

Dentofacial deformities in this plane are commonly defects in width, usually of the maxilla i.e. posterior crossbites, unilateral or bilateral. This discrepancy is often combined with antero-posterior and vertical problems and deviation of the mandible in centric occlusion. The correction of these problems can be adequately dealt with by means of orthodontic treatment in the growing child, as the midpalatal suture only fuses at the approximate age of 15 years. However, in the adult patient where the required maxillary expansion is greater than 3 mm, a surgical orthodontic approach should be considered. It may be more stable and has a shorter treatment time (see Case 7).

Orthodontic preparation is required, followed by surgical intervention. The palate is widened, or narrowed, from the superior aspect after Le Fort I down fracture. Alternatively, crossbites may be corrected by posterior maxillary segmental osteotomies. An alternative treatment approach is to perform expansion of the upper dental arch by surgical assisted expansion of the maxilla. With this technique the surgeon will perform the Le Fort I osteotomies; however, the maxilla is not down fractured. The maxilla is then slowly expanded by means of an orthodontic expansion appliance.

Facial asymmetry

Facial asymmetry usually manifest as a discrepancy in all three planes of space, and may be associated with Class I, but is a more frequently seen together with Class II and III dental occlusions. In some instances the asymmetry is secondary to condylar hyperplasia, TMJ ankylosis, displaced condylar fractures, hemifacial microsomia, hemifacial hypertrophy, and Romberg syndrome.

Vertical asymmetry

The left and right sides of the maxilla and mandible are at different levels and there is a cant in the occlusal plane. When a tongue depressor is held between the patient's teeth the asymmetry is particularly noticeable.

Sagittal asymmetry

One side of the maxilla and mandible is placed further forward than the other (typical in hemifacial microsomia and cleft palate deformities).

Transverse asymmetry

The maxilla and/or mandible have different widths relative to the mid sagittal plane.

Treatment

Presurgical orthodontics involves alignment of teeth with the bony base. No attempt should be made to correct the cant of the occlusal plane. The surgical correction of the occlusal cant enhances the correction

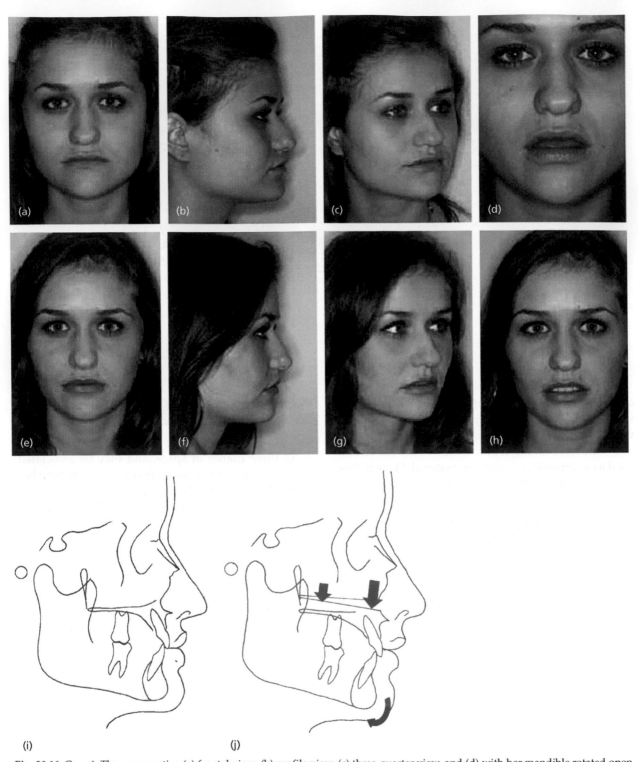

Fig. 30.16 Case 6. The preoperative (a) frontal view, (b) profile view, (c) three-quarter view, and (d) with her mandible rotated open upper incisors are not visible. The postoperative (e) frontal view, (f) profile view, (g) three-quarter view, and (h) the increased incisor show is apparent following down grafting of the maxilla. (i) The pre-surgical cephalometric tracing and the (j) surgical prediction tracing indicating the hard and soft tissue changes after 6mm down graft of the anterior maxilla.

of the asymmetry of the face. Maxillary width deficiencies may be corrected orthodontically in the growing child, but, in general, problems of asymmetry are more effectively dealt with by a surgical approach, directed at the area of the deformity and in all three planes of space.

Distraction osteogenesis

Distraction osteogenesis is the slow, controlled application of force to a planned osteotomized bone gap, resulting in the generation of new bone and soft tissue. A unique feature of distraction osteogenesis is

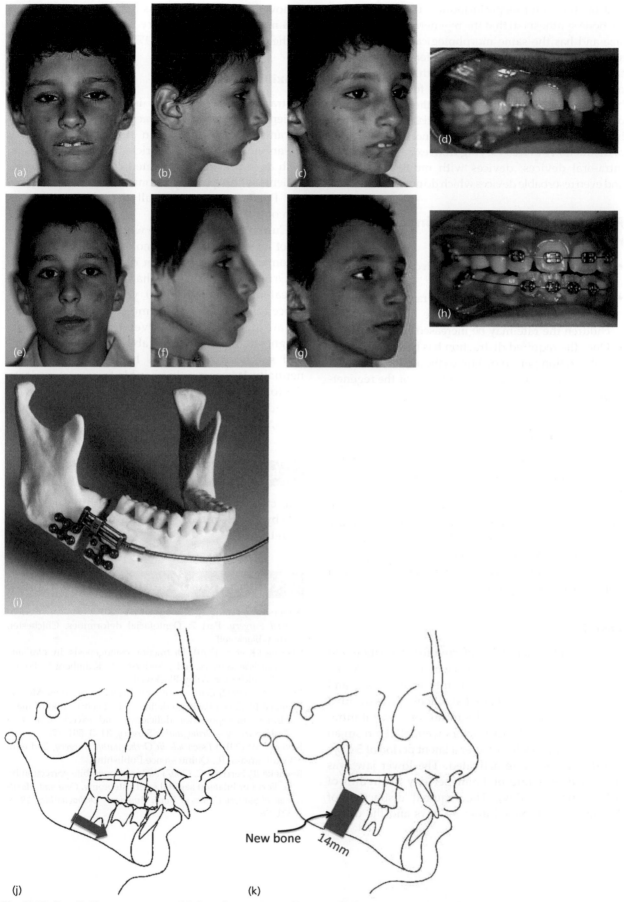

Fig. 30.17 Case 7. The pre-treatment (a) frontal view, (b) profile view, (c) three-quarter view, and (d) occlusion. Post-treatment (e) frontal view, (f) profile view, (g) three-quarter view, and (h) occlusion. (i) An intra-oral distraction device. The pre-treatment cephalometric tracing (j) and post-distraction tracing (k). Source: Reproduced from Reyneke (2010) with permission. © Quintessence Publishing Co Inc, Chicago.

that the bone and its periosteum act as the template for bone synthesis so that the regeneration is the same size and has the same morphological characteristics as the native bone. Distraction offers a few advantages over conventional orthognathic surgical techniques: (1) there is no requirement for bone grafting hence no donor site morbidity; (2) there is simultaneous expansion of surrounding soft tissues. There have been exciting and innovative advances in the design of distraction devices varying from extra-oral devices, intra-oral devices, devices with multivector forces and even resorbable devices which do not need removal.

Protocol for distraction in the maxillofacial region:

- The distraction device is activated 5–7 days after placement.
- Facial bones are distracted at a rate of 1 mm/day with a rhythm of 0.5 mm twice daily. In young children the rate may be increased to 1.5 mm/day.
- Once the required distraction has been achieved, a stabilization period of 3 times the active distraction time is necessary for consolidation of the regenerated bone.

Mandibular distraction

Mandibular distraction is mostly used to lengthen the mandible in patients with severe skeletal and soft tissue deficiency. Distraction of the lower jaw is indicated in the treatment of syndromic cases such as hemifacial microsomia, Pierre Robin sequence, Treacher Collins syndrome, Nager syndrome and other congenital micrognathia. Case 7 (see Fig. 30.17) demonstrates the successful treatment of a patient with Pierre Robin syndrome.

Case 7

A 7-year-old patient was referred for evaluation and treatment of a severely deficient mandible. As an infant he suffered from difficulty in breathing and feeding. He was now teased at school. It was decided to advance his mandible by means of bilateral intra-oral distractors. The distractors were placed from an extra-oral approach and after a latent period of 5 days the distractors were activated. The lower jaw was distracted at a rate of 1 mm per day (a rhythm of 0.5 mm twice a day). The required distraction of 14 mm was completed after 14 days and the driver

removed. The distractor was removed after a period of 3 months and preliminary orthodontic alignment of the teeth started (Fig. 30.17).

Maxillary distraction

Distraction of the maxilla is mostly indicated in patients with severe mid-face deficiency requiring advancements of more than 10 mm or if maxillary advancement may be restricted by fibrous tissue, such as in previously operated cleft palate patients. Patients with Aperts syndrome, Crouzon syndrome, and Pfieffer syndrome usually benefit from distraction of the maxilla.

Currently researchers are working on the possibility of remote controlled technology for distractors and automatic driver systems for distractor appliances.

Orthognathic surgery has evolved from life-threatening procedures 60 years ago to surgical procedures that can, in some cases, be performed on an outpatient basis. Over time the clinician's diagnostic skills, technical ability, instrumentation, and special investigations have improved exponentially. It is currently possible to correct intricate dentofacial deformities successfully and with confidence. Orthognathic surgery not only change faces, it also changes lives.

Acknowledgment

This chapter was written expressly for this Essentials title by Professor Johan Reyneke and Professor Carlo Ferretti.

Recommended reading

Anderson L, Kahnberg K, Pogrel MA. (2010) *Oral and Maxillofacial Surgery*. Part 7: Dentofacial deformities. Chichester, Wiley-Blackwell.

Cheung LK *et al.* (2010) Distraction osteogenesis. In: *Oral and Maxillofacial Surgery*. (eds, Anderson L, Kahnberg K, Pogrel MA). Chichester, Wiley-Blackwell.

Proffit WR. (1992) *Contemporary Orthodontics*. St Louis, Mosby.

Reyneke JP. (2007) Basic guidelines for the correction of mandibular anteroposterior deficiency and excess. *Clinics in Plastic Surgery – Orthognathic Surgery*, **34**, 3, 501–17.

Reyneke JP. (2010) *Essentials in Orthognathic Surgery*, 2nd edn. Carol Stream, IL, Quintessence Publishing.

Reyneke JP, Ferrretti C. (2007) Anterior open bite correction by Le Fort I or bilateral sagittal split osteotomy. *Oral and Maxillofacial Surgery Clinics of North America – Orthognathics*, **19**, 3, 321–38.

Chapter 31

Mandibular Reconstruction

Whenever a portion of the mandible is resected, consideration must be given to subsequent reconstruction. Although most patients do receive mandibular reconstruction following resection, there is still a minority for whom no reconstruction may be the most practical alternative. These cases particularly include shorter lateral defects, not involving the symphysis and parasymphysis areas, in elderly or medically compromised patients. The subsequent deformity in the absence of reconstruction is often acceptable under these circumstances. However, at present, the "gold standard" for reconstruction is autogenous bone.

Marginal resection

Marginal resection of the mandible may be indicated for the excision of a benign tumor, a superficial malignant tumor involving periosteum only, or for infection. In this case mandibular continuity is not disrupted. However, the mandible is at risk for subsequent fracture, particularly if radiation therapy has to be given. For this reason, reconstruction is often performed. Bony reconstruction will also enable subsequent insertion of osseointegrated implants, if indicated, to complete prosthodontic reconstruction. In a young patient reconstruction may not be necessary since some spontaneous regeneration of bone may occur, particularly if the periosteum is retained. However, the mandible may need to be reinforced with a reconstruction plate (usually around 2.4mm in thickness with appropriate screws) to minimize the risk of fracture. Following marginal resection, reconstruction can be with corticocancellous blocks from the iliac crest (full thickness or partial thickness), which can be contoured so that they will mortice into place with minimal or no fixation (Fig. 31.1). For a lesion less than about 3cm in size this can be carried out immediately from an intraoral approach; for defects greater than this, consideration should be given to carrying this out secondarily and possibly from an extraoral approach, to avoid the risk of graft failure due to infection secondary to salivary contamination. Subsequent soft tissue grafting is often necessary to supply attached mucosa for denture or implant insertion. This is often carried out by means of a split-thickness skin graft, and normally done as a secondary procedure following incorporation of the bone graft.

Segmental resection

Segmental resection of the mandible with loss of mandibular continuity may be necessary for benign or malignant lesions, as well as for chronic infection. Temporary immediate reconstruction is often carried out by means of a reconstruction plate, but these are rarely satisfactory for long-term use. The usual history is for the plate to either exteriorize itself and become secondarily infected, or for screw loosening and mobility to occur. Depending on the forces placed on it, these problems will normally occur after some 18 months or 2 years. Plate fracture has also been reported (Fig. 31.2). In particular, reconstruction plates fail most frequently in the anterior mandible, but can survive in the long-term in the body and posterior parts of the mandible, particularly if these have adequate soft tissue coverage, which may have to be in the form of a soft tissue flap, such as a pectoralis major flap.

Nevertheless, it is generally more appropriate to reconstruct the mandible with non-vascularized autogenous bone. Non-vascularized autogenous bone is normally used as a secondary procedure.

Essentials of Oral and Maxillofacial Surgery, First Edition. Edited by M. Anthony Pogrel, Karl-Erik Kahnberg and Lars Andersson.
© 2014 John Wiley & Sons, Ltd. Published 2014 by John Wiley & Sons, Ltd.
Companion website: www.wiley.com/go/pogrel/oms

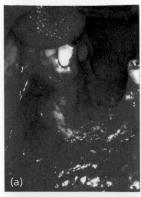
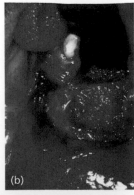

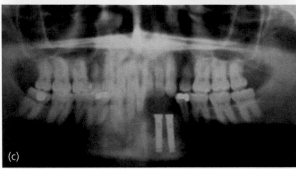

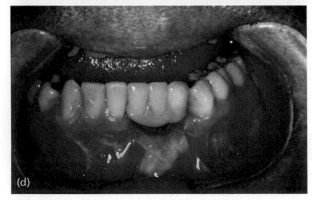

Fig. 31.1 A marginal resection of the mandible for a fibro-osseous lesion (a) reconstructed with an iliac crest bone graft mortised into place intraorally at the time of the primary resection (b) and secondarily skin grafted and implants inserted and an implant supported restoration placed (c, d).

Immediate segmental reconstruction with non-vascularized autogenous bone from an intraoral approach has been associated with a high failure rate, although it was recommended by Obwegeser amongst others. The reasons for failure are generally wound breakdown intraorally and contamination of the wound with saliva, or primary infection due to oral contamination. Reconstruction is therefore more normally carried out secondarily. The most appropriate time to carry this out would appear to be some 6–8 weeks following primary resection for the following reasons:

- this gives the intraoral wound time to heal and gain some tensile strength;
- the wound bed has time to self-decontaminate;
- scarring and fibrosis have not had an opportunity to develop.

Resection is often carried out from a combined intraoral and extraoral approach, and temporary reconstruction is carried out with a titanium reconstruction plate (usually a 2.4 mm plate is adequate). Some 6–8 weeks later, definitive reconstruction is carried out from an extraoral approach using autogenous bone. Depending on the circumstances, this can be by the use of autogenous ribs (usually in a younger patient) (Fig. 31.3), corticocancellous blocks from the iliac crest (full thickness or partial thickness) (Fig. 31.4), or cancellous bone marrow in a carrier tray. The tray can be of titanium mesh or an allogenic bone tray (Fig. 31.5), or in exceptional circumstances, it may be an autogenous bone tray, since it may be possible to carry out a segmental resection of the mandible for a benign lesion, excise the lesion from the mandible, and reinsert it as its own carrier tray.

Over the years, many attempts have been made to reconstruct the mandible using the actual autogenous mandible that was previously resected. In the case of a benign lesion, it may be possible to resect the mandible, remove the lesion, and reinsert the mandible. In most cases this does mean hollowing the mandible out to resemble a tray, perforating the tray, and

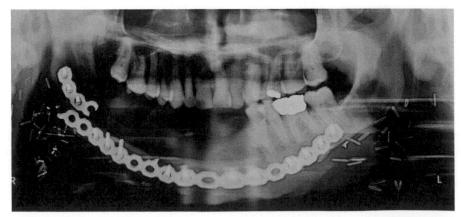

Fig. 31.2 A fractured reconstruction plate used to span a segmental defect, which had not received a bone graft.

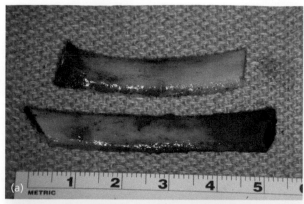

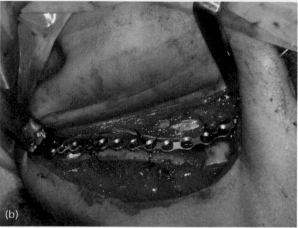

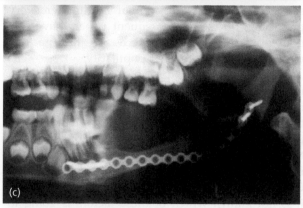

Fig. 31.3 Two ribs (a) used to reconstruct the mandible following resection of a desmoplastic fibroma in a 4-year-old (b). Same patient at 6 years of age (c).

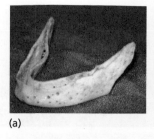 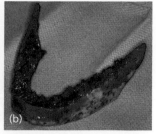

Fig. 31.5 Segmental mandibular reconstruction utilizing a freeze-dried allogenic mandibular crib (a) packed with autogenous bone marrow (b).

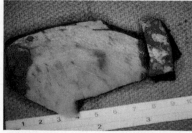

Fig. 31.4 Corticocancellous full thickness iliac crest bone graft used for secondary reconstruction of a segmental defect of the mandible. The graft is secured to the reconstruction plate with screws.

securing it with a reconstruction plate, and then completing the reconstruction with autogenous marrow within the tray. This gives the most esthetic reconstruction, since it is the patient's own mandible and therefore the contour is the most acceptable. Figure 31.6 shows this technique used for a high-flow vascular malformation of the mandible. When this treatment is contemplated for aggressive lesions, or even malignant lesions, the resected mandible must be "sterilized" in some way to kill unwanted cells. In most cases the technique is just as described, in removing the lesion from the resected mandible, reducing the mandible to an autogenous tray and perforating it. Three different methods of sterilizing the mandible have been described. The first involves autoclaving the mandible; this will render the mandible non-vital, but most studies have shown that even with autogenous marrow grafting, excessive resorption normally occurs, and this technique is not widely practiced today. An alternative technique is to devitalize the mandible by means of cryotherapy, and for this the mandibular tray is immersed in liquid nitrogen at −196°C for 10 minutes. The mandible is then allowed to thaw and is refrozen. Studies have shown that liquid nitrogen predictably causes cell death below −20°C and that the most satisfactory results are achieved with a rapid freeze and a slow thawing process. Although described in the literature, the technique does not appear to be widely practiced today. The third technique involves gamma irradiation of the mandible which will successfully devitalize the mandible, and does not appear to result in excessive resorption when it is reinserted and rigidly fixed and grafted. If a source of radiation is locally available, this technique can be carried out in one session while the patient is asleep and at the same time as the initial resection. The mandible can be cleaned, placed in a sterile autoclave bag and receive around 50 Gy of radiation in less than 1 hour, in time for reinsertion into the patient. Otherwise, the procedure must be staged. Any of these techniques may result in a more acceptable contour than using an autogenous graft from another part of the body.

Studies have shown that segmental resections of up to 6 cm are associated with a high success rate when reconstructed by any of these techniques.

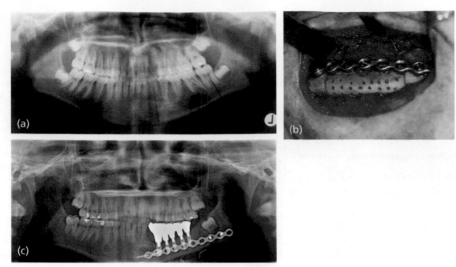

Fig. 31.6 A vascular malformation of the left posterior mandible (a) which was resected, the lesion curetted out and the mandible recontoured as an autogenous tray which was reinserted, secured, and packed with autogenous marrow (b) into which implants were later inserted (c). (Courtesy of Janice S. Lee DDS, MD, MS.)

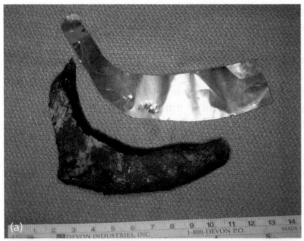

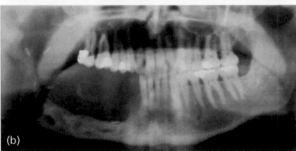

Fig. 31.7 (a) A 10 cm non-vascularized full-thickness iliac crest bone graft to reconstruct a hemimandible including the condyle on removal from the hip. (b) Nine months later, after removal of the bone plate.

Above 6 cm the failure rate starts to increase and when the resected area exceeds 9 cm the failure rate from a non-vascularized graft may be as high as 75%. Figure 31.7 shows a successful 10 cm non-vascularized graft even though it has undergone considerable resorption. Failure usually occurs because of failure of the bone graft to become vascularized and reincorporate, with subsequent infection and wound breakdown.

A number of factors have been identified which may improve or compromise bone healing and the incorporation of bone grafts on reconstruction. Platelet rich plasma (PRP), and possibly other platelet-derived and other growth factors, may enhance incorporation of bone grafts and also may enhance soft tissue healing. Early initial results were very promising, but some subsequent papers have cast doubts on the long-term success of these factors, which have decreased their popularity.

Bone morphogenic proteins (BMPs) have been identified but have only recently become commercially available. They have the ability to induce bone formation by recruiting osteoblastic stem cells to produce bone, thus possibly avoiding a bone graft. In the USA only BMP-2 is currently available, although in Europe BMP-7 (also known as osteoprotein or OP1) is also available. Although these show promise, it is not known which of these factors is going to prove the most effective, and whether more than one factor is necessary to get the maximum enhancement of bone incorporation, and even whether there is a cascade process involved. At the current time, BMP-2 can only be utilized on an acellular bovine collagen sponge which is compressible and limits its usefulness to procedures such as sinus grafting for implants.

When the bone graft has taken successfully, subsequent staged procedures include removal of the bone plate. This may be necessary to allow subsequent vestibuloplasty and implant insertion. It may be necessary if the patient can feel the plate or screws beneath the tissue, if the plate appears to be in danger of exteriorizing itself, or if subsequent resorption of the bone graft is anticipated due to the effects of stress shielding. Stress shielding remains controversial in the maxillofacial regions. In the long bones, particularly the humerus, this has been shown to be a real issue, in that when a rigid bone plate is removed after healing of a fracture of the humerus, it is not uncommon for refracture to occur since the bone plate has shielded the humerus from excessive forces, and therefore it has never fully remodeled and gained its premorbid strength. Although some studies have shown that stress shielding may be a factor in the healing of mandibular fractures, other studies have shown that it does not appear to be an issue. Nevertheless, there are some patients who do seem to show excessive resorption following bone grafting, and it is felt that the presence of a rigid reconstruction plate may mean that the bone graft is not subjected to physiological forces, and therefore resorbs at an excessive rate. In these cases, removal of the bone plate may be advisable before the resorptive process becomes too pronounced. Timing of the removal of the plate is often critical, since one cannot remove it prior to the bone graft incorporating, but one wishes to remove it before excessive resorption has occurred. A time of between 4 and 9 months is normally quoted following the grafting procedure before removal of the bone plate. Occasionally bone plates also have to be removed for other reasons, including infection, screw loosening, plate fracture, and exteriorization of the plate or the patient being able to feel the plate through the soft tissues. Occasionally plates also cause discomfort with extremes of temperature. Following removal of the bone plate, it would be possible to carry out vestibuloplasty if necessary and to allow for subsequent osseointegrated implant insertion.

Non-vascularized bone grafting for mandibular reconstruction

Multiple sites have been advocated for obtaining bone that might be used for maxillofacial reconstruction. Some sites, such as the radius and ulna, are rarely used today. Cranial bone is used for posttraumatic reconstruction of the mid and upper face, but quantities are generally insufficient for mandibular reconstruction. The main sites used for nonvascularized mandibular reconstruction are ribs, the iliac bone, and the proximal tibia.

Ribs

Ribs can be used with a cartilage cap from the costochondral junction if they are required for temporomandibular joint (TMJ) reconstruction, or without cartilage for mandibular reconstruction, particularly in children. In an adult, a considerable length of rib can be obtained (often up to 15cm) accepting the curvature of the rib. Ribs are normally taken between the fifth and eighth ribs (avoiding the ribs with considerable attachment of the pectoralis major muscle and also avoiding the free floating ribs). Ribs can be taken from either side with equal ease.

This procedure is normally only carried out under intubated general anesthesia with the ability to administer positive pressure ventilation in the event of a pneumothorax. The surgical procedure involves identifying the rib or ribs to be taken and an incision is made directly over the rib. In females, the incision is normally placed beneath the breast or developing breast so that it will be hidden beneath the breast in the erect position. The incision is taken through the superficial musculature down to the periosteum and perichondrium. No major structures are encountered and only superficial bleeding vessels should be encountered. Once the periosteum of the rib has been identified, it is incised sharply down to the rib itself. If cartilage is to be taken, the incision should continue over the costochondral junction down to the cartilage.

At the anterior end of the incision through periosteum and perichondrium a T-junction should be made to limit the anterior extent of the perichondrial stripping, but to allow 4 or 5mm of cartilage to be taken. A periosteal elevator is now used to strip the periosteum off the superior surface of the rib and cartilage. With great care, one then turns the corner and starts stripping periosteum from the superior and inferior surfaces of the rib. It must be remembered that the neurovascular bundle supplying the rib runs in a groove on the inner aspect of the inferior surface of the rib. It is crucial that the dissection be subperiosteal at all times. The dissection is then continued with care on the inferior surface of the rib. Although normal periosteal elevators can be used for this dissection, special instruments are available, such as the elevator (Fig. 31.8).

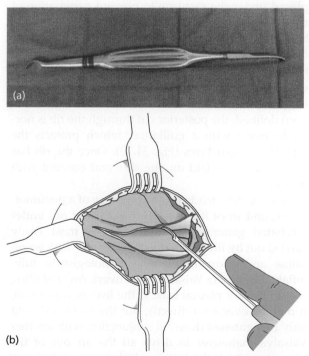

Fig. 31.8 (a) An Overholt periosteal stripper to raise periosteum around a rib. (b) Note the T-shaped incision through the periosteum.

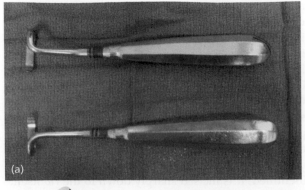

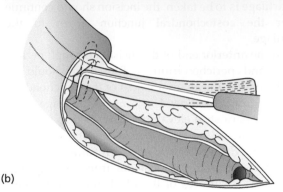

Fig. 31.9 (a) Doyen retractor (b) placed under a rib to elevate periosteum, protecting the underlying pleura.

Once the subperiosteal dissection has been completed and the rib isolated, an instrument such as the appropriate Doyen retractor can be placed under the rib and the subperiosteal dissection confirmed and continued (Fig. 31.9). The rib is always sectioned at the anterior end first. If this is in cartilage, it can be carried out with a scalpel, but an instrument must be placed under the cartilage to prevent penetration of the pleura. If the anterior sectioning is to be in rib bone itself, then a guillotine or rib shears can be used. Once the anterior cut has been made, the rib can then be raised and, with ease, the subperiosteal dissection can continue as far posteriorly as required for the length of rib needed. Once the posterior limit has been defined, the posterior cut through the rib is normally made with a guillotine, which protects the underlying structures (Fig. 31.10). Once the rib has been taken, it is laid on one side and covered with moist gauze.

A test is now made for the presence of a pneumothorax, and since the procedure is carried out under intubated general anesthesia, this is most easily carried out by filling the chest wall cavity with warm saline and allowing the anesthesiologist to fully inflate the chest (a Valsalva maneuver). Any bubbling will indicate a pleural leak. If the leak is very small, it may be oversewn directly, but the sutures should only be tightened down in conjunction with another Valsalva maneuver to drive all the air out of the pleural cavity. If the leak is a little larger, a drainage tube can be placed, and then a purse-string suture placed around it; the drainage tube is withdrawn as

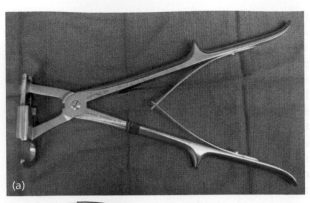

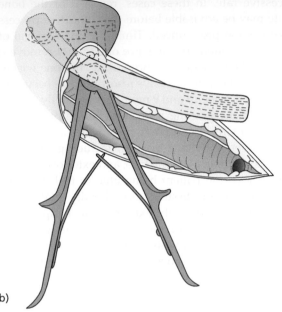

Fig. 31.10 (a) A guillotine rib cutter (b) used to cut the posterior end of the rib.

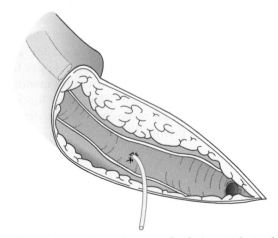

Fig. 31.11 A pursestring suture round a drainage tube to close a small pneumothorax.

the purse-string suture is tightened on another Valsalva maneuver and this may give good closure of the hole (Fig. 31.11). If closure cannot be obtained, then an underwater sealed drain must be inserted, and this will normally go from the opening and emerge high in the chest in order to drain air. This drain will be placed to low-volume wall suction and left in place for 24–36 hours.

If more than one rib is required, then the adjacent rib can normally also be harvested in the same way through the same incision. If more than two ribs are required, then it is necessary to leave alternate ribs so that the patient does not develop a flail chest. Sometimes this requires a second chest wall incision, but sometimes it can be obtained through the one incision if it is correctly placed. Closure is carried out in layers and postoperatively an upright chest radiograph is obtained as soon as possible to check for the presence of a pneumothorax. With any pneumothorax occupying more than about 15% of the lung volume, an opinion should be obtained with regard to placement of an underwater sealed drain. At the completion of the surgery, a long-acting local anesthetic, either given as a single injection or via a subcutaneous infusion device, can make postoperative physical therapy and chest movement more acceptable to the patient. Chest wall discomfort is to be expected on deep inspiration for some time after this procedure. Postoperative physical therapy with inspiratory spirometry is often indicated.

When the wound is closed, attention can now be turned to the harvested ribs. If it is required to include costochondral cartilage, this can now be shaped with a scalpel to leave a cap of about 2 mm of cartilage on the end of the rib (Fig. 31.12). This approximates well to a TMJ. If more cartilage is left, there is a risk of it separating from the rib on pressure, and also more risk of overgrowth occurring from the cartilage. The rib can be effectively straightened with a rib morcellizer, but care must be taken not to splinter the rib. Ribs from younger people will straighten more easily than ribs from older patients. When securing ribs in place with screws, they generally require a washer of some kind to prevent the screw from splintering the rib. In some cases it is preferable to use a bone plate and put the plates and screws through the plate, or even titanium mesh and place the screws through the mesh, so the pressure is spread more evenly.

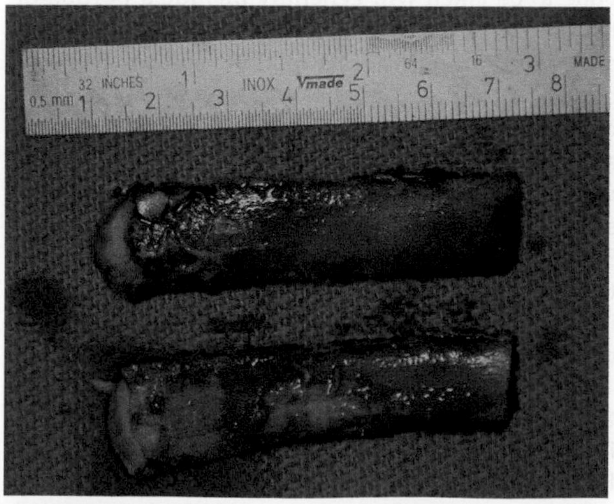

Iliac crest

Anterior iliac crest

This donor site is the workhorse of the reconstructive oral and maxillofacial surgeon. The landmark of the anterior iliac spine can normally be identified by palpation on all but the most obese patients and the outline of the crest of the ilium can also be mapped out on the skin. The initial incision should not be placed right over the crest since this can be uncomfortable postoperatively with some clothing. It is also advisable to hide the incision below the crest of the ridge in connection with various items of clothing. The normal technique is to pull the skin upwards by depressing the soft tissues superior to the crest with the palm of the hand. This will allow an incision to be made directly over the crest of the ilium, but when the tension is released from the incision, it will lie 3–4 cm below the iliac crest (Fig. 31.13). The incision can be made directly through skin, subcutaneous tissue, Scarpa's fascia, any superficial rectus muscle, and down to the iliac crest. If one approaches the iliac crest directly, virtually no major muscle attachments are encountered. Incisions from the lateral side will

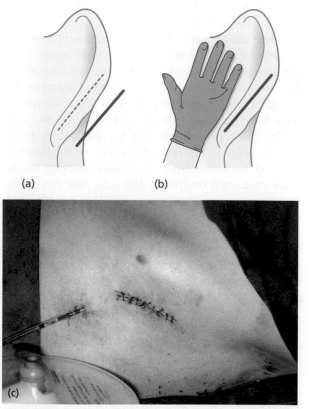

Fig. 31.12 Two ribs with cartilage caps to reconstruct the temporomandibular joints.

Fig. 31.13 Site of the incision to approach the anterior iliac crest. Note the palm of the hand to provide tension so the incision is over the iliac crest (a) so that the final scar is below the iliac crest (b, c).

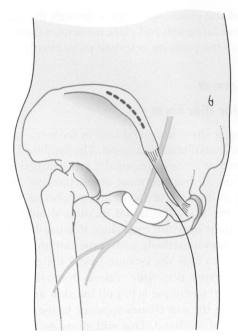

Fig. 31.14 The tubercle (with dotted line over it) has the largest source of cancellous bone in the anterior ilium. It is 5–6 cm posterior to the anterior superior iliac spine.

entail sectioning of the gluteal muscles. There is a number of superficial sensory nerves passing over the crest of the ridge, and in particular, the iliohypogastric nerve is normally at risk and often leaves patients with a palm-sized area of paresthesia on the lateral side of the iliac crest. The lateral cutaneous nerve of the thigh is normally placed more anterior.

Once the crest has been identified, the incision can be taken down to the bone itself and subperiosteal elevation can be commenced. In most cases, it is advisable to formally identify the anterior limit of the iliac crest and the origin of the inguinal ligament. As one goes more posteriorly, the tubercle is identified some 5–6 cm posterior to the anterior spine, and this is the most productive site for harvesting bone marrow (Fig. 31.14). If medial cortex of the ilium is required, then the subperiosteal dissection only needs to be continued on the medial side, and this strips away easily, since the iliacus muscle is not attached to the ilium superiorly, and there are no other muscle attachments or vital structures in this area. On the lateral side, however, the gluteal muscles are attached, and if full-thickness grafts are required, these will need to be stripped away resulting in short-term discomfort and stiffness.

To obtain marrow

This is normally obtained directly over the iliac tubercle, since this is the widest point of the ilium (some 5–6 cm posterior to the anterior iliac spine), although it can be obtained elsewhere in the ilium. A lid from the superior surface of the iliac crest is normally raised, centered over the tubercle. This can take the form of bone cuts anteriorly and posteriorly joined by a cut directly along the middle of the iliac crest to raise small trap doors medially and laterally to expose the crest. If this is to be carried out, periosteum should remain attached laterally and medially so that these trap doors do not become totally free grafts. On completion of the procedure, these trap doors can be replaced. Cuts can be made with chisels, drills, or reciprocating saw. Alternatively, a single coffin lid type bone flap can be raised based either laterally or medially; again, periosteum should be retained at the site of the hinge so that it does not become a totally free flap (Fig. 31.15). Marrow is now exposed and can be curetted with suitable size curettes. One should start with the largest curette possible to fit between the lateral and medial plates of bone, and curettage may need to be quite aggressive. As one descends inferiorly, the size of curette may need to be decreased to fit between the lateral and medial plates. Care should be taken to attempt to avoid perforation, which normally occurs on the medial side. Small perforations can be accepted, the main risk is to underlying structures. Amounts vary, but 20–30 mL of compressed bone can normally be obtained from the average ilium. If necessary, both left and right sides can be used at a single operation. On completion of taking the marrow, the bone flap can be replaced and is normally self-retaining, though if required a suture can be placed through holes drilled in the bone. The marrow that is taken is normally placed in a container and covered with a moist gauze. Closure is in layers, starting with the periosteum and including Scarpa's fascia, and the wound does not normally need to be drained.

Corticocancellous blocks

The anterior iliac crest lends itself to taking corticocancellous blocks for more extensive reconstruction. If bone is to be taken from the medial surface of the iliac crest, then the periosteum and iliacus muscle are retracted with an abdominal retractor and the area of bone to be taken is outlined with a drill or reciprocating saw. The inferior margin of the bone to be taken only needs to be outlined through the cortex. The bone to be taken will generally include a portion of the iliac crest, and so the anterior and posterior cuts are made through approximately 50% of the iliac crest, and are then joined along the center of the iliac crest. The block of bone is then removed utilizing appropriate sized straight and curved chisels. In this way, copious amounts of bone can be removed in strips approximately 2–3 cm in width (Fig. 31.16). Strips wider than this tend to fracture. On completion, a suction drain is often placed over the harvesting site and left in place for 24–36 hours, or until drainage is less than 20 mL in 8 hours.

For major mandibular reconstruction, through and through corticocancellous blocks can be taken to include both lateral and medial cortices of the ilium, leaving a hole in the ilium. For this, extensive periosteal stripping needs to take place on both the medial and lateral surfaces to identify the iliac ligament,

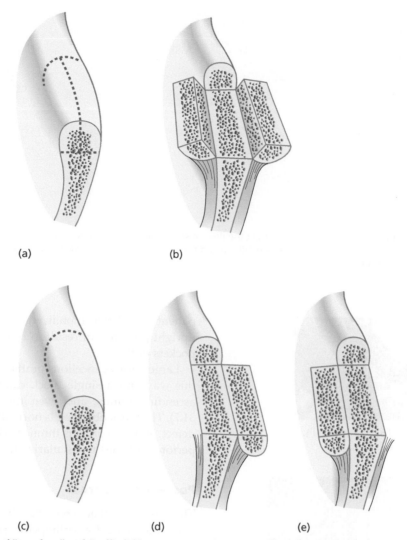

(a)   (b)

(c)   (d)   (e)

Fig. 31.15 The variety of "trapdoor" and "coffin lid" type incisions, based laterally and medially, that are used to access the cancellous bone in the iliac tubercle.

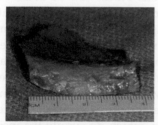

Fig. 31.16 Corticocancellous strips of bone taken from the medial surface of the ilium.

anterior notch, and posteriorly towards the sacroiliac joint, which should not be entered. This defines the area of bone that can be taken. A template is often helpful depicting the shape of bone required, and this can be made from sterilized aluminum from a soft drink can. A flexible plastic surgical ruler can also be used. The easiest way to take the size of block required is to remove the associated iliac crest. If this is carried out, the iliac crest is removed as a single block, starting at least 1 cm posterior to the anterior superior iliac spine, to prevent its fracture, and proceeding poste-

riorly, 1 cm posterior to the posterior limit of the block. In this way, the crest can be removed and then wired or plated back in place once the block has taken, and it will mortise into place nicely (Fig. 31.17). The corticocancellous full-thickness block can now be taken from above, with appropriate drills and saws. However, this does weaken the crest considerably, and may cause more postoperative morbidity. A preferable technique is to leave the iliac crest intact and to take the full-thickness portion of bone from below it (Fig. 31.18). These blocks are normally taken from the ipsilateral side of the patient, since the curvature is more appropriate to the mandible on the same side. If the crest is to be left intact, the approach is normally from the medial side where access is better, and is with a combination of reciprocal saw, oscillating saw, and drills. Once the block has been taken, some marrow can usually be obtained from around the edges, and is often helpful in the reconstruction to augment any defects.

The wound is normally drained with a suction drain and closure is then carried out in the normal

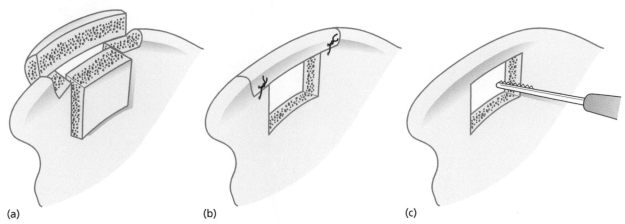

(a)   (b)   (c)

Fig. 31.17 (a, b) The technique of removing and rewiring the iliac crest to remove corticocancellous blocks of bone from below the crest, similar to the one seen in Fig. 31.4. (c) By using oscillating and reciprocating saws the crest can often be left intact for greater strength and decreased morbidity.

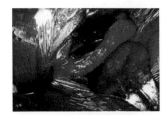

Fig. 31.18 The residual defect seen clinically.

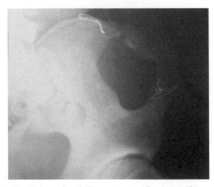

Fig. 31.19 Radiograph of ilium 6 months post iliac crest graft showing residual asymptomatic defect.

way in layers. Long-term postoperative radiographs show that a corticocancellous block less than 2–3 cm will normally form new bone, whereas a larger one will leave a permanent defect in the ilium, although herniation does not occur (Fig. 31.19). However, if it is felt that it may be necessary to go back again to obtain more bone for subsequent reconstructions, it is not necessary to drain the site and in this case blood will accumulate in the defect and, if periosteum is intact, may form new bone that can be reharvested. This does, however, run the risk of extensive hematoma formation. A drain placed in a full-thickness donor site will normally drain a total of 100–200 ml of blood over 24–36 hours, and should be removed when drainage is below 20 mL in 8 hours. It is often helpful not to remove the drain until the

patient has been mobilized, since assuming the upright posture can result in drainage of additional pockets of fluid.

Large corticocancellous grafts can be harvested in this way and a single block can include the body, ascending ramus, and even the condyle (see Fig. 31.7). The block obtained is normally shaped to fit the defect, and the cortex is thinned with a large bur and perforated to aid revascularization.

Posterior iliac crest

The posterior iliac crest has been advocated for obtaining bone for orthopedic procedures on the spine, but has also been suggested as a donor site for oral and maxillofacial surgical procedures. Large amounts of marrow can be obtained (up to 40–50 mL of compressed marrow from each side), and small corticocancellous blocks can be obtained. The incision runs over the posterior iliac crest which can normally be palpated and starts approximately 3 cm lateral to the midline of the center of the spine, and as it goes superiorly, it moves laterally at about 15° to stay over the posterior iliac crest. The incision is deepened down to the posterior crest, and no major structures are identified en route, except for the cluneal nerves, which do supply the ipsilateral skin around the anus itself and can give an area of paresthesia in this region. They can normally be retracted with the soft tissues.

The main complications of this technique are possible involvement of the sacroiliac joint, and postoperative back discomfort, which is often difficult to separate from any other cause of back pain. The main disadvantage of this technique, however, is that it is necessary to turn the patient over to obtain the bone, and this is technically difficult to perform (particularly on an obese patient), and may provide some difficulties in staging the procedure and keeping the recipient site sterile if it has been opened first. This wound does not normally need to be drained.

Tibia

The proximal end of the tibia has been advocated as a donor site for bone marrow, and small pieces of cortex only. Both lateral and medial approaches have been suggested. Both approaches are fairly straight-forward. In the lateral approach, Gerdy's tubercle is identified and the incision carried down at 45° from it inferiorly for 2–3 cm and by blunt dissection can be carried straight down to the tibia. There are normally no major vessels or nerves encountered in this approach. Similarly, the medial approach entails a vertical incision 1 cm medial to the anterior prominence of the tibia, and blunt dissection down to the tibia itself. The major complication from tibial bone harvest is tibial plateau fracture, which has been noted in connection with maxillofacial procedures, and can be a major long-term complication. For this reason, no bone should be taken (either cortical or cancellous) within 1 cm of the tibial plateau.

An oval window is made through the cortical bone of the tibia. This is normally approximately 2 cm by 1 cm, and is performed with a drill (Fig. 31.20). It should be oval without sharp edges to prevent any stress fractures developing from the corners of the window. The window can either be removed completely (and used as a cortical graft), or replaced at the end of the procedure, or swung out on attached periosteum, either laterally or medially. Once through the cortical bone, marrow can be curetted with ease, although one should stay at least 1 cm below the plateau. Twenty milliliters of compressed marrow can often be obtained from the tibia, although it is always of a more fatty appearance than marrow from the hip. Nevertheless, it does perform well clinically when used in a carrier tray for mandibular reconstruction.

The wound is normally repaired in layers. Postoperative weightbearing precautions vary widely. In practice, the medial epicondyle of the tibia takes approximately 55% of the body weight, whilst the lateral epicondyle takes approximately 45% of the weight. Therefore, one would assume that tibial plateau fractures were more likely to happen from the medial approach, and more weightbearing precautions may need to be taken. Both in orthopedic and oral and maxillofacial surgery, however, weightbearing precautions following tibial grafting vary widely, from some centers advocating no precautions at all and letting the patient walk immediately, to those that provide a cane, or walker, or even instructing the patient not to be weightbearing on the knee for 3–4 weeks. In practice, the complication rate does not seem to vary, so it would appear that in most cases, minimal weightbearing precautions are necessary.

Bone-containing microvascular free flaps

An alternative technique for reconstruction following segmental resection is with a microvascular free flap. Possible donor sites include the fibula (Fig. 31.21), iliac crest or scapula. The radius was previously used for this purpose, but it is associated with a high incidence of subsequent fracture of the radius, and this technique is rarely employed today. To be successful, there need to be suitable feeding vessels; these would normally be the facial vessels, but, if necessary, other vessels can be used. If the length of the vascular pedicle is in doubt, intervening vein grafts can be used to enable successful anastomosis. Conceptually, the advantages of a microvascular reconstruction are:

- soft tissue can be transferred at the same time as the bone;
- all procedures can be performed primarily;
- this technique can be used in areas of poor vascularity, including previous radiation therapy;
- success rate remains high for longer-span reconstructions.

The disadvantages of reconstruction with a vascularized graft may include:

- The bulk of soft tissue transferred with the bone is often too thick for subsequent prosthodontic reconstruction and subsequent procedures must be carried out to thin the soft tissues.
- The bulk of bone is often suboptimal for later implant insertion, though the initial graft can be augmented or modified in some way to make implant insertion more feasible. For example, a fibular bone graft can be doubled over on itself to create a double thickness (a single fibula is approximately 10–12 mm in thickness) (Fig. 31.22) to ensure that more bone is present for implant insertion.

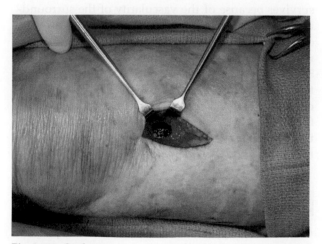

Fig. 31.20 Oval window in the lateral tibia and bone removed.

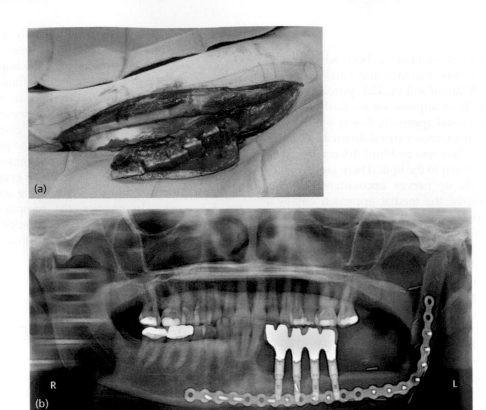

Fig. 31.21 (a) Mandibular reconstruction including the condyle with a segmentalized free fibula bone graft. (b) It was subsequently secondarily restored with osseointegrated implants following thinning of the intraoral soft tissue component of the graft.

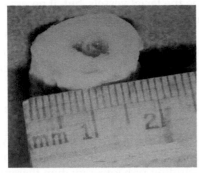

Fig. 31.22 Cross-section of a fibula showing the thick cortical bone with a smaller area of predominately yellow, fatty, marrow with an overall diameter of 10–12 mm.

Staged techniques

Reconstruction of the mandibular condyle, ramus of mandible, and body of mandible is associated with particular problems. Primary reconstruction with a non-vascularized bone graft is associated with a high failure rate, normally from wound breakdown in the mandibular body section associated with thin intraoral mucosa and wound contamination. Breakdown rarely occurs over the ascending ramus of the mandible or condyle area since these are not normally contaminated by saliva and have covering from the medial pterygoid muscle medially and the masseter muscle laterally, providing a bulk of vascu-

larized soft tissue. However, secondary reconstruction, even carried out after 6 or 8 weeks, is problematic, since it is difficult to gain secondary access to the glenoid fossa to insert a non-vascularized graft, such as a rib graft secondarily. Although temporary alloplastic condyles are available, they are sometimes difficult to insert, and are very often difficult to remove, since fibrosis often forms around the condyle head making subsequent removal and replacement with a rib graft difficult (Fig. 31.23). For this reason, a staged reconstruction has been advocated. In this technique, following resection, immediate reconstruction of the condyle and ascending ramus is carried out with a rib graft (Fig. 31.24). This maintains the articulation of the glenoid fossa, and generally survives because of the vascularity of the surrounding musculature and the adequacy of the intraoral closure. Temporary reconstruction of the body of the mandible is with a titanium reconstruction plate. Some 6–8 weeks later, the body of the mandible is then reconstructed from an extraoral approach, as detailed previously, using corticocancellous blocks from the ilium. In this way, the reconstruction of both the condyle and the body of the mandible is optimized, and high success rates have been reported.

Radiation therapy

Radiation therapy to the mandibular area complicates reconstruction. Radiation therapy causes an endar-

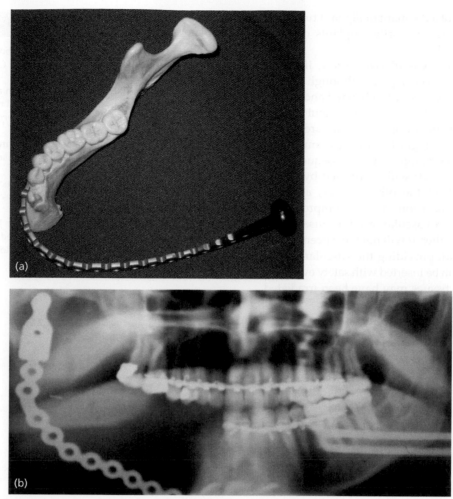

Fig. 31.23 A temporary alloplastic titanium condyle attached to a reconstruction plate. Removal of the condyle for secondary autogenous reconstruction can be difficult due to fibrosis and scarring.

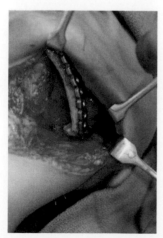

Fig. 31.24 A rib graft attached to a reconstruction plate for primary reconstruction of the condyle. The mandibular body will be reconstructed secondarily with a corticocancellous block graft from the iliac crest.

teritis, which decreases the vascularity, cellularity, and tissue oxygenation of the associated tissues. The endarteritis and hypocellularity usually commence some 3–4 months following the radiation therapy and are continuous in nature; they are well established by 6 months. The tendency is for the endarteritis and

hypocellularity to become more pronounced with time. There is no evidence that it is a reversible process. There is, however, a so-called "golden window" up to 3–4 months following radiation therapy during which bone grafting can be carried out in a normal way. From a practical point of view, the immediate local complications of radiation therapy will often preclude the bone graft during the first 6 weeks following radiation therapy, while the mucositis, etc. resolve, and therefore the "golden window" is really from 6 weeks to 3–4 months following radiation therapy. After this time, the failure rate from non-vascularized bone grafts is generally felt to be unacceptably high due to the avascular tissue bed. If it is intended to carry out mandibular reconstruction in an area that has received more than 55 Gy of radiation, it should either be with a vascularized graft or possibly following a course of hyperbaric oxygen therapy to increase the vascularity and cellularity of the tissue bed. There is good evidence that hyperbaric oxygen (30–40 dives at 2.4 atmospheres pressure for approximately 90 minutes) can produce a tissue bed in which a non-vascularized bone graft can survive. There is no evidence that hyperbaric oxygen can reactivate a dormant malignant tumor or cause recurrence of a dormant malignant tumor. If the bone graft takes satisfactorily, implants can subsequently be inserted.

In the case of a vascularized graft, if previous radiation therapy has been given, although the nature of the recipient vessels may be changed and they may have a greater element of fibrosis, successful anastomosis, and re-establishment of vascularity are possible.

If a microvascular graft is inserted immediately and then radiation therapy given subsequently, then the microvascular graft will be affected by radiation therapy just like all the other tissues, and subsequently implant insertion may be compromised. If, however, the microvascular graft is inserted after radiation therapy, then it will not have been subjected to irradiation, and, providing the vascularity is adequate, implants can be inserted with safety even though the surrounding tissues may have been irradiated.

Recommended reading

Marx RE. (1994) Clinical application of bone biology to mandibular and maxillary reconstruction. *Clinics in Plastic Surgery*, **21**, 377.

Obwegeser HL. (1966) Simultaneous resection and reconstruction of parts of the mandible via the intraoral route in patients with and without gross infections. *Oral Surgery, Oral Medicine, Oral Pathology*, **21**, 693.

Pogrel MA. (1989) The marginal mandibularectomy for the treatment of mandibular tumours. *British Journal of Oral and Maxillofacial Surgery*, **27**, 132.

Pogrel MA, Schmidt BL. (2010) Mandibular reconstruction. In: *Oral and Maxillofacial Surgery* (eds, Andersson L, Kahnberg K-E, Pogrel MA). Oxford, Wiley-Blackwell.

Pogrel MA, Podlesh S, Anthony JP, Alexander J. (1997) A comparison of vascularized and nonvascularized bone grafts for reconstruction of mandibular continuity defects. *Journal of Oral and Maxillofacial Surgery*, **55**, 1200.

Part 7: Temporomandibular Joint Disorders

(Section Editor: Tony Pogrel)

Chapter 32

Diagnosis and Non-surgical Management of Orofacial Pain

There are multiple causes of orofacial pain separate from temporomandibular disorders, including a number of medical and dental conditions.

Medical conditions which can mimic orofacial pain

Intracranial disorders

Disorders of the intracranial structures, such as neoplasia, aneurysm, abscess, hemorrhage or hematoma, and edema can usually be easily differentiated from orofacial pain (Fig. 32.1). They should be considered first in the diagnostic process, because they can be life-threatening and require immediate attention. The characteristics of serious intracranial disorders include new or abrupt onset of pain, pain that increases in severity, interruption of sleep by pain, pain precipitated by exertion or positional change, and neurologic deficits. One vascular pain disorder, temporal arteritis – a giant cell arteritis – may be misdiagnosed as myofascial pain involving the temporalis muscle. If treatment is delayed, temporal arteritis can lead to a sudden loss of vision.

Neurovascular headache disorders

Headache is a common complaint reported by patients suffering from musculoskeletal jaw disorders.

Primary headache

Primary headache disorders associated with orofacial pain include migraine headaches, migraine-variant headaches, cluster headaches, chronic paroxysmal hemicrania, and tension-type headaches.

Secondary headache

Secondary headache disorders are defined as headaches that develop secondary to another condition or mechanism. These could include physical exertion, cold stimuli, trauma, infection, metabolic disorders, or substance withdrawal.

Neuropathic pain disorders

Neuropathic pain is a disorder resulting from injury, peripheral and/or central, in the pain transmission system and is usually present in the absence of an ongoing primary source for the pain. Neuropathic pain disorders are divided into either paroxysmal (episodic) or continuous painful conditions.

Paroxysmal disorders

The paroxysmal conditions associated with orofacial pain include: trigeminal neuralgia, glossopharyngeal neuralgia, and the more rare conditions of nervous intermedius neuralgia and superior laryngeal neuralgia.

Continuous disorders

The continuous neuropathic pain disorders associated with orofacial pain are primarily deafferentation pain syndromes related to compression or distortion, demyelination, infarction, or inflammation of the cranial nerves. Acute herpes zoster, chronic postherpetic

Essentials of Oral and Maxillofacial Surgery, First Edition. Edited by M. Anthony Pogrel, Karl-Erik Kahnberg and Lars Andersson.
© 2014 John Wiley & Sons, Ltd. Published 2014 by John Wiley & Sons, Ltd.
Companion website: www.wiley.com/go/pogrel/oms

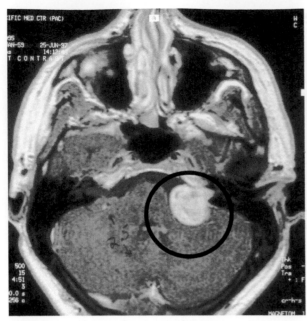

Fig. 32.1 Acoustic neuroma can initially present as face and jaw pain.

neuralgia, diabetic neuropathy, and neuromas are examples of continuous neuropathic pain syndromes.

Headache attributed to associated extracranial pain disorders

Extracranial pain disorders associated with orofacial pain include pain related to the eyes, ears, nose, sinuses, throat, intraoral structures, neck, jaw, and cranial bones.

Intraoral pain disorders

Intraoral pain disorders include odontogenic pain, and pain conditions associated with mucogingival tissues, tongue, and salivary glands.

Musculoskeletal, cervical and temporomandibular disorders

Musculoskeletal conditions affecting the jaw (TMD) and neck are the major cause of non-odontogenic pain in the orofacial region. They include cervical spine and temporomandibular joint (articular) disorders; and cervical and masticatory muscle (non-articular) disorders.

Temporomandibular disorders

Temporomandibular disorders (TMD) were referred to as a syndrome in the past. Common terms were "TMJ", "TMJ syndrome", or "TMJ pain–dysfunction syndrome". Presently they are considered to be a collection of various distinct articular or muscular conditions affecting the jaw, often with similar signs and symptoms, but different underlying mechanisms. The common clinical presentation is any combination of jaw, face, head, or ear pain, TMJ noises such as clicking, popping or crepitus, or grating, and/or limited jaw opening, jaw catching, and locking. Related symptoms, without proven cause and effect, include global headaches, neck pain, tinnitus, ear fullness or perceived hearing loss, and dizziness. Pain in the TMJ region is reported in approximately 10% of the population over 18 years of age (8–15% for women and 3–10% for men). The gender ratio varies between cross-sectional studies from anywhere from 4:1 to 2:1 female to male. The peak age is approximately 35–45 years (the child-bearing years of females).

Although the etiology of the various subsets of TMD was in the past thought to directly relate to occlusal discrepancies and improper jaw relationships, presently the number of related contributing factors for each specific diagnosis is uncertain and many times unknown. It is now generally felt that malocclusion is not directly correlated to the various subsets of TMD. Contributing etiologic factors include trauma, possibly parafunction, gender and hormonal factors, systemic factors, overuse of the masticatory system, and psychosocial and behavioral factors. Recent evidence suggests a specific gene expression, primarily in females, implicated as a risk factor for persistent orofacial pain.

Classification of articular disorders

TMJ disorders include congenital, developmental, or acquired disorders, disc derangement disorders, condylar dislocation, inflammatory disorders, non-inflammatory disorders, ankylosis, and fracture of the condylar process.

Disc derangements

Disc derangement disorders represent an abnormal anatomical relationship or misalignment of the articular disc and condyle. Recent studies are revealing, however, that there is a great deal of variation in the disc position even in individuals without joint pain, joint noise, or jaw dysfunction. Stretched or torn collateral discal ligaments are thought to be the reason why discs become displaced, although there is still uncertainty regarding the natural history of these derangement conditions. Articular discs are typically displaced anteriorly and medially (Fig. 32.2), but can also be positioned laterally, or even posteriorly.

Condylar dislocation

Condylar dislocation or open lock is a hypermobility condition of the jaw. It occurs when the condyle inadvertently becomes positioned anterior and superior to the articular eminence, during jaw opening or protrusion, and is unable to return to a closed position. It can be caused by trauma, extended periods of mouth opening such as a long dental appointment, or can be a manifestation of joint hypermobility.

Inflammatory and non-inflammatory disorders

Inflammatory joint disorders can occur as an inflammation of the synovium (synovitis) and/or joint capsule (capsulitis). This may be the result of trauma, infection, or cartilage degeneration, or the sequelae of a systemic polyarthritic or collagen disease (rheumatoid arthritis, lupus, Reiter's syndrome).

Non-inflammatory joint disorders include primary and secondary osteoarthritis. Osteoarthritis (OA) is defined as a non-inflammatory degenerative condition of the joint characterized by deterioration and abrasion of articular tissue and concomitant remodeling of the underlying subchondral bone due to overload of the remodeling mechanism. OA is classified as primary OA when the etiology is unknown and secondary OA when an etiologic event or factor can be identified (e.g. gout, Cushing's disease, osteonecro-

sis, infections, Charcot's neuropathic pain). It can be further categorized into active OA or stable OA, sometimes referred to as osteoarthrosis. Active OA is related to an active change or degeneration in the articular tissues, whereas stable OA refers to the recortication of the articular osseous structure with a lack of any further structural change (Fig. 32.3).

Muscular disorders

The underlying mechanisms that cause masticatory muscle pain are similar to those that cause skeletal muscle disorders throughout the rest of the body. Some mechanisms thought to be related to muscle pain include overuse, localized ischemia, spontaneous activity of deep nociceptors, sympathetic nervous system hemodynamic perfusion changes, and changes in descending anti-nociceptive modulation.

Myofascial pain

Myofascial pain is characterized by a regional or local dull, aching muscle pain that increases during function. Clinically there are localized tender sites or trigger points in the muscle, tendon, or fascia. Palpation of the trigger point provokes pain referral to a distant site such as the teeth, ear, or head and this must be present to meet the criteria for myofascial pain. Patients may also report muscle stiffness, ear symptoms such as tinnitus, decreased mouth opening that can be passively stretched by more than 4 mm, and hyperalgesia in the region of the referred pain. Myofascial pain is not considered an inflammatory process; whereas tendonitis is an inflammation and/or soreness in the tendinous attachments of masticatory muscles.

Centrally mediated myalgia

Fibromyalgia, a type of general or global muscle pain involved with central nervous system upregulation, can be confused with local or regional muscle pain if the clinician is not comprehensive with the history taking and physical assessment process. Fibromyalgia

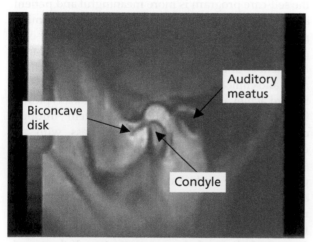

Fig. 32.2 MRI sagittal view of an anterior disc displacement without reduction.

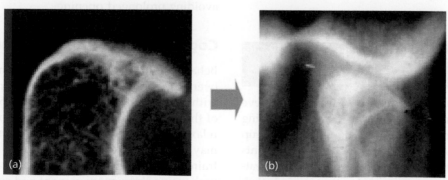

Fig. 32.3 (a) Active osteoarthritis is an active change or degeneration in the articular hard tissues. The cortical outline is no longer intact and there are erosions and subchondral bone cyst formation. (b) Stable osteoarthritis is a recortication (smooth surface) of the articular hard tissues and a probable end to any further structural change.

is characterized by a continuous, aching pain in many areas of the body. It is associated with generalized fatigue, chronic headache, irritable bowel syndrome, sleep disturbance, and emotional distress including anxiety, depression, and somatization.

Assessment of musculoskeletal disorders

Comprehensive history and examination

The gold standard for diagnosis of TMD is the interpretation of findings from a comprehensive history and comprehensive physical examination. Psychological and psychosocial assessment can be effectively incorporated as part of the pain history with standardized self-report questionnaires.

Imaging

Imaging of the TMJ and orofacial structures may be necessary to rule out structural disorders of the jaw and other medical conditions that may be masquerading as a jaw disorder. After a panorex type radiograph, cone-beam computed tomography is the most accurate method for radiographically examining patients with suspected TMJ degenerative disease or other osseous pathology and structural aberrations.

MRI has diverse capabilities for the examination of suspected TMJ soft tissue disorders and pathology, i.e. disc displacement, effusion, and tumors. As the resolution improves and technical advancement occurs, MRI is clearly becoming the study of choice for complex problem solving.

Adjunctive diagnostic devices

There are a number of electronic devices marketed to diagnose jaw disorders (TMD) including electromyography testing, jaw tracking, thermography, sonography, and vibration analysis. However, the sensitivity (percentage of correctly diagnosed patients) and specificity (percentage of correctly diagnosed normals) of these technical diagnostic TMD tests is open to question.

Management of musculoskeletal disorders

The majority of patients with jaw disorders achieve good symptomatic relief with a medical model using non-invasive management. Long-term follow-up studies show that 85% to more than 90% of patients have few or no symptoms after conservative treatment. Jaw disorders are similar to other musculoskeletal disorders, but currently not enough is known about the natural course of most jaw disorders and which signs and symptoms will progress to more serious conditions. As in other musculoskeletal conditions, the TMD signs and symptoms vary and may be transient and self-limiting, resolving without serious long-term effects. Untreated disc displacement without reduction may also undergo a natural resolution of symptoms over time, as may degenerative joint disease. For these reasons a special effort should be made to avoid aggressive, irreversible therapy for articular and non-articular jaw disorders.

A multidisciplinary medical model that includes patient education and self-care, cognitive behavioral intervention, pharmacologic therapy, physical rehabilitation, and/or orthopedic appliance therapy is endorsed for the management of nearly all patients. The management goals should be diagnosis specific. The common goals are reduction of pain, reduction of adverse loading, improvement of mobility and function, and restoration of activities of daily living.

Patient education and self-care

The success of a self-care program depends on patient motivation, cooperation, and adherence. A successful program begins with a thorough explanation of the patient's diagnosis and a discussion about the prognosis. Once the patient understands their condition, the self-care program is more meaningful and patient adherence is higher. When the jaw disorder is mild, patient education and instruction in a self-care program may be all that is required. The self-care instructions should be specific for the patient's diagnosis and clinical presentation; and should be directed toward achievable goals. These instructions typically include resting the masticatory system through correct relaxed jaw posture awareness with an emphasis on not contacting opposing teeth unless swallowing, i.e. preventing awake clenching and grinding of the teeth. Patients need to be mindful of any other oral habits that may be delaying their recovery such as jaw protrusion, cheek sucking, or tongue bracing behaviors. Patients generally benefit from a soft diet and slower mastication. If they need joint protection, as in the case of joint inflammation or disc instability, patients benefit from chewing on the affected side, limiting incising their food and avoiding prolonged opening.

Cognitive behavioral intervention

Behavioral intervention is an important part of the overall medical management program for patients with jaw disorders. Simply making patients aware of their jaw habits is often enough to improve jaw relaxation skills, but changing persistent habits may require a structured program with a clinician trained in behavior modification strategies. Comprehensive stress management and counseling programs using a combination of EMG biofeedback, progressive relaxation, diaphragmatic breathing, and self-directed changes in lifestyle appear to be more effective than any one behavioral treatment procedure in isolation.

Pharmacologic therapy

The indicated classes of pharmacologic agents include analgesics, non-steroidal anti-inflammatory drugs (NSAIDs), corticosteroids, anxiolytics, muscle relaxants, lowdose (pain-dosing) antidepressants, and nerve membrane stabilizers. The non-opiate analgesics, such as acetaminophen, are effective for mild to moderate pain, whereas the opioid narcotics, such as codeine, Ultram, hydrocodone, and Demerol, should only be used short term for controlling more severe acute pain. Opioid narcotics produce tolerance and dependence and should be used on a time-contingent basis. NSAIDs, such as ibuprofen, naproxen, or nabumetone, are effective analgesics and anti-inflammatory agents. They are prescribed for painful articular inflammatory disorders, not usually for muscle disorders.

The benzodiazepines, such as alprazolam, lorazepam, and diazepam, are most commonly prescribed for their anti-anxiety effects. These drugs act as depressants when used long-term; thus they should only be used short-term for acute muscle pain/spasm (trismus), to relax patients prior to jaw manipulation for acute disc displacement without reduction, or for sleep disturbances associated with anxiety. Muscle relaxants, such as cyclobenzaprine, metaxolone, and tizanidine, are useful for acute and/or chronic muscle pain.

Membrane stabilizers or anti-seizure drugs, such as carbamazepine and phenytoin, have been replaced with improved medications such as gabapentin and pregabalin for persistent pain conditions including neuropathic atypical odontalgia pain. These second-generation medications have less significant side-effect profiles than the former drugs.

Physical therapy

Treatment goals commonly include pain control, optimizing joint biomechanics and range of motion, restoring functional muscle strength and endurance, and restoring the ability to perform activities of daily living, such as talking, chewing, yawning, and singing; or of the cervical and upper quarter regions such as sitting, reading, driving, lifting, and reaching.

The management begins with patient education and instructions in a structured self-care program. The next goal is to reduce pain as efficiently as possible, so the patient can begin exercising their jaw, neck, and upper quarter as appropriate. Physical agents such as moist heat, cold packs, transcutaneous electrical nerve stimulators (TENS), iontophoresis, ultrasound (Fig. 32.4), and vapocoolants may be used initially for pain control.

Soft-tissue mobilization and myofascial release techniques are commonly used to increase local cir-

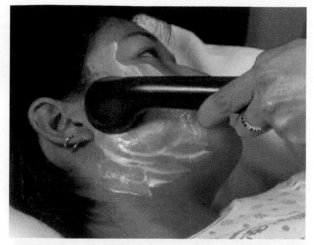

Fig. 32.4 Ultrasound application to the right masseter region.

culation, restore normal muscle tone, and deactivate myofascial trigger points. Once the patient has better pain control, the therapist can mobilize the joints as needed, and begin a range-of-motion and muscle conditioning program.

Orthopedic appliance therapy

Orthopedic appliances, also referred to as orthoses, occlusal splints, bite splints, bite plates, night guards, or bruxism appliances, have been commonly used in the management of jaw disorders. There is general agreement that some patients with myofascial pain, articular disc instability, and joint inflammation sustain their symptoms with bruxism at night. These patients may benefit from appliances worn during sleep. Also, appliances have dental benefits with regard to protecting the teeth and/or restorations from wear and fracture, as well as decreasing tooth sensitivity and mobility. Appliances should only be worn during sleep in order to limit the amount of time the appliance masks the periodontal proprioceptive input that allows the patient to return to their intercuspal position when the appliance is removed. Eventually random wear at night, during periods of increased stress, should be all that is necessary.

There still is great debate about how to design an appliance for the greatest efficacy. Appliance design, i.e. specific types of occlusal interfaces and/or jaw positions, does not appear to be a very critical factor for the management of bruxism or masticatory muscle pain. Most dentists agree, however, that orthopedic appliances should cover all the teeth on either the maxillary or mandibular arch in order to prevent irreversible changes in the occlusion (Fig. 32.5). Partial coverage appliances can allow teeth to extrude or intrude and/or cause condyles to reposition themselves within the articular fossae. The type of material, hard acrylic or soft vinyl, is no longer felt to be an important consideration.

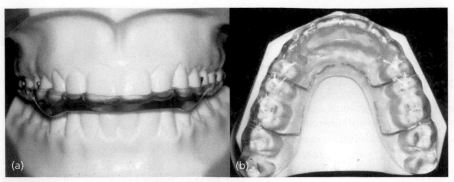

Fig. 32.5 (a, b) Frontal and occlusal views of a maxillary orthosis.

Conclusion

Utilizing the philosophies and modalities described in this chapter, over 85% of orofacial pain sufferers can obtain complete or meaningful resolution of symptoms. Surgery is only rarely indicated.

Recommended reading

Garefis P, Grigoriadou E, Zarifi A, Koidis PT. (1994) Effectiveness of conservative treatment for craniomandibular disorders: a 2-year longitudinal study. *Journal of Orofacial Pain*, **8**, 309–14.

LeResche L. (1997) Epidemiology of temporomandibular disorders: implications for the investigation of etiologic factors. *Critical Reviews in Oral Biology and Medicine*, **8**, 291–305.

McNeil C, Rudd PA. (2010) Diagnosis and non-surgical management of orofacial pain. In: *Oral and Maxillofacial Surgery* (eds, Andersson L, Kahnberg K-E, Pogrel MA). Oxford, Wiley-Blackwell.

Stohler CS. (2007) The end of an era: orofacial pain enters the genomic age219–28. In: *The Puzzle of Orofacial Pain* (eds, Turp JC, Sommer C, Hugger A), pp. 2007. Basel, Karger AG.

Chapter 33

Temporomandibular Joint Surgery (Including Arthroscopy)

Arthroscopy

Modern arthroscopy started with the commercial introduction of the flexible fiber-light cable in the early 1970s. Another invention, the Hopkins rod-lens telescope, also introduced commercially in the 1970s, constituted a significant improvement in the optics, and arthroscopy of the temporomandibular joint (TMJ) began shortly afterwards. TMJ arthroscopy provides unique possibilities for simultaneous intra-articular diagnosis and surgical treatment.

Anatomic considerations

The joint is divided by the disc into an upper and a lower compartment. The volume of the upper compartment is about twice as large as that of the lower compartment. Puncture of the upper compartment involves only trocar penetration of the lateral capsule, while puncture of the lower compartment involves penetration of both the capsule and the disc ligament. Thus, puncture of the lower compartment always involves the slight risk of damaging the lateral disc attachment, which may, in turn, cause displacement of the disc medially. For these reasons arthroscopy is usually restricted to the upper joint space. It is relatively safe to insert the instruments from the lateral side between the temporal vessels posteriorly and the temporal branch of the facial nerve anteriorly.

Diagnostic arthroscopy

The advent of high resolution MRI has decreased the need for diagnostic arthroscopy. One advantage of arthroscopy is that, depending on the condition, diagnosis and therapy can be performed simultaneously.

Possible indications for arthroscopic examination (Fig. 33.1) are:

- disc derangements;
- osteoarthritis;
- rheumatic joint disease;
- crystal-induced arthritis;
- synovial pseudotumors.

Arthroscopic examination can also show discal perforations which are not visible on MRI.

Contraindications

Absolute contraindications include:

- bony ankylosis;
- advanced resorption of the glenoid fossa;
- infection in the joint area;
- malignant tumors.

Relative contraindications include:

- patients at increased risk for hemorrhage;
- patients at increased risk for infection;
- fibrous ankylosis.

Arthroscopy equipment

Figure 33.2 shows a suitable set of instruments. Most telescopes have a diameter of about 2 mm but ultrathin telescopes have been developed with a diameter of about 0.7 mm. Such a reduction in diameter results in a loss of optical quality. There is also an increased risk that the instrument will break. The telescope should have a direction of view of 30°. This allows the field of vision to be increased simply by rotating the instrument. A 1.2 mm disposable standard needle is suitable for outflow. For triangulation purposes a twin sheath is used. This allows for switching the position of the working instruments

Essentials of Oral and Maxillofacial Surgery, First Edition. Edited by M. Anthony Pogrel, Karl-Erik Kahnberg and Lars Andersson.
© 2014 John Wiley & Sons, Ltd. Published 2014 by John Wiley & Sons, Ltd.
Companion website: www.wiley.com/go/pogrel/oms

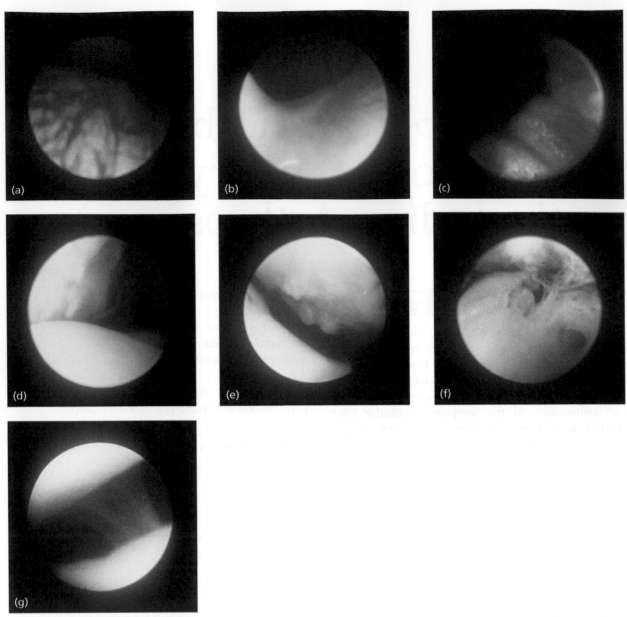

Fig. 33.1 Arthroscopic features of inflammation, osteoarthritis, and adhesions. (a) Right joint, upper compartment: increased vascularity in the posterior disc attachment. (b) Left joint, upper compartment: capillary hyperemia in the posterior disc attachment. (c) Left joint, upper compartment: synovial hyperplasia and capillary hyperemia in the posterior disc attachment. (d) Left joint, upper compartment: fibrillation in the temporal fibrocartilage, disc unaffected below. (e) Right joint, upper compartment: lesion in the temporal fibrocartilage, disc unaffected below. (f) Left joint, upper compartment: small disc perforation in posterior part of the disc. (g) Left joint, upper compartment: single fibrotic band (adhesion) between temporal fibrocartilage and disc in the medial part.

and telescope. A Xenon cold-light source provides a light with accurate color purity.

Instruments for arthroscopic surgery are:

- forceps, knives, and scissors;
- suction punch;
- mini-shavers;
- bipolar cautery;
- surgical lasers (most frequently Holmium/YAG).

Arthroscopic procedures

Arthroscopy can be performed under local or general anesthesia.

Puncture

First, the upper compartment is distended with 2 mL of lidocaine which is injected slowly until resistance is felt. The so-called inferolateral approach gains good access to the posterior part of the upper compartment of the TMJ (Fig. 33.3). This is also the best approach for puncturing the lower compartment. The anterolateral and endaural approaches are mainly used when arthroscopic surgery is intended.

Correct placement of the arthroscope should be confirmed through the telescope. An outflow portal is then created (inferolateral approach) about 5 mm anterior to and slightly below the arthroscopic sheath. Continuous irrigation is performed, to ensure a clear

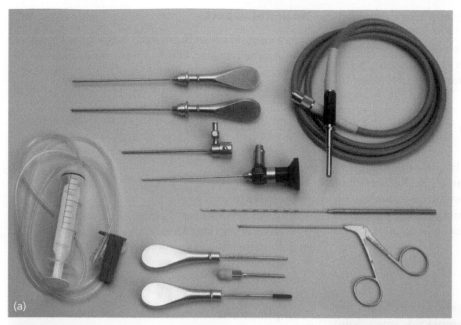

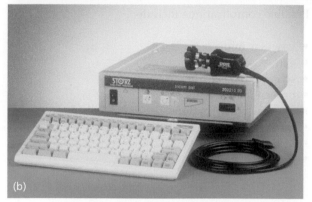

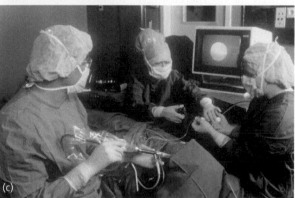

Fig. 33.2 Arthroscopic equipment. (a) Telescope, arthroscopic sheath, trocars, biopsy forceps, irrigation syringe, and light cable. (b) Camera and light source. (c) Arthroscopy in action.

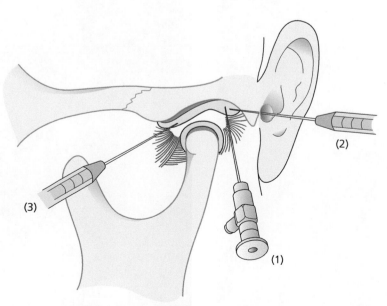

Fig. 33.3 Puncture directions for the TMJ. (1) Inferolateral. (2) Endaural. (3) Anterolateral.

field of vision and to keep the joint space extended, using isotonic saline solution. For more prolonged arthroscopic surgery, Ringer's solution may be a better alternative because it has been found to protect the chondrocytes and maintain the synthesis of proteoglycans.

Arthroscopic examination (diagnostic arthroscopy)

The arthroscopic examination begins with identification of the arthroscopic landmarks – i.e. the boundary between the disc and the posterior disc attachment, the medial capsule, and the inferior part of the eminence, followed by a methodical examination of the joint compartment.

Arthroscopic surgery

In the field of orthopedic surgery, arthroscopic procedures have increasingly replaced open joint surgery. The duration of the postoperative period and the frequency of complications have thereby been reduced.

However, arthroscopic surgery of the TMJ is more difficult. The anatomic position limits the possibilities for surgery and the small size and the anatomy of the joint often give limited access for the instruments. The introduction of new instruments with fine dimensions and the surgical laser has increased the possibilities for arthroscopic surgery of the TMJ.

Technical aspects

Minor surgical procedures, such as lysis and lavage or partial synovectomy, can be performed under local anesthesia with or without sedation. The surgical procedures are best performed under direct visual control either with a double cannula or with triangulation.

The following surgical procedures can currently be performed:

* biopsy;
* lavage (Fig. 33.4);
* lysis (Fig. 33.5) ;
* disc repositioning;
* synovectomy (Fig. 33.6) ;
* debridement and abrasion;
* restriction;
* intra-articular pharmacotherapy.

Complications

Possible complications include:

* vascular injury;
* extravasation;
* scuffing of cartilage;
* broken instruments;
* otologic complications;
* intracranial damage;
* infection;
* nerve injury.

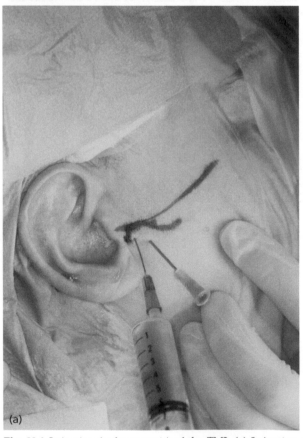
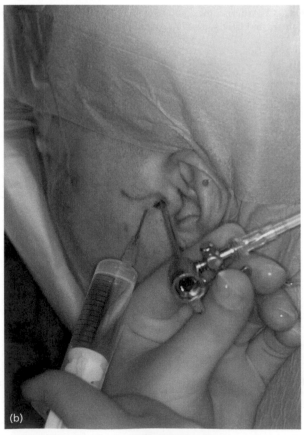

Fig. 33.4 Irrigation (arthrocentesis) of the TMJ. (a) Irrigation using two needles. (b) During arthroscopy using the arthroscopic sheath for outflow providing effective irrigation.

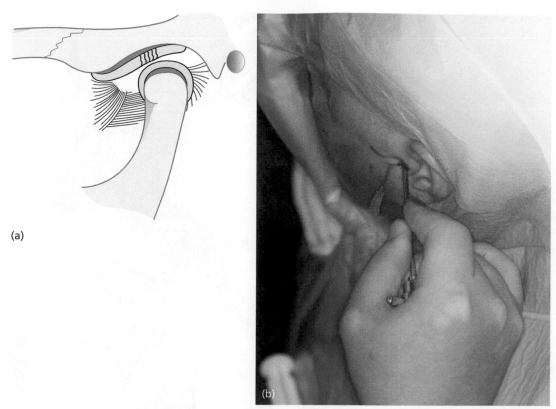

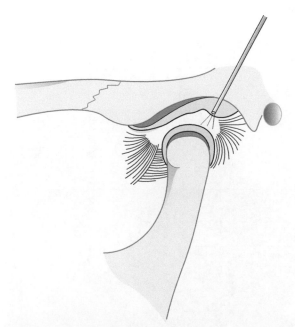

(a)

Fig. 33.5 Lysis of adhesions. (a) Simplified drawing of adhesion between the temporal fibrocartilage and the disc. (b) Semi-blind release of adhesions in the joint.

Fig. 33.6 Simplified drawing of laser synovectomy in the TMJ. In patients with hypermobility, the laser may also be used in a coagulating mode to create scar tissue, thereby limiting translation of the disc–condyle complex.

Concluding remarks

Similar to developments in the field of orthopedic surgery, TMJ arthroscopy has become an important method for diagnosis and treatment. Its accuracy in diagnosing TMJ diseases is high and simultaneous biopsy can be performed to improve diagnosis. Complications are minor and infrequent. However, high resolution MRI has made diagnostic arthroscopy less needed, and the small size and complexity of the joint, together with the small size of the instruments has hindered the development of therapeutic arthroscopy.

Open temporomandibular joint surgery

Overall, open joint surgery is indicated in less than 5% of patients with TMJ symptoms. The remainder can be treated non-surgically, or with arthroscopic procedures.

Conditions that may require open TMJ surgery

- Mechanical disorders:
  - disc displacement;
  - mandibular dislocation.
- Degenerative joint disease.
- TMJ trauma.
- TMJ abnormalities:
  - congenital;
  - acquired.
- TMJ tumors.

Surgical approaches to the TMJ

Preparation of the surgical site

The standard approach to the TMJ is the preauricular approach (Fig. 33.7). It uses the preauricular skin fold

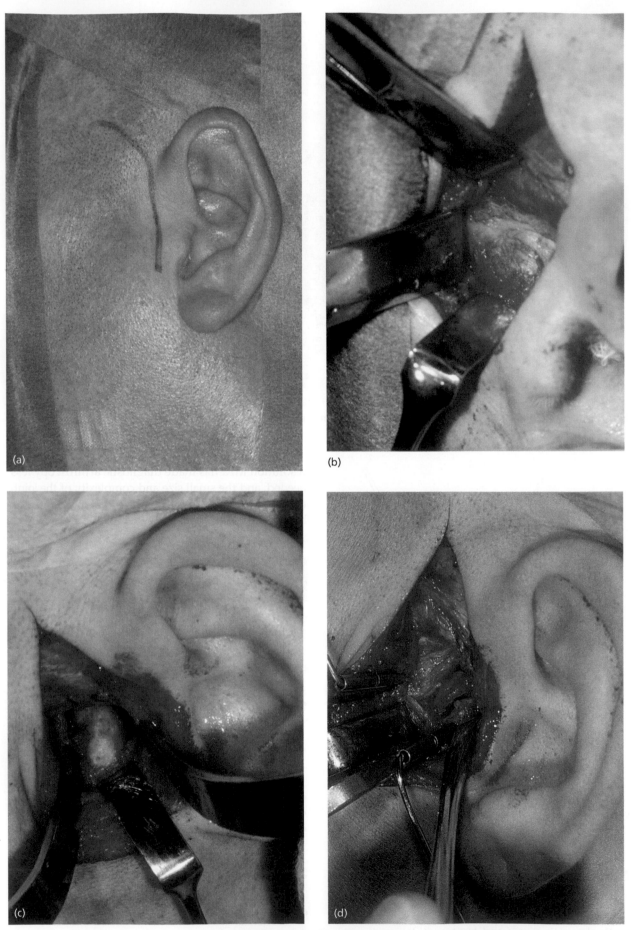

Fig. 33.7 Surgical dissection of the TMJ. (a) Preauricular incision line. (b) Zygomatic arch and lateral capsule exposed. (c) Lateral capsule opened and condylar retractors placed. (d) Kirschner wires drilled into the eminence and condyle and a Wilkes self-retaining retractor (W. Lorenz Surgical, Jacksonville, FL) applied to increase access to the joint.

and, if needed, may be extended superiorly and slightly anteriorly. Normally, when an intra-articular procedure is intended there is no need for a superior or anterior extension of the incision but in cases where access to the area anterior to the eminence is needed such an extension of the incision is practical.

The dissection continues in layers down to the capsule of the joint, taking care to avoid the zygomatico-temporal branch of the facial nerve. The temporalis fascia is exposed and any vessels running posteriorly are ligated or cauterized. The fascia is then followed inferiorly down to the superior part of the zygomatic arch. The temporal artery and vein may be ligated if they interfere with the exposure of the joint. The auriculotemporal nerve usually runs together with the artery and vein and may be dissected free and retracted anteriorly. The dissection is then continued with an anteriosuperior incision through the superficial layer of the temporalis fascia, which is then extended inferiorly. The scissors are used to identify the zygomatic arch. An almost constant finding is a fairly large vein running over the zygomatic arch in a superior direction. This vein is a useful landmark for the anatomical location of the glenoid fossa. After exposure of the zygomatic arch, the lateral capsule is easily found inferiorly. The structures anterior and inferior to the capsule are protected with retractors. A horizontal incision in the superior part of the capsule provides access to the upper compartment, to perform the definitive surgery. Closure of the incision is made in the usual manner beginning with the lateral capsule and the temporal fascia and then a few sutures in the deeper subcutaneous tissue and finally a running 4/0 subcuticular suture to close the skin.

Surgical procedures

Disc repositioning

Disc repositioning means that the anteriorly displaced disc is surgically repositioned back to its original position on the condyle (Fig. 33.8).

Modified condylotomy

The hypothesis of this method is that if the position of the condyle is altered, the load on the posterior disc attachment will be reduced, which in turn will facilitate a spontaneous repositioning of the disc on the condyle (Fig. 33.9). In the knee, the same method has been used in the past by performing an osteotomy of the tibia, thereby changing the load on the meniscus.

The technique comprises an intraoral vertical ramus osteotomy via an incision of the buccal fold posteriorly. The posterior segment containing the condyle is allowed to drop a few millimeters but the

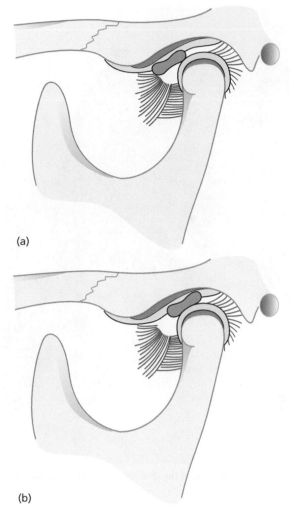

(a)

(b)

Fig. 33.8 Simplified drawing showing surgical repositioning of the disc. (a) Displaced disc. (b) Disc after surgical repositioning.

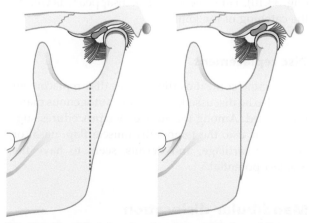

Fig. 33.9 Simplified drawing showing modified condylotomy of the TMJ.

segment is not fixed to the distal portion of the mandible. The wound is sutured and intermaxillary fixation with elastics is then applied and held for 2 weeks, and an occlusal splint is often utilized to create an open bite on the operated side.

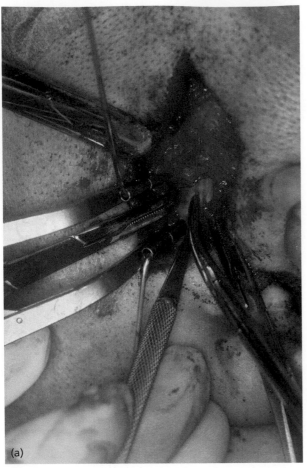
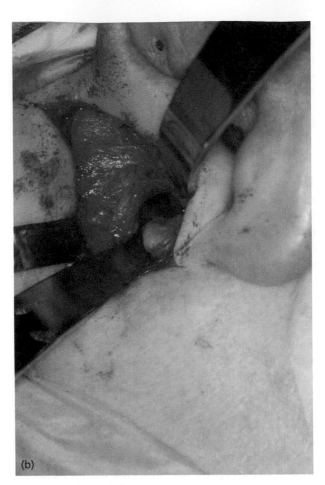

Fig. 33.10 (a) Excision of the disc. (b) Exposure of an interfering osteophyte on the condyle.

Discectomy

Discectomy treats both the displaced disc and the problematic callus in the disc and does it effectively (Fig. 33.10). Thus, the loud click disappears as well as the catching of the joint.

Disc replacement

In the same context as discectomy, disc replacement must also be discussed. Today only autogenous material is used. Among the autogenous procedures suggested for use, the temporalis muscle flap, nasal or auricular cartilage, and dermis, seem to have the greatest potential.

Mandibular dislocation

Epidemiological studies have revealed an increased incidence of general joint hypermobility in children, in women compared with men, and in some racial groups (Eskimos and Chinese).

Clinical diagnosis

Clinical diagnosis is usually not a problem. In bilateral dislocations there is a frontal open bite, in unilateral dislocations there is a deviation of the mandible to the opposite side and a lateral open bite on the same side. The condyle is not seated in the glenoid fossa and thus the area anterior to the tragus appears "empty". Radiographic examination confirms the dislocated mandibular condyles.

Surgical treatment

Acute dislocation is best managed with manual repositioning which is easy and quick provided that a proper technique is used. The so called Hippocratic technique is normally employed (Fig. 33.11).

Several methods for management of recurrent dislocation have been proposed through the years, such as blocking procedures, anchoring procedures, methods inducing scar tissue, myotomy, eminectomy, and discectomy. Both open surgery and arthroscopic procedures have been described and all appear to enjoy a high success rate.

Chronic closed lock and osteoarthritis

Chronic closed lock and osteoarthritis are described under the same heading as they frequently occur together.

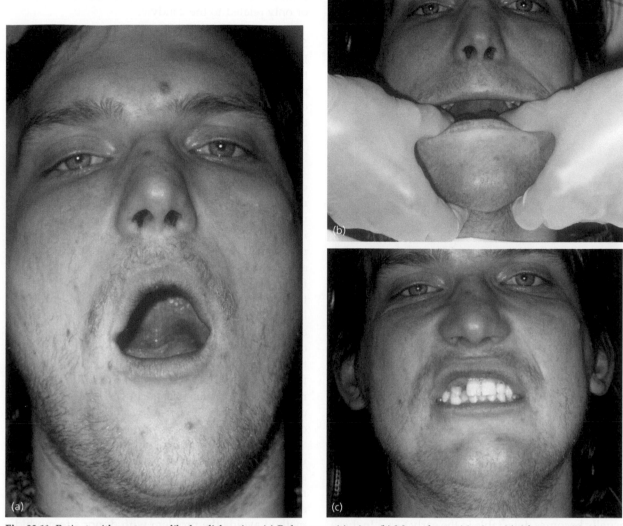

Fig. 33.11 Patient with acute mandibular dislocation. (a) Before repositioning. (b) Manual repositioning. (c) After repositioning.

In its early phase, chronic closed lock may show no lesions in the fibrocartilage but sooner or later they will appear. Osteoarthritis (also called degenerative joint disease) is thought to be a primarily degenerative disease of the cartilage. Synovial inflammation may occur secondary to the primary disease process. Cartilage debris and inflammatory mediators are thought to provoke the synovitis. Osteoarthritis may also occur in a generalized form.

In chronic closed lock, the disc is permanently displaced, resulting in a load on the vascularized and innervated posterior disc attachment. The translation will be impaired by the displaced disc as well as adhesions resulting from the chronic synovitis. The reduced translation, in turn, impairs the vascular supply to the posterior disc attachment and, if this is prolonged, the nutrition and lubrication of the joint will be affected, aggravating the degenerative process.

The TMJ has a marked capacity for adaptation and repair. Thus, the TMJ may develop a spontaneous remission similar to that seen in other joints. Until more is known about the disease mechanisms for chronic closed lock and osteoarthritis, we can at best prevent further development of the disease, improve mandibular function, and reduce the pain.

Surgical procedures advocated include discectomy, modified condylotomy, arthroplasty and even joint replacement (Fig. 33.12).

Ankylosis

For ankylosis, several surgical techniques have been suggested, such as gap osteotomy, chostochondral graft, auricular graft, dermis, alloplastic grafts, TMJ prostheses, and distraction osteogenesis. The suggested wide variety of methods indicates that there is still not a satisfactory treatment.

Acquired abnormalities

Condylar hyperplasia

Excessive growth of the mandible may affect only the condyle, the condyle and the ramus, or the whole

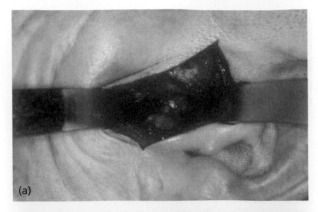

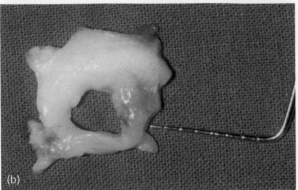

Fig. 33.12 Patient with osteoarthritis. (a) Interfering osteophyte on the condyle. (b) Excised disc with a large perforation.

mandible. The condition is usually unilateral. Several thorough reviews have been published but it is still unclear how the condition develops and progresses. It is more common in females than in males and it usually becomes detectable in the early teens. In these patients the excessive growth usually ceases when normal growth has ended. However, there are also cases where a recurrence of growth takes place after cessation of normal growth. In these patients the growing condyle is not only hyperplastic but also shows asymmetric growth. In some cases the overgrowth may result from the development of an osteochondroma.

Diagnosis

It is most important to determine whether the condition is in a residual (inactive) stage or not. Repeated occlusal assessments may be one method of detecting growth. However, compensatory growth of the maxilla may occur concealing the actual growth. Radiographic examination may reveal a size difference of the condyle between the right and left sides which may indicate condylar hyperplasia. However, it has to be remembered that the condyle normally shows variation in size and form. Especially when only a panoramic radiograph is taken the distortion can be considerable depending on the angle of the long axis of the condyle. A CT scan is therefore more reliable. Bone scintigraphy, especially when combined with CT, is a reliable method for detection of

metabolic activity in the condyle and may also show if the activity is found in other parts of the mandible or only related to the condyle.

Surgical treatment

In the growing child there are two options. If the child has a mild anomaly and is close to when cessation of normal growth is predicted, observation may be an option. However, if the anomaly is considerable and there is a long time until cessation of growth, a resection of the abnormal growth center in the superior part of the condyle is recommended (Fig. 33.13). Another important thing to understand is that mandibular hyperplasia is a disease of the mandible. This means that the disc and the temporal component are not affected. Another thing that can be advantageous is that the condylar neck is frequently thicker than normal and may therefore be large enough to act as a new condyle. This observation has formed the basis for an elegant and simple solution to the reconstruction task. The condyle is first resected via a preauricular approach. The lateral part of the ramus is then exposed via a submandibular approach and a vertical osteotomy performed in the posterior part. This posterior segment may be regarded as a bone–muscle flap as it has muscle attached to it medially. The superior part is smoothened and pushed up against the disc. Fixation to the remaining part of the ramus is done with miniplates (Fig. 33.14).

Another method for hemifacial microsomia is to use distraction osteogenesis. The condyle is resected and an L-osteotomy is then performed in the posterior part of the ramus. The segment is then gradually advanced superiorly to form the new condyle. The method avoids the problem with donor site morbidity but it is complicated and expensive.

The condyle can also be reconstructed using a costochondral graft. It involves a certain risk of donor site morbidity and asymmetric excessive growth of the graft, which in turn can result in a mandibular asymmetry.

In cases with the rotational form, simultaneous orthognathic surgery is frequently required as well as pre- and postoperative orthodontic treatment.

Ankylosis

Ankylosis, by definition, means that the joint is fused with bone. However, the term has often been broadened to also comprise fibro-osseous or fibrous fusion of the joint. The condition may occur after trauma (most frequently intra-articular), infection, chronic polyarthritis, or as a result of radiation therapy. It occurs both in adults and children.

Surgical treatment

The surgical protocol involves resection of the bone mass, creating a gap of about 10 mm both laterally and medially. If interincisal opening is still limited after this procedure, an osteotomy (or ostectomy) of

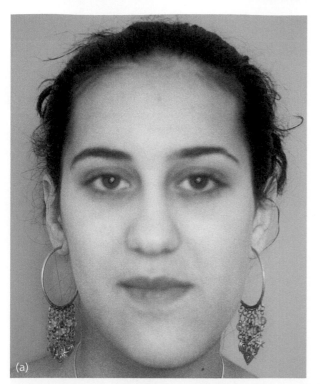

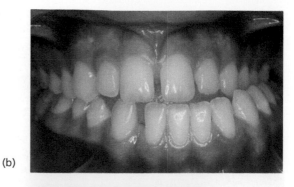

(b)

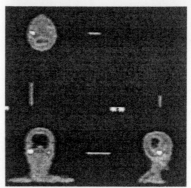

(a)

(c)

Fig. 33.13 A 14-year-old girl with an actively growing condylar hyperplasia. (a) Clinical picture showing deviation of the chin to the opposite side. (b) Occlusal view showing crossbite on the opposite side. (c) SPECT-SCAN showing increased uptake in the right TMJ.

the coronoid process may be performed as well. This will usually lead to an interincisal opening of about 35 mm or more (Fig. 33.15).

The TMJ may then be reconstructed in several ways. In the past costochondral graft was the method of choice. However, excessive growth of the graft can result in mandibular asymmetry. This occurs most frequently in the child but may also occur in adults. The costochondral graft may be used with or without an interpositional material. Several such materials have been used in the past, autogeneous such as auricular cartilage, dermis, temporalis fascia, and temporalis muscle. Another suggested method is to use distraction osteogenesis (see under Condylar hyperplasia).

The most disturbing complication after TMJ ankylosis operations is reankylosis. The reported figures vary from 0–37%. Complications with costochondral grafts are overgrowth of the graft, malocclusion, persistent pain, and donor site morbidity, in addition to re-ankylosis. Gap osteotomy may have the least complications. Temporalis muscle flap may create muscle symptoms at the donor site. In patients with TMJ prostheses, joint failure, Frey's syndrome, and persistent pain seem to be most common.

Synovial chondromatosis

The disease is not a true neoplasm but is better regarded as a metaplastic activity within the synovial membrane. For unknown reasons, the synovial membrane starts to produce small cartilage particles which are then released into the joint cavity. The number of free bodies may be as many as 200. Interestingly, the disease seems to be limited to the upper compartment. If free bodies are found in the lower compartment there is always a disc perforation present allowing the particles to slip into the lower compartment.

A CT scan usually displays free bodies in the TMJ as at least some of the fragments are calcified. However, there are also exceptional cases where no calcified bodies are seen and where the free bodies are also difficult to depict on MRI, because of the high water content of the cartilage fragments.

Arthroscopy is very accurate in diagnosing synovial chondromatosis. Symptomatic relief can also be obtained by flushing out the majority of the smaller fragments and the excess synovial fluid that creates the swelling. However, the bigger fragments cannot be removed arthroscopically and open surgery is therefore often necessary (Fig. 33.16). Recurrences are rare.

Temporomandibular joint reconstruction

When severe destruction or ankylosis of the temporomandibular joint occurs, joint replacement may be necessary. Although there are a number of autogenous sites that have been used over the years, the

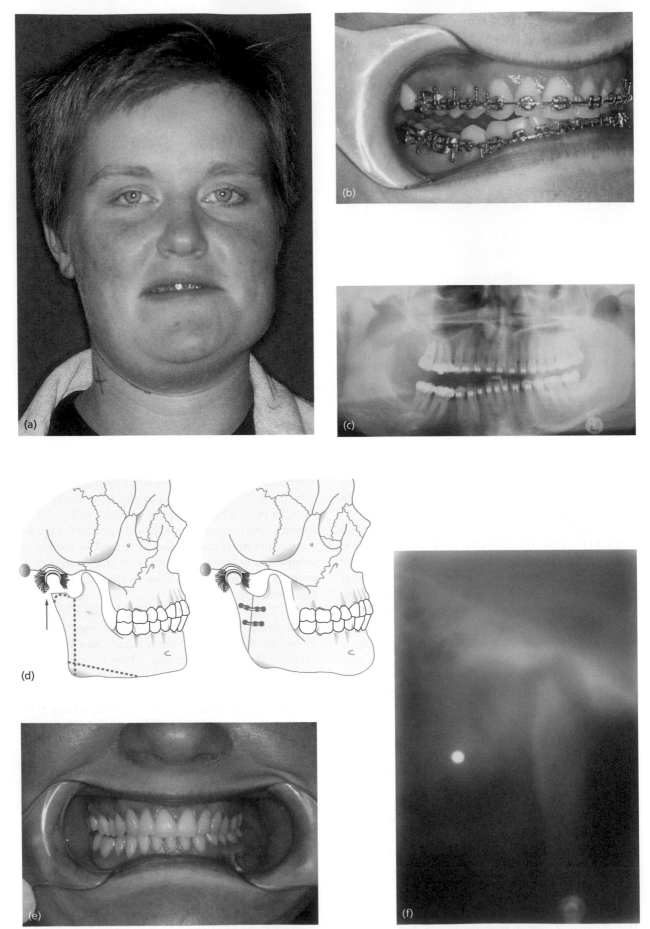

Fig. 33.14 Patient with a rotational type of condylar hyperplasia. (a) Clinical picture. (b) Intraoral view showing open bite on the right side. (c) Radiograph showing enlarged condyle, collum, and ramus. (d) Simplified drawing showing the surgical technique used to reconstruct the TMJ. (e) Occlusion 5 years postoperatively. (f) Radiograph 5 years postoperatively.

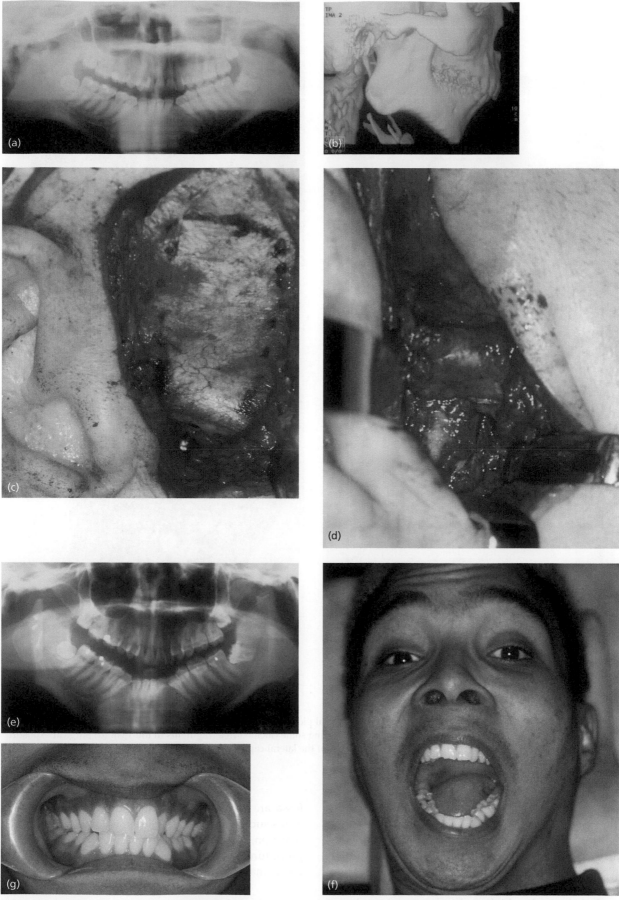

Fig. 33.15 Patient with ankylosis of the right TMJ after trauma. (a) Preoperative panoramic radiograph. (b) Preoperative three-dimensional CT (notice the elongated coronoid process on the right side). (c) The right TMJ after resection of the ankylotic bone. The temporalis muscle/fascia flap is outlined. (d) The flap rotated down and sutured into the joint. The condylar stump is advanced superiorly below the interposed muscle flap after a vertical ramus osteotomy. (e) Postoperative panoramic radiograph. (f) Maximum opening of 41 mm at 3-year follow-up examination (compares with preoperative opening of 10 mm). (g) Occlusion at 3-year follow-up examination.

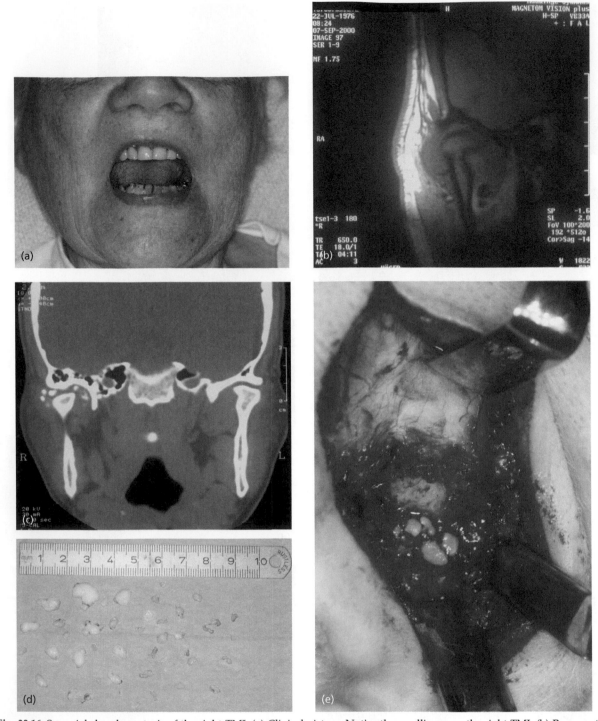

Fig. 33.16 Synovial chondromatosis of the right TMJ. (a) Clinical picture. Notice the swelling over the right TMJ. (b) Preoperative MRI showing an expanded TMJ capsule and fluid. (c) CT showing some calcified free fragments in the TMJ. (d) Surgical exposure of the right TMJ. Fragments emerge from the joint on incision of the lateral capsule. (e) The fragments found in the joint. Some of them are almost 10 mm in diameter.

costochondral graft is the one that is most frequently employed. Alloplastic joints are now available and there are a handful of different types that are manufactured and commercially available. Most are similar to orthopedic alloplastic joints in that they are often made of titanium with a chrome/cobalt surfaced head and an ultra-high molecular weight polymer (UHMWP) glenoid fossa.

The term TMJ reconstruction should be reserved for the situations when both the condyle and the fossa are reconstructed. Otherwise, one should use terms such as condylar replacement and fossa reconstruction, respectively. In various reconstructive procedures of the TMJ one can choose between autogenous material and alloplastic devices.

Autogenous reconstruction

In 1927 Wassmund described the use of free metatarsal grafts for condylar replacement. Other donor

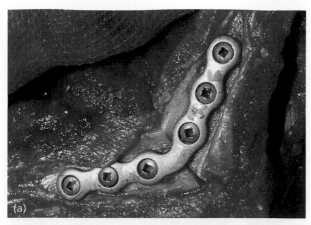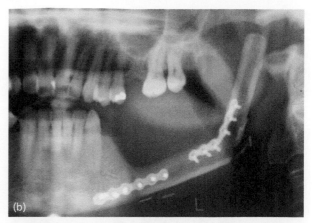

Fig. 33.17 (a) A triangular piece of a fibula graft has been cut out to permit contouring of the fibula to match both the body and ramus of the mandible. If a locking plate system is used, one can refrain from stripping the periosteum under the plate. (b) A vascularized fibula graft reconstructing both the body and ramus of the mandible. Note the bony fusion between the fibula and the native mandible.

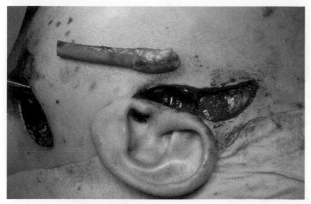

Fig. 33.18 After harvest, the cartilage of the costochondral graft has been cut to fit the contour of the reshaped fossa.

tissues that have been used for condylar replacement include clavicle, iliac crest, and vascularized fibula (Fig. 33.17). Of all the autogenous donor sites, however, ribs have been used more than anything else. Rib grafts can be used either as free or vascularized costochondral grafts. The costochondral graft consists of both bone and hyaline cartilage.

The popularity of costochondral grafts for condylar replacement is based on several factors. Ribs are relatively easy to harvest. The size of the graft usually fits the native TMJ dimensions (Fig. 33.18) , and it is rather easy to adapt the rib and its cartilage to the local conditions (Figs 33.19, 33.20). In patients who are not skeletally mature, the costochondral graft may have some persisting growth potential.

The growth potential is, however, a potential disadvantage of the costochondral graft. The graft may grow too much, too little, or not at all. Children who have had condylar replacement with rib grafts may have to undergo further surgical procedures to correct the jaw position later on.

The downside of costochondral grafts also includes things they have in common with other autogenous grafts, such as ankylosis/reankylosis, resorption, and donor site morbidity. While costochondral grafts for

condylar replacement do relatively well in many instances, they are not reliable in the treatment of TMJ ankylosis since reankylosis can occur.

Prosthetic reconstruction of the TMJ

TMJ prostheses can be divided into two major categories: custom made and stock products. A custom-made prosthesis is one that is made on a model of the patient's skeletal components. Thus, the prosthesis is made to match the patient's individual anatomy. A stock product, on the other hand, is a standard design that comes in various sizes, small, medium, and large. For a stock prosthesis, the bone contour is adjusted to fit the prosthesis. These two types of prostheses have one thing in common. They both have a fossa made of UHMWP (Fig. 33.21) and the actual cup of the fossa has only one size. In both types, the fossa component is attached to the zygomatic arch with 2.0 mm titanium screws.

Surgical considerations in prosthetic TMJ reconstruction

The surgical approaches are basically the same as for costochondral condylar replacement. It is important to keep the surgical fields free from oral contamination. Thus, the oral cavity should be excluded from the surgical field with a surgical drape.

The preauricular incision can usually be made somewhat lower than when a costochondral graft is installed, since there is no need to swing down a temporal fascia flap to line the fossa. For the approach to the lateral aspect of the ramus, personal preferences, just as much as anything else, may guide the approach of choice. The dissection should create a subperiosteal tunnel between the two incisions. This tunnel should be wide enough for a little finger to pass through. That is approximately the width required to pass the prosthetic mandibular component through, as well. If this tunnel turns out to be

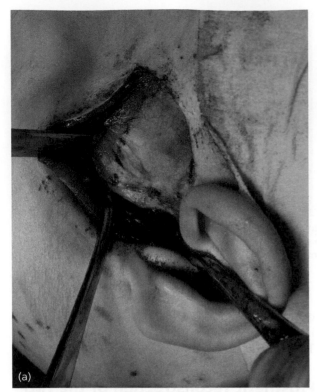

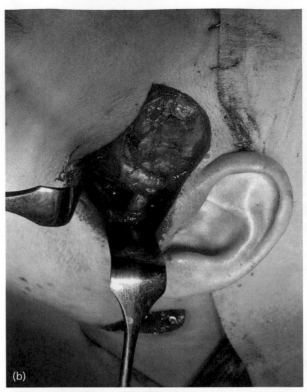

Fig. 33.19 (a) A 3-year-old boy has developed a unilateral TMJ ankylosis following urosepsis. After release of the ankylosis and preparation of the fossa region, a temporalis fascia flap is designed to line out the fossa. (b) The temporalis fascia flap has been brought around the base of the zygomatic arch, and is sutured medially in the fossa cavity. The cartilaginous part of the costochondral graft is resting on the soft tissue lining created by the temporal fascia flap.

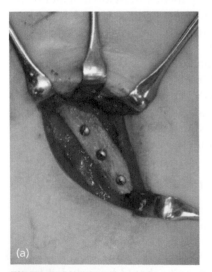

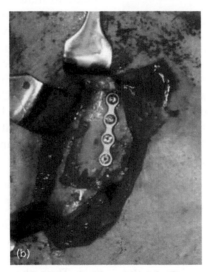

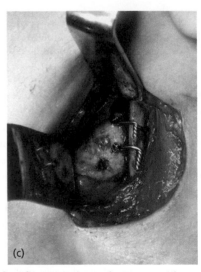

Fig. 33.20 (a) A costochondral graft in a 5-year-old, attached with screws only. Care must be taken not to insert the screws with too much force. If the rib is very soft, a plate must be added as a washer, such as in (b). (b) A four-hole miniplate serves as a washer for the osteosynthesis of a costochondral graft to the mandibular angle. (c) Same patient as in Figs 33.18 and 33.19. In this case the costochondral graft has been placed along the posterior border of the mandibular ramus, and is attached with steel wire osteosynthesis.

too narrow, it will be much more difficult to widen it once the fossa component has been installed (Fig. 33.22).

One advantage with prosthetic reconstruction over costochondral or other autogenous reconstruction, is that the patient can, and actually should, exercise right after surgery. Another advantage with prosthetic reconstruction of the TMJ is that the pros-

thetic devices can withstand the reactive forces that will arise in cases where the mandible is advanced at the time of TMJ reconstruction. Such situations may occur in patients whose joints are severely destroyed by rheumatoid arthritis (RA). One typical feature of a patient with longstanding RA is the bird face, with a variably severe mandibular micrognathia and retrognathia (Fig. 33.23). In such cases an aggressive

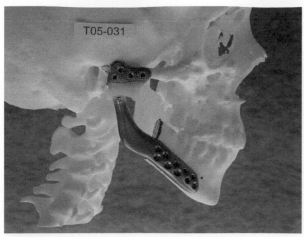

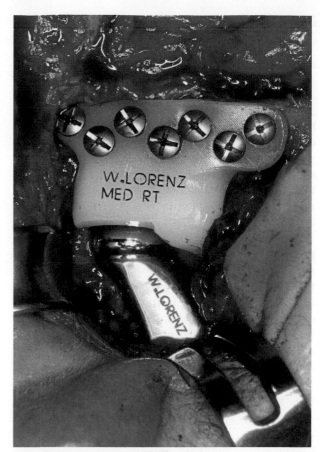

Fig. 33.21 An individual three-dimensional model of a patient where a critical size defect has been created in the preparation for a custom-made prosthesis by TMJ Concepts (Ventura, California, USA). The mandibular component is machined out of titanium, and has a condylar head of CoCr pressed on top. The fossa component is, just like in the Biomet device, made of UHMWP, but is attached to a titanium mesh plate formed according to the individual anatomy of the patient. (Reproduced from Westermark A, Koppel D, Leiggener C. (2007) Condylar replacement alone is not sufficient for prosthetic reconstruction of the temporomandibular joint. *International Journal of Oral and Maxillofacial Surgery* 35, 488–92. Copyright © 2007 Elsevier.)

Fig. 33.22 A Biomet® total joint prosthesis has been installed. The signs on the fossa component verify that it is a right-sided, medium-size component. All screw holes have been used. Note that the condylar head is seated in the posterior part of the fossa cup. (Reproduced from Westermark A, Koppel D, Leiggener C. (2007) Condylar replacement alone is not sufficient for prosthetic reconstruction of the temporomandibular joint. *International Journal of Oral and Maxillofacial Surgery* 35, 488–92. Copyright © 2007 Elsevier.)

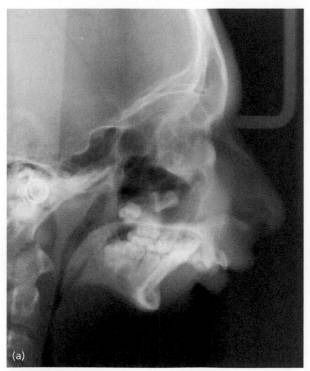

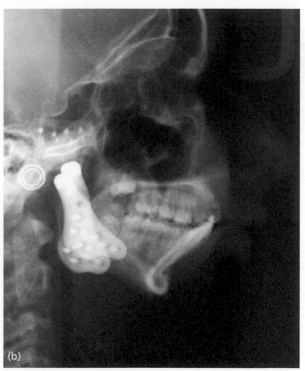

Fig. 33.23 (a) Profile radiograph of a 15-year-old patient who has been ankylosed since a very early age. The resulting growth impairment has been so severe that the patient can no longer defend her airway. Shortly after this radiograph was obtained, the patient had a tracheostomy to secure the airway. (b) Resection of bilateral ankylosis followed by installation of TMJ Concepts patient-fitted total TMJ prostheses has resulted in improved pharyngeal airway space. The patient is released from the tracheostomy. The prosthetic devices withstand the posterior pressure put upon them by the suprahyoid muscles. The mandible was advanced as much as the dentition allowed. A genioplasty will follow, to further improve both the airway space and the patient's profile.

mandibular advancement can be combined with installation of the total joint prostheses. A costochondral graft will not give the same postoperative stability. Similar situations may occur in patients who have been ankylosed from an early age. TMJ ankylosis in early childhood will dramatically impair mandibular growth. The resulting micrognathia may become so severe that the patient cannot defend the airway. With the release of the ankylosis and the advancement of the mandible, the pharyngeal airway will increase.

For the ankylosed TMJ, reankylosis is a risk after prosthetic reconstruction of the joint. The prosthetic reconstruction requires a rather large gap between the fossa and the ramus. The gap can reach the width of a critical size defect; in this area such a defect is considered to be 2–2.5 cm. Recently, fat grafting has been introduced as a treatment modality to further reduce the risk of reankylosis. A free fat graft can be harvested from just under the umbilicus. The fat graft is packed around the joint components to fill empty spaces, before the wounds are closed.

Treatment expectations after prosthetic reconstruction of the TMJ

TMJ reconstruction is a treatment option for the joint that is no longer a functioning joint. Sometimes TMJ reconstruction is, actually, TMJ construction, such as in cases with congenital absence of joint components. A long-standing ankylosis means that surrounding muscles and soft tissues have adapted to the immobilized joint, sometimes with severely impaired mobility as a result. In congenital deficiencies there may be total absence of muscles to perform the joint movements. Also, because of loss of function of the lateral pterygoid muscle in most TMJ reconstruction cases, translation is severely impaired. There may be some translational movement because of the lowered rotation point. This inferior hinge axis gives a false translational image to the joint movement. A realistic expectation of opening capacity after TMJ reconstruction is around 35 mm. It should be emphasized, however, that the opening capacity to a large extent

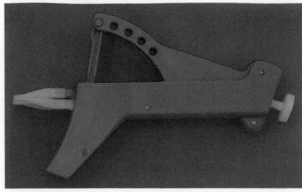

Fig. 33.24 The TheraBite® (Cranio Mandibular Rehab Inc., Denver, Colorado, USA) is an example of a useful device for jaw exercise.

depends on the patients' compliance with their postoperative physiotherapy. Patients who have suffered from ankylosis must be prepared to maintain a lifelong exercise program to maintain a good opening capacity. There are physical therapy appliances to support these exercises (Fig. 33.24). With respect to pain one must remember that, while most of the joint-related pain will be reduced by the installation of a TMJ prosthesis, muscle pain and myofascial pain may persist. As long as one maintains the correct indications for treatment, one can expect an overall improvement of the patient's quality-of-life scores.

Recommended reading

Bradley PA, Al-Kayat A. (1979) A modified approach to the temporomandibular joint and malar arch. *British Journal of Oral Surgery*, **17**, 91–103.

Holmlund A. (2010) Arthroscopy and arthroscopic surgery. In: *Oral and Maxillofacial Surgery* (eds, Andersson L, Kahnberg K-E, Pogrel MA). Oxford, Wiley-Blackwell.

Holmlund A. (2010) Temporomandibular joint surgery. In: *Oral and Maxillofacial Surgery* (eds, Andersson L, Kahnberg K-E, Pogrel MA). Oxford, Wiley-Blackwell.

Wassmund M. (1927) *Frakturen und Luxationen des Gesichtsschädels*, pp. 335–40. Leipzig, Verlag von Hermann Meusser.

Westermark A. (2010) Temporomandibular joint reconstruction. In: *Oral and Maxillofacial Surgery* (eds, Andersson L, Kahnberg K-E, Pogrel MA). Oxford, Wiley-Blackwell.

Index

Page numbers in *italic* refer to figures.
Page numbers in **bold** refer to tables.

Essentials of Oral and Maxillofacial Surgery, First Edition. Edited by M. Anthony Pogrel, Karl-Erik Kahnberg and Lars Andersson.
© 2014 John Wiley & Sons, Ltd. Published 2014 by John Wiley & Sons, Ltd.
Companion website: www.wiley.com/go/pogrel/oms

Printed and bound by CPI Group (UK) Ltd, Croydon, CR0 4YY

27/10/2024

14580196-0001